New Frontiers in Clinical Drug Research: Anti-Cancer and Anti-HIV Agents

New Frontiers in Clinical Drug Research: Anti-Cancer and Anti-HIV Agents

Editor: Horatio Finley

AMERICAN
MEDICAL PUBLISHERS
www.americanmedicalpublishers.com

AMERICAN
MEDICAL PUBLISHERS
www.americanmedicalpublishers.com

Cataloging-in-Publication Data

New frontiers in clinical drug research : anti-cancer and anti-HIV agents / edited by Horatio Finley.
p. cm.
Includes bibliographical references and index.
ISBN 979-8-88740-323-6
1. Antineoplastic agents. 2. HIV Infections--Chemotherapy. 3. Cancer--Chemotherapy.
4. AIDS (Disease)--Chemotherapy. 5. Drugs--Research. 6. Clinical pharmacology.
7. Clinical trials. I. Finley, Horatio.
RS431.A64 N49 2023
615.798--dc23

American Medical Publishers,
41 Flatbush Avenue,
1st Floor, New York,
NY 11217, USA

ISBN 979-8-88740-323-6 (Hardback)

Contents

Preface

Every book is initially just a concept; it takes months of research and hard work to give it the final shape in which the readers receive it. In its early stages, this book also went through rigorous reviewing. The notable contributions made by experts from across the globe were first molded into patterned chapters and then arranged in a sensibly sequential manner to bring out the best results.

Anti-cancer agents are the chemicals that are utilized for arresting the growth of cancer cells. These chemicals affect the abnormal growth of cancer cells but they also impact the normal cells such as the cells in the bone marrow, skin, gonads and gastrointestinal tract. Various drugs that are utilized for inhibiting the growth of cancer cells include hydroxyurea, platinum-based drugs and L-asparaginase. Anti-HIV agents on the other hand, are those compounds which decrease the viral load and probability of transmitting HIV to others. Various compounds that are utilized for the treatment of HIV infections include nucleotide reverse transcriptase inhibitors (NtRTIs), and nucleoside reverse transcriptase inhibitors (NRTIs). The NtRTIs are developed to fight virus resistance as they are phosphorylated and require less cellular processing. A significant role is played by secondary metabolites produced by living organisms in the drug development and discovery, as they have biological and structural diversity. They hold the potential for developing anti-cancer and anti-HIV drugs. This book unfolds the innovative aspects of clinical drug research on anti-cancer and anti-HIV agents which will be crucial for the progress of this field in the future. It will serve as a valuable source of reference for graduate and post graduate students.

It has been my immense pleasure to be a part of this project and to contribute my years of learning in such a meaningful form. I would like to take this opportunity to thank all the people who have been associated with the completion of this book at any step.

Editor

1

Apple Peel Flavonoid Fraction 4 Suppresses Breast Cancer Cell Growth by Cytostatic and Cytotoxic Mechanisms

Chao-Yu Loung [1,†], Wasundara Fernando [1,†], H.P. Vasantha Rupasinghe [1,2] and David W. Hoskin [3,*]

1 Department of Pathology, Faculty of Medicine, Dalhousie University, Halifax, NS B3H 4R2, Canada; joe.loung@dal.ca (C.-Y.L.); wasufer@dal.ca (W.F.); vrupasinghe@dal.ca (H.P.V.R.)
2 Department of Plant, Food, and Environmental Sciences, Faculty of Agriculture, Dalhousie University, Truro, NS B2N 5E3, Canada
3 Department of Pathology, Department of Microbiology and Immunology, Department of Surgery, Faculty of Medicine, Dalhousie University, Halifax, NS B3H 4R2, Canada
* Correspondence: d.w.hoskin@dal.ca
† These authors contribute equally to this work.

Abstract: Many dietary flavonoids possess anti-cancer activities. Here, the effect of apple peel flavonoid fraction 4 (AF4) on the growth of triple-negative (MDA-MB-231, MDA-MB-468), estrogen receptor-positive (MCF-7), and HER2-positive (SKBR3) breast cancer cells was determined and compared with the effect of AF4 on normal mammary epithelial cells and dermal fibroblasts. AF4 inhibited breast cancer cell growth in monolayer cultures, as well as the growth of MCF-7 spheroids, without substantially affecting the viability of non-malignant cells. A sub-cytotoxic concentration of AF4 suppressed the proliferation of MDA-MB-231 cells by inhibiting passage through the G_0/G_1 phase of the cell cycle. AF4-treated MDA-MB-231 cells also exhibited reduced in vitro migration and invasion, and decreased Akt (protein kinase B) signaling. Higher concentrations of AF4 were selectively cytotoxic for MDA-MB-231 cells. AF4 cytotoxicity was associated with the intracellular accumulation of reactive oxygen species. Importantly, intratumoral administration of AF4 suppressed the growth of MDA-MB-231 xenografts in non-obese diabetic severe combined immunodeficient (NOD-SCID) female mice. The selective cytotoxicity of AF4 for breast cancer cells, combined with the capacity of sub-cytotoxic AF4 to inhibit breast cancer cell proliferation, migration, and invasion suggests that flavonoid-rich AF4 (and its constituents) has potential as a natural therapeutic agent for breast cancer treatment.

Keywords: apoptosis; breast cancer; cell cycle; flavonoids; reactive oxygen species; tumor suppression

---

1. Introduction

The regular consumption of fruits and vegetables that are rich in flavonoids and other bioactive molecules is associated with a reduced risk of developing various types of cancers [1–5]. It is unlikely that any single natural source-derived compound is responsible for this beneficial effect since multiple bioactive molecules in flavonoid-rich foods are likely to act in a synergistic fashion. Numerous studies on phytochemicals as potential anti-cancer agents have found that these natural compounds affect many different signaling pathways involved in cancer development and progression [6,7]. It is hoped that further research on the anti-cancer properties of phytochemicals will lead to the development of plant-based therapeutics for the prevention or treatment of cancer.

Apples, which are a common source of dietary flavonoids, have been widely investigated for their disease-fighting properties [8–11]. Apple peel flavonoid fraction 4 (AF4) is a flavonoid-rich ethanolic extract of the Northern Spy apple cultivar [12]. AF4 contains a number of polyphenolic compounds, including flavonols, anthocyanins, dihydrochalcones, phenolic acids, and flavan-3-ols. Quercetin glycosides (quercetin-3-*O*-galactoside, quercetin-3-*O*-rutinoside, quercetin-3-*O*-glucoside and quercetin-3-*O*-rhamnoside) comprise approximately 70% of the phenolic content of AF4. Previous studies have established the neuroprotective and anti-inflammatory properties of AF4 in different mouse models [12,13]. AF4 also inhibits the growth of hepatocellular carcinoma (HepG2) cells by causing cell cycle arrest and apoptosis, as well as acting as a topoisomerase toxicant [14].

Breast cancer is the most common cancer among North American women and the second highest cause of cancer-related deaths [15]. The poor prognosis of metastatic breast cancer mandates the development of novel treatment strategies. The impact of AF4 treatment on breast cancer cells has not yet been determined. In the current study we used in vitro and in vivo approaches to elucidate the selective cytotoxic, anti-proliferative, anti-migratory and tumor suppressor effects of AF4 on breast cancer cells.

2. Results

2.1. Apple Peel Flavonoid Fraction 4 (AF4) Selectively Inhibits the Growth of Breast Cancer Cells

Exposure to AF4 reduced the number of viable triple-negative (MDA-MB-231, MDA-MB-468), estrogen receptor-positive (MCF-7), and HER2 receptor-positive (SKBR3) breast cancer cells in monolayer cultures in a dose- and time-dependent manner, as indicated by reduced cellular metabolic activity measured by 3-(4,5-dimethythiazol-2-yl)-2,5-diphenyltetrazolium bromide (MTT) assays (Figure 1A). Sensitivity to AF4 (100 μg/mL) at 72 h was as follows: MDA-MB-231 (39% ± 3% viable) and MDA-MB-468 (38% ± 3% viable) > SKBR3 (48% ± 2% viable) > MCF-7 (56% ± 2% viable). AF4 was selective for breast cancer cells since a concentration of AF4 (100 μg/mL) that was cytotoxic for breast cancer cells had little effect on the viability of nonmalignant human mammary epithelial cells (HMEC) and MCF-10A mammary epithelial cells (Figure 1B).

In comparison to quercetin, AF4 was a less potent inhibitor of breast cancer cell growth but had greater selectivity (Figure S1). MCF-7 spheroids that were grown in the presence of AF4 (100 μg/mL) were smaller than vehicle-treated control spheroids (Figure 1C). In addition, numerous floating cells with morphology characteristic of dead or dying cells were present in AF4-treated cultures, and there was a significant decrease in the number of viable MCF-7 cells, as indicated by reduced phosphatase activity, within spheroids treated with AF4 (100 μg/mL) relative to vehicle-treated controls. Therefore, AF4 inhibited breast cancer cell growth in both 2-dimensional and 3-dimensional culture systems. Subsequent experiments focused on the effect of AF4 on MDA-MB-231 cells as this breast cancer cell line was most sensitive to AF4 and readily forms tumors in immune-deficient mice.

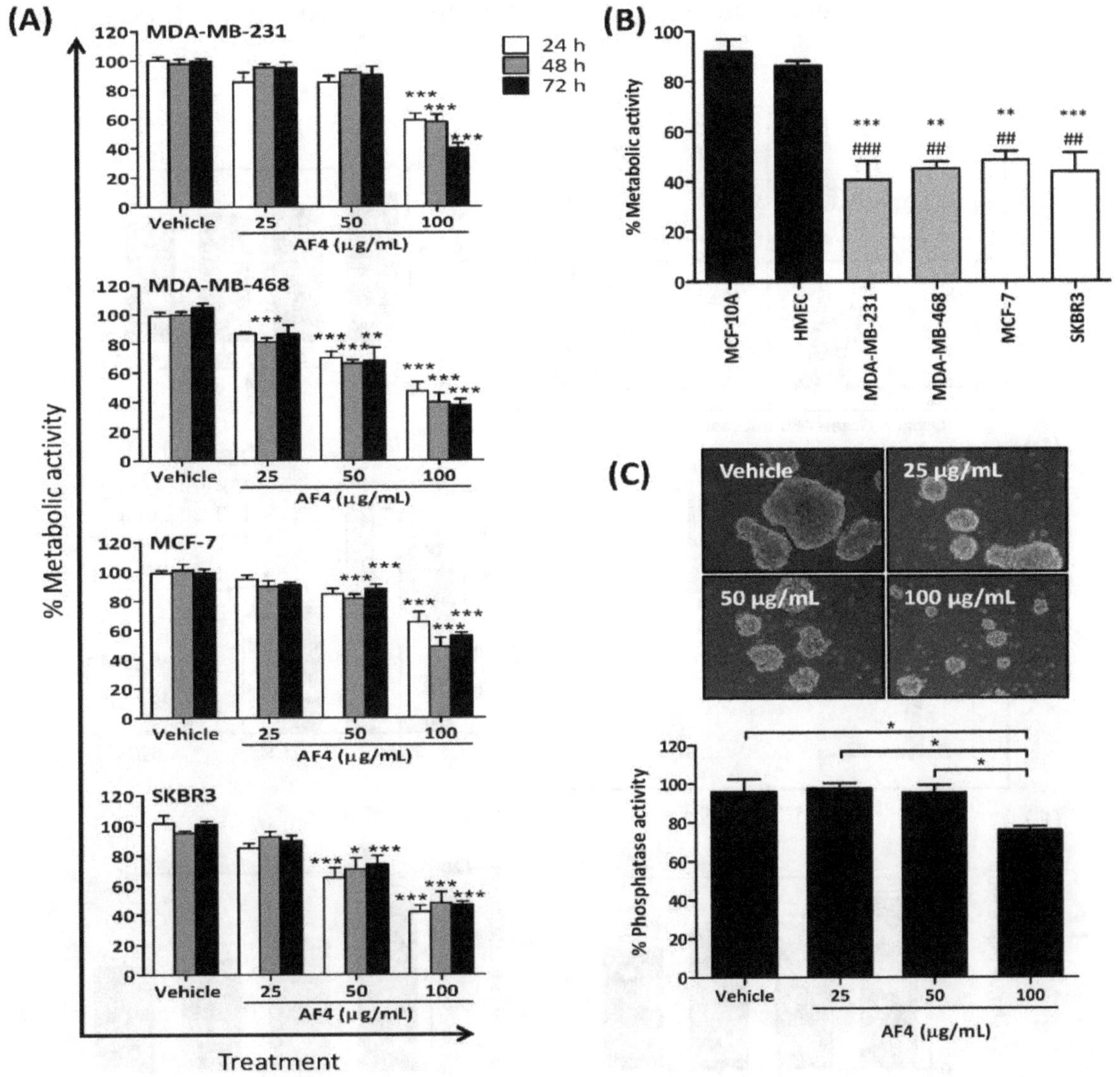

Figure 1. Apple peel flavonoid fraction 4 (AF4) is selectively cytotoxic to breast cancer cells. (**A**) MDA-MB-231, MDA-MB-468, MCF-7 and SKBR3 cells were cultured in the absence or presence of the indicated concentrations of AF4 for the indicated times. The % metabolic activity of AF4-treated cells was determined using an MTT (3-(4,5-dimethythiazol-2-yl)-2,5-diphenyltetrazolium bromide) assay. Data are expressed as mean ± standard error of the mean (SEM). (**B**) The % metabolic activity of AF4-treated (100 μg/mL) breast cancer cells was compared to MCF-10A cells (#) and HMECs (*) cells. Data from MTT assays are expressed as mean ± SEM. (**C**) MCF-7 spheroids were cultured for 72 h in the absence or presence of the indicated concentrations of AF4. Relative cell number of viable cells was determined by acid phosphatase assay. Data are shown as mean ± SEM. (A–C) Statistical analysis of 3 independent experiments was performed using analysis of variance (ANOVA) and Tukey's multiple comparisons test; * $p < 0.05$, ** and ## $p < 0.01$, *** and ### $p < 0.001$.

2.2. *AF4 Suppresses the Proliferation of MDA-MB-231 Cells*

Next, we determined whether a non-cytotoxic concentration of AF4 could impact breast cancer cell growth. As shown in Figure 2, flow cytometric analysis of Oregon Green 488-stained MDA-MB-231 cells that were treated with a sub-cytotoxic dose of AF4 (40 μg/mL) revealed a significant reduction in the number of cell divisions (Figure 2A). In addition, cell cycle analysis showed that AF4-treated MDA-MB-231 cells accumulated in the G_0/G_1 phase of the cell cycle, with a corresponding reduction in the number of MDA-MB-231 cells in the S phase of the cell cycle (Figure 2B). The same effect was observed in AF4-treated MDA-MB-468 cells (Figure S2). Consistent with an AF4-induced partial block at G_0/G_1, there was reduced expression of CDK4 and cyclin D3 in AF4-treated MDA-MB-231 cells (Figure 2C).

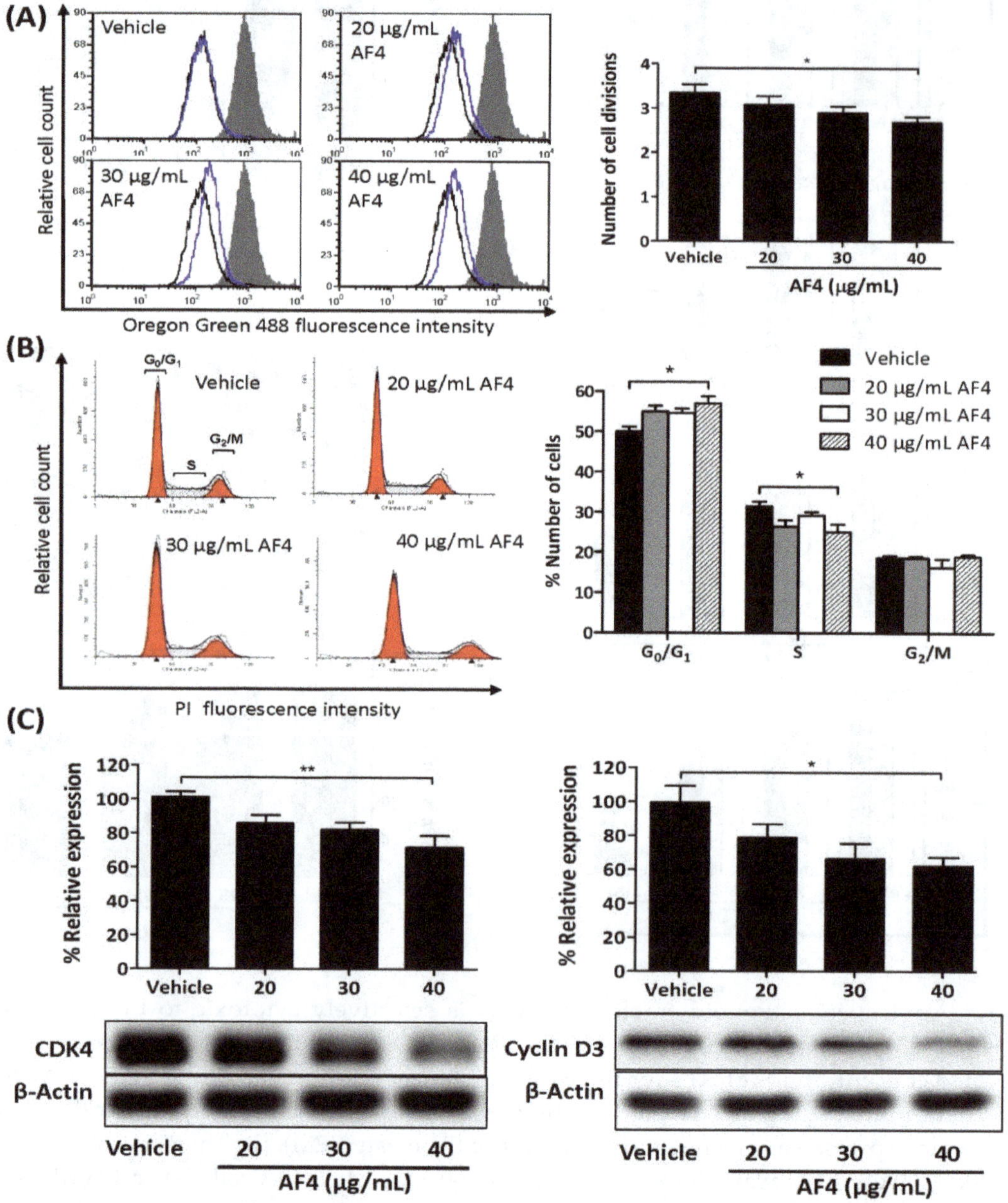

Figure 2. AF4 inhibits breast cancer cell proliferation. (**A**) MDA-MB-231 cells were stained with Oregon Green 488 dye and then cultured for 72 h in the absence or presence of the indicated concentrations of AF4. Fluorescence was measured by flow cytometry. Data are shown as representative histograms (filled peak, non-proliferating cells; black peak, vehicle; blue peak, AF4) and mean number of cell divisions ± SEM. (**B**) MDA-MB-231 cells were cultured for 72 h in the absence or presence of the indicated concentrations of AF4. Cells were stained with propidium iodide (PI) and cell cycle analysis was performed by flow cytometry. Data are shown as representative histograms and mean % number of cells ± SEM in each phase of the cell cycle. (**C**) MDA-MB-231 cells were cultured for 24 h in the absence or presence of the indicated concentrations of AF4. The relative expression of CDK4 and cyclin D3 was determined using Western blot analysis. Equal protein loading was confirmed by probing for β-actin. Data shown are representative blots and mean % relative expression ± SEM. (A–C) Statistical analysis of 3 independent experiments was performed using ANOVA and Tukey's multiple comparisons test; * $p < 0.05$, ** $p < 0.01$.

2.3. *AF4 Inhibits the Migration and Invasion of MDA-MB-231 Cells*

Gap closure and trans-well migration assays were used to determine the effect of sub-cytotoxic AF4 on the migration and invasion capacity of MDA-MB-231 cells. These experiments used AF4 at a final concentration of 20 μg/mL in order to ensure that there would be no AF4-associated cytotoxic activity. As shown in Figure 3, a sub-cytotoxic concentration of AF4 (20 μg/mL) inhibited the migration of MDA-MB-231 cells by 65% in gap closure assays and by 87% in trans-well migration assays (Figure 3A and B, respectively). In addition, the invasion of MDA-MB-231 cells through a fibronectin-coated porous membrane was reduced by 80% in the presence of sub-cytotoxic AF4 (Figure 3C). Expression of invasion-promoting matrix metalloproteinase 2 (MMP2) was also significantly reduced when MDA-MB-231 cells were cultured in the presence of sub-cytotoxic AF4 (Figure 3D).

2.4. *AF4-Induced Apoptosis Is Associated with Oxidative Stress*

To determine the mechanism by which AF4 killed breast cancer cells, MDA-MB-231 cells were stained with Annexin V-488 and propidium iodide (PI) prior to culture for 24 h in the presence of a cytotoxic concentration of AF4 (100 μg/mL). As shown in Figure 4A, flow cytometric analysis revealed that a high concentration of AF4 caused MDA-MB-231 cells to die by apoptosis (Figure 4A). In contrast, neither MCF-10A epithelial cells nor dermal fibroblasts were sensitive to AF4, suggesting a selective cytotoxic effect on neoplastic cells. As shown in Figure 4B,C, treatment of MDA-MB-231 cells with an apoptosis-inducing concentration of AF4 resulted in the generation of reactive oxygen species (ROS), as indicated by Amplex Red assays and flow cytometric analysis of cells stained with the ROS-sensitive dye 5-(and-6)-chloromethyl-2′,7′-dichlorodihydrofluorescein diacetate, acetyl ester (CM-H_2DCFDA). MCF-10A cells that were cultured in the presence of AF4 (100 μg/mL) also exhibited increased levels of intracellular ROS (Figure S3). Oxidative stress was at least in part responsible for the cytotoxic action of AF4 since apoptosis of AF4-treated MDA-MB-231 cells was reduced in the presence of the antioxidant N-acetyl cysteine (NAC). In comparison to MDA-MB-231 cells, non-malignant MCF-10A epithelial cells were relatively resistant to oxidative stress (Figure S4).

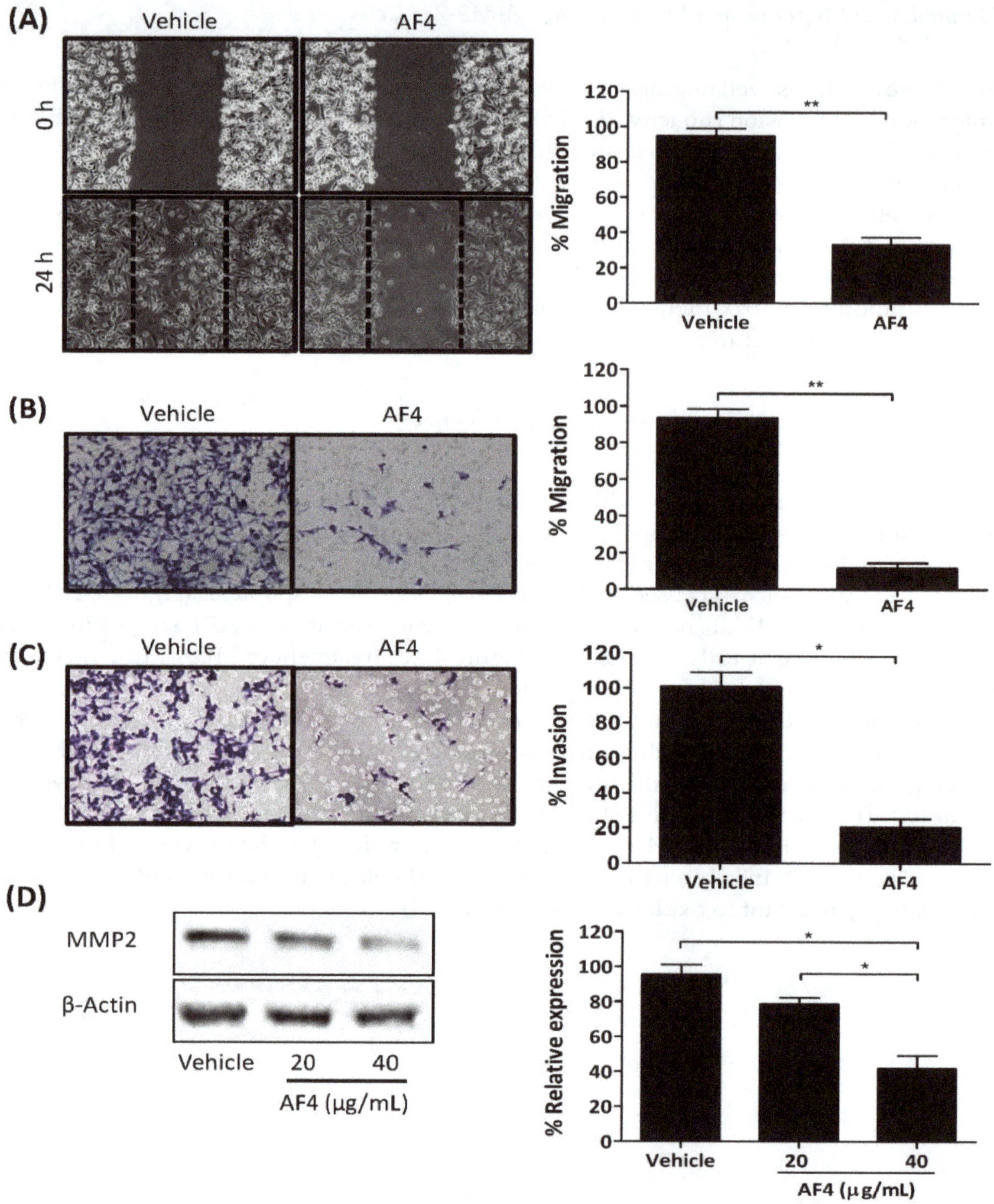

Figure 3. AF4 inhibits breast cancer cell motility and invasion. (**A**) Mitomycin C-treated MDA-MB-231 cells were cultured in wells containing cell culture inserts, which were removed at 0 h. After 24 h culture in the absence or presence of 20 μg/mL AF4 cultures were photographed. Representative images and mean % migration ± SEM of 3 independent experiments are shown. (**B**) Serum-starved MDA-MB-231 cells were treated with 20 μg/mL AF4 for 24 h. Mean % migration ± SEM through an 8 μm porous membrane and (**C**) mean % invasion ± SEM through a fibronectin-coated 8 μm porous membrane were determined as described in the Methods. (**D**) MDA-MB-231 cells were cultured for 24 h in the absence or presence of the indicated concentrations of AF4. Relative expression of MMP2 was determined using Western blot analysis. Equal protein loading was confirmed by probing for β-actin expression. Data shown are representative blots and mean % relative expression ± SEM. Statistical analysis of 3 independent experiments was performed using (A–C) Student's *t*-test or (D) ANOVA and Tukey's multiple comparisons test; * $p < 0.01$, ** $p < 0.001$.

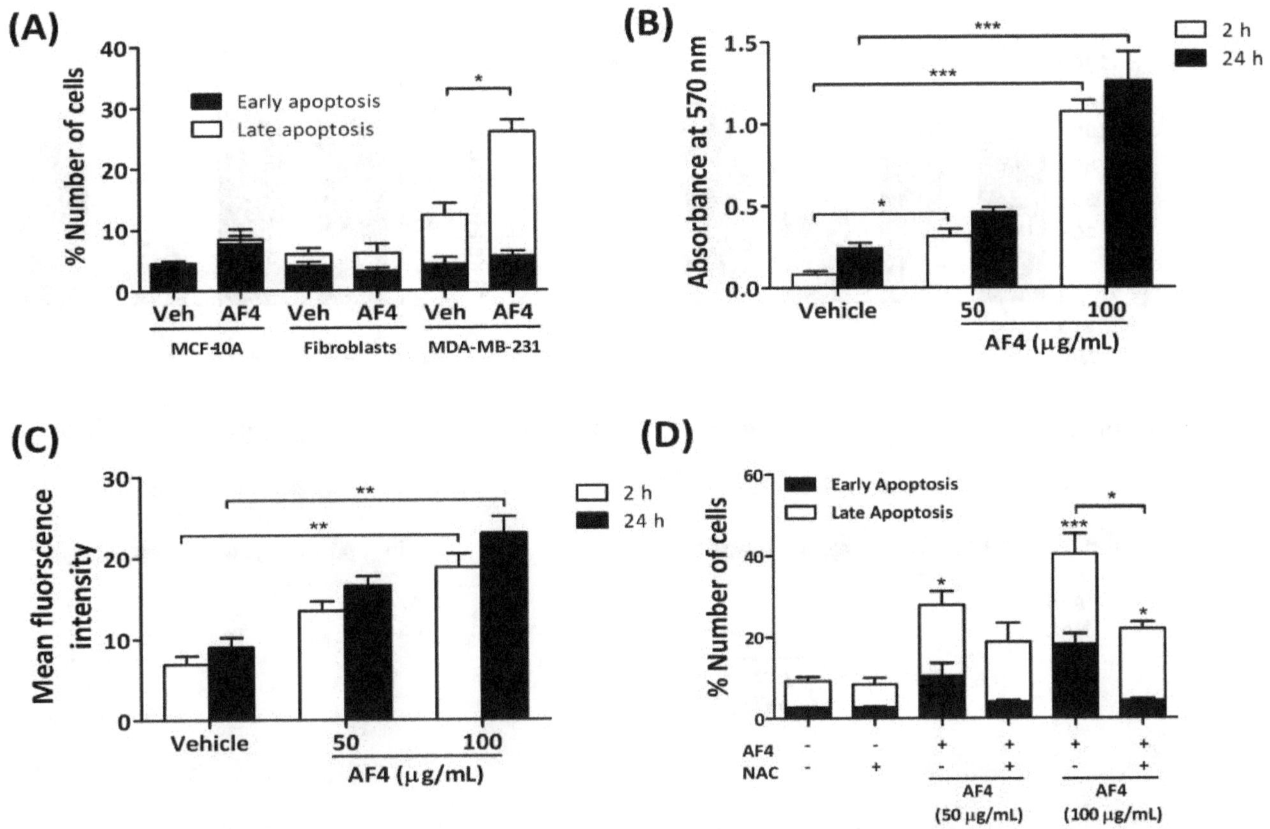

Figure 4. AF4-induced apoptosis of breast cancer cells is reactive oxygen species (ROS)-dependent. (**A**) MCF-10A cells, fibroblasts and MDA-MB-231 cells were cultured for 24 h in the absence or presence of 100 μg/mL AF4, and then stained with Annexin-V-488 and propidium iodide (PI) for flow cytometric analysis. Data are shown as mean % cell number ± SEM of 3 independent experiments. (**B**) MDA-MB-231 cells were cultured in the absence or presence of the indicated concentrations of AF4 for 2 h or 24 h and relative ROS in cultures was determined by Amplex Red assay. Data are shown as mean absorbance at 570 nm ± SEM of 3 independent experiments. (**C**) CM-H_2DCFDA-stained MDA-MB-231 cells were cultured in the absence or presence of the indicated concentrations of AF4 for 2 h or 24 h and the relative amount of intracellular ROS was determined by fluorescence at 529 nm. Data are shown as mean fluorescence intensity ± SEM of 3 independent experiments. (**D**) MDA-MB-231 cells were cultured for 24 h in the absence or presence of 100 μg/mL AF4 without or with 5 mM N-acetyl cysteine (NAC), and then stained with Annexin-V-488 and PI for flow cytometric analysis. Data are shown as mean % cell number ± SEM of 3 independent experiments. (A–D) Statistical analysis was performed using ANOVA and Tukey's multiple comparisons test; * $p < 0.05$, ** $p < 0.01$, *** $p < 0.001$.

2.5. AF4 Inhibits Akt Signaling

To determine a possible mechanism to account for the growth inhibitory effect of AF4, we examined the impact of AF4 on Akt (protein kinase B) signaling in MDA-MB-231 cells. A sub-cytotoxic concentration of AF4 (40 μg/mL) was used in these experiments in order to obtain sufficient protein for western blot analysis. Figure 5 shows that AF4 inhibited the phosphorylation-induced activation of Akt at Thr308. AF4 also suppressed Ser380 phosphorylation of phosphatase and tensin homolog (PTEN), which is the upstream inhibitor of Akt. Both PTEN and Akt phosphorylation were restored when AF4-treated MDA-MB-231 cells were cultured in the presence of the antioxidant NAC. The importance of the Akt signaling pathway for the growth and survival of MDA-MB-231 cells was confirmed using 2 different Akt inhibitors (MK2206 and SC66). Figure S5 shows that the percentage of apoptotic MDA-MB-231 cells increased significantly when Akt activation was inhibited.

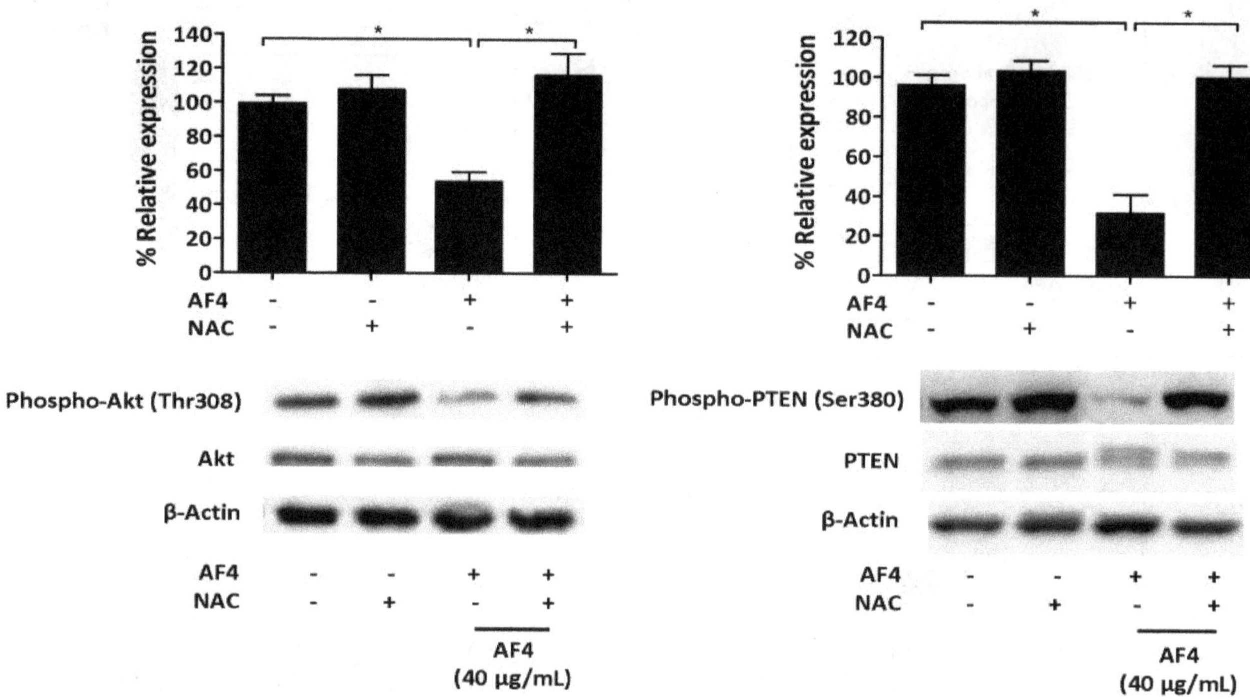

Figure 5. AF4 inhibits Akt and phosphatase and tensin homolog (PTEN) phosphorylation in breast cancer cells. MDA-MB-231 cells were cultured for 24 h in the absence or presence of 40 μg/mL AF4 without or with 5 mM NAC. Relative expression of phospho-Akt (Thr308), total Akt, phospho-PTEN (Ser380), and total PTEN was determined using Western blot analysis. Equal protein loading was confirmed by probing for β-actin expression. Data are shown as representative blots and mean % relative expression ± SEM of 3 independent experiments. Statistical analysis was performed using ANOVA and Tukey's multiple comparisons test; * $p < 0.05$.

2.6. AF4 Suppresses Growth of MDA-MB-231 Xenografts

The effect of AF4 on in vivo tumor growth was determined by intratumoral administration of AF4 (0.5 mg/kg) to MDA-MB-231 xenografts grown in female non-obese diabetic severe combined immunodeficient (NOD-SCID) mice. Dosage that was predicted to suppress MDA-MB-231 tumor growth was based on the total concentration of quercetin, quercetin glycosides, catechin, epicatechin, cyanidin-3-*O*-galactoside, phloridzin, chlorogenic acid and cafeic acid within AF4. Consistent with our in vitro findings regarding the anti-proliferative and cytotoxic activities of AF4, Figure 6A shows that treatment with AF4 significantly slowed the growth of MDA-MB-231 xenografts. Examination of tumor sections stained with hematoxylin and eosin revealed larger areas of necrosis in AF4-treated tumors (Figure 6B). Moreover, in comparison to saline-treated tumors, expression of the endothelial cell marker CD31 was reduced in the interior and periphery of AF4-treated tumors. No adverse effects were noted in AF4-treated mice, including no significant difference in average body weight between the treatment groups at day 15 (saline-treated group, 24.5 ± 0.6 g; AF4-treated group, 26.3 ± 0.5 g; $p > 0.05$ by Student's *t*-test).

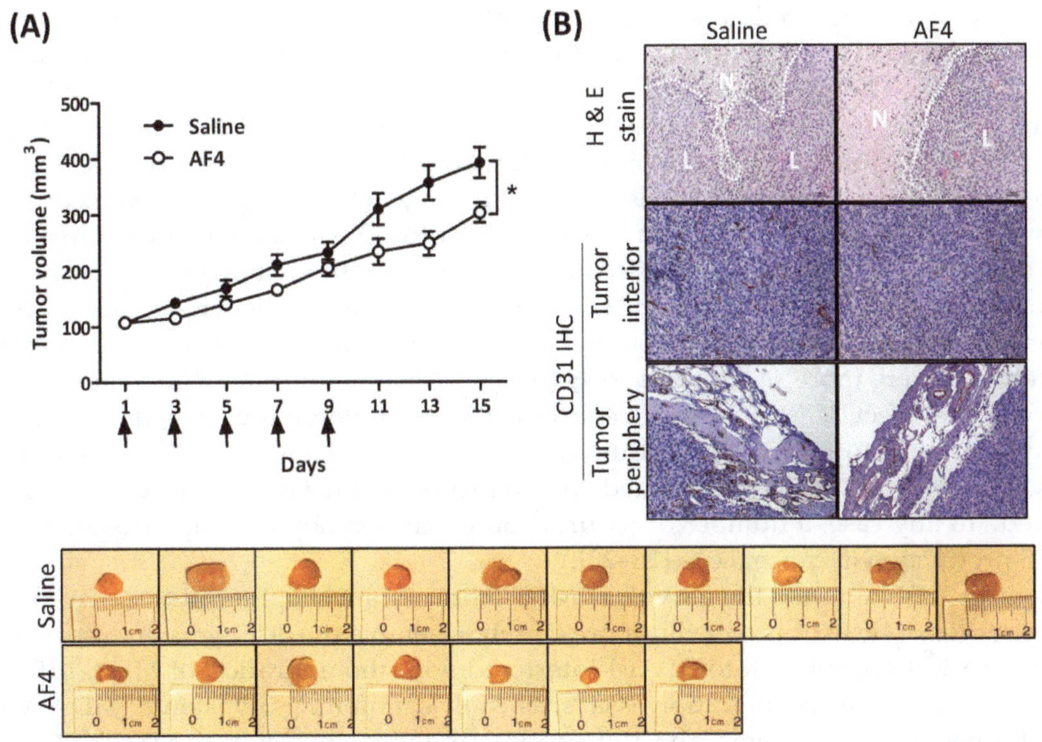

Figure 6. AF4 suppresses MDA-MB-231 xenograft growth. MDA-MB-231 cells were xenografted into the left flank of non-obese diabetic severe combined immunodeficient (NOD-SCID) female mice and AF4 (0.5 mg/kg) or saline was injected directly into the resulting tumors every second day (day 1, 3, 5, 7 and 9, indicated by arrows) for 9 days. The control group consisted of 10 animals and the AF4 treatment group was 7 animals. (**A**) Mean tumor volume ± SEM was determined every second day. Statistical analysis was determined by Student's *t*-test; * $p < 0.05$. Excised tumors from each treatment group at day 15 are shown. (**B**) At day 15 mice were euthanized and tumors were excised, fixed, and sectioned for staining with hematoxylin and eosin (H&E) and detection of CD31 expression by immunohistochemistry (IHC). Representative sections are shown; N denotes areas of necrosis and L denotes live cells.

3. Discussion

Dietary phytochemicals have received unique attention in the search for novel and safer cancer treatment options in light of widely documented findings that many of these natural sourced compounds kill cancer cells but are relatively non-toxic to healthy cells [14,16–19]. In this study, we used MTT assays to show that AF4 suppressed the growth of triple-negative (MDA-MB-231 and MDA-MB-468), estrogen receptor-positive (MCF-7) and HER2 receptor-positive (SKBR3) breast cancer cells but had little effect on the growth of non-malignant mammary epithelial cells (HMECs and MCF-10A), suggesting a pronounced selectivity for neoplastic cells. In contrast, quercetin, which is a minor component of AF4 [12], exhibited less selectivity for breast cancer cells.

MDA-MB-231 cells that were exposed to a low concentration of AF4 tended to accumulate at G_0/G_1, likely as a result of reduced expression of cyclin D3 and CDK4 that promote gene expression needed for G_1 progression [20]. AF4-treated MDA-MB-468 cells also arrested at G_0/G_1. This effect of AF4 on 2 different breast cancer cell lines differed from the G_2/M cell cycle arrest seen in cultures of AF4-treated HepG2 hepatocarcinoma cells [14], suggesting that the anti-proliferative activity of AF4 may be cell type-dependent. Treatment with a higher concentration of AF4 induced MDA-MB-231 cells to undergo apoptosis; however, the viability of non-malignant fibroblasts and MCF-10A mammary epithelial cells was not affected. AF4-induced apoptosis of breast cancer cells was consistent with an earlier report of apoptotic death of liver cancer cells following treatment with AF4 [14]. We demonstrate here, for the first time, that AF4-induced cytotoxicity was at least partially due to the accumulation of intracellular ROS because the antioxidant NAC protected MDA-MB-231 cells from the cytotoxic effect of AF4. In contrast, quercetin-induced apoptosis of MDA-MB-231 cells is reported to be ROS-independent [21], which argues against a major role for quercetin in the cytotoxic effect of AF4. Interestingly, non-malignant MCF-10A cells also showed increased levels of intracellular ROS following AF4 treatment, even though these cells were refractory to the cytotoxic effect of AF4. Multiple mechanisms exist to either prevent oxidative stress or manage the negative consequences of this condition; however, excessive production and accumulation of ROS can overwhelm these defenses [22]. In line with evidence that neoplastic cells are more sensitive to ROS than are their non-malignant counterparts [23], we found that MDA-MB-231 breast cancer cells were more sensitive to ROS than non-malignant MCF-10A mammary epithelial cells. The selective effect of AF4 on breast cancer cells may involve the capacity of healthy cells to defend against endogenous ROS [24]. Although certain components of AF4 possess anti-oxidant capabilities [25], the ability of unfractionated AF4 to protect against oxidative stress has not yet been demonstrated. In any case, a number of natural source antioxidants, at high doses, are capable of causing ROS production in cancer cells [26–28].

Importantly, AF4 inhibited the growth of MCF-7 breast cancer spheroids that, in comparison to monolayer cultures of breast cancer cells, more closely resemble the 3-dimensional structure of solid tumors [29]. In addition, sub-cytotoxic AF4 interfered with the migration of MDA-MB-231 cells in gap closure and trans-well cell migration assays, as well as inhibiting invasion of MDA-MB-231 cells through a fibronectin-coated membrane and suppressing the expression of MMP2. These findings suggest that AF4 may be able to interfere with breast cancer metastasis since tumor cell locomotion and the ability to degrade extracellular matrix components via the synthesis of proteolytic enzymes such as MMP2 play essential roles in the metastatic process [30].

Decreased phosphorylation of Akt in the presence of AF4 may account for its anti-proliferative and cytotoxic effects on MDA-MB-231 cells since the growth, survival, and metabolism of breast cancer cells involves activation of Akt [31]. The important role played by the Akt signaling pathway in the growth and survival of MDA-MB-231 cells was confirmed by the observation that Akt inhibition resulted in apoptosis of MDA-MB-231 cells. Phosphorylation of PTEN, which is a tumor suppressor protein that downregulates Akt signaling [32], was downregulated in AF4-treated MDA-MB-2312 cells. Decreased activation of inhibitory PTEN is consistent with the finding that AF4 did not completely block Akt activation. AF4-induced ROS production is likely to be involved in the effects of AF4 on Akt and PTEN since ROS can directly inhibit Akt via the phosphorylation of thiol groups within the protein, whereas phosphatases such as PTEN are deactivated by ROS [33]. Restoration of Akt and PTEN phosphorylation to control levels when NAC was added to cultures of AF4-treated MDA-MB-231 cells confirmed the involvement of AF4-induced ROS in modulation of the Akt signaling pathway.

Intratumoral administration of AF4 suppressed the growth of MDA-MB-231 xenografts in immune-deficient mice, most likely due to the combination of anti-proliferative and cytotoxic effects of AF4 that were revealed by our in vitro studies. In this regard, AF4-treated tumors contained larger areas of necrosis relative to saline-treated tumors. In addition, decreased expression of the endothelial cell marker CD31 in the periphery and interior of AF-4 treated tumors suggested that AF4 may inhibit angiogenesis. Notably, AF4 did not cause any distress or adverse side effects such as weight loss in treated animals. Injection of AF4 directly into the tumor was employed to eliminate potential issues of AF4 bioavailability following oral dosing. Therefore, it will be important in future studies to assess the effectiveness of oral or intraperitoneal administration of AF4 to tumor-bearing mice. Delivery of an optimal concentration of AF4 to the tumor microenvironment via the oral or intraperitoneal route will likely require a nanoparticle delivery vehicle of the type that has been reported to greatly enhance the bioavailability of other bioactive phytochemicals such as curcumin [34,35]. In this regard, nanoparticles have also been employed to deliver plant extracts with anticancer properties to various types of cancer cells [36]. Identification of the components of AF4 that are responsible for its anticancer activity could allow for the development of nanoparticles containing one or more pure compounds with greater bioactivity relative to the AF4 extract; however, it is important to note that such an approach risks the loss of any potential synergy between major and minor components of AF4. Nevertheless, demonstration of AF4-mediated in vivo tumor suppressor activity, as well as reduced proliferation/survival and motility/invasion of MDA-MB-231 triple-negative breast cancer cells following AF4 treatment, suggests that AF4 and its bioactive components warrant further investigation as potential selective natural-source agents for the treatment of triple-negative breast cancer.

4. Materials and Methods

4.1. Reagents

AF4 was extracted from the peels of the apple cultivar Northern Spy, as previously described [12]. AF4 in ethanol was filter-sterilized and stored at −80 °C. Prior to use in this study, ethanol was evaporated under nitrogen gas and the AF4 residue was dissolved in sterile pyrogen-free water and aliquots of the resulting AF4 stock (10 mg/mL) were stored at −20 °C. Amplex Red reagent, Annexin-V-488, Dulbecco's modified Eagle's medium (DMEM), DMEM/F12, horse serum, fetal calf serum, CM-H_2DCFDA, and PI were from Life Technologies Inc. (Burlington, ON, Canada). Hydroxyethyl piperazineethanesulfonic acid (HEPES)- and bicarbonate-buffered mammary epithelial cell medium, mammary epithelial cell growth supplement, penicillin/streptomycin solution and poly-L-lysine were purchased from ScienCell Research Laboratories Inc. (Carlsbad, CA, USA). DMEM, phenol red-free DMEM, recombinant human insulin, hydrocortisone, phosphatase substrate, Triton X-100, mitomycin C, NAC, MTT, quercetin, MK2206, and SC66 were from Sigma-Aldrich (Oakville, ON, Canada). Paraformaldehyde was from Bioshop Canada Inc. (Burlington, ON, Canada). Fibroblast cell growth medium and supplements were from Lonza Inc. (Walkersville, MD, USA). DNase-free RNase A was from Qiagen Inc. (Mississauga, ON, Canada). Recombinant epidermal growth factor and basic fibroblast growth factor were from PeproTech (Rocky Hill, NJ). Diff-Quik staining kit was from Siemens Healthcare Diagnostics (Los Angeles, CA, USA). Rodent M block, anti-rabbit horse 6 radish peroxidase (HRP)-polymer and HRP/DAB detection system were from Biocare Medical (Markham, ON, Canada). HRP-conjugated anti-β-actin monoclonal antibody (Ab), anti-cyclin D3 monoclonal Ab, anti-CDK4 rabbit Ab, anti-phospho-PTEN (Ser380) monoclonal Ab, anti-PTEN monoclonal Ab, anti-Akt monoclonal Ab, and anti-phospho-Akt (Thr308) monoclonal Ab were from Cell Signaling Technology (Beverly, MA, USA). Anti-MMP2 Ab and anti-CD31 Ab were from Abcam Inc. (Toronto, ON, Canada). HRP-conjugated-goat anti-mouse IgG Ab and HRP-conjugated-donkey anti-rabbit IgG Ab were from Santa Cruz Biotechnology (Santa Cruz, CA, USA).

4.2. Cell Culture

The MDA-MB-231 breast cancer cell line was provided by Dr. S. Drover (Memorial University of Newfoundland, St. John's, NL, Canada). MDA-MB-468, MCF-7, and SKBR3 breast cancer cell lines were from Dr. P. Lee, Dr. K. Goralski and Dr. G. Dellaire, respectively (Dalhousie University, Halifax, NS, Canada). Breast cancer cell lines were authenticated by short tandem repeat analysis conducted by ATCC (Manassas, VA, USA). All breast cancer cell lines were cultured in DMEM supplemented with 10% heat-inactivated fetal calf serum, 5 mM HEPES buffer (pH 7.4), 2 mM L-glutamine, 100 U/mL penicillin, and 100 μg/mL streptomycin, and were maintained at 37 °C in a humidified incubator supplied with 10% CO_2. HMECs from ScienCell Research Laboratories Inc. were grown in serum-free, HEPES- and bicarbonate-buffered mammary epithelial cell medium supplemented with 1% mammary epithelial cell growth supplement and 1% penicillin/streptomycin solution, and maintained for a maximum of seven passages at 37 °C in a humidified incubator supplied with 5% CO_2. The MCF-10A normal mammary epithelial cell line was from Dr. P. Marcato (Dalhousie University, Halifax, NS, Canada). MCF-10A cells were cultured in DMEM/F12 supplemented with 10% heat-inactivated horse serum, 10 μg/mL human insulin, 20 μg/mL EGF, 0.5 μg/mL hydrocortisone, 100 U/mL penicillin, and

100 μg/mL streptomycin. MDF-10A cultures were maintained at 37 °C in a humidified incubator supplied with 10% CO_2. Human dermal fibroblasts from Lonza Inc. (Walkersville, MD, USA) were maintained as per the supplier's instructions.

4.3. MTT (3-(4,5-Dimethythiazol-2-yl)-2,5-Diphenyltetrazolium Bromide) Assay for Cell Viability

Cells were plated in quadruplicate into 96-well flat-bottom plates at a density of 5×10^3 cells/well and cultured in the absence or presence of the indicated concentrations of AF4 for desired time. At the end of culture, MTT was added to each well to a final concentration of 0.5 μg/mL. Plates were then incubated for 2 h at 37 °C, after which supernatant was removed and formazan crystals in each well were solubilized in 100 μL of dimethyl sulfoxide (DMSO). Absorbance was measured at 570 nm using an Asys Expert Microplate Reader (Biochrom Ltd., Cambridge, UK). Results are expressed as % metabolic activity relative to the medium control.

4.4. Acid Phosphatase Assay of Spheroid Growth

MCF-7 cells in F12 medium containing 20 ng/mL basic fibroblast growth factor, 20 ng/mL epidermal growth factor, 100 U/mL penicillin, 100 μg/mL streptomycin and B27 serum-free supplement were cultured for 48 h in ultra-low adherent cell culture plates and then treated with the indicated concentrations of AF4 or vehicle for 72 h. Spheroids were photographed, washed with phosphate-buffered saline, resuspended in 100 μL acid phosphatase assay solution (0.1 M sodium acetate at pH 5.5, 0.1% Triton-X-100, 4 mg/mL phosphatase substrate) and incubated for 2 h at 37 °C in the dark. The reaction was stopped by adding 25 μL 1 N NaOH to each well. Absorbance was measured at 405 nm using an Asys Expert Microplate Reader and % acid phosphatase activity was determined.

4.5. Flow Cytometric Cell Proliferation Assay

MDA-MB-231 cell cultures were synchronized by serum starvation for 20 h and then seeded into 6-well plates and allowed to form monolayers. Cells were stained with 1.25 μM Oregon Green 488 dye in serum-free DMEM and a sample of stained cells was retained for use as a non-proliferative control. The remaining cells were cultured for 72 h in the absence or presence of the indicated concentrations of AF4. Cellular fluorescence was then measured using a FACSCalibur instrument (BD Bioscience, Mississauga, ON, Canada). The fluorescence of control and AF4-treated cells was compared to that of the non-proliferative control and the number of cell divisions (n) was calculated as follows: $MCF_{baseline} = (2^n)(MCF_{sample})$; where n denotes the number of cell divisions and MCF denotes mean channel fluorescence.

4.6. Cell-Cycle Analysis

MDA-MB-231 and MBA-MB-468 cell cultures were synchronized by serum starvation for 20 h and then cultured for 72 h in the absence or presence of the indicated concentrations of AF4. Cells were then collected, washed with ice-cold phosphate-buffered saline, and ice-cold 70% ethanol was added drop-wise to the cells under constant agitation. Cells were then stored at −20°C for 24 h, washed, and resuspended in phosphate-buffered saline containing 0.02 mg/mL PI, 0.1% Triton X-100, and 0.2 mg/mL DNase-free RNase A. After incubation for 30 min at room temperature in the dark, cellular fluorescence was determined using a FACSCalibur instrument. Data were analyzed using ModFitLT V2.0 software (Becton Dickson, CA, US).

4.7. Gap-Closure Assay

MDA-MB-231 cells were seeded at a density of 1×10^4 cells/mL into wells containing culture inserts. After 18 h of culture, cells were treated with 10 μg/mL of mitomycin C in serum-free DMEM for 2 h at 37 °C to prevent cell division. After 12 h, cells were washed with complete DMEM and cultured in the absence or presence of 20 μg/mL AF4. At 0 h and 24 h, culture inserts were removed and the gaps were photographed.

4.8. *Trans-Well Migration/Invasion Assay*

MDA-MB-231 cells were treated with 20 μg/mL AF4 for 24 h and serum-starved for 6 h, after which 5×10^4 cells in serum-free DMEM were placed into wells of the upper chamber of the trans-well cell migration apparatus. The bottom chamber wells contained DMEM plus 10% fetal calf serum as a chemoattractant. Migration of cells through an 8 μm porous membrane (uncoated or coated with fibronectin) was detected by Diff-Quik staining. Migrated cells were imaged under a light microscope.

4.9. *Flow Cytometric Measurement of Apoptosis*

MDA-MB-231 cells were seeded at a density of 1×10^5 cells/well into 6-well plates and cultured in the absence or presence of the indicated concentrations of AF4 without or with 5 mM NAC for the desired time. In separate experiments, MDA-MB-231 cells were cultured for 48 h in the absence or presence of the Akt inhibitors MK2206 and SC66. At the end of culture cells were harvested, washed and stained with Annexin-V-488 and PI (1 μg/mL) for 15 min at room temperature. Flow cytometric analysis was performed using a FACSCalibur instrument.

4.10. *Reactive Oxygen Species (ROS) Measurements*

Measurement of ROS by Amplex Red assay was performed in 96-well flat-bottom plates containing quadruplicate cultures of MDA-MB-231 cells without or with AF4 at 50 μg/mL. In the dark, 100 μL of master mix containing 25 μM Amplex Red reagent and 0.005 U/mL HRP in phenol red-free cDMEM was added to each culture. After incubation at 37 °C for 2 or 24 h, absorbance was measured at 570 nm with an Asys Expert Microplate Reader. Measurement of ROS by fluorescence was performed by staining quadruplicate cultures of MDA-MB-231 cells or MCF-10A cells with 5 μM CM-H_2DCFDA in serum- and phenol-red free DMEM. Cells were then cultured for 2 or 24 h in the absence or presence of the indicated concentrations of AF4 in phenol-red free DMEM containing 1% fetal calf serum. Fluorescence at 529 nm was measured with a Spectramax M2 Microplate Reader (Molecular Devices, San Jose, CA, USA).

4.11. *Western Blot Analysis*

MDA-MB-231 cells were cultured in the absence or presence of the indicated concentrations of AF4 for 24 h, and then placed in ice-cold lysis buffer (50 mM Tris at pH 7.5, 150 mM NaCl, 50 mM disodium hydrogen phosphate, 0.25% sodium deoxycholate, 0.1% Nonidet P-40, 100 μM Na_3VO_4, 10 mM NaF, 5 mM ethylenediaminetetraacetic acid and 5 mM ethylene glycol tetraacetic acid) containing freshly added protease inhibitors (1 mM phenylmethylsulfonylfluoride, 10 μg/mL aprotinin, 5 μg/mL leupeptin, 10 μM phenylarsine oxide, 1 mM dithiothreitol and 5 μg/mL pepstatin). After 15 min, cell lysates were cleared by centrifugation and the protein concentration was determined by Bradford assay. Equal amounts of protein (20 μg) were loaded into 12% or 15% sodium dodecyl sulfate polyacrylamide gels. Separated proteins were transferred onto nitrocellulose membranes, which were then blocked by 1 h incubation in 5% non-fat milk or 5% bovine serum albumin in Tween-Tris buffered saline (TBS) solution (0.25 M Tris at pH 7.5, 150 mM NaCl, 0.2% Tween-20). Blots were probed overnight at 4 °C with an optimal concentration of primary Ab, and then washed thoroughly with Tween-TBS and probed with HRP-conjugated donkey anti-rabbit IgG Ab or anti-mouse IgG Ab, as appropriate, for 1 h at room temperature. Even protein loading was confirmed by probing the blots with HRP-conjugated rabbit anti-β actin Ab. Proteins of interest were visualized by chemiluminescence.

4.12. Xenograft Breast Cancer Model

Six to eight week-old female NOD-SCID mice were purchased from Charles River Canada (Lasalle, QC, Canada) and housed under sterile conditions and fed a sterilized rodent diet and water supplied ad libitum. Pathogen-free MDA-MB-231 cells (5×10^7) were implanted by subcutaneous injection into the right hind flank. Starting two weeks after xenografting, tumor sizes and body weights were recorded every other day until the last day (day 15) of the experiment. Tumor volume was calculated according to the equation, $(L \times P^2)/2$ where L is tumor length and P is perpendicular to tumor length. Intratumoral injection of AF4 commenced once the tumors reached a volume of 100 mm^3 (recorded as day 1). A total of 5 intratumoral injections of AF4 at 0.5 mg/kg in 20 µL saline (7 mice) or saline alone (10 mice) were administered every other day for 9 days. Mice were monitored for an additional 6 days and their tumor sizes and body weights were recorded. Mice were euthanized at day 15, after which the tumors were excised and photographed. Tumors were fixed in buffered formalin, embedded in paraffin and cut into 5 µm thick sections. Tumor sections were mounted onto glass slides and stained with hematoxylin and eosin for detection of necrotic and live cells. Immunohistochemistry was performed to detect CD31 expression. Ethics approval for animal use was obtained from the Dalhousie University Committee on Laboratory Animals, and was in accordance with Canadian Council on Animal Care guidelines.

Supplementary Materials:
Figure S1: AF4 is a more selective but less potent inhibitor of breast cancer cell growth, Figure S2: AF4 induces G_0/G_1 cell cycle arrest in MDA-MB-468 breast cancer cells, Figure S3: AF4 treatment causes ROS accumulation in non-malignant MCF-10A mammary epithelial cells, Figure S4: MDA-MB-231 breast cancer cells are more sensitive than non-malignant MCF-10A mammary epithelial cells to oxidative stress, Figure S5: Akt inhibition causes apoptosis of MDA-MB-231 breast cancer cells.

Author Contributions: Conceptualization, D.W.H. and H.P.V.R.; methodology, C.-Y.L. and W.F.; formal analysis, C.-Y.L. and W.F.; writing-original draft preparation, C.-Y.L. and W.F.; writing-review and editing, D.W.H.; supervision, D.W.H.; project administration, D.W.H. and H.P.V.R.; funding acquisition, D.W.H. and H.P.V.R.

Acknowledgments: W.F. was supported by a trainee award from the Beatrice Hunter Cancer Research Institute with funds provided by the Harvey Graham Cancer Research Fund as part of The Terry Fox Strategic Health Research Training Program in Cancer Research at the Canadian Institutes for Health Research.

References

1. Bamia, C.; Lagiou, P.; Jenab, M.; Aleksandrova, K.; Fedirko, V.; Trichopoulos, D.; Overvad, K.; Tjønneland, A.; Olsen, A.; Clavel-Chapelon, F.; et al. Fruit and vegetable consumption in relation to hepatocellular carcinoma in a multi-centre, European cohort study. *Br. J. Cancer* **2015**, *112*, 1273–1282. [CrossRef] [PubMed]
2. Núñez-Sánchez, M.A.; González-Sarrías, A.; Romo-Vaquero, M.; García-Villalba, R.; Selma, M.V.; Tomás-Barberán, F.A.; García-Conesa, M.-T.; Espín, J.C. Dietary phenolics against colorectal cancer. From promising preclinical results to poor translation into clinical trials: Pitfalls and future needs. *Mol. Nutr. Food Res.* **2015**, *59*, 1274–1291. [CrossRef] [PubMed]
3. Khan, N.; Mukhtar, H. Dietary agents for prevention and treatment of lung cancer. *Cancer Lett.* **2015**, *359*, 155–164. [CrossRef] [PubMed]
4. Liu, H.; Wang, X.-C.; Hu, G.-H.; Guo, Z.-F.; Lai, P.; Xu, L.; Huang, T.-B.; Xu, Y.-F. Fruit and vegetable consumption and risk of bladder cancer. *Eur. J. Cancer Prev.* **2015**, *24*, 508–516. [CrossRef] [PubMed]
5. Bradbury, K.E.; Appleby, P.N.; Key, T.J. Fruit, vegetable, and fiber intake in relation to cancer risk: Findings from the European Prospective Investigation into Cancer and Nutrition (EPIC). *Am. J. Clin. Nutr.* **2014**, *100*, 394S–398S. [CrossRef] [PubMed]
6. Kale, A.; Gawande, S.; Kotwal, S. Cancer phytotherapeutics: Role for flavonoids at the cellular level. *Phytother. Res.* **2008**, *577*, 567–577. [CrossRef]
7. Yao, H.; Xu, W.; Shi, X.; Zhang, Z. Dietary flavonoids as cancer prevention agents. *J. Environ. Sci. Health Part C* **2011**, *29*, 1–31. [CrossRef] [PubMed]
8. Vineetha, V.P.; Girija, S.; Soumya, R.S.; Raghu, K.G. Polyphenol-rich apple (*Malus domestica* L.) peel extract attenuates arsenic trioxide induced cardiotoxicity in H9c2 cells via its antioxidant activity. *Food Funct.* **2014**, *5*, 502–511. [CrossRef]

9. Ribeiro, F.A.P.; Gomes de Moura, C.F.; Aguiar, O.; de Oliveira, F.; Spadari, R.C.; Oliveira, N.R.C.; Oshima, C.T.F.; Ribeiro, D.A. The chemopreventive activity of apple against carcinogenesis. *Eur. J. Cancer Prev.* **2014**, *23*, 477–480. [CrossRef]
10. Balasuriya, N.; Rupasinghe, H.P.V. Antihypertensive properties of flavonoid-rich apple peel extract. *Food Chem.* **2012**, *135*, 2320–2325. [CrossRef]
11. Tow, W.W.; Premier, R.; Jing, H.; Ajlouni, S. Antioxidant and antiproliferation effects of extractable and nonextractable polyphenols isolated from apple waste using different extraction methods. *J. Food Sci.* **2011**, *76*, T163–T172. [CrossRef] [PubMed]
12. Keddy, P.G.W.; Dunlop, K.; Warford, J.; Samson, M.L.; Jones, Q.R.D.; Rupasinghe, H.P.V.; Robertson, G.S. Neuroprotective and anti-inflammatory effects of the flavonoid-enriched fraction AF4 in a mouse model of hypoxic-ischemic brain injury. *PLoS ONE* **2012**, *7*, e51324. [CrossRef] [PubMed]
13. Warford, J.; Jones, Q.R.D.; Nichols, M.; Sullivan, V.; Rupasinghe, H.P.V.; Robertson, G.S. The flavonoid-enriched fraction AF4 suppresses neuroinflammation and promotes restorative gene expression in a mouse model of experimental autoimmune encephalomyelitis. *J. Neuroimmunol.* **2014**, *268*, 71–83. [CrossRef] [PubMed]
14. Sudan, S.; Rupasinghe, H.P.V. Flavonoid-enriched apple fraction AF4 induces cell cycle arrest, DNA topoisomerase II inhibition, and apoptosis in human liver cancer HepG2 cells. *Nutr. Cancer* **2014**, *66*, 1237–1246. [CrossRef] [PubMed]
15. Siegel, R.L.; Miller, K.D.; Jemal, A. Cancer statistics, 2018. *CA Cancer J. Clin.* **2018**, *68*, 7–30. [CrossRef] [PubMed]
16. Cheng, S.; Gao, N.; Zhang, Z.; Chen, G.; Budhraja, A.; Ke, Z.; Son, Y.-O.; Wang, X.; Luo, J.; Shi, X. Quercetin induces tumor-selective apoptosis through downregulation of Mcl-1 and activation of Bax. *Clin. Cancer Res.* **2010**, *16*, 5679–5691. [CrossRef] [PubMed]
17. Matsuo, M.; Sasaki, N.; Saga, K.; Kaneko, T. Cytotoxicity of flavonoids toward cultured normal human cells. *Biol. Pharm. Bull.* **2005**, *28*, 253–259. [CrossRef] [PubMed]
18. Romanouskaya, T.V.; Grinev, V.V. Cytotoxic effect of flavonoids on leukemia cells and normal cells of human blood. *Bull. Exp. Biol. Med.* **2009**, *148*, 57–59. [CrossRef] [PubMed]
19. Yadegarynia, S.; Pham, A.; Ng, A.; Nguyen, D.; Lialiutska, T.; Bortolazzo, A.; Sivryuk, V.; Bremer, M.; White, J.B. Profiling flavonoid cytotoxicity in human breast cancer cell lines: Determination of structure-function relationships. *Nat. Prod. Commun.* **2012**, *7*, 1295–1304. [CrossRef]
20. Takaki, T.; Echalier, A.; Brown, N.R.; Hunt, T.; Endicott, J.A.; Noble, M.E.M. The structure of CDK4/cyclin D3 has implications for models of CDK activation. *Proc. Natl. Acad. Sci. USA* **2009**, *106*, 4171–4176. [CrossRef]
21. Chien, S.Y.; Wu, Y.C.; Chung, J.G.; Yang, J.S.; Lu, H.F.; Tsou, M.F.; Wood, W.G.; Kuo, S.J.; Chen, D.R. Quercetin-induced apoptosis acts through mitochondrial- and caspase-3-dependent pathways in human breast cancer MDA-MB-231 cells. *Hum. Exp. Toxicol.* **2009**, *28*, 493–503. [CrossRef] [PubMed]
22. McEligot, A.J.; Yang, S.; Meyskens, F.L., Jr. Redox regulation by intrinsic species and extrinsic nutrients in normal and cancer cells. *Annu. Rev. Nutr.* **2005**, *25*, 261–295. [CrossRef] [PubMed]
23. Reczek, C.R.; Chandel, N.S. The two faces of reactive oxygen species in cancer. *Annu. Rev. Cancer Biol.* **2017**, *1*, 79–98. [CrossRef]
24. Han, Y.; Chen, J.Z. Oxidative stress induces mitochondrial DNA damage and cytotoxicity through independent mechanisms in human cancer cells. *Biomed. Res. Int.* **2013**, *2013*, 825065. [CrossRef] [PubMed]
25. Rice-Evans, C.A.; Miller, N.J.; Paganga, G. Structure-antioxidant activity relationships of flavonoids and phenolic acids. *Free Radic. Biol. Med.* **1996**, *20*, 933–956. [CrossRef]
26. Polyakov, N.E.; Leshina, T.V.; Konovalova, T.A.; Kispert, L.D. Carotenoids as scavengers of free radicals in a Fenton reaction: Antioxidants or pro-oxidants? *Free Radic. Biol. Med.* **2001**, *31*, 398–404. [CrossRef]
27. Lambert, J.D.; Elias, R.J. The antioxidant and pro-oxidant activities of green tea polyphenols: A role in cancer prevention. *Arch. Biochem. Biophys.* **2010**, *501*, 65–72. [CrossRef]
28. Fernando, W.; Rupasinghe, H.P.V.; Hoskin, D.W. Dietary phytochemicals with anti-oxidant and pro-oxidant activities: A double-edged sword in relation to adjuvant chemotherapy and radiotherapy? *Cancer Lett.* **2019**, *452*, 168–177. [CrossRef]
28. Fernando, W.; Rupasinghe, H.P.V.; Hoskin, D.W. Dietary phytochemicals with anti-oxidant and pro-oxidant activities: A double-edged sword in relation to adjuvant chemotherapy and radiotherapy? *Cancer Lett.* **2019**, *452*, 168–177. [CrossRef]

29. Weigelt, B.; Ghajar, C.M.; Bissell, M.J. The need for complex 3D culture models to unravel novel pathways and identify accurate biomarkers in breast cancer. *Adv. Drug Deliv. Rev.* **2014**, *69–70*, 42–51. [CrossRef]
30. Liotta, L.A. Gene products which play a role in cancer invastion and metastasis. *Breast Cancer Res. Treat.* **1988**, *11*, 113–124. [CrossRef]
31. Dey, N.; De, P.; Leyland-Jones, B. PI3K-AKT-mTOR inhibitors in breast cancers: From tumor cell signaling to clinical trials. *Pharmacol. Ther.* **2017**, *175*, 91–106. [CrossRef] [PubMed]
32. Song, G.; Ouyang, G.; Bao, S. The activation of Akt/PKB signaling pathway and cell survival. *J. Cell. Mol. Med.* **2005**, *9*, 59–71. [CrossRef] [PubMed]
33. Leslie, N.R.; Bennett, D.; Lindsay, Y.E.; Stewart, H.; Gray, A.; Downes, C.P. Redox regulation of PI 3-kinase signalling via inactivation of PTEN. *EMBO J.* **2003**, *22*, 5501–5510. [CrossRef] [PubMed]
34. Camargo, L.E.A.; Brustolin Ludwig, D.; Tominaga, T.T.; Carletto, B.; Favero, G.M.; Mainardes, R.M.; Khalil, N.M. Bovine serum albumin nanoparticles improve the antitumor activity of curcumin in a murine melanoma model. *J. Microencapsul.* **2018**, *35*, 467–474. [CrossRef] [PubMed]
35. Ban, C.; Jo, M.; Park, Y.H.; Kim, J.H.; Han, J.Y.; Lee, K.W.; Kweon, D.H.; Choi, Y.J. Enhancing the oral bioavailability of curcumin using solid lipid nanoparticles. *Food Chem.* **2019**, *302*, 125328. [CrossRef] [PubMed]
36. Armendáriz-Barragán, B.; Zafar, N.; Badri, W.; Galindo-Rodríguez, S.A.; Kabbaj, D.; Fessi, H.; Elaissari, A. Plant extracts: From encapsulation to application. *Expert Opin. Drug Deliv.* **2016**, *13*, 1165–1175. [CrossRef] [PubMed]

2

Anticancer Potential of Resveratrol, β-Lapachone and their Analogues

Danielly C. Ferraz da Costa [1,†], Luciana Pereira Rangel [2,†], Mafalda Maria Duarte da Cunha Martins-Dinis [3,†], Giulia Diniz da Silva Ferretti [3,†], Vitor F. Ferreira [4] and Jerson L. Silva [3,*]

1 Departamento de Nutrição Básica e Experimental, Instituto de Nutrição, Universidade do Estado do Rio de Janeiro, Rio de Janeiro 20550-013, Brazil; danielly.costa@uerj.br
2 Faculdade de Farmácia, Universidade Federal do Rio de Janeiro, Rio de Janeiro 21941-902, Brazil; lprangel@pharma.ufrj.br
3 Programa de Biologia Estrutural, Instituto de Bioquímica Médica Leopoldo de Meis, Instituto Nacional de Ciência e Tecnologia de Biologia Estrutural e Bioimagem, Universidade Federal do Rio de Janeiro, Rio de Janeiro 21941-902, Brazil; mafaldamariamartins@gmail.com (M.M.D.d.C.M.-D.); giuliadiniz@hotmail.com (G.D.d.S.F.)
4 Departamento de Tecnologia Farmacêutica, Faculdade de Farmácia, Universidade Federal Fluminense, Rio de Janeiro 24241-000, Brazil; vitorferreira@id.uff.br
* Correspondence: jerson@bioqmed.ufrj.br
† These authors contributed equally to this work.

Abstract: This review aims to explore the potential of resveratrol, a polyphenol stilbene, and beta-lapachone, a naphthoquinone, as well as their derivatives, in the development of new drug candidates for cancer. A brief history of these compounds is reviewed along with their potential effects and mechanisms of action and the most recent attempts to improve their bioavailability and potency against different types of cancer.

Keywords: resveratrol; β-lapachone; cancer

---

1. Introduction

Cancer is a critical public health problem worldwide, with more than 18 million new cases and 9.6 million deaths estimated in 2018 [1]. Cancer therapeutics involves multiple combined approaches and requires the development of strategies based on the design and synthesis of promising compounds to improve treatment response. The search for new molecules with antitumor activity is still necessary and pursued by the pharmaceutical industry and many different research groups. Natural compounds have long been used for this purpose, leading to the development of new drugs, or as templates for new molecules with similar structures and effects [2]. Historically, bioactive compounds derived from animals and plants have been extensively used to treat diseases, which explain the scientific interest in natural products for drug discovery [3]. Both resveratrol and β-lapachone have been used with this purpose, leading to the development of new derivatives and the production of delivery systems aimed at improving the bioavailability of these compounds. In this review, we describe the potential of resveratrol, a polyphenol stilbene, and β-lapachone, a napthoquinone (Figure 1), as well as their derivatives, in the development of new drug candidates for cancer. We begin with a brief history of these compounds and move further to the discussion of their potential effects and mechanisms of action and the most recent attempts to improve their bioavailability and potency against different types of cancer.

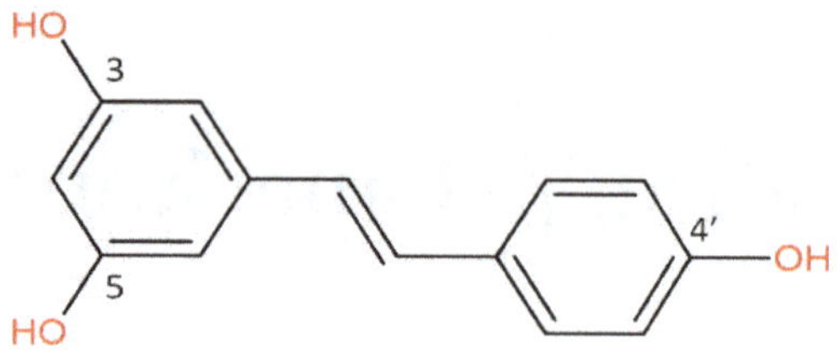

Resveratrol
(3,4′,5-trihydroxy-trans-stilbene)

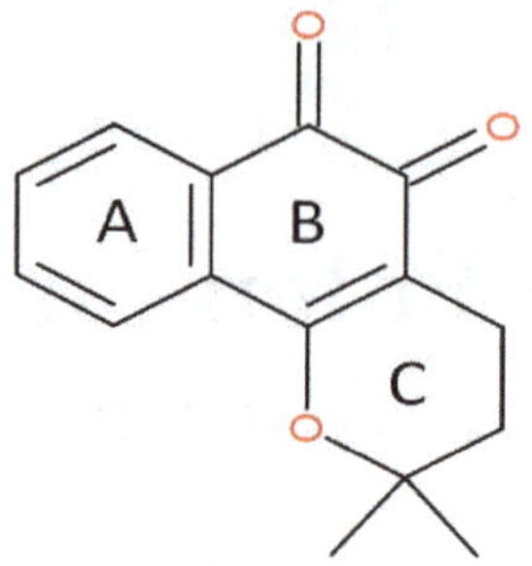

β-Lapachone
(3,4-dihydro-2,2-dimethyl-2H-naphthol[1,2-b]pyran-5,6-dione)

Figure 1. Structures of resveratrol and β-lapachone.

2. Resveratrol and Stilbene-Based Compounds

Stilbenes are phytochemicals with small molecular weights (approximately 200–300 g/mol) found in a wide range of plants and dietary supplements [4]. Stilbene-based compounds have become of particular interest because of their wide range of biological activities. Among them, resveratrol (3,4′,5-trihydroxy-*trans*-stilbene) is a natural nonflavonoid polyphenol, classified as a phytoalexin, which can be naturally produced by more than 70 plant species (including grapes, blueberries, raspberries, mulberries and peanuts) in response to stressful conditions, such as fungal infection and ultraviolet radiation. In plants, the molecule exists as *trans*-resveratrol and *cis*-resveratrol isomers, and their glucosides, *trans*-piceid and *cis*-piceid. Since resveratrol is efficiently extracted from grape skin during the wine-making process, red wine is the most important dietary source of this bioactive compound [5–7]. Resveratrol has attracted scientific attention since 1997, when Jang et al. first demonstrated its ability to modulate in vivo carcinogenesis by inhibiting tumor initiation, promotion and progression in mice [8]. After that, the number of published papers regarding the role of resveratrol in blocking the multistep process of carcinogenesis increased substantially [9,10].

Currently, resveratrol is well characterized as a potent chemopreventive and chemotherapeutic agent in different cancer experimental models and clinical trials (for a review, see our recent publication) [11]. Several cell processes are targeted by this phytoalexin by upregulation or downregulation of multiple molecular pathways involved in cancer. Resveratrol modulates xenobiotic metabolism by inhibiting phase I cytochrome P450 enzymes responsible for carcinogen activation and by inducing phase II carcinogen detoxifying enzymes; reduces oxidative stress and inflammation by decreasing reactive oxygen species (ROS) generation and downregulating cyclooxygenase (COX) and inflammatory cytokines; promotes cell proliferation arrest by modulating cell cycle regulatory machinery such as cyclins and cyclin-dependent kinases (CDKs); induces apoptosis of damaged or transformed cells by different mechanisms, including upregulation of the p53 tumor suppressor protein and BAX and downregulation of Bcl2 and survivin; suppresses angiogenesis, invasion and metastasis by inhibiting hypoxia-induced factor-1α (HIF-1α) and matrix metalloproteinases; targets hormone signaling due to its relevant antiestrogenic activity in hormone-dependent cancers; and reduces the risk of multidrug resistance (MDR) via multiple targets related to carcinogenesis and chemo/radioresistance [12,13]. Resveratrol has also been proposed as a pro-oxidant agent depending on the concentration, exposure time and cell type. The oxidative damage caused by this compound represents one of the cytotoxic mechanisms involved in tumor cell death [14,15].

Mutant p53 is associated with aggregation, which results in negative dominance and gain-of-function effects [16–19]. Novel compounds can directly target the interaction of p53 mutant aggregates with their p63 and p73 paralogues and with other transcription factors [17,20]. New compounds capable of intervening in the formation of aggregates can range from natural molecules such as resveratrol analogues, synthetic molecules such as Michael acceptors, small synthetic peptides, aptamers of nucleic acids and glycosaminoglycans [17]. These new drugs have great potential to represent radical innovation. In our recently published paper, we demonstrated that resveratrol inhibits the aggregation of p53 mutants *in vitro*, in tumor cells and in xenotransplants implanted in nude mouse models (Figure 2) [21]. However, very high doses were required to exert the effect. We intend to use synthetic chemistry to produce resveratrol analogs with higher potency that can be used as pharmaceuticals.

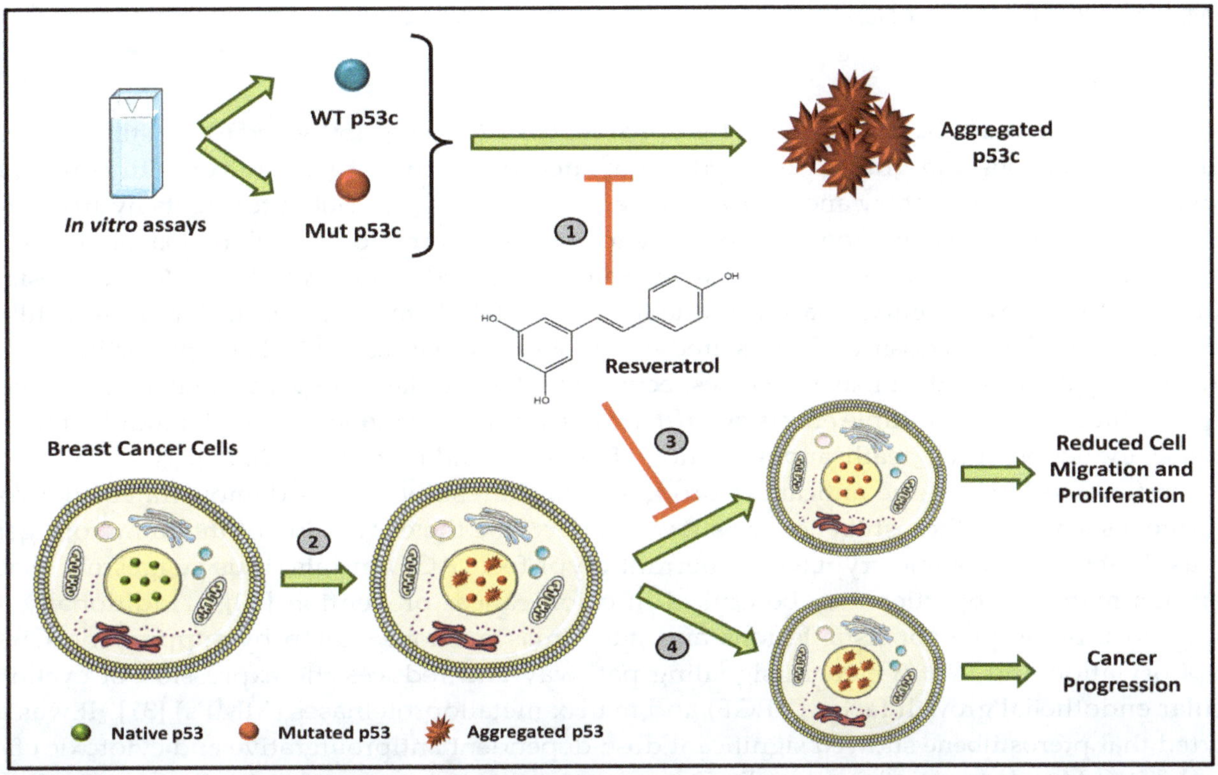

Figure 2. Schematic representation of p53 inhibition by resveratrol. In (**1**), the resveratrol in vitro capacity of inhibition of both WT and mutant p53 aggregation is described. (**2**) When mutations in the TP53 gene appear, the protein produced is less stable and forms aggregates. These aggregates are related to a direct effect in cancer proliferation and migration that is inhibited by treatment with resveratrol (**3**). Otherwise, cancer progression occurs (**4**). Extracted from Ferraz da Costa, 2018 [21].

In another study, we described that transient transfection of the wild-type p53 gene causes H1299 cells (null to p53) to become more sensitive and responsive to the pro-apoptotic properties of resveratrol, similar to what was observed in MCF-7 cells. It was proposed that resveratrol could be used therapeutically in combination with other methods of promoting p53 activity in cells, such as gene therapy using the wild-type (WT) p53 gene or chemicals that restore p53 function [22].

In mammalian experimental models, resveratrol is extensively metabolized and quickly eliminated, resulting in poor bioavailability. After oral administration, resveratrol is absorbed by passive diffusion or by membrane transporters at the intestinal level and is then released in the bloodstream, where it can be detected as an unmodified or metabolized molecule [13,23]. Although 75% of resveratrol is absorbed through the oral route, only 1% is detected in the blood plasma after the whole metabolism [24]. In recent years, different methodological approaches and synthetic derivatives have been developed to improve resveratrol bioavailability. Many studies have been performed to synthesize new and more effective resveratrol analogs that display better pharmacokinetic properties, low toxicity and minimum side effects. The methoxylated, hydroxylated and halogenated resveratrol derivatives are more explored due to their beneficial biological activities and increased oral bioavailability [25]. Previous studies showed that methoxylation increases metabolic stability and the time length required for the molecules to reach the plasma concentration peak. Moreover, the substitution of hydroxyl groups of resveratrol to methoxyl groups substantially potentiated its therapeutic versatility. It was also reported that the introduction of additional hydroxyl groups significantly increased the biological activity of resveratrol analogs [23,25]. In this review, we collect and present recent evidence in the literature regarding resveratrol derivatives and their anticancer effects, with an emphasis on the molecular mechanisms involved.

2.1. *Methoxylated Resveratrol Derivatives*

2.1.1. Pterostilbene

Pterostilbene (*trans*-3,5-dimethoxy-40-hydroxystilbene) is a naturally occurring stilbene, found mainly in blueberries and grapes. It is a dimethylated derivative of resveratrol with comparable antioxidant, anti-inflammatory and anticarcinogenic properties [26]. Substituting its hydroxyl for a methoxyl group enhances the lipophilicity of pterostilbene, adding to its in vivo bioavailability and, thus, improving the biological activity of this compound compared to resveratrol [27]. A study designed to compare the bioavailability, pharmacokinetics and metabolism of resveratrol and pterostilbene following equimolar oral dosing administered in rats showed that resveratrol and pterostilbene were approximately 20% and 80% bioavailable, respectively [28]. Cumulative experimental data have noted that pterostilbene exerts multiple effects against a variety of cancer models through modulation of the cell cycle, induction of cell death, and inhibition of invasion and metastasis [26,29].

The first evidence of the anticancer properties of pterostilbene was demonstrated in a colon tumorigenesis model. Pterostilbene was shown to decrease the expression of inflammatory genes, such as iNOS in the colonic crypts and aberrant crypt foci (ACF) in rats, thus suggesting that its anti-inflammatory properties may be critical in colon cancer prevention [30]. Additionally, this compound inhibits preneoplastic lesions and adenomas in mouse colon by suppressing GSK3β phosphorylation and Wnt/β-catenin signaling pathway and reduces the expression of cyclin D1, vascular endothelial growth factor (VEGF) and matrix metalloproteinases (MMPs) [31]. It was also reported that pterostilbene showed significant dose-dependent antiproliferative and cytotoxic effects and inhibited Myc, beta-catenin and cyclin D gene expression in human colon cancer Caco-2 cells [32]. In gastric adenocarcinoma cells, pterostilbene inhibits cellular proliferation and leads cells to apoptosis by different pathways, such as caspase cascade activation and modulation of cell-cycle regulating proteins [33]. In a human model of hepatocellular carcinoma, pterostilbene suppresses tumor growth by interfering in the signal transduction pathways of NF-κB and on the expression of VEGF, matrix metalloproteinase-9 (MMP-9), AP-1 and mitogen-activated protein kinase (MAPK) [34,35]. Breast cancer stem cells isolated from MCF-7, which expresses the surface antigen CD44+/CD24–, were selectively eliminated by pterostilbene. Furthermore, this compound induces necrosis and inhibits mammosphere formation, increases the activity of paclitaxel, decreases CD44 expression, induces β-catenin phosphorylation through the inhibition of hedgehog/Akt/GSK3β signaling and decreases the expression of c-Myc and cyclin D1 [36]. More recent studies showed that pterostilbene is a promising agent against human papillomavirus (HPV) E6+ tumors tested in vitro and in vivo. In vitro, this compound downregulates the viral oncogene E6. On the other hand, in mouse TC1 tumors, in addition to inhibiting E6, pterostilbene suppressed VEGF and tumor development [37]. In acute lymphoblastic leukemia cell lines Jurkat and Molt-4, the potential of pterostilbene to modulate Fas, a member of the death-inducing family of tumor necrosis factor (TNF), was investigated. Pterostilbene increased both Fas mRNA and its cell surface levels, thus leading to apoptosis [38].

2.1.2. Trimethoxystilbene

Trimethoxystilbene (*trans*-3,4′,5-trimethoxystilbene) is also a methylated resveratrol derivative, described as a potent chemopreventive agent, which promotes the induction of cell cycle arrest, reduces angiogenesis, inhibits cancer cell proliferation, increases apoptosis and decreases metastasis [25]. In MCF-7 breast cancer cells, this compound acts by inhibiting epithelial–mesenchymal transition (EMT), negatively modulating β-catenin nuclear translocation and phosphatidylinositol 3-kinase (PI3K)/protein kinase B (AKT) signaling [39]. Its anticancer mechanisms on lung cancer cells involve apoptosis induction by activation of caspases 3 and 9 and poly (ADP-ribose) polymerase interruption [40]. Additionally, in human lung cancer (A549), trimethoxystilbene promotes a decrease in invasive, migratory and adhesive characteristics of these cells and modulates the mRNA levels that encode for MMP-2 protein [41]. When evaluating the effect of this resveratrol derivative in rat C6 and human T98G glioma cells, a massive accumulation of cells at the G2/M phase of the cell cycle and apoptosis via caspase-3 related to p53 tumor suppressor protein induction were observed [42]. Trimethoxystilbene is a more effective derivative than resveratrol in suppressing the growth of HepG2 hepatocellular carcinoma cells via induction of G2/M cell cycle arrest (by upregulation of cyclin B1) and apoptosis (by downregulation of Bcl-2) [43].

2.1.3. Tetramethoxystilbene

The modification of the resveratrol structure that generates its analogue tetramethoxystilbene improved its bioactivity by suppressing cell growth in prostate, colon, ovarian and hepatocellular cancer cells. This analogue demonstrates a higher activity on human melanoma A375 by decreasing cell proliferation after treatment using a lower dose (IC_{50} = 0.7 μM) than resveratrol (IC_{50} = 100 μM) [44]. Compared with the *trans* form of the 3,4,5,4′-tetramethoxystilbene resveratrol derivative compound, the *cis* form is ten times more potent at decreasing the growth of human WI38VA virally transformed fibroblasts [45]. Using a xenograft of human ovarian cancer (A2780 and SKOV-3) as a model to study the effect of *trans*-3,4,5,4′-tetramethoxystilbene, it was observed that treatment with this derivative is able to reduce tumor cell growth [46,47]. For breast cancer, it was demonstrated that proapoptotic proteins and voltage-dependent anion channel 1 (VDAC-1) expression were increased after treatment [48]. As a new approach to treat osteosarcoma cells resistant to paclitaxel and cisplatin, the use of tetramethoxystilbene decreases, in vitro and in vivo, the viability of resistant cells and induces massive apoptosis [49].

2.1.4. Pentamethoxystilbene

Pentamethoxystilbene is a hybrid molecule chemically synthesized and, similar to resveratrol, has low oral bioavailability but presents high intravenous bioavailability. In breast carcinoma cells (MCF-7), this derivative is a good antiproliferative candidate that acts through different pathways as a G1 cell cycle regulator, modulating cyclins E and D and retinoblastoma protein (pRb). It is a better suppressor agent for breast cancer cells than resveratrol or other methoxylated derivatives. At the IC_{50} concentration of this derivative (37.8 μM), treatment with resveratrol only reduces cell survival 20% [50]. In colon cancer, a better response was reached with this compound, with activation of apoptosis through cell cycle arrest in G2/M phase, polymerization of microtubules and finally caspase-induced apoptosis. Beyond apoptosis, the compound may decrease iNOS, β-catenin and cell proliferation [51,52]. No further studies have been published with this derivative since 2012.

2.2. *Hydroxylated Resveratrol Derivatives*

2.2.1. Dihydroxystilbene

The resveratrol analogue 4,4′-dihydroxy-*trans*-stilbene (4,4′-DHS) was designed to improve resveratrol efficiency, both as an antioxidant and antiproliferative agent. 4,4′-DHS exhibits remarkably higher cytotoxicity than resveratrol against human promyelocytic leukemia (HL-60) cells [53]. 4,4′-DHS also inhibits the clonogenic efficiency of fibroblasts nine times more potently than resveratrol, although with a different mechanism. 4,4′-DHS predominantly induces an accumulation of cells in G1 phase, whereas resveratrol disturbs the G1/S phase transition. Furthermore, 4,4′-DHS increases p21 and p53 protein levels, whereas resveratrol leads to phosphorylation of the S-phase checkpoint protein Chk1 [54]. In a mouse lung cancer model, 2,3- and 4,4′-dihydroxystilbene (at 10 and 25 mg/kg, administered twice daily) inhibited tumor growth and metastasis. The antitumor and antimetastatic effects of these compounds were partly due to anti-lymphangiogenesis and the regulation of M2 macrophage activation and differentiation [55]. The cytotoxic action of 4,4′-DHS was also investigated in vitro in human neuroblastoma cell lines and in a mouse xenograft model of human neuroblastoma. The pharmacological action of 4,4′-DHS in the human neuroblastoma IMR32 cells was mediated by the destabilization of mitochondrial and lysosomal membranes, associated with modulation of several related pro- and anti-apoptotic cascades of proteins. Additionally, in the animal model, the oral administration of 4,4′-DHS for one month was well tolerated and demonstrated a greater therapeutic potential than resveratrol [56]. More recently, Saha et al. demonstrated that in melanoma cells, 4,4′-DHS acts by inducing apoptosis and cell cycle arrest in G1 phase and inhibiting cell proliferation. A significant reduction of melanoma tumors in a preclinical murine model was observed, and the antimetastatic effect of 4,4′-DHS was shown in a melanoma-mediated lung metastasis model in vivo [57]. In vivo assays performed in different mouse models of tumor xenografts demonstrated that 4,4′-DHS was able to disrupt the DNA replication pathway, leading to the apoptosis of pancreatic, ovarian and colorectal cancer cells [58].

2.2.2. Tetrahydroxystilbene

Tetrahydroxystilbene is a natural resveratrol analogue with multiple biological activities. In SK-Mel-28 melanoma cells, treatment with this compound induced apoptosis and inhibited cell proliferation [59,60]. In prostate cancer, its anticancer mechanisms involve JAK1 leading to STAT3 activation, which leads to a cytokine signal transduction pathway [61]. In liver and colon cancer cells, tetrahydroxystilbene arrests the cell cycle at G1 phase by modulating the cyclins pathway [62,63]. In human leukemia cells (U937), this compound induces massive apoptosis and leads to cell cycle arrest in G1 phase by regulating Bcl-2 and cIAP-2 (anti-apoptotic proteins). In cervix cancer, it acts by modulating p53 protein, thus leading cells to apoptosis [64,65]. In the last year, the 2,3,5,4′-tetrahydroxystilbene-2-O-β-D-glucoside (THSG) derivative was the major compound studied. In HT-29 colon adenocarcinoma cells, treatment with this compound reduced cell migration, invasion and adhesion, thus inhibiting metastasis. This is possible because THSG inhibits NF-κB pathway activation and consequently suppresses proteins involved in migration and invasion, such as MMP-2 and p-VE-cadherin, and ICAM-1 proteins involved in cell adhesion [66]. In vivo assays with THSG, using azoxymethane-induced colorectal cancer in rats, induced a 50% reduction in total colonic aberrant crypt foci by the inhibition of NF-κB pathway activation [67]. In MCF-7 breast cancer cells exposed to adriamycin and THSG, the vascular endothelial growth factor/phosphatidylinositol 3-kinase/Akt pathway was inhibited, triggering apoptosis by modulating Bcl-2 and caspase-3 [68].

2.2.3. Hexahydroxystilbene

Hexahydroxystilbene is a synthetic resveratrol derivative with higher biological activity [69]. When tested in breast cancer cells, hexahydroxystilbene induced apoptosis and inhibited cell proliferation by p53 protein accumulation and downregulation of mitochondrial superoxide dismutase [70]. In human colon cancer cells (HT-29), treatment with this compound leads to apoptosis and cell cycle arrest [71]. Similar results were observed in leukemia cells, with apoptosis induction by caspase activation pathways [72]. In vivo assays in a melanoma mouse model also demonstrate the induction of apoptosis pathway by upregulation of p21, downregulation of CDK-2 and cell cycle arrest at the G2/M phase [73]. Hexahydroxystilbene demonstrates an antiproliferative effect and accelerates senescence in cultured human peritoneal mesothelial cells by an oxidative stress-dependent mechanism. Treatment with 10 μM hexahydroxystilbene promoted an increase in 8-OHdG levels, a product of DNA oxidation, and a time-dependent increase in ROS release was also reported. On the other hand, soluble factors released by human peritoneal mesothelial cells that senesced prematurely in response to treatment promoted the growth of colorectal and pancreatic carcinomas in vitro [74]. No further studies have used this compound since 2013.

Although many studies have reported that stilbene compounds could play essential roles as chemotherapeutic agents by regulating multiple mechanisms and acting on different targets, further translational research is required to determine if the preclinical anticancer properties of these compounds, either alone or as part of combined therapies, are applicable in a clinical setting. The IC_{50} values for resveratrol and its derivatives vary in a wide range, as indicated in Table 1.

Table 1. IC_{50} values of resveratrol and derivatives in different study models.

Compound	2D Structure	IC_{50}	Study Model	References
Resveratrol and Resveratrol Methoxylated Derivatives				
Resveratrol	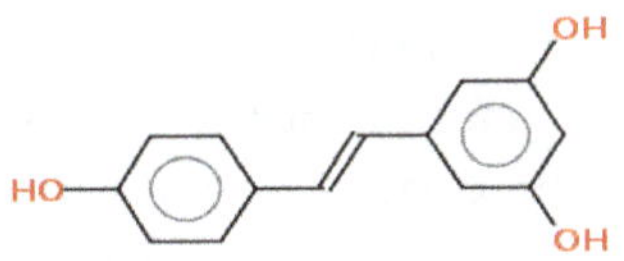	15–145 μM	Breast (MCF-7, MDA-MB-231, MDA-MB-468, MDA-MB-453), lung (A549, H460), pancreatic (Colo-357, Panc-1), prostate (LNCap, DU145) and colon (HCT116, Caco2) cancer cells; cervix carcinoma (HeLa); hepatocarcinoma (HepG2); melanoma (A357, SK-MEL-31); glioma (C6, T98G)	[22,42,75–78]
Pterostilbene	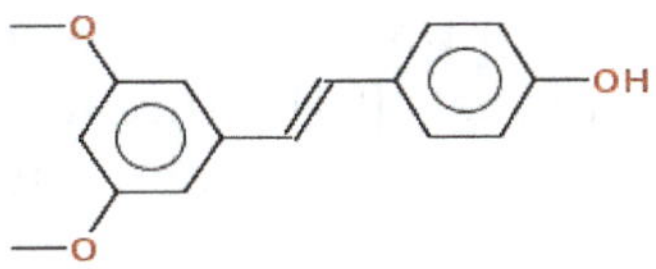	4.1–108 μM	Acute lymphoblastic leukemia (Molt-4), acute T cell leukemia (Jurkat), breast (MDA-MB-231), colon (COLO 205, HCT-116, HT-29) and endometrial (HEC-1A, ECC-1) cancer cells; melanoma (A357); hepatocarcinoma (HepG2); cervix carcinoma (HeLa, SiHa); epidermoid carcinoma (CaSki);	[27,38,79–81]
Trimethoxystilbene	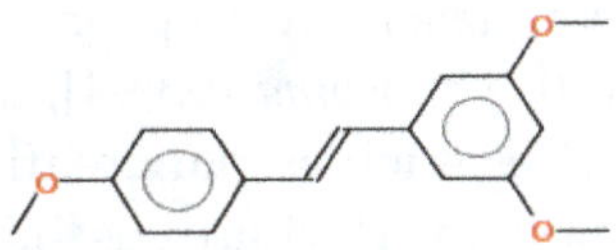	0.08–80.3 μM	Colon (Caco2, SW480), head and neck (KB), lymphoma (TK6) and breast (MCF-7) cancer cells; glioma (C6, T98G)	[39,42,82]
Tetramethoxystilbene	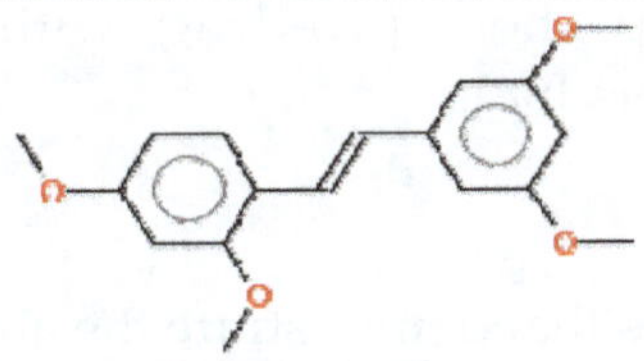	4-60–μM	Leukemia (HL-60) and breast (BT-459) cancer cells, melanoma (SK-MEL); cervix carcinoma (HeLa)	[83]
Pentamethoxystilbene	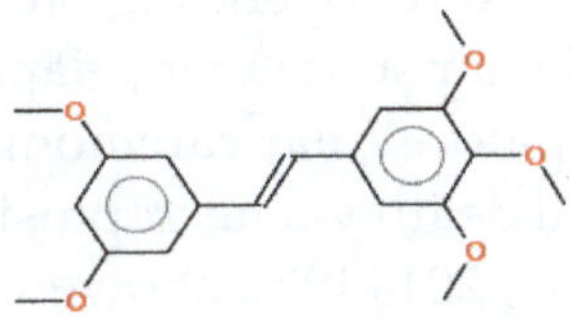	29.2–37.8 μM	Breast (MCF-7) and colon (Colon26) cancer cells	[50,52]
Hydroxylated Resveratrol Derivatives				
Dihydroxystilbene	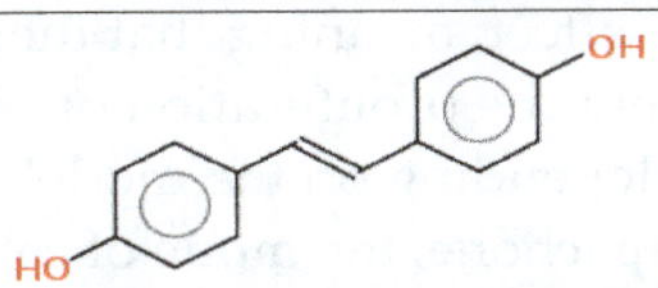	2.3–6.5 μM	Leukemia (HL-60), colon (HCT-116) and breast (MDA-MB-231) cancer cells; osteosarcoma (U2OS)	[57]
Tetrahydroxystilbene	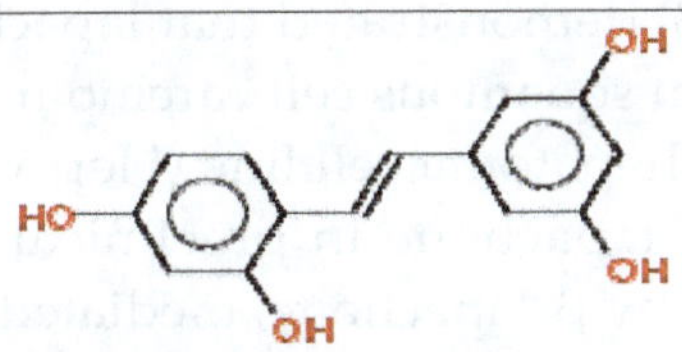	58.4–620.6 μM	Acute T cell leukemia (Jurkat), breast (MCF-7), lung (H1299, A549) and prostate (LNC) cancer cells;	[68,72,84]
Hexahydroxystilbene	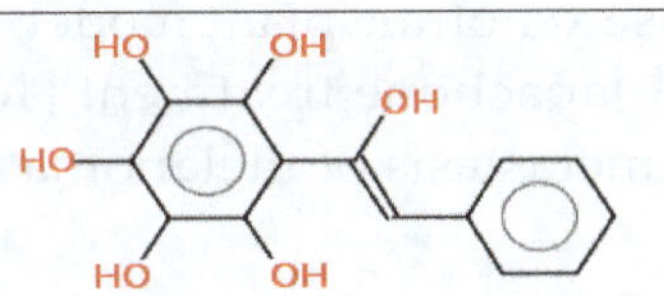	6.25–127.8 μM	Breast (T47D, ZR-75-1, MDA-MB-231), colon (HT-29), leukemia (HL-60) cancer cells; melanoma (M24met)	[69–71,73]

3. β-Lapachone and Its Derivatives: The South American Promise for Cancer

Quinones are widely distributed in nature, products of the secondary metabolism of several different species, with an incredible variety of biological responses [85,86]. Quinones may act as vitamins, antioxidants and are capable of stimulating antibacterial, antiallergic and anticancer effects, among others [87], which motivate their investigation as a therapeutic tool. Quinones can be cytotoxic through several mechanisms of action, including redox cycles, arylation of the thiol groups of proteins, intercalation, induction of breaks in the DNA chain, generation of free radicals and other ROS and bioreductive alkylation of critical cellular proteins and DNA via the formation of quinone methide. Besides basic research studies, quinone-based compounds are already used in the clinic. For instance, in cancer, doxorubicin, mitoxantrone and mitomycin C are used, among others [88,89]. Among all naphthoquinones described to date, three of them are widely known, mostly due to their anticancer effects and the story of their discovery—lapachol, β-lapachone and α-lapachone—of which lapachol (2-hydroxy-3-(3-methyl-2-butenyl-)-1,4-naphthoquinone, $C_{15}H_{14}O_3$), with a molecular weight of 242.2738 g/mol, was isolated first from the heartwood of *Tabebuia impetiginosa*, a widespread tree species in Brazil and other South American countries [90]. No antitumor properties were reported for lapachol until Rao et al., in 1962, described a potent anticancer effect in rats [91]. Since then, a great interest in the research of the anticancer properties of lapachol and its derivatives, or structural isomers, α- and β-lapachone, has risen [92].

β-lapachone (3,4-dihydro-2,2-dimethyl-2H-naphthol[1,2-b]pyran-5,6-dione, $C_{15}H_{14}O_3$), molecular weight 242.2738 g/mol, is an isomer of lapachol and has been described to promote several biological effects, such as anti-inflammatory, antibacterial and anti-*Trypanosoma* [93,94], and most important for this review, anticancer properties in different cancer types such as pancreatic cancer [95], breast cancer [96], hepatocellular carcinoma [97] and others. Several derivatives have been developed throughout the years, and it is noteworthy that a β-lapachone pro-drug, with commercial name ARQ-761, is in phase I/II of clinical studies for solid tumors [98].

3.1. *Anticancer Effects*

As mentioned previously, there is a plethora of studies that demonstrate the ability of β-lapachone to induce cell death in several cancer cell lines, [95–97,99–101], but depending on the type of cancer, it is able to induce different types of cell death. Many studies demonstrate that β-lapachone is capable of inducing apoptosis [96,101,102] in cells such as HepG2, a hepatocellular carcinoma cell line [103], but, on the other hand, others demonstrate an ability to induce cell death via necroptosis, which is a type of organized necrosis [104–106]. As another example, Park et al., 2014 [97], showed that β-lapachone is capable of inducing this type of cell death in SK-Hep1, another hepatocellular carcinoma cell line.

Most anti-neoplastic drugs demonstrate a cytostatic effect, meaning that they are able to inhibit cell proliferation, and the ability of β-lapachone to prevent the proliferation of cancer cells has long been described [107]. IC_{50} values vary in a wide range, depending on the model tested (Table 2). As observed for the type of cell death that is induced by β-lapachone, the mode of cell cycle arrest is also dependent on the cell type under study. Dias et al. (2018) demonstrated that lapachone and its iodine derivatives induce cell cycle arrest in G2/M in human oral squamous cell carcinoma cells, and Lai et al. (1998) [108] showed cell cycle arrest in the S phase for a hepatoma cell line (HepA2).

There is also evidence of antitumoral effects of β-lapachone in preclinical studies. Wu et al. reported the promotion of heat shock protein 90 cleavage by β-lapachone, mediated by oxidative stress in NQO1-expressing cell lines. In the same work, in a mouse xenotransplant model, human lung cancer xenograft growth and angiogenesis were inhibited by β-lapachone treatment [109]. Kee et al. also demonstrated that β-lapachone is able to suppress lung metastasis of melanoma in an experimental mouse model [102].

Table 2. IC_{50} values of β-lapachone and derivatives in different study models.

Compound	2D Structure	IC_{50}	Study Model	References
Lapachol	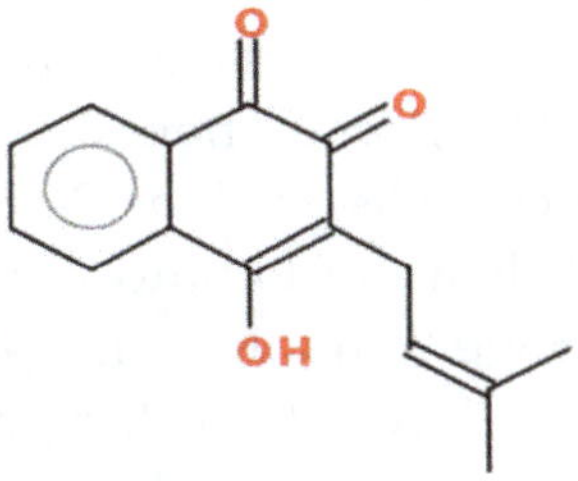	16.04–72.3 μM	Human chronic myelogenous leukemia (K562, Lucena), Burkitt's lymphoma (Daudi), Breast cancer (MCF-7, SK-BR3)	[110,111]
ß-lapachone	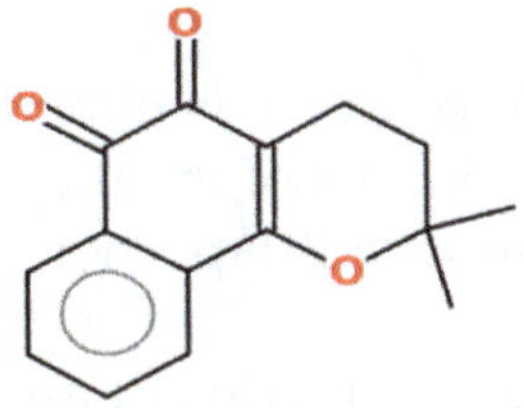	0.03–70.13 μM	Lung cancer cells (A549 cell line); Tongue squamous cell carcinoma (HSC-3, SCC4, SCC9, SCC15, SCC25), hepatocellular carcinoma (HEPG2), HL-60, K562, Gastric adenocarcinoma (AGP-01, ACP-02, ACP-03), colon adenocarcinoma (HT-29, HCT-116).	[112,113]
α-lapachone	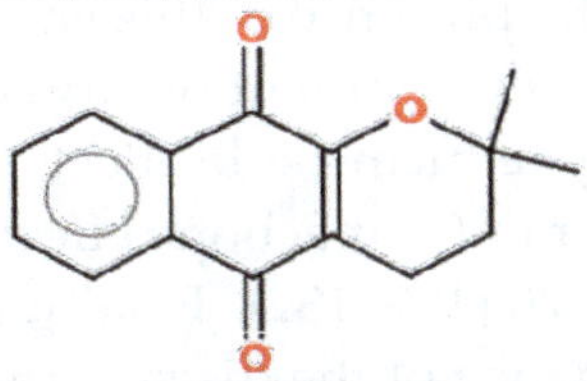	38–69 μM	K562, Lucena, Daudi, MCF-7	[111]
3-iodo-ß-lapachone	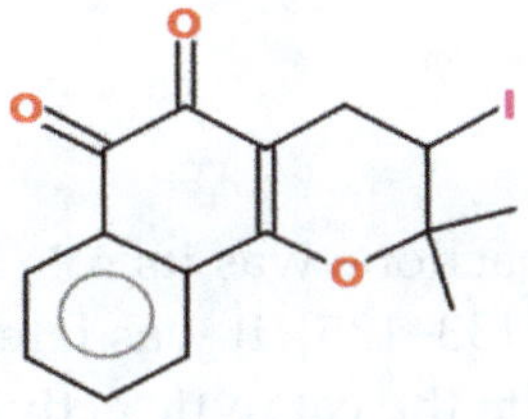	0.02–5.61 μM	Tongue squamous cell carcinoma (HSC-3, SCC4, SCC9, SCC15, SCC25), hepatocellular carcinoma (HEPG2), HL-60, K562, Gastric adenocarcinoma (AGP-01, ACP-02, ACP-03), colon adenocarcinoma (HT-29, HCT-116).	[113]
3-I-α-lapachone	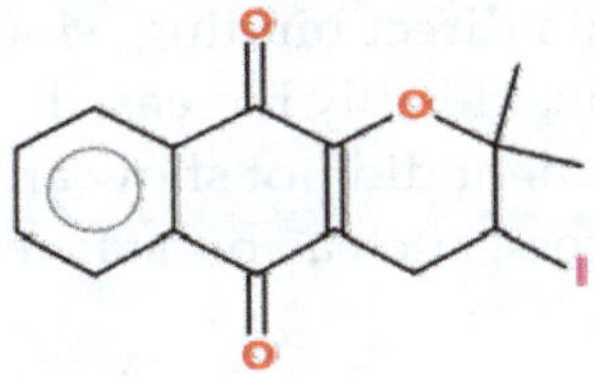	0.77–14.65 μM		
naphtho[2,1-d]oxazole-4,5-diones	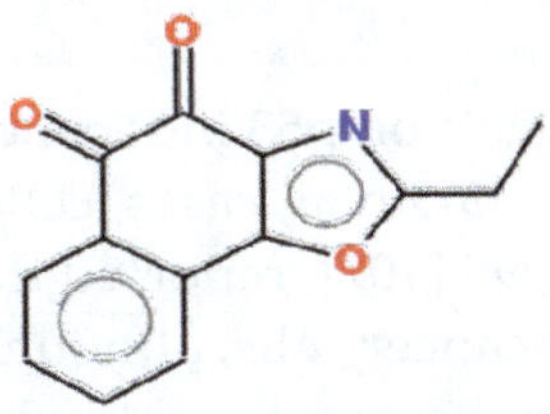	4.6–20 μM *	Lung cancer cells (A549 cell line)	[112]

* IC_{50} values range for all derivatives shown in reference [112].

3.2. Mechanisms of Action

3.2.1. ROS and NQO1

The primary mechanism of action of β-lapachone and its derivatives is the formation of ROS [92] through its processing by NAD(P)H quinone oxidoreductase 1 (NQO1). This enzyme is able to catalyze a futile redox cycle, leading to the formation of unstable hydroquinone, which is rapidly oxidized back to the original quinone under aerobic conditions [114]. The continuous redox cycles eventually oxidize a large number of reduced pyridine nucleotides, which form ROS [115]. This effect is quite robust, since one mol of β-lapachone is capable of generating 120 mol of superoxide in two min, consuming 60 mol of NAD(P)H [106], which results in a rapid depletion of intracellular NAD+ pool over 20 to 30 min [116]. This abnormal production of ROS leads to an increase in Ca^{++}, depolarization of the mitochondrial membrane and a decrease in ATP synthesis. Therefore, in a general way, the activation of β-lapachone by NQO1 leads to cell death by apoptosis [117,118]. There are several studies that show that β-lapachone leads to the formation of ROS in cancer cells, such as Park et al., in 2014, who report that the increase of ROS is capable of inducing cell death of hepatocellular carcinoma cells (SK-Hep1) [97]. In 2011, the same group showed that ROS were involved in β-lapachone-induced autophagy in glioma cells (U87 MG). Bey et al. (2013) showed that H_2O_2 is the primary obligate ROS species necessary for β-lapachone breast cancer cell cytotoxicity through lipid peroxidation, which damages cellular membranes and organelles [106].

It is important to note that several types of solid tumors, such as cholangiocarcinoma [119], lung [120], pancreas [121], breast [122] and squamous cell carcinoma of the uterine cervix [123], have high expression of NQO1, and there are studies that demonstrate a β-lapachone preferential tropism for NQO1-positive cells [124].

Liver tumors are a very interesting case, since normal hepatocytes do not express NQO1 [125,126], but preneoplastic lesions and hepatic tumors demonstrate the presence of this enzyme [127,128]. Thus, this differentiated expression may be very important in the development of targeted therapies since it induces cell death of neoplastic or preneoplastic cells, greatly reducing side effects on healthy liver cells. Additionally, hyperthermia has been reported as an enhancer of β-lapachone effects due to the increase in NQO1 levels after heat shock and its stabilization by HSP70 [129–132]. Finally, it is noteworthy that NQO1-positive breast cancer cells correlate with the malignancy of the disease and could be used as a prognostic biomarker for breast cancer [124].

3.2.2. Topoisomerase Inhibition

One of the first mechanisms of action reported for β-lapachone was its role as a topoisomerase I modulator. Earlier thought of as a topoisomerase activator [133–135], it was later shown to act as an inhibitor, through the demonstration that β-lapachone inhibits the catalytic activity of topoisomerase I (purified from calf thymus and human cells), through its direct binding, since the incubation of topoisomerase I with β-lapachone (before adding DNA) considerably increased its inhibition, but the incubation of topoisomerase I with DNA prior to the treatment did not show any effect [136]. Other studies refer to similar effects in cell lines of different cancers, such as prostate cancer, breast cancer and leukemia [96,137,138].

3.2.3. p53

A number of studies have demonstrated β-lapachone effects on p53 independently of the cell p53 status (no expression or expression of wild-type or mutant p53); in all cases, cells can be sensitive to the effects of β-lapachone [107,139,140]. Huang Pardee, in 1999 [107], reported that β-lapachone had the ability to drastically reduce levels of mutant p53 in colon cancer cells, although it did not alter the expression levels of wild-type p53. In addition, p53 can also be regulated by β-lapachone through its phosphorylation and consequent activation, with no modification in its expression levels [141]. Finally, Pink et al. (2000) reported the β-lapachone-mediated activation of a cysteine-protease capable of digesting several cellular proteins, including p53 [142].

3.2.4. Other Cellular or Molecular Pathways

Yu et al. demonstrated the anti-tumor effect of β-lapachone on breast cancer tumors with a variation in the phosphorylation of AKT, 4EBP-1 and S6, which are related to the mTOR pathway and is also related to the apoptotic activity of this compound in gastric carcinoma cells [101]. Additionally, Wu et al., in 2016 [109], demonstrated that the effect of β-lapachone on reducing the growth of lung cancer cell tumors is related to AKT. In addition to the mTOR pathway, E-cadherin was altered in tumors, and Kim et al. (2007) [102] suggested that β-lapachone inhibits the progression and metastasis of hepatocellular carcinoma by increasing the expression of this protein and other proteins of the mTOR pathway. Additionally, the inactivation of the Akt/mTOR pathway was again attributed to β-lapachone, promoting the inhibition of EMT transition in NQO1-positive cells.

3.3. Strategies to Overcome β-Lapachone Bioavailability and Toxicity Issues: Drug Delivery and Derivatives Synthesis

Even though β-lapachone is a promising anticancer drug, its low bioavailability represents a limitation for clinical use due to low solubility in water and gastrointestinal fluids [143]. There is also a concern with the low concentration reached in the target cells and systemic toxicity, since β-lapachone displays a general distribution pattern and a dose limitation because of the risk of methemoglobinemia through the generation of nonspecific ROS at high doses [116,143].

As mentioned before, β-lapachone (Table 2) has a molecular weight of 242.29 g/mol; it is a small molecule, nonionized in the intestinal system, with pH-independent solubility. The experimental solubility value is very similar to the theoretical value of 48.33 μg/mL [112,144]. β-lapachone has the potential to be orally administered; its estimated oral fraction absorbed and intestinal effective permeability value is 85% [145]; however, a bioavailability of 15.5% through oral administration was shown in rats, probably due to broad metabolic first-pass degradation in the liver, intestines and low solubility in water, with a slow dissolution rate in the intestinal tissue [144]. Moreover, preclinical studies demonstrate that, to promote a better absorption of β-lapachone, different formulations would be necessary, and due to these findings, along with its first-pass metabolism, it was considered a difficult drug for oral administration [144,146].

Due to the low availability and unspecific toxicity of β-lapachone, there is a constant need for the development of new drug delivery systems to increase bioavailability to promote its use. There are two classical systems of β-lapachone delivery, cyclodextrin inclusion complexes and liposomes, although most studies are concerned with physical–chemical and absorption properties without any cancer therapy approach. A thorough review on this subject was written by Ferreira et al., 2016 [147]. Here, we focus on anticancer approaches.

The intricate structure of cyclodextrin allows the formation of β-lapachone/cyclodextrin inclusion complexes because of its hydrophobic core [145,148]. These inclusion complexes are capable of increasing drug bioavailability, altering their permeability, dissolution properties or both [149]. Seoane et al. (2013) used a methylated-β-cyclodextrin/poloxamer 407 mixture to create a delivery system of β-lapachone and evaluated its antitumoral activity. This system has the particularity of forming a gel above 29 °C, which facilitates intratumoral and extended drug delivery. MCF-7 tumor-bearing mice treated with this system, by intratumoral injection, showed a reduction of tumor volume without apparent liver and kidney toxicity [150].

Liposomes (one or multiple layers of phospholipids) are very interesting delivery systems because they can be used for both hydrophobic and hydrophilic drugs and display remote drug loading, homogeneous particle size, long-circulating stability, specific release and the ability to lower drug toxicity [151]. Liposomes with β-lapachone, in different mixed micellar formulations of phosphatidylcholine, sodium deoxycholate and sodium lauryl sulfate (SLS), showed the ability to increase gastrointestinal absorption at different sites (particularly in the large intestines) due to β-lapachone solubilization and interaction with the intestinal membrane [152].

Recently, there has been an increased exploration of nanosystems or nanoparticle delivery systems to surpass the limitations of these delivery systems and increase specificity and cytotoxicity to cancer cells. Dai et al. (2019) [153] developed a nanosystem with a charge-reversal ability and self-amplifiable drug release system that encapsulated β-lapachone in a pH/ROS cascade-responsive polymeric prodrug micelle. They showed that this system is capable of effectively increasing cell uptake and specific delivery through acidity-activating charge conversion and ROS-response drug release. Upon the uptake of β-lapachone, ROS formation was increased (NQO1-mediated), which lowered the cell ATP levels and consequently reduced P-gp-mediated drug efflux, decreasing multidrug resistance (MDR). This caused a massive reduction of MCF-7 tumors treated with this β-lapachone delivery system and low systemic toxicity [153].

Another strategy to increase the therapeutic efficacy of β-lapachone, through the reduction of MDR, is to promote its codelivery with another drug, such as doxorubicin. This was an option used by Li et al., demonstrating that a nanostructured lipid carrier (NLC) codelivering β-lapachone and doxorubicin had a higher therapeutic efficacy in breast cancer tumor-bearing mice, leading the authors to propose this as a possible strategy to overcome MDR in breast cancer [154].

A nanoparticle developed by Yin et al., a ROS-responsive block copolymer prodrug that self-assembles into polymeric micelles that encapsulate β-lapachone, increased tumor-specific ROS formation after intravenous administration in tumor-bearing mice. This increased ROS level and triggered drug release, allowing maximization of therapeutic efficacy, suppression of tumor growth and minimization of systemic toxicity [155].

There are three main strategies to develop β-lapachone derivatives or analogues—A- and C-ring modifications and redox center modifications—which can be obtained by copper-catalyzed azide-alkalyne cycloaddition, palladium-catalyzed cross couplings and heterocyclization reactions [156]. The great progress seen in this field is due to essential contributions from Brazilian research groups, such as Vitor Francisco Ferreira and Eufrânio Nunes da Silva Júnior [156–161]. However, most studies of β-lapachone derivatives or analogues are composed of a series of compounds with different modifications and analysis of the possible anticancer effect in cancer cell lines [89,156,161]. Nevertheless, there are more in-depth studies that attempt to understand the mechanisms of action of the compounds and eventually test them on experimental tumor models.

Recently, Dias et al. (2018) [113] showed that β-lapachone and its 3-iodine derivatives (3-I-α-lapachone and 3-I-β-lapachone) were able to induce significant cytotoxicity against different types of cancer cells (Table 2), with cell cycle arrest in G2/M, DNA fragmentation, increase in apoptosis protein levels and morphology, and production of ROS. This work also demonstrated that these compounds were able to reduce tumor burden for mice xenotransplanted with breast adenocarcinoma cells, without any alteration of biochemical, hematological or histological parameters of the treated mice, showing a nonsignificant systemic toxicity. Li et al. described a new class of β-lapachone derivatives, naphtho[2,1-d]oxazole-4,5-diones (Table 2), with higher solubility and comparable activities, both in vitro and in vivo (xenotransplants), against NQO1-positive A549 lung cancer cells [112]. The compounds β-lap-dC3 and -dC6 are prodrug diester derivatives of β-lapachone. When encapsulated in PEG-β-PLA micelles, they were described to be more efficient in loading micelles than β-lapachone itself, and β-lap-dC3 improved the survival rate of NSCLC xenograft-bearing mice, increasing β-lapachone concentration in the target tissues, which makes it a promising therapy to be developed against NQO1-positive cells [162].

Finally, the sensitization of cells promoted by different energy sources, such as light or radiation, in combination with β-lapachone and its derivatives has also been described. Lamberti et al. (2018) showed the synergism between halogenated derivatives of β-lapachone and photodynamic therapy in melanoma cells with positive results due to the upregulation of NQO1 expression [163]. Ionizing radiation at low doses was applied in combination with sublethal doses of β-lapachone in non-small-cell lung cancer (NSCLC) cell lines and in xenograft models in vivo [164]. Additionally, the massive release of ROS promoted by ionizing radiation was applied together with nontoxic β-lapachone doses to head and neck patient samples [165]. These results suggested the use of this combination to increase the efficacy of radiotherapy in NQO1-positive tumors and shall be tested in clinical trials in the near future.

4. Conclusions

Both of the molecules reviewed here, β-lapachone and resveratrol, are paradoxical. While they are naturally occurring products, or at least derived from natural sources, they can be radically improved by human manipulation. They represent a case study for natural products that can be enhanced by structural manipulation and/or delivery systems. In this paper, we intended to compile the available information about β-lapachone and resveratrol, with a special focus on what has been found in recent years and on the possible impact in cancer therapy, also showing how a bioactive compound/molecule can be found in natural resources, which are a possible reservoir of new therapies. However, it is essential not to be dismissive of the importance of manipulating natural molecules to increase their efficiency and specificity. The results obtained with β-lapachone, resveratrol and their analogues for cancer therapy are promising, especially if we manage to improve their specificity for cancer cells, with less systemic toxicity (a major problem for most chemotherapies) and their delivery, particularly by making them orally bioavailable for patient comfort. The similarities and differences between the two groups of compounds can be observed through the comparison between the values shown in Tables 1 and 2 and the properties listed in the supplementary material tables (Tables S1–S4).

Supplementary Materials: Table S1: Bioactivity prediction (druglikeness*) of β-lapachone and its derivatives for specific biological activities; Table S2: Bioactivity prediction (druglikeness*) of resveratrol and its derivatives for specific biological activities; Table S3: Chemical and pharmacological properties of Lapachol, β-lapachone and derivatives; Table S4: Chemical and pharmacological properties of resveratrol and derivatives.

Author Contributions: D.C.F.d.C., L.P.R., V.F.F. and J.L.S. wrote and edited the text. M.M.D.d.C.M.-D. and G.D.d.S.F. wrote the text. All authors have read and agreed to the published version of the manuscript.

References

1. The International Agency for Research on Cancer (IARC). *Latest Global CANCER Data: Cancer Burden Rises to 18.1 Million New Cases and 9.6 Million Cancer Deaths in 2018*; IARC: Lyon, France, 2018.
2. Newman, D.J.; Cragg, G.M. Natural products as sources of new drugs over the 30 years from 1981 to 2010. *J. Nat. Prod.* **2012**, *75*, 311–335. [CrossRef] [PubMed]
3. Harvey, A.L.; Edrada-Ebel, R.; Quinn, R.J. The re-emergence of natural products for drug discovery in the genomics era. *Nat. Rev. Drug Discov.* **2015**, *14*, 111–129. [CrossRef] [PubMed]
4. Roupe, K.; Remsberg, C.; Yanez, J.; Davies, N. Pharmacometrics of Stilbenes: Seguing Towards the Clinic. *Curr. Clin. Pharmacol.* **2008**, *1*, 81–101. [CrossRef] [PubMed]
5. Siemann, E.H.; Creasy, L.L. Concentration of the phytoalexin resveratrol in wine. *Am. J. Enol. Vitic.* **1992**, *43*, 49–52.
6. Signorelli, P.; Ghidoni, R. Resveratrol as an anticancer nutrient: Molecular basis, open questions and promises. *J. Nutr. Biochem.* **2005**, *16*, 449–466. [CrossRef] [PubMed]
7. Ali, K.; Maltese, F.; Choi, Y.H.; Verpoorte, R. Metabolic constituents of grapevine and grape-derived products. *Phytochem. Rev.* **2010**, *9*, 357–378. [CrossRef]
8. Jang, M.; Cai, L.; Udeani, G.O.; Slowing, K.V.; Thomas, C.F.; Beecher, C.W.W.; Fong, H.H.S.; Farnsworth, N.R.; Kinghorn, A.D.; Mehta, R.G.; et al. Cancer chemopreventive activity of resveratrol, a natural product derived from grapes. *Science* **1997**, *275*, 218–220. [CrossRef]
9. Baur, J.A.; Sinclair, D.A. Therapeutic potential of resveratrol: The in vivo evidence. *Nat. Rev. Drug Discov.* **2006**, *5*, 493–506. [CrossRef]
10. Pezzuto, J.M. Resveratrol as an inhibitor of carcinogenesis. *Pharm. Biol.* **2008**, *46*, 443–573. [CrossRef]
11. Da Costa, D.C.F.; Fialho, E.; Silva, J.L. Cancer chemoprevention by resveratrol: The P53 tumor suppressor protein as a promising molecular target. *Molecules* **2017**, *22*, 1014. [CrossRef]
12. Kundu, J.K.; Surh, Y.J. Cancer chemopreventive and therapeutic potential of resveratrol: Mechanistic perspectives. *Cancer Lett.* **2008**, *269*, 243–261. [CrossRef] [PubMed]
13. Varoni, E.M.; Lo Faro, A.F.; Sharifi-Rad, J.; Iriti, M. Anticancer Molecular Mechanisms of Resveratrol. *Front. Nutr.* **2016**, *3*, 8. [CrossRef] [PubMed]
14. De la Lastra, C.A.; Villegas, I. Resveratrol as an antioxidant and pro-oxidant agent: Mechanisms and clinical implications. *Biochem. Soc. Trans.* **2007**, *35*, 1156–1160. [CrossRef]
15. Martins, L.A.M.; Coelho, B.P.; Behr, G.; Pettenuzzo, L.F.; Souza, I.C.C.; Moreira, J.C.F.; Borojevic, R.; Gottfried, C.; Guma, F.C.R. Resveratrol Induces Pro-oxidant Effects and Time-Dependent Resistance to Cytotoxicity in Activated Hepatic Stellate Cells. *Cell Biochem. Biophys.* **2014**, *68*, 247–257. [CrossRef] [PubMed]

16. Silva, J.L.; Vieira, T.C.R.G.; Gomes, M.P.B.; Ano Bom, A.P.; Lima, L.M.T.R.; Freitas, M.S.; Ishimaru, D.; Cordeiro, Y.; Foguel, D. Ligand binding and hydration in protein misfolding: Insights from studies of prion and p53 tumor suppressor proteins. *Acc. Chem. Res.* **2010**, *43*, 271–279. [CrossRef] [PubMed]
17. Silva, J.L.; Cino, E.A.; Soares, I.N.; Ferreira, V.F.; De Oliveira, G. Targeting the Prion-like Aggregation of Mutant p53 to Combat Cancer. *Acc. Chem. Res.* **2018**, *51*, 181–190. [CrossRef]
18. Ano Bom, A.P.D.; Rangel, L.P.; Costa, D.C.F.; De Oliveira, G.A.P.; Sanches, D.; Braga, C.A.; Gava, L.M.; Ramos, C.H.I.; Cepeda, A.O.T.; Stumbo, A.C.; et al. Mutant p53 aggregates into prion-like amyloid oligomers and fibrils: Implications for cancer. *J. Biol. Chem.* **2012**, *287*, 28152–28162. [CrossRef]
19. Silva, J.L.; Gallo, C.V.D.M.; Costa, D.C.F.; Rangel, L.P. Prion-like aggregation of mutant p53 in cancer. *Trends Biochem. Sci.* **2014**, *39*, 260–267. [CrossRef]
20. Xu, J.; Reumers, J.; Couceiro, J.R.; De Smet, F.; Gallardo, R.; Rudyak, S.; Cornelis, A.; Rozenski, J.; Zwolinska, A.; Marine, J.C.; et al. Gain of function of mutant p53 by coaggregation with multiple tumor suppressors. *Nat. Chem. Biol.* **2011**, *7*, 285–295. [CrossRef]
21. Ferraz Da Costa, D.C.; Campos, N.P.C.; Santos, R.A.; Guedes-Da-Silva, F.H.; Martins-Dinis, M.M.D.C.; Zanphorlin, L.; Ramos, C.; Rangel, L.P.; Silva, J.L. Resveratrol prevents p53 aggregation in vitro and in breast cancer cells. *Oncotarget* **2018**, *9*, 29112–29122.
22. Ferraz da Costa, D.C.; Casanova, F.A.; Quarti, J.; Malheiros, M.S.; Sanches, D.; dos Santos, P.S.; Fialho, E.; Silva, J.L. Transient Transfection of a Wild-Type p53 Gene Triggers Resveratrol-Induced Apoptosis in Cancer Cells. *PLoS ONE* **2012**, *7*, e48746. [CrossRef] [PubMed]
23. Chimento, A.; De Amicis, F.; Sirianni, R.; Sinicropi, M.S.; Puoci, F.; Casaburi, I.; Saturnino, C.; Pezzi, V. Progress to improve oral bioavailability and beneficial effects of resveratrol. *Int. J. Mol. Sci.* **2019**, *20*, 1381. [CrossRef] [PubMed]
24. Walle, T. Bioavailability of resveratrol. *Ann. N. Y. Acad. Sci.* **2011**, *1215*, 9–15. [CrossRef] [PubMed]
25. Nawaz, W.; Zhou, Z.; Deng, S.; Ma, X.; Ma, X.; Li, C.; Shu, X. Therapeutic versatility of resveratrol derivatives. *Nutrients* **2017**, *9*, 1188. [CrossRef] [PubMed]
26. McCormack, D.; McFadden, D. Pterostilbene and cancer: Current review. *J. Surg. Res.* **2012**, *173*, e53–e61. [CrossRef]
27. Kosuru, R.; Rai, U.; Prakash, S.; Singh, A.; Singh, S. Promising therapeutic potential of pterostilbene and its mechanistic insight based on preclinical evidence. *Eur. J. Pharmacol.* **2016**, *789*, 229–243. [CrossRef]
28. Kapetanovic, I.M.; Muzzio, M.; Huang, Z.; Thompson, T.N.; McCormick, D.L. Pharmacokinetics, oral bioavailability, and metabolic profile of resveratrol and its dimethylether analog, pterostilbene, in rats. *Cancer Chemother. Pharmacol.* **2011**, *68*, 593–601. [CrossRef]
29. Ma, Z.; Zhang, X.; Xu, L.; Liu, D.; Di, S.; Li, W.; Zhang, J.; Zhang, H.; Li, X.; Han, J.; et al. Pterostilbene: Mechanisms of its action as oncostatic agent in cell models and in vivo studies. *Pharmacol. Res.* **2019**, *145*, 104265. [CrossRef]
30. Suh, N.; Paul, S.; Hao, X.; Simi, B.; Xiao, H.; Rimando, A.M.; Reddy, B.S. Pterostilbene, an active constituent of blueberries, suppresses aberrant crypt foci formation in the azoxymethane-induced colon carcinogenesis model in rats. *Clin. Cancer Res.* **2007**, *13*, 350–355. [CrossRef]
31. Chiou, Y.S.; Tsai, M.L.; Wang, Y.J.; Cheng, A.C.; Lai, W.M.; Badmaev, V.; Ho, C.T.; Pan, M.H. Pterostilbene inhibits colorectal aberrant crypt foci (ACF) and colon carcinogenesis via suppression of multiple signal transduction pathways in azoxymethane-treated mice. *J. Agric. Food Chem.* **2010**, *58*, 8833–8841. [CrossRef]
32. Wawszczyk, J.; Kapral, M.; Hollek, A.; Węglarz, L. In vitro evaluation of antiproliferative and cytotoxic properties of pterostilbene against human colon cancer cells. *Acta Pol. Pharmacol.* **2014**, *71*, 1051–1055.
33. Pan, M.H.; Chang, Y.H.; Badmaev, V.; Nagabhushanam, K.; Ho, C.T. Pterostilbene induces apoptosis and cell cycle arrest in human gastric carcinoma cells. *J. Agric. Food Chem.* **2007**, *55*, 7777–7785. [CrossRef] [PubMed]
34. Pan, M.H.; Chiou, Y.S.; Chen, W.J.; Wang, J.M.; Badmaev, V.; Ho, C.T. Pterostilbene inhibited tumor invasion via suppressing multiple signal transduction pathways in human hepatocellular carcinoma cells. *Carcinogenesis* **2009**, *30*, 1234–1242. [CrossRef]
35. Huang, C.S.; Ho, C.T.; Tu, S.H.; Pan, M.H.; Chuang, C.H.; Chang, H.W.; Chang, C.H.; Wu, C.H.; Ho, Y.S. Long-term ethanol exposure-induced hepatocellular carcinoma cell migration and invasion through lysyl oxidase activation are attenuated by combined treatment with pterostilbene and curcumin analogues. *J. Agric. Food Chem.* **2013**, *61*, 4326–4335. [CrossRef] [PubMed]

36. Wu, C.H.; Hong, B.H.; Ho, C.T.; Yen, G.C. Targeting cancer stem cells in breast cancer: Potential anticancer properties of 6-shogaol and pterostilbene. *J. Agric. Food Chem.* **2015**, *63*, 2432–2441. [CrossRef] [PubMed]
37. Chatterjee, K.; Mukherjee, S.; Vanmanen, J.; Banerjee, P.; Fata, J.E. Dietary polyphenols, resveratrol and pterostilbene exhibit antitumor activity on an HPV E6-positive cervical cancer model: An in vitro and in vivo analysis. *Front. Oncol.* **2019**, *9*, 352. [CrossRef] [PubMed]
38. Ramezani, G.; Pourgheysari, B.; Shirzad, H.; Sourani, Z. Pterostilbene increases Fas expression in T-lymphoblastic leukemia cell lines. *Res. Pharmacol. Sci.* **2019**, *14*, 55.
39. Tsai, J.H.; Hsu, L.S.; Lin, C.L.; Hong, H.M.; Pan, M.H.; Way, T.D.; Chen, W.J. 3,5,4′-Trimethoxystilbene, a natural methoxylated analog of resveratrol, inhibits breast cancer cell invasiveness by downregulation of PI3K/Akt and Wnt/β-catenin signaling cascades and reversal of epithelial-mesenchymal transition. *Toxicol. Appl. Pharmacol.* **2013**, *272*, 746–756. [CrossRef]
40. Weng, C.J.; Yang, Y.T.; Ho, C.T.; Yen, G.C. Mechanisms of apoptotic effects induced by resveratrol, dibenzoylmethane, and their analogues on human lung carcinoma cells. *J. Agric. Food Chem.* **2009**, *57*, 5235–5243. [CrossRef]
41. Yang, Y.T.; Weng, C.J.; Ho, C.T.; Yen, G.C. Resveratrol analog-3,5,4′-trimethoxy-*trans*-stilbene inhibits invasion of human lung adenocarcinoma cells by suppressing the MAPK pathway and decreasing matrix metalloproteinase-2 expression. *Mol. Nutr. Food Res.* **2009**, *53*, 407–416. [CrossRef]
42. Zielińska-Przyjemska, M.; Kaczmarek, M.; Krajka-Kuźniak, V.; Łuczak, M.; Baer-Dubowska, W. The effect of resveratrol, its naturally occurring derivatives and tannic acid on the induction of cell cycle arrest and apoptosis in rat C6 and human T98G glioma cell lines. *Toxicol. In Vitro* **2017**, *43*, 69–75. [CrossRef] [PubMed]
43. Wang, G.; Guo, X.; Chen, H.; Lin, T.; Xu, Y.; Chen, Q.; Liu, J.; Zeng, J.; Zhang, X.K.; Yao, X. A resveratrol analog, phoyunbene B, induces G2/M cell cycle arrest and apoptosis in HepG2 liver cancer cells. *Bioorg. Med. Chem. Lett.* **2012**, *22*, 2114–2118. [CrossRef] [PubMed]
44. Androutsopoulos, V.P.; Fragiadaki, I.; Spandidos, D.A.; Tosca, A. The resveratrol analogue, 3,4,5,4′-trans-tetramethoxystilbene, inhibits the growth of A375 melanoma cells through multiple anticancer modes of action. *Int. J. Oncol.* **2016**, *49*, 1305–1314. [CrossRef] [PubMed]
45. Gosslau, A.; Pabbaraja, S.; Knapp, S.; Chen, K.Y. Trans- and cis-stilbene polyphenols induced rapid perinuclear mitochondrial clustering and p53-independent apoptosis in cancer cells but not normal cells. *Eur. J. Pharmacol.* **2008**, *587*, 25–34. [CrossRef]
46. Piotrowska, H.; Myszkowski, K.; Abraszek, J.; Kwiatkowska-Borowczyk, E.; Amarowicz, R.; Murias, M.; Wierzchowski, M.; Jodynis-Liebert, J. DMU-212 inhibits tumor growth in xenograft model of human ovarian cancer. *Biomed. Pharmacol.* **2014**, *68*, 397–400. [CrossRef]
47. Piotrowska-Kempisty, H.; Rucinski, M.; Borys, S.; Kucinska, M.; Kaczmarek, M.; Zawierucha, P.; Wierzchowski, M.; Lazewski, D.; Murias, M.; Jodynis-Liebert, J. 3′-hydroxy-3,4,5,4′-tetramethoxystilbene, the metabolite of resveratrol analogue DMU-212, inhibits ovarian cancer cell growth in vitro and in a mice xenograft model. *Sci. Rep.* **2016**, *6*, 32627. [CrossRef]
48. Hong, M.; Park, N.; Chun, Y.J. Role of annexin A5 on mitochondria-dependent apoptosis induced by tetramethoxystilbene in human breast cancer cells. *Biomol. Ther.* **2014**, *22*, 519–524. [CrossRef]
49. Xu, H. (Z)-3,4,3′,5′-Tetramethoxystilbene, a natural product, induces apoptosis and reduces viability of paclitaxel-And cisplatin-resistant osteosarcoma cells. *J. Cancer Res. Ther.* **2016**, *12*, 1261. [CrossRef]
50. Pan, M.H.; Lin, C.L.I.; Tsal, J.H.; Ho, C.T.; Chen, W.J. 3,5,3′,4′,5′ -Pentamethoxystilbene (MR-5), a synthetically methoxylated analogue of resveratrol, inhibits growth and induces G1 cell cycle arrest of human breast carcinoma MCF-7 Cells. *J. Agric. Food Chem.* **2010**, *58*, 226–234. [CrossRef]
51. Li, H.; Wu, W.K.K.; Zheng, Z.; Che, C.T.; Yu, L.; Li, Z.J.; Wu, Y.C.; Cheng, K.W.; Yu, J.; Cho, C.H.; et al. 2,3′,4,4′,5′-Pentamethoxy-*trans*-stilbene, a resveratrol derivative, is a potent inducer of apoptosis in colon cancer cells via targeting microtubules. *Biochem. Pharmacol.* **2009**, *78*, 1224–1232. [CrossRef]
52. Li, H.; Wu, W.K.K.; Li, Z.J.; Chan, K.M.; Wong, C.C.M.; Ye, C.G.; Yu, L.; Sung, J.J.Y.; Cho, C.H.; Wang, M. 2,3′,4,4′,5′-Pentamethoxy-*trans*-stilbene, a resveratrol derivative, inhibits colitis-associated colorectal carcinogenesis in mice. *Br. J. Pharmacol.* **2010**, *160*, 1352–1361. [CrossRef]
53. Fan, G.J.; Liu, X.D.; Qian, Y.P.; Shang, Y.J.; Li, X.Z.; Dai, F.; Fang, J.G.; Jin, X.L.; Zhou, B. 4,4′-Dihydroxy-*trans*-stilbene, a resveratrol analogue, exhibited enhanced antioxidant activity and cytotoxicity. *Bioorg. Med. Chem.* **2009**, *17*, 2360–2365. [CrossRef]

54. Savio, M.; Coppa, T.; Bianchi, L.; Vannini, V.; Maga, G.; Forti, L.; Cazzalini, O.; Lazzè, M.C.; Perucca, P.; Prosperi, E.; et al. The resveratrol analogue 4,4′-dihydroxy-*trans*-stilbene inhibits cell proliferation with higher efficiency but different mechanism from resveratrol. *Int. J. Biochem. Cell Biol.* **2009**, *41*, 2493–2502. [CrossRef]
55. Kimura, Y.; Sumiyoshi, M.; Baba, K. Antitumor and antimetastatic activity of synthetic hydroxystilbenes through inhibition of lymphangiogenesis and M2 macrophage differentiation of tumor-associated macrophages. *Anticancer Res.* **2016**, *36*, 137–148.
56. Saha, B.; Patro, B.S.; Koli, M.; Pai, G.; Ray, J.; Bandyopadhyay, S.K.; Chattopadhyay, S. *trans*-4,4′-Dihydroxystilbene (DHS) inhibits human neuroblastoma tumor growth and induces mitochondrial and lysosomal damages in neuroblastoma cell lines. *Oncotarget* **2017**, *8*, 73905. [CrossRef]
57. Saha, B.; Pai, G.B.; Subramanian, M.; Gupta, P.; Tyagi, M.; Patro, B.S.; Chattopadhyay, S. Resveratrol analogue, *trans*-4,4′-dihydroxystilbene (DHS), inhibits melanoma tumor growth and suppresses its metastatic colonization in lungs. *Biomed. Pharmacol.* **2018**, *107*, 1104–1114. [CrossRef]
58. Chen, C.W.; Li, Y.; Hu, S.; Zhou, W.; Meng, Y.; Li, Z.; Zhang, Y.; Sun, J.; Bo, Z.; DePamphilis, M.L.; et al. DHS (trans−4,4′-dihydroxystilbene) suppresses DNA replication and tumor growth by inhibiting RRM2 (ribonucleotide reductase regulatory subunit M2). *Oncogene* **2019**, *38*, 2364–2379. [CrossRef]
59. Larrosa, M.; Tomás-Barberán, F.A.; Espín, J.C. Grape polyphenol resveratrol and the related molecule 4-hydroxystilbene induce growth inhibition, apoptosis, S-phase arrest, and upregulation of cyclins A, E, and B1 in human SK-Mel-28 melanoma cells. *J. Agric. Food Chem.* **2003**, *51*, 4576–4584. [CrossRef]
60. Larrosa, M.; Tomás-Barberán, F.A.; Espín, J.C. The grape and wine polyphenol piceatannol is a potent inducer of apoptosis in human SK-Mel-28 melanoma cells. *Eur. J. Nutr.* **2004**, *43*, 275–284. [CrossRef]
61. Barton, B.E.; Karras, J.G.; Murphy, T.F.; Barton, A.; Huang, H.F.S. Signal transducer and activator of transcription 3 (STAT3) activation in prostate cancer: Direct STAT3 inhibition induces apoptosis in prostate cancer lines. *Mol. Cancer Ther.* **2004**, *3*, 11–20.
62. Wolter, F.; Clausnitzer, A.; Akoglu, B.; Stein, J. Piceatannol, a Natural Analog of Resveratrol, Inhibits Progression through the S Phase of the Cell Cycle in Colorectal Cancer Cell Lines. *J. Nutr.* **2002**, *132*, 298–302. [CrossRef]
63. Kuo, P.L.; Hsu, Y.L. The grape and wine constituent piceatannol inhibits proliferation of human bladder cancer cells via blocking cell cycle progression and inducing Fas/membrane bound Fas ligand-mediated apoptotic pathway. *Mol. Nutr. Food Res.* **2008**, *52*, 408–418. [CrossRef]
64. Liu, W.H.; Chang, L. Sen Piceatannol induces Fas and FasL up-regulation in human leukemia U937 cells via Ca2+/p38α MAPK-mediated activation of c-Jun and ATF-2 pathways. *Int. J. Biochem. Cell Biol.* **2010**, *42*, 1498–1506. [CrossRef]
65. Füllbeck, M.; Huang, X.; Dumdey, R.; Frommel, C.; Dubiel, W.; Preissner, R. Novel curcumin- and emodin-related compounds identified by in silico 2D/3D conformer screening induce apoptosis in tumor cells. *BMC Cancer* **2005**, *5*, 97. [CrossRef] [PubMed]
66. CL, L.; SL, H.; Leung, W.; JH, J.; GC, H.; CT, L.; CC, W. 2,3,5,4′-tetrahydroxystilbene-2-*O*-β-D-glucoside suppresses human colorectal cancer cell metastasis through inhibiting NF-κB activation. *Int. J. Oncol.* **2016**, *49*, 629–638.
67. Lin, C.L.; Jeng, J.H.; Wu, C.C.; Hsieh, S.L.; Huang, G.C.; Leung, W.; Lee, C.T.; Chen, C.Y.; Lee, C.H. Chemopreventive Potential of 2,3,5,4′-Tetrahydroxystilbene-2-*O*-β-*D*-glucoside on the Formation of Aberrant Crypt Foci in Azoxymethane-Induced Colorectal Cancer in Rats. *Biomed Res. Int.* **2017**, *2017*, 3634915. [CrossRef]
68. Shen, J.; Zhang, Y.; Shen, H.; Pan, H.; Xu, L.; Yuan, L.; Ding, Z. The synergistic effect of 2,3,5,4′-Tetrahydroxystilbene-2-*O*-β-*D*-glucoside combined with Aadriamycin on MCF-7 breast cancer cells. *Drug Des. Dev. Ther.* **2018**, *12*, 4083–4094. [CrossRef]
69. Szekeres, T.; Saiko, P.; Fritzer-Szekeres, M.; Djavan, B.; Jäger, W. Chemopreventive effects of resveratrol and resveratrol derivatives. *Ann. N. Y. Acad. Sci.* **2011**, *1215*, 89–95. [CrossRef]
70. Murias, M.; Luczak, M.W.; Niepsuj, A.; Krajka-Kuzniak, V.; Zielinska-Przyjemska, M.; Jagodzinski, P.P.; Jäger, W.; Szekeres, T.; Jodynis-Liebert, J. Cytotoxic activity of 3,3′,4,4′,5,5′-hexahydroxystilbene against breast cancer cells is mediated by induction of p53 and downregulation of mitochondrial superoxide dismutase. *Toxicol. In Vitro* **2008**, *22*, 1361–1370. [CrossRef]

71. Saiko, P.; Pemberger, M.; Horvath, Z.; Savinc, I.; Grusch, M.; Handler, N.; Erker, T.; Jaeger, W.; Fritzer-Szekeres, M.; Szekeres, T. Novel resveratrol analogs induce apoptosis and cause cell cycle arrest in HT29 human colon cancer cells: Inhibition of ribonucleotide reductase activity. *Oncol. Rep.* **2008**, *19*, 1621–1626.
72. Kucinska, M.; Piotrowska, H.; Luczak, M.W.; Mikula-Pietrasik, J.; Ksiazek, K.; Wozniak, M.; Wierzchowski, M.; Dudka, J.; Jäger, W.; Murias, M. Effects of hydroxylated resveratrol analogs on oxidative stress and cancer cells death in human acute T cell leukemia cell line: Prooxidative potential of hydroxylated resveratrol analogs. *Chem. Biol. Interact.* **2014**, *209*, 96–110. [CrossRef] [PubMed]
73. Paulitschke, V.; Schicher, N.; Szekeres, T.; Jäger, W.; Elbling, L.; Riemer, A.B.; Scheiner, O.; Trimurtulu, G.; Venkateswarlu, S.; Mikula, M.; et al. 3,3′,4,4′,5,5′-hexahydroxystilbene impairs melanoma progression in a metastatic mouse model. *J. Investig. Dermatol.* **2010**, *130*, 1668–1679. [CrossRef] [PubMed]
74. Mikuła-Pietrasik, J.; Sosińska, P.; Wierzchowski, M.; Piwocka, K.; Ksiazek, K. Synthetic resveratrol analogue, 3,3′,4,4′,5,5′-hexahydroxy-*trans*-stilbene, accelerates senescence in peritoneal mesothelium and promotes senescence-dependent growth of gastrointestinal cancers. *Int. J. Mol. Sci.* **2013**, *14*, 22483–22498. [CrossRef]
75. Kotha, A.; Sekharam, M.; Cilenti, L.; Siddiquee, K.; Khaled, A.; Zervos, A.S.; Carter, B.; Turkson, J.; Jove, R. Resveratrol inhibits Src and Stat3 signaling and induces the apoptosis of malignant cells containing activated Stat3 protein. *Mol. Cancer Ther.* **2006**, *5*, 621–629. [CrossRef]
76. Fouad, M.A.; Agha, A.M.; Merzabani, M.A.; Shouman, S.A. Resveratrol inhibits proliferation, angiogenesis and induces apoptosis in colon cancer cells: Calorie restriction is the force to the cytotoxicity. *Hum. Exp. Toxicol.* **2013**, *32*, 1067–1080. [CrossRef]
77. Li, P.; Yang, S.; Dou, M.; Chen, Y.; Zhang, J.; Zhao, X. Synergic effects of artemisinin and resveratrol in cancer cells. *J. Cancer Res. Clin. Oncol.* **2014**, *140*, 2065–2075. [CrossRef]
78. Wu, Z.; Liu, B.; Cailing, E.; Liu, J.; Zhang, Q.; Liu, J.; Chen, N.; Chen, R.; Zhu, R. Resveratrol inhibits the proliferation of human melanoma cells by inducing G1/S cell cycle arrest and apoptosis. *Mol. Med. Rep.* **2015**, *11*, 400–404. [CrossRef]
79. Shin, H.J.; Han, J.M.; Choi, Y.S.; Jung, H.J. Pterostilbene suppresses both cancer cells and cancer stem-like cells in cervical cancer with superior bioavailability to resveratrol. *Molecules* **2020**, *25*, 228. [CrossRef]
80. Wen, W.; Lowe, G.; Roberts, C.M.; Finlay, J.; Han, E.S.; Glackin, C.A.; Dellinger, T.H. Pterostilbene, a natural phenolic compound, synergizes the antineoplastic effects of megestrol acetate in endometrial cancer. *Sci. Rep.* **2017**, *7*, 1–10. [CrossRef]
81. Cheng, T.C.; Lai, C.S.; Chung, M.C.; Kalyanam, N.; Majeed, M.; Ho, C.T.; Ho, Y.S.; Pan, M.H. Potent anti-cancer effect of 39-hydroxypterostilbene in human colon xenograft tumors. *PLoS ONE* **2014**, *9*, e111814. [CrossRef]
82. Schneider, Y.; Chabert, P.; Stutzmann, J.; Coelho, D.; Fougerousse, A.; Gossé, F.; Launay, J.F.; Brouillard, R.; Raul, F. Resveratrol analog (Z)-3,5,4′-trimethoxystilbene is a potent anti-mitotic drug inhibiting tubulin polymerization. *Int. J. Cancer* **2003**, *107*, 189–196. [CrossRef]
83. Zaki, M.A.; Balachandran, P.; Khan, S.; Wang, M.; Mohammed, R.; Hetta, M.H.; Pasco, D.S.; Muhammad, I. Cytotoxicity and modulation of cancer-related signaling by (Z)- and (E)-3,4,3′,5′-tetramethoxystilbene isolated from *Eugenia rigida*. *J. Nat. Prod.* **2013**, *76*, 679–684. [CrossRef]
84. Xu, M.; Wang, C.; Zhu, M.; Wang, X.; Zhang, L.; Zhao, J. 2, 3, 5, 4-tetrahydroxy diphenylethylene-2-O-glucoside inhibits the adhesion and invasion of A549 human lung cancer cells. *Mol. Med. Rep.* **2017**, *16*, 8900–8906.
85. Bolton, J.L.; Trush, M.A.; Penning, T.M.; Dryhurst, G.; Monks, T.J. Role of quinones in toxicology. *Chem. Res. Toxicol.* **2000**, *13*, 135–160. [CrossRef]
86. El-Najjar, N.; Gali-Muhtasib, H.; Ketola, R.A.; Vuorela, P.; Urtti, A.; Vuorela, H. The chemical and biological activities of quinones: Overview and implications in analytical detection. *Phytochem. Rev.* **2011**, *10*, 353. [CrossRef]
87. Tseng, C.H.; Cheng, C.M.; Tzeng, C.C.; Peng, S.I.; Yang, C.L.; Chen, Y.L. Synthesis and anti-inflammatory evaluations of β-lapachone derivatives. *Bioorg. Med. Chem.* **2013**, *21*, 523–531. [CrossRef]
88. Bolton, J.L.; Dunlap, T. Formation and biological targets of quinones: Cytotoxic versus cytoprotective effects. *Chem. Res. Toxicol.* **2017**, *30*, 13–37. [CrossRef]

89. Cardoso, M.F.C.; Rodrigues, P.C.; Oliveira, M.E.I.M.; Gama, I.L.; Da Silva, I.M.C.B.; Santos, I.O.; Rocha, D.R.; Pinho, R.T.; Ferreira, V.F.; De Souza, M.C.B.V.; et al. Synthesis and evaluation of the cytotoxic activity of 1,2-furanonaphthoquinones tethered to 1,2,3-1H-triazoles in myeloid and lymphoid leukemia cell lines. *Eur. J. Med. Chem.* **2014**, *84*, 708–717. [CrossRef]
90. Thomson, R.H. Distribution and Biogenesis. In *Naturally Occurring Quinones*; Elsevier: Amsterdam, The Netherlands, 1971.
91. Rao, K.V.; Mcbride, T.J.; Oleson, J.J. Recognition and Evaluation of Lapachol as an Antitumor Agent. *Cancer Res.* **1968**, *28*, 1952–1954.
92. Hussain, H.; Green, I.R. Lapachol and lapachone analogs: A journey of two decades of patent research (1997–2016). *Expert Opin. Ther. Pat.* **2017**, *27*, 1111–1121. [CrossRef]
93. Salas, C.; Tapia, R.A.; Ciudad, K.; Armstrong, V.; Orellana, M.; Kemmerling, U.; Ferreira, J.; Maya, J.D.; Morello, A. *Trypanosoma cruzi*: Activities of lapachol and α- and β-lapachone derivatives against epimastigote and trypomastigote forms. *Bioorg. Med. Chem.* **2008**, *16*, 668–674. [CrossRef]
94. Boveris, A.; Stoppani, A.O.M.; Docampo, R.; Cruz, F.S. Superoxide anion production and trypanocidal action of naphthoquinones on *Trypanosoma cruzi*. *Comp. Biochem. Physiol. Part C Comp.* **1978**, *61*, 327–329. [CrossRef]
95. Silvers, M.A.; Deja, S.; Singh, N.; Egnatchik, R.A.; Sudderth, J.; Luo, X.; Beg, M.S.; Burgess, S.C.; DeBerardinis, R.J.; Boothman, D.A.; et al. The NQO1 bioactivatable drug, β-lapachone, alters the redox state of NQO1 pancreatic cancer cells, causing perturbation in central carbon metabolism. *J. Biol. Chem.* **2017**, *292*, 18203–18216. [CrossRef]
96. Wuerzberger, S.M.; Pink, J.J.; Planchon, S.M.; Byers, K.L.; Bornmann, W.G.; Boothman, D.A. Induction of apoptosis in MCF-7: WS8 breast cancer cells by β-Lapachone. *Cancer Res.* **1998**, *58*, 1876–1885. [PubMed]
97. Park, E.J.; Min, K.J.; Lee, T.J.; Yoo, Y.H.; Kim, Y.S.; Kwon, T.K. β-Lapachone induces programmed necrosis through the RIP1-PARP-AIF-dependent pathway in human hepatocellular carcinoma SK-Hep1 cells. *Cell Death Dis.* **2014**, *5*, e1230. [CrossRef] [PubMed]
98. Gerber, D.E.; Beg, M.S.; Fattah, F.; Frankel, A.E.; Fatunde, O.; Arriaga, Y.; Dowell, J.E.; Bisen, A.; Leff, R.D.; Meek, C.C.; et al. Phase 1 study of ARQ 761, a β-lapachone analogue that promotes NQO1-mediated programmed cancer cell necrosis. *Br. J. Cancer* **2018**, *119*, 928. [CrossRef]
99. Don, M.J.; Chang, Y.H.; Chen, K.K.; Ho, L.K.; Chau, Y.P. Induction of CDK inhibitors (p21WAF1 and p27Kip1) and BAK in the β-lapachone-induced apoptosis of human prostate cancer cells. *Mol. Pharmacol.* **2001**, *59*, 784–794. [CrossRef]
100. Liu, T.J.; Lin, S.Y.; Chau, Y.P. Inhibition of poly(ADP-ribose) polymerase activation attenuates β-lapachone-induced necrotic cell death in human osteosarcoma cells. *Toxicol. Appl. Pharmacol.* **2002**, *182*, 116–125. [CrossRef]
101. Yu, H.Y.; Kim, S.O.; Jin, C.Y.; Kim, G.Y.; Kim, W.J.; Yoo, Y.H.; Choi, Y.H. β-lapachone-induced apoptosis of human gastric carcinoma AGS cells is caspase-dependent and regulated by the PI3K/Akt pathway. *Biomol. Ther.* **2014**, *22*, 184. [CrossRef]
102. Kee, J.Y.; Han, Y.H.; Kim, D.S.; Mun, J.G.; Park, S.H.; So, H.S.; Park, S.J.; Park, R.; Um, J.Y.; Hong, S.H. β-Lapachone suppresses the lung metastasis of melanoma via the MAPK signaling pathway. *PLoS ONE* **2017**, *12*, e0176937. [CrossRef]
103. Woo, H.J.; Park, K.Y.; Rhu, C.H.; Lee, W.H.; Choi, B.T.; Kim, G.Y.; Park, Y.M.; Choi, Y.H. β-lapachone, a quinone isolated from Tabebuia avellanedae, induces apoptosis in HepG2 hepatoma cell line through induction of Bax and activation of caspase. *J. Med. Food* **2006**, *9*, 161–168. [CrossRef]
104. Bey, E.A.; Bentle, M.S.; Reinicke, K.E.; Dong, Y.; Yang, C.R.; Girard, L.; Minna, J.D.; Bornmann, W.G.; Gao, J.; Boothman, D.A. An NQO1- and PARP-1-mediated cell death pathway induced in non-small-cell lung cancer cells by β-lapachone. *Proc. Natl. Acad. Sci. USA* **2007**, *104*, 11832–11837. [CrossRef]
105. Huang, X.; Dong, Y.; Bey, E.A.; Kilgore, J.A.; Bair, J.S.; Li, L.S.; Patel, M.; Parkinson, E.I.; Wang, Y.; Williams, N.S.; et al. An NQO1 substrate with potent antitumor activity that selectively kills by PARP1-induced programmed necrosis. *Cancer Res.* **2012**, *72*, 3038–3047. [CrossRef] [PubMed]
106. Bey, E.A.; Reinicke, K.E.; Srougi, M.C.; Varnes, M.; Anderson, V.E.; Pink, J.J.; Li, L.S.; Patel, M.; Cao, L.; Moore, Z.; et al. Catalase abrogates β-lapachone-induced PARP1 hyperactivation-directed programmed necrosis in NQO1-positive breast cancers. *Mol. Cancer Ther.* **2013**, *12*, 2110–2120. [CrossRef] [PubMed]

107. Huang, L.; Pardee, A.B. β-lapachone induces cell cycle arrest and apoptosis in human colon cancer cells. *Mol. Med.* **1999**, *5*, 711–720. [CrossRef] [PubMed]
108. Lai, C.; Liu, T.; Ho, L.; Don, M.; Chau, Y. Beta-lapachone induced cell death in human hepatoma (HepA2) cells. *Histol. Histopathol.* **1998**, *13*, 89–97. [PubMed]
109. Wu, Y.; Wang, X.; Chang, S.; Lu, W.; Liu, M.; Pang, X. β-lapachone induces NAD(P)H:quinone oxidoreductase-1- and oxidative stress-dependent heat shock protein 90 cleavage and inhibits tumor growth and angiogenesiss. *J. Pharmacol. Exp. Ther.* **2016**, *357*, 466–475. [CrossRef]
110. Silva, E.O.; de Carvalho, T.C.; Parshikov, I.A.; dos Santos, R.A.; Emery, F.S.; Furtado, N.A.J.C. Cytotoxicity of lapachol metabolites produced by probiotics. *Lett. Appl. Microbiol.* **2014**, *59*, 108–114. [CrossRef]
111. Salustiano, E.J.S.; Netto, C.D.; Fernandes, R.F.; Da Silva, A.J.M.; Bacelar, T.S.; Castro, C.P.; Buarque, C.D.; Maia, R.C.; Rumjanek, V.M.; Costa, P.R.R. Comparison of the cytotoxic effect of lapachol, α-lapachone and pentacyclic 1,4-naphthoquinones on human leukemic cells. *Investig. New Drugs* **2010**, *28*, 139–144. [CrossRef]
112. Li, X.; Bian, J.; Wang, N.; Qian, X.; Gu, J.; Mu, T.; Fan, J.; Yang, X.; Li, S.; Yang, T.; et al. Novel naphtho[2,1-d]oxazole-4,5-diones as NQO1 substrates with improved aqueous solubility: Design, synthesis, and in vivo antitumor evaluation. *Bioorg. Med. Chem.* **2016**, *24*, 1006–1013. [CrossRef]
113. Dias, R.B.; de Araújo, T.B.S.; de Freitas, R.D.; Rodrigues, A.C.B.D.C.; Sousa, L.P.; Sales, C.B.S.; de Valverde, L.F.; Soares, M.B.P.; dos Reis, M.G.; Coletta, R.D.; et al. β-Lapachone and its iodine derivatives cause cell cycle arrest at G2/M phase and reactive oxygen species-mediated apoptosis in human oral squamous cell carcinoma cells. *Free Radic. Biol. Med.* **2018**, *126*, 87–100.
114. Ross, D.; Siegel, D. Functions of NQO1 in cellular protection and CoQ10 metabolism and its potential role as a redox sensitive molecular switch. *Front. Physiol.* **2017**, *8*, 595. [CrossRef] [PubMed]
115. Siegel, D.; Yan, C.; Ross, D. NAD(P)H:quinone oxidoreductase 1 (NQO1) in the sensitivity and resistance to antitumor quinones. *Biochem. Pharmacol.* **2012**, *83*, 1033–1040. [CrossRef] [PubMed]
116. Chakrabarti, G.; Moore, Z.R.; Luo, X.; Ilcheva, M.; Ali, A.; Padanad, M.; Zhou, Y.; Xie, Y.; Burma, S.; Scaglioni, P.P.; et al. Targeting glutamine metabolism sensitizes pancreatic cancer to PARP-driven metabolic catastrophe induced by ß-lapachone. *Cancer Metab.* **2015**, *3*, 12. [CrossRef] [PubMed]
117. Tagliarino, C.; Pink, J.J.; Reinicke, K.E.; Simmers, S.M.; Wuerzberger-Davis, S.M.; Boothman, D.A. μ-calpain activation in β-lapachone-mediated apoptosis. *Cancer Biol. Ther.* **2003**, 2, 141–152. [CrossRef] [PubMed]
118. Li, L.S.; Bey, E.A.; Dong, Y.; Meng, J.; Patra, B.; Yan, J.; Xie, X.J.; Brekken, R.A.; Barnett, C.C.; Bornmann, W.G.; et al. Modulating endogenous NQO1 levels identifies key regulatory mechanisms of action of β-lapachone for pancreatic cancer therapy. *Clin. Cancer Res.* **2011**, *17*, 275–285. [CrossRef] [PubMed]
119. Buranrat, B.; Chau-In, S.; Prawan, A.; Puapairoj, A.; Zeekpudsa, P.; Kukongviriyapan, V. NQO1 expression correlates with Cholangiocarcinoma prognosis. *Asian Pac. J. Cancer Prev.* **2012**, *13*, 131–136.
120. Siegel, D.; Franklin, W.A.; Ross, D. Immunohistochemical detection of NAD(P)H:Quinone oxidoreductase in human lung and lung tumors. *Clin. Cancer Res.* **1998**, *4*, 2065–2070.
121. Awadallah, N.S.; Dehn, D.; Shah, R.J.; Russell Nash, S.; Chen, Y.K.; Ross, D.; Bentz, J.S.; Shroyer, K.R. NQO1 expression in pancreatic cancer and its potential use as a biomarker. *Appl. Immunohistochem. Mol. Morphol.* **2008**, *16*, 24–31. [CrossRef]
122. Yang, Y.; Zhang, Y.; Wu, Q.; Cui, X.; Lin, Z.; Liu, S.; Chen, L. Clinical implications of high NQO1 expression in breast cancers. *J. Exp. Clin. Cancer Res.* **2014**, *33*, 14. [CrossRef]
123. Ma, Y.; Kong, J.; Yan, G.; Ren, X.; Jin, D.; Jin, T.; Lin, L.; Lin, Z. NQO1 overexpression is associated with poor prognosis in squamous cell carcinoma of the uterine cervix. *BMC Cancer* **2014**, *14*, 414. [CrossRef]
124. Yang, Y.; Zhou, X.; Xu, M.; Piao, J.; Zhang, Y.; Lin, Z.; Chen, L. β-Lapachone suppresses tumour progression by inhibiting epithelial-to-mesenchymal transition in NQO1-positive breast cancers. *Sci. Rep.* **2017**, *7*, 2681. [CrossRef] [PubMed]
125. Siegel, D.; Ross, D. Immunodetection of NAD(P)H:quinone oxidoreductase 1 (NQO1) in human tissues. *Free Radic. Biol. Med.* **2000**, *29*, 246–253. [CrossRef]
126. Strassburg, A.; Strassburg, C.P.; Manns, M.P.; Tukey, R.H. Differential gene expression of NAD(P)H:Quinone oxidoreductase and NRH:Quinone oxidoreductase in human hepatocellular and biliary tissue. *Mol. Pharmacol.* **2002**, *61*, 320–325. [CrossRef]
127. Schor, N.A.; Morris, H.P. The activity of the D T diaphorase in experimental hepatomas. *Cancer Biochem. Biophys.* **1977**, *2*, 5–9.

128. Cresteil, T.; Jaiswal, A.K. High levels of expression of the NAD(P)H:Quinone oxidoreductase (NQO1) gene in tumor cells compared to normal cells of the same origin. *Biochem. Pharmacol.* **1991**, *42*, 1021–1027. [CrossRef]
129. Hori, T.; Kondo, T.; Lee, H.; Song, C.W.; Park, H.J. Hyperthermia enhances the effect of β-lapachone to cause γh2AX formations and cell death in human osteosarcoma cells. *Int. J. Hyperth.* **2011**, *27*, 53–62. [CrossRef]
130. Dong, G.Z.; Youn, H.; Park, M.T.; Oh, E.T.; Park, K.H.; Song, C.W.; Kyung Choi, E.; Park, H.J. Heat shock increases expression of NAD(P)H:quinone oxidoreductase (NQO1), mediator of β-lapachone cytotoxicity, by increasing NQO1 gene activity and via Hsp70-mediated stabilisation of NQO1 protein. *Int. J. Hyperth.* **2009**, *25*, 477–487. [CrossRef]
131. Song, C.W.; Chae, J.J.; Choi, E.K.; Hwang, T.S.; Kim, C.; Lim, B.U.L.; Park, H.J. Anti-cancer effect of bio-reductive drug β-lapachon is enhanced by activating NQO1 with heat shock. *Int. J. Hyperth.* **2008**, *24*, 161–169. [CrossRef]
132. Park, H.J.; Choi, E.K.; Choi, J.; Ahn, K.J.; Kim, E.J.; Ji, I.M.; Kook, Y.H.; Ahn, S.D.; Williams, B.; Griffin, R.; et al. Heat-induced up-regulation of NAD(P)H:quinone oxidoreductase potentiates anticancer effects of β-lapachone. *Clin. Cancer Res.* **2005**, *11*, 8866–8871. [CrossRef]
133. Boothman, D.A.; Trask, D.K.; Pardee, A.B. Inhibition of Potentially Lethal DNA Damage Repair in Human Tumor Cells by β-Lapachone, an Activator of Topoisomerase I. *Cancer Res.* **1989**, *49*, 605–612.
134. Jones, J.C.; Stevnsner, T.; Mattern, M.R.; Bohr, V.A. Effect of specific enzyme inhibitors on replication, total genome DNA repair and on gene-specific DNA repair after UV irradiation in CHO cells. *Mutat. Res. Repair* **1991**, *255*, 155–162. [CrossRef]
135. Katz, E.J.; Vick, J.S.; Kling, K.M.; Andrews, P.A.; Howell, S.B. Effect of topoisomerase modulators on cisplatin cytotoxicity in human ovarian carcinoma cells. *Eur. J. Cancer Clin. Oncol.* **1990**, *26*, 724–727. [CrossRef]
136. Li, C.J.; Averboukh, L.; Pardee, A.B. β-Lapachone, a novel DNA topoisomerase I inhibitor with a mode of action different from camptothecin. *J. Biol. Chem.* **1993**, *268*, 22463–22468.
137. Li, C.J.; Wang, C.; Pardee, A.B. Induction of Apoptosis by β-Lapachone in Human Prostate Cancer Cells. *Cancer Res.* **1995**, *55*, 3712–3715. [PubMed]
138. Furuya, Y.; Ohta, S.; Ito, H. Apoptosis of androgen-independent mammary and prostate cell lines induced by topoisomerase inhibitors: Common pathway of gene regulation. *Anticancer Res.* **1997**, *17*, 2089–2093.
139. Planchon, S.M.; Wuerzberger, S.; Boothman, D.A.; Church, D.R.; Wilding, G.; Frydman, B.; Witiak, D.T.; Hutson, P. β-Lapachone-mediated Apoptosis in Human Promyelocytic Leukemia (HL-60) and Human Prostate Cancer Cells: A p53-independent Response. *Cancer Res.* **1995**, *55*, 3706–3711.
140. Li, Y.; Sun, X.; LaMont, J.T.; Pardee, A.B.; Li, C.J. Selective killing of cancer cells by β-lapachone: Direct checkpoint activation as a strategy against cancer. *Proc. Natl. Acad. Sci. USA* **2003**, *100*, 2674–2678. [CrossRef]
141. Choi, Y.H.; Ho, S.K.; Yoo, M.A. Suppression of human prostate cancer cell growth by β-lapachone via down-regulation of pRB phosphorylation and induction of Cdk inhibitor P21 WAF1/CIP1. *J. Biochem. Mol. Biol.* **2003**, *36*, 223–229. [CrossRef]
142. Pink, J.J.; Wuerzberger-Davis, S.; Tagliarino, C.; Planchon, S.M.; Yang, X.H.; Froelich, C.J.; Boothman, D.A. Activation of a cysteine protease in MCF-7 and T47D breast cancer cells during β-lapachone-mediated apoptosis. *Exp. Cell Res.* **2000**, *255*, 144–145. [CrossRef]
143. Ough, M.; Lewis, A.; Bey, E.A.; Gao, J.; Ritchie, J.M.; Bornmann, W.; Boothman, D.A.; Oberley, L.W.; Cullen, J.J. Efficacy of β-lapachone in pancreatic cancer treatment: Exploiting the novel, therapeutic target NQO1. *Cancer Biol. Ther.* **2005**, *4*, 102–109. [CrossRef]
144. Kim, I.; Kim, H.; Ro, J.; Jo, K.; Karki, S.; Khadka, P.; Yun, G.; Lee, J. Preclinical pharmacokinetic evaluation of β-lapachone: Characteristics of oral bioavailability and first-pass metabolism in rats. *Biomol. Ther.* **2015**, *23*, 296. [CrossRef] [PubMed]
145. Mangas-Sanjuan, V.; Gutiérrez-Nieto, J.; Echezarreta-López, M.; González-Álvarez, I.; González-Álvarez, M.; Casabó, V.G.; Bermejo, M.; Landin, M. Intestinal Permeability of β-Lapachone and Its Cyclodextrin Complexes and Physical Mixtures. *Eur. J. Drug Metab. Pharmacokinet.* **2016**, *41*, 795–806. [CrossRef] [PubMed]
146. Blanco, E.; Bey, E.A.; Khemtong, C.; Yang, S.G.; Setti-Guthi, J.; Chen, H.; Kessinger, C.W.; Carnevale, K.A.; Bornmann, W.G.; Boothman, D.A.; et al. β-lapachone micellar nanotherapeutics for non-small cell lung cancer therapy. *Cancer Res.* **2010**, *70*, 3896–3904. [CrossRef] [PubMed]

147. Ferreira, V.; Nicoletti, C.; Ferreira, P.; Futuro, D.; da Silva, F. Strategies for Increasing the Solubility and Bioavailability of Anticancer Compounds: β-Lapachone and Other Naphthoquinones. *Curr. Pharm. Des.* **2016**, *22*, 5899–5914. [CrossRef]
148. Szejtli, J. *Cyclodextrin Technology*; Springer: Berlin, Germany, 2013; ISBN 9788578110796.
149. Dahan, A.; Lennernäs, H.; Amidon, G.L. The fraction dose absorbed, in humans, and high jejunal human permeability relationship. *Mol. Pharm.* **2012**, *9*, 1847–1851. [CrossRef]
150. Seoane, S.; Díaz-Rodríguez, P.; Sendon-Lago, J.; Gallego, R.; Pérez-Fernández, R.; Landin, M. Administration of the optimized β-Lapachone-poloxamer-cyclodextrin ternary system induces apoptosis, DNA damage and reduces tumor growth in a human breast adenocarcinoma xenograft mouse model. *Eur. J. Pharm. Biopharm.* **2013**, *84*, 497–504. [CrossRef]
151. Allen, T.M.; Cullis, P.R. Liposomal drug delivery systems: From concept to clinical applications. *Adv. Drug Deliv. Rev.* **2013**, *65*, 36–48. [CrossRef]
152. Jang, S.B.; Kim, D.; Kim, S.Y.; Park, C.; Jeong, J.H.; Kuh, H.J.; Lee, J. Impact of micellar vehicles on in situ intestinal absorption properties of β-lapachone in rats. *Korean J. Physiol. Pharmacol.* **2013**, *17*, 9–13. [CrossRef]
153. Dai, L.; Li, X.; Duan, X.; Li, M.; Niu, P.; Xu, H.; Cai, K.; Yang, H. A pH/ROS Cascade-Responsive Charge-Reversal Nanosystem with Self-Amplified Drug Release for Synergistic Oxidation-Chemotherapy. *Adv. Sci.* **2019**, *6*, 1801807. [CrossRef]
154. Li, X.; Jia, X.; Niu, H. Nanostructured lipid carriers co-delivering lapachone and doxorubicin for overcoming multidrug resistance in breast cancer therapy. *Int. J. Nanomed.* **2018**, *13*, 4107–4119. [CrossRef]
155. Yin, W.; Ke, W.; Chen, W.; Xi, L.; Zhou, Q.; Mukerabigwi, J.F.; Ge, Z. Integrated block copolymer prodrug nanoparticles for combination of tumor oxidative stress amplification and ROS-responsive drug release. *Biomaterials* **2019**, *195*, 63–74. [CrossRef]
156. Da Silva Júnior, E.N.; Jardim, G.A.M.; Jacob, C.; Dhawa, U.; Ackermann, L.; de Castro, S.L. Synthesis of quinones with highlighted biological applications: A critical update on the strategies towards bioactive compounds with emphasis on lapachones. *Eur. J. Med. Chem.* **2019**. [CrossRef]
157. Di Rosso, M.E.; Barreiro Arcos, M.L.; Elingold, I.; Sterle, H.; Baptista Ferreira, S.; Ferreira, V.F.; Galleano, M.; Cremaschi, G.; Dubin, M. Novel o-naphthoquinones induce apoptosis of EL-4 T lymphoma cells through the increase of reactive oxygen species. *Toxicol. In Vitro* **2013**, *27*, 2094–2104. [CrossRef]
158. Araújo, A.J.; de Souza, A.A.; da Silva Júnior, E.N.; Marinho-Filho, J.D.B.; de Moura, M.A.B.F.; Rocha, D.D.; Vasconcellos, M.C.; Costa, C.O.; Pessoa, C.; de Moraes, M.O.; et al. Growth inhibitory effects of 3′-nitro-3-phenylamino nor-beta-lapachone against HL-60: A redox-dependent mechanism. *Toxicol. In Vitro* **2012**, *26*, 585–594. [CrossRef]
159. Da Rocha, D.R.; De Souza, A.C.G.; Resende, J.A.L.C.; Santos, W.C.; Dos Santos, E.A.; Pessoa, C.; De Moraes, M.O.; Costa-Lotufo, L.V.; Montenegro, R.C.; Ferreira, V.F. Synthesis of new 9-hydroxy-α- and 7-hydroxy-β-pyran naphthoquinones and cytotoxicity against cancer cell lines. *Org. Biomol. Chem.* **2011**, *9*, 4315–4322. [CrossRef]
160. Bortolot, C.S.; da S.M. Forezi, L.; Marra, R.K.F.; Reis, M.I.P.; Sá, B.V.F.; Filho, R.I.; Ghasemishahrestani, Z.; Sola-Penna, M.; Zancan, P.; Ferreira, V.F.; et al. Design, Synthesis and Biological Evaluation of 1H-1,2,3-Triazole-Linked-1H-Dibenzo[b,h]xanthenes as Inductors of ROS-Mediated Apoptosis in the Breast Cancer Cell Line MCF-7. *Med. Chem.* **2018**, *15*, 119–129.
161. Da Cruz, E.H.G.; Silvers, M.A.; Jardim, G.A.M.; Resende, J.M.; Cavalcanti, B.C.; Bomfim, I.S.; Pessoa, C.; De Simone, C.A.; Botteselle, G.V.; Braga, A.L.; et al. Synthesis and antitumor activity of selenium-containing quinone-based triazoles possessing two redox centres, and their mechanistic insights. *Eur. J. Med. Chem.* **2016**, *122*, 1–16. [CrossRef]
162. Ma, X.; Huang, X.; Moore, Z.; Huang, G.; Kilgore, J.A.; Wang, Y.; Hammer, S.; Williams, N.S.; Boothman, D.A.; Gao, J. Esterase-activatable β-lapachone prodrug micelles for NQO1-targeted lung cancer therapy. *J. Control. Release* **2015**, *200*, 201–211. [CrossRef]
163. Lamberti, M.J.; Morales Vasconsuelo, A.B.; Chiaramello, M.; Ferreira, V.F.; Macedo Oliveira, M.; Baptista Ferreira, S.; Rivarola, V.A.; Rumie Vittar, N.B. NQO1 induction mediated by photodynamic therapy synergizes with β-Lapachone-halogenated derivative against melanoma. *Biomed. Pharmacother.* **2018**, *108*, 1553–1564. [CrossRef]

164. Motea, E.A.; Huang, X.; Singh, N.; Kilgore, J.A.; Williams, N.S.; Xie, X.J.; Gerber, D.E.; Beg, M.S.; Bey, E.A.; Boothman, D.A. NQO1-dependent, tumor-selective radiosensitization of non-small cell lung cancers. *Clin. Cancer Res.* **2019**, *25*, 2601–2609. [CrossRef]
165. Li, L.S.; Reddy, S.; Lin, Z.H.; Liu, S.; Park, H.; Chun, S.G.; Bornmann, W.G.; Thibodeaux, J.; Yan, J.; Chakrabarti, G.; et al. NQO1-Mediated tumor-selective lethality and radiosensitization for head and neck cancer. *Mol. Cancer Ther.* **2016**, *15*, 1757–1767. [CrossRef] [PubMed]

3

Eradication of Human Immunodeficiency Virus Type-1 (HIV-1)-Infected Cells

Nejat Düzgüneş * and Krystyna Konopka

Department of Biomedical Sciences, Arthur A. Dugoni School of Dentistry, University of the Pacific, 155 Fifth Street, Room 412, San Francisco, CA 94103, USA; kkonopka@pacific.edu
* Correspondence: nduzgunes@pacific.edu

Abstract: Predictions made soon after the introduction of human immunodeficiency virus type-1 (HIV-1) protease inhibitors about potentially eradicating the cellular reservoirs of HIV-1 in infected individuals were too optimistic. The ability of the HIV-1 genome to remain in the chromosomes of resting CD4+ T cells and macrophages without being expressed (HIV-1 latency) has prompted studies to activate the cells in the hopes that the immune system can recognize and clear these cells. The absence of natural clearance of latently infected cells has led to the recognition that additional interventions are necessary. Here, we review the potential of utilizing suicide gene therapy to kill infected cells, excising the chromosome-integrated HIV-1 DNA, and targeting cytotoxic liposomes to latency-reversed HIV-1-infected cells.

Keywords: suicide gene therapy; CRISPR/Cas9; broadly neutralizing antibodies; cytotoxic liposomes; lentivirus

---

1. Antiretroviral Therapy

Following cell entry, human immunodeficiency virus type 1 (HIV-1) integrates its genome into the host cell chromosome. While some infected cells produce new virions, others are infected latently and do not express any viral envelope glycoproteins (Env; gp120/gp41) on their surface [1,2]. Treatment with antiviral drugs can inhibit the binding of the viral glycoproteins to the co-receptors on host cells (e.g., maraviroc), the fusion of the viral membrane with host cells (e.g., enfuvirtide), reverse transcription of the RNA genome of the virus (e.g., abacavir, lamivudine), integration of the reverse transcribed, double-stranded DNA into the host cell chromosome (e.g., raltegravir), and the viral protease involved in viral polyprotein cleavage and virus maturation (e.g., indinavir, darunavir). These treatments, however, do not eliminate the source of the virus, which is the HIV provirus integrated into the cellular chromosome.

Various therapeutic approaches have been tried in an attempt to eradicate the source of the virus. Soon after the introduction of protease inhibitors for HIV therapy, a mathematical analysis of the decay of blood levels of the virus following the co-administration of nelfinavir, zidovudine, and lamivudine suggested that cell-free virions and productively infected CD4+ T cells would be eliminated in less than two months [3]. The analysis also suggested that lymphocytes latently infected with an infectious provirus could be "completely eliminated after 2.3–3.1 years of treatment with a 100%-inhibitory antiretroviral regimen." Nevertheless, the possibility was raised that longer treatment periods might be needed because of the "possible existence of undetected viral compartments or sanctuary sites", as well as the persistence of infected mononuclear cells that could not be activated to produce virions [3]. Therapeutic interventions have also included early antiretroviral treatment during seroconversion, structured treatment interruptions, and targeted toxins; however, these approaches have not been able to eradicate the virus [4,5].

2. HIV-1 Latency

HIV-1 remains latent in some infected cells. These cells do not express any viral proteins on their surface, and they do not present any peptides in association with Class I major histocompatibility (MHC) molecules [6–8]. These latently infected cells, widely believed to be memory CD4+ T cells, and possibly cells of the monocyte-macrophage lineage [9–11], are hidden from recognition by the cellular immune system and render HIV infection intrinsically incurable with current antiretroviral therapy alone [12]. It is thought that the low-level viremia that continues despite therapy and the short-term viral blips (RNA below 200 copies/mL) do not depend on the presence of new drug-resistance mutations due to active replication but rather arise from viral release from stable reservoirs [12,13].

HIV latency is a multifactorial process. In most cases, the HIV-1 proviral DNA, reverse transcribed from the viral RNA genome, integrates into the host cell genome in regions that are being transcribed actively. It is ironic that most latent proviral DNA in patients who are on combination antiretroviral therapy (cART) and have suppressed viral replication are found in actively transcribed segments of the cellular chromosomes [13]. Several mechanisms of transcriptional interference may be involved in suppressing the expression of the proviral DNA: (i) the cytoplasmic sequestration of transcription factors, including NF-κB and NFAT, may inhibit viral gene expression; (ii) if the host promoter is located upstream of the provirus, the RNA polymerase (Pol II) may "read through" the HIV-1 promoter (5′-LTR) and displace the transcription factors necessary for viral transcription; (iii) if the proviral DNA has integrated into the host chromosome in the opposite orientation of the host gene, the RNA Pol II complexes of the provirus and the host may collide, and RNA transcription stops; (iv) resting CD4+ T cells have low levels of Cyclin T1, which would otherwise form P-TEFb and also play a role in HIV-1 transcription and Tat-mediated transactivation—this would therefore result in a lack of transcription of proviral DNA; (v) methylation of DNA and compaction of chromatin may also contribute to transcriptional silencing and hence HIV-1 latency [13].

A groundbreaking study by Lehrman et al. [14] showed that inhibition of histone deacetylase (the chromatin remodeling enzyme that helps maintain the latency of integrated HIV-1) by valproic acid, together with cART supplemented with enfuvirtide (ENF), reduced the frequency of resting cell infection. This finding suggested that, with new approaches, it may be possible to reduce or eliminate the reservoir of HIV in infected individuals. A subsequent study employing raltegravir or enfuvirtide in addition to standard cART and valproic acid in a slightly larger patient pool showed, however, that there was no effect on the low-level viremia measured by single-copy plasma HIV RNA [15]. This approach relied on cell death upon activation of the latently infected cells, or by recognition and destruction by the immune system. Margolis et al. [16] indicated that "a major approach to HIV eradication envisions antiretroviral suppression, paired with targeted therapies to enforce the expression of viral antigen from quiescent HIV-1 genomes, *and immunotherapies to clear latent infection*." Sengupta and Siliciano [17] reiterated this point, stating "neither viral cytopathic effects nor CTL-mediated lysis may occur upon latency reversal *without additional interventions*." In this mini-review, we describe most of these "additional interventions", including some approaches from our laboratory.

3. Latency Reversal

Richman et al. [9] emphasized that latency is likely to be established and maintained by blocks at different steps in the HIV-1 replicative cycle, which may complicate efforts to eradicate these cells. One of these blocks was inhibited by the administration of the histone deacetylase inhibitor, vorinostat, to HIV-infected patients, as shown by cellular acetylation and an increase in HIV RNA expression in resting CD4+ cells [18]. Thus, the latency of HIV-1 in resting CD4+ cells in patients can be reversed by a tolerable dose of vorinostat. The low number of latently infected cells in patients has hindered studies on HIV-1 activation. Latently infected T cell lines are thus useful in experiments identifying the agents that can activate latent HIV-1. Another problem with the activation of latently infected cells is the percentage of cells that are actually induced to synthesize viral proteins. The site of chromosomal insertion of HIV-1 DNA affects the response to activating agents; for example, phytohemagglutinin and vorinostat reactivated proviruses at distinct genomic locations [19]. Since the activation of the cells will produce infectious virions, it will be necessary to concomitantly employ a cART regimen used in the studies of Lehrman et al. [20] (2005) and Archin et al. [15].

Latency reversing agents include various protein kinase C activators, such as diacylglycerol lactones [21], anti-tumor-promoting phorbol esters [4,22] histone deacetylase inhibitors [23], interleukin-7 [14], toll-like receptor-1 and-7 agonists [24], bryostatin analogs [25] and other compounds [26,27]. Spina et al. [26] compared the response to numerous activators of primary T cell models, J-Lat cell lines, and patient-derived infected cells, and found that the different cellular systems responded differently to the activators than the latently infected T cells obtained from patients. Nevertheless, protein kinase C agonists and phytohemagglutinin were able to activate latent HIV in all the cellular models developed in different laboratories. A library of marine natural products was used to identify four latency reversing agents, including aplysiatoxin, which induced the expression of HIV-1 provirus in cell lines and primary cell models at concentrations 900-fold lower than that of prostratin without significant effects on cell viability [28]. The expression of provirus-derived RNA in single cells upon the reversal of latency—even before the synthesis of viral proteins—may be useful in delineating the mechanisms of these agents [29].

Another approach to reversing latency is the use of the CRISPR/Cas9-derived systems [SunTag and synergistic activation mediator (SAM) systems] that recruit several transcriptional activation domains to an optimal target region within the HIV 5′ long terminal repeat (LTR) [30]. Transcriptional activation of proviral genomes was observed in various latently infected cell lines at levels comparable to or higher than treatment with established latency reversal agents and led to the production of infectious virions. A similar system that comprised an RNA-guided dCas9-VP64 activator targeting the junction between two NF-κB transcription factor-binding sites within the LTR enhancer region induced transcriptional activation of latent HIV-1 infection in all latency models tested [31].

In the "shock and kill" studies described above, it was expected that HIV-1-specific CD8+ cytotoxic T lymphocytes would recognize HIV-1 antigens on the activated CD4+ T cells and kill them. However, some latency reversal agents were found to also adversely affect the function of CD8+ cells [32,33]. Another consideration in this approach, which is also relevant to the other methods described below, is the potential of stimulating a deleterious, systemic inflammatory response [33]. Huang et al. [34] showed that following the ex vivo exposure of CD4+ T lymphocytes from ART-treated individuals to several latency-reversing agents and autologous CD8+ T lymphocytes reduced cellular HIV DNA but could not deplete the replication-competent virus. This observation may indicate that cells containing replication-competent HIV are resistant to cytotoxic T cells.

4. Suicide Gene Therapy

The insertion of potentially cytotoxic genes that can be activated by characteristic proteins of HIV-1 may be a useful approach to eliminating HIV-1-infected cells. Plasmids expressing the diphtheria toxin A-fragment (DT-A) under the control of HIV-1 LTR sequences (−167 to +80) could be *trans*-activated by the viral Tat protein, but the toxin gene was also expressed to some extent without Tat [35]. When *cis*-acting negative regulatory elements from the *env* region of the viral genome were incorporated in the 3′ untranslated region of these plasmids, basal expression from the LTR was minimized. The DT-A gene could then be *trans*-activated at a maximal level in the presence of both Tat and Rev proteins from the virus. CD4+ H9 cells that were transduced with a retrovirus to express this gene construct and then infected with HIV-1 could limit HIV-1 production [36]. The intracellularly "immunized" cells were protected against clinical HIV-1 strains up to 59 days [37]. Co-transfection of HeLa cells with the plasmid expressing DT-A and the proviral HIV-1 clone, HXBΔBgl, completely inhibited virus production by the cells [38].

Our laboratory is working on developing an HIV-1-specific promoter that minimizes basal expression (e.g., in the absence of the HIV-1 transactivator, Tat) and that drives the expression of suicide genes that would induce cell death specifically in HIV-1-infected cells. As an initial attempt at modifying the LTR, we generated several clones with deletions in parts of the LTR (Figure 1). For example, LTR2 had the modulatory region deleted, whereas in LTR3, the NF-κB binding site was deleted. In a model system employing Tat-expressing HeLa cells and luciferase-expressing, wild-type, and mutant LTR-driven plasmids, we showed that the mutant LTR2, from which the modulatory elements at the 5′ end of the LTR were deleted, was 100-fold more responsive to the presence of Tat (which would only be present in infected cells that are actively producing the virus) than in control cells not expressing any Tat (e.g., uninfected cells or quiescent, latently-infected cells) [39] (Figure 2). The LTR2 promoter may now be used to drive the expression of the herpes simplex virus thymidine kinase (HSV-*tk*) gene preferentially in infected cells, resulting in cytotoxicity upon administration of the anti-herpesvirus drug, ganciclovir (Figure 3). To enable this construct to be delivered to all HIV-1-infected cells, it would most likely have to be incorporated into an HIV-1-based lentiviral vector. The advantage of this system over the DT-A-based plasmid described above is that it can be turned on and off. Thus, "treatment" can be initiated by the administration of ganciclovir and interrupted by ceasing it. We previously studied cytotoxicity induced by the HSV-*tk* system in oral squamous cell carcinoma and cervical carcinoma cells [40–43], as well as in an animal model of oral cancer [44,45].

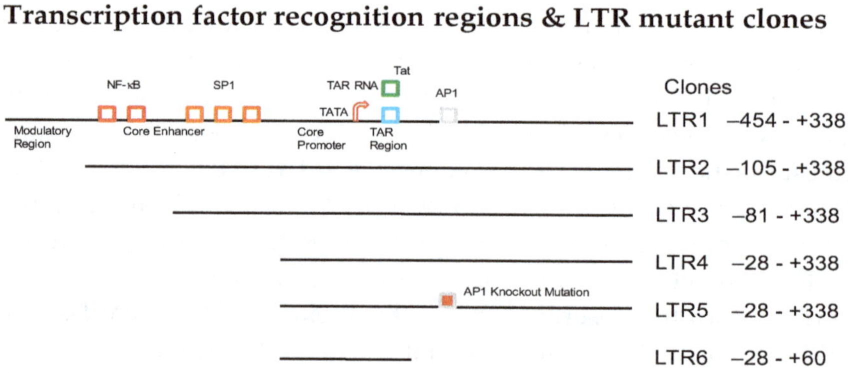

Figure 1. Transcription factor recognition regions of human immunodeficiency virus type-1 (HIV-1) long terminal repeat (LTR) and mutated LTR sequences used in HIV-1-specific gene expression studies shown in Figure 2.

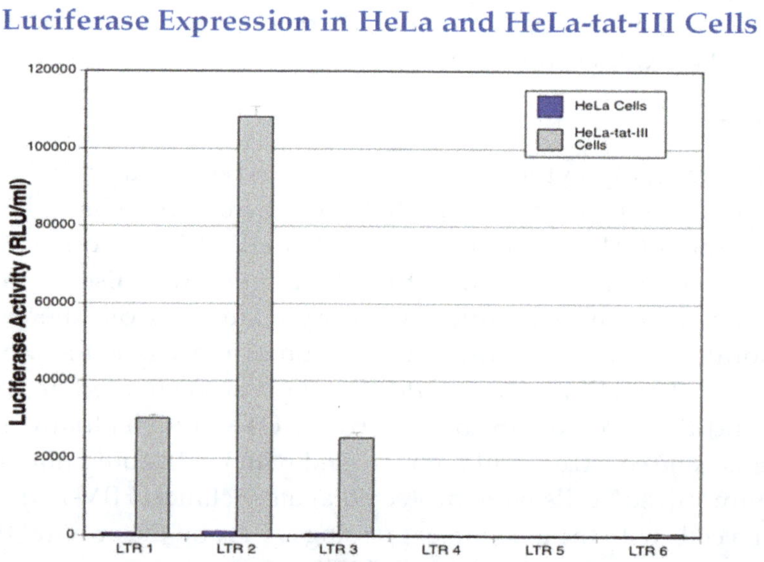

Figure 2. Comparison of luciferase gene expression from wild type LTR and LTR mutant clones (shown in Figure 1) in HeLa cells and HeLa-tat-III cells that constitutively express the HIV-1 Tat protein (data from [39]).

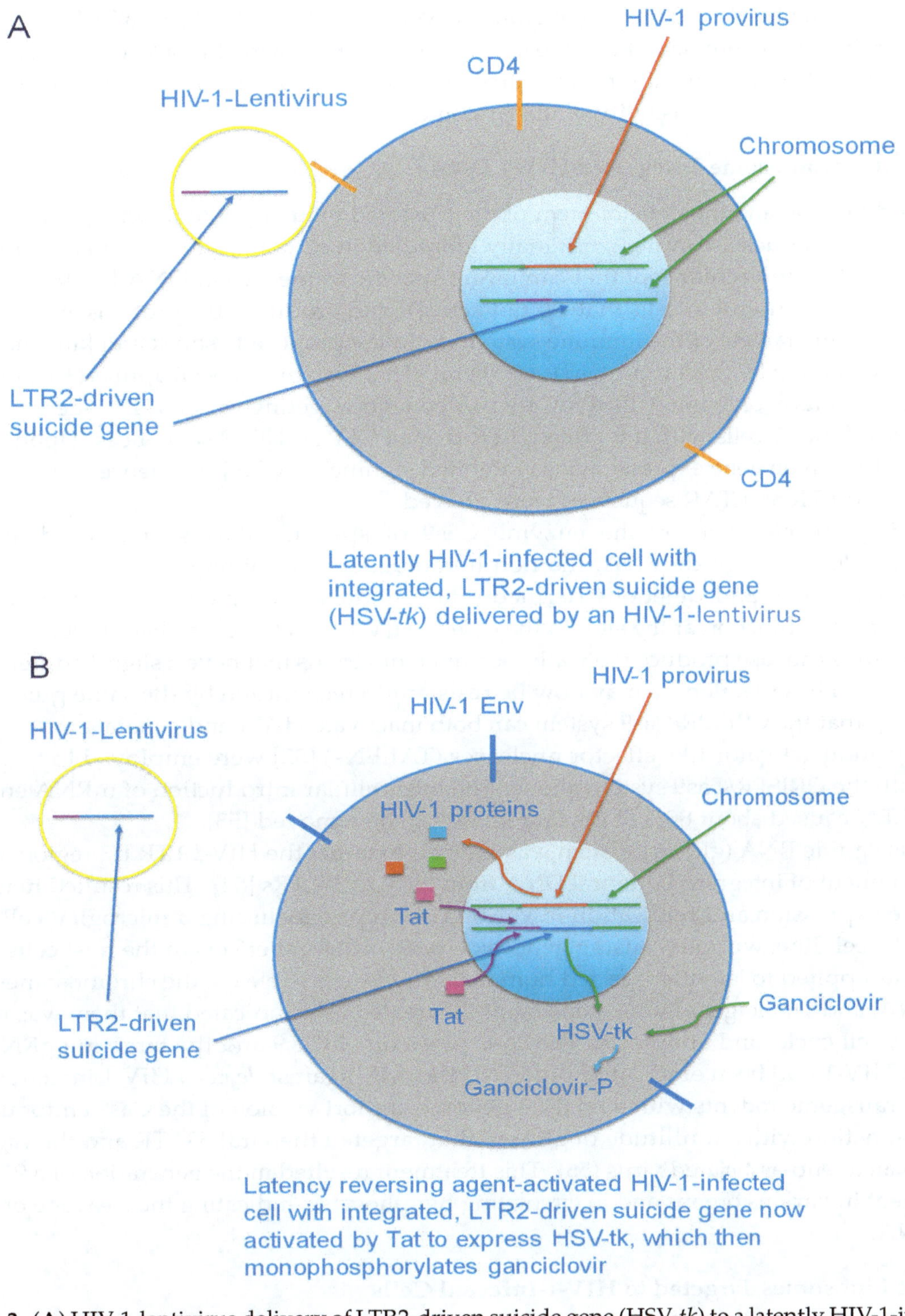

Figure 3. (**A**) HIV-1-lentivirus delivery of LTR2-driven suicide gene (HSV-*tk*) to a latently HIV-1-infected CD4+ cell. The suicide gene is then integrated into the chromosome of the cell. (**B**) Latency reversing agent-activated HIV-1-infected cell with integrated LTR2-driven suicide gene. The cell produces viral proteins, including Tat, which activates the LTR2 to express HSV-*tk*, which then monophosphorylates ganciclovir that has been delivered to the cell.

There is still a finite amount of luciferase expression from LTR1, LTR2, and LTR3 in the absence of Tat (Figure 2). Further genetic engineering of the HIV-1 promoter will be necessary to eliminate even this basal level of gene expression.

Garg and Joshi [46] cloned the *tk* gene into the vector, pNL-GFPRRESA, which includes the full LTR promoter that also expresses GFP in the presence of Tat. Following the selection of cells expressing GFP and treatment with ganciclovir, virus production and the number of virus-infected cells was reduced, demonstrating the feasibility of this system.

5. Excision of Chromosome-Integrated HIV-1 DNA

The modification and the development of the clustered regularly interspaced palindromic repeat (CRISPR)/Cas9 endonuclease system, originally identified in certain bacteria as an adaptive immune system, has led to a molecular tool that can target specific sequences in DNA [47,48]. This method could be particularly useful in cells that are not activated to produce HIV proteins and hence are not amenable to become targets of the immune system (as in the proposed "shock and kill" method), or in suicide gene activation by the Tat protein (*vide supra*). This system has been applied to alter the HIV-1 genome and block its expression. CRISPR/Cas9 components targeting various HIV1-derived sequences were transfected into T cells with integrated, LTR-driven GFP and TAR sequences. Upon stimulation of the cells, LTR-driven gene expression was inhibited significantly [49]. Sequence analysis confirmed that the targeted LTR and TAR sequences were cleaved.

Following the cleavage by the enzyme Cas9 of specific DNA sequences determined by intracellularly delivered guide RNA, the non-homologous end joining (NHEJ) machinery of the cells causes insertions and deletions (termed "indels") at the cleaved site, thereby causing the impairment of DNA function at the site. In the case of HIV-1-infected cells, these indels can inactivate the virus, but they can also produce replication-competent virions that have a slightly different proviral DNA sequence. These sequences may now be resistant to recognition by the same guide RNA [50], demonstrating that the CRISPR/Cas9 system can both inactivate HIV-1 and generate mutant virus [51].

Transcription activator-like effector nucleases (TALENs) [52] were employed to target the LTR site used with the CRISPR/Cas9 system above. The intracellular introduction of mRNA encoding the specific TALEN caused about 80% of the target DNA to be removed [53].

The Cas9/guide RNA (gRNA) system was utilized to target the HIV-1 LTR U3 region and excised a 9709 bp fragment of integrated proviral DNA from its 5′ to 3′ LTRs [54]. This resulted in inactivation of viral gene expression and replication in various cell types, including a microglial cell line and a promonocytic cell line, without causing genotoxicity or off-target effects in the host cells. The same approach was applied to latently infected human CD4+ T-cells to cleave the chromosome-integrated proviral DNA, and whole-genome sequencing of the treated cells indicated that there was no effect on cell viability, cell cycle, and apoptosis. The co-expression of Cas9 and the targeting gRNAs in cells from which HIV-1 had been eradicated protected the cells against *de novo* HIV-1 infection [55]. In a study with transgenic rodents with the HIV-1 genome, a short version of the Cas9 endonuclease was used in conjunction with a multitude of gRNAs that targeted the viral 5′-LTR and the *gag* gene and delivered in an adeno-associated virus [56]. This treatment resulted in the generation of a 978 bp HIV-1 DNA fragment in various organs and in circulating lymphocytes, indicating the cleavage of part of the proviral DNA.

6. Cytotoxic Liposomes Targeted to HIV-1-Infected Cells

In addition to the delivery of an HIV-1-activated suicide gene into latently-infected cells, our laboratory is focusing on the killing of such cells by targeting liposomes encapsulating cytotoxic drugs to infected cells whose latency has been reversed and that now express Env on their surface. For this purpose, we are coupling broadly neutralizing anti-Env antibodies (bNAb) [57–59], CD4-immunoadhesin [60], or CD4-derived peptides [61] as ligands to target the activated cells (Figure 4). Such liposomes are expected to be internalized, as shown for liposomes targeted to cancer cells [62,63] (*vide infra*) and kill the infected cells. To prevent an immune reaction to the antibodies, they can be engineered to be "humanized" for eventual clinical use, as in the case of a number of antibody-based drugs, including anti-HER2 [64].

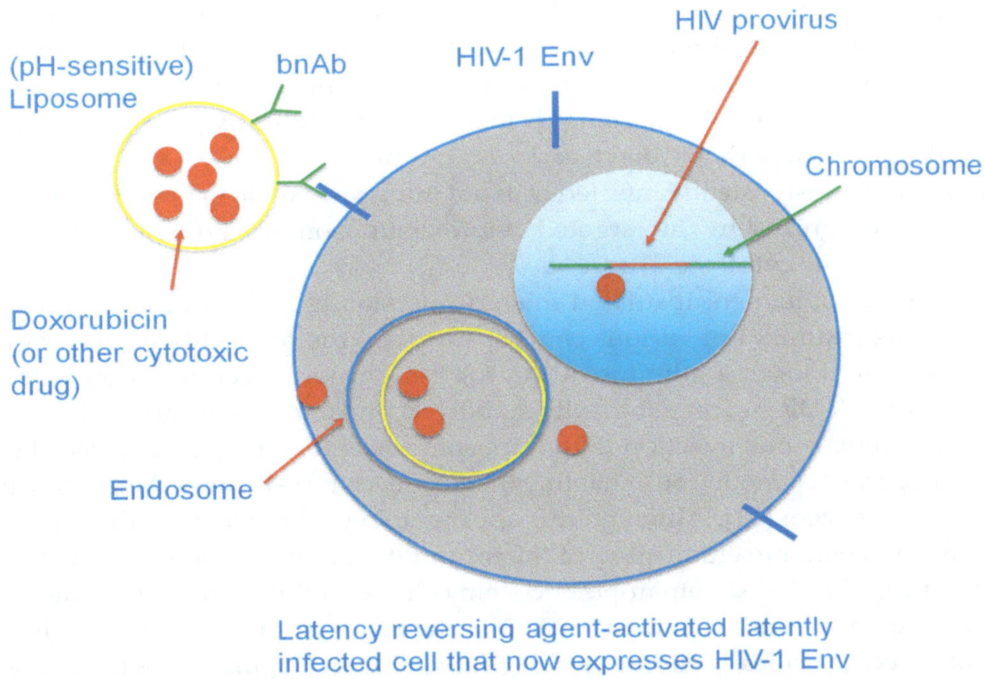

Figure 4. Cytotoxic liposome targeted to cell surface Env, which is expressed following treatment of a latently infected cell with a latency reversing agent. The targeting ligand is a broadly neutralizing anti-Env antibody. The liposome is endocytosed after binding to cell surface Env. The liposome may be engineered to be pH-sensitive so as to destabilize the endosome membrane at mildly acidic pH achieved in the endosome lumen and to enhance drug delivery to the cytoplasm.

Sterically stabilized liposomes containing poly(ethylene glycol) (PEG)-conjugated lipids and loaded with the cytotoxic DNA-intercalating anticancer drug, doxorubicin, are currently approved for the treatment of Kaposi's sarcoma, ovarian cancer, breast cancer, and multiple myeloma [65]. These liposomes have prolonged circulation in the bloodstream and can extravasate into tissues, including lymph nodes [66]. Liposomes administered subcutaneously are cleared via the local lymph nodes [66,67], thus localizing in tissues where HIV-1 is either replicating or hiding in latently infected cells [68–70]. Subcutaneous injection of liposomes carrying indinavir resulted in a 21–126 fold higher accumulation of the drug in all tissues compared to the free drug [71]. Indinavir delivered subcutaneously in liposomes to HIV-1-infected macaques localized in lymph nodes and caused a significant reduction in viral load [72]. Liposomes encapsulating the HIV-1 protease inhibitor, L-689,502, reduced the EC_{50} of the drug by 3-5-fold in infected macrophages [73]. The protease inhibitor PI1 encapsulated in liposomes targeted to gp120 expressed on infected cells via the antibody F105 had a 10-fold higher anti-HIV activity than the free drug at 100 nM [74]. However, it should be noted that, although the activity of antiviral agents can be enhanced by delivery in liposomes, and passive targeting to lymph nodes may reduce the need for daily administration of the drugs, this approach will not lead to the eradication of HIV-1-infected cells.

Nevertheless, liposomes containing cytotoxic drugs and targeted via anti-HER2 (ErbB2) monoclonal antibody fragments have been utilized in cancer chemotherapy. For example, they enhanced doxorubicin uptake in HER2-overexpressing cells in culture by up to 700-fold and resulted in tumor regression in five different tumor xenograft animal models [62], indicating their superior ability to kill tumor cells. Doxorubicin liposomes targeted to cell surface CD44 receptors on B16F10 melanoma cells had a 5-6-fold higher rate constant of cell killing than the free drug for a given amount of intracellular doxorubicin [63], showing the effectiveness of targeting. Sterically stabilized liposomes can also be rendered pH-sensitive to facilitate or enhance the intracellular delivery of cytotoxic drugs [75,76].

Since latently infected cells do not express the viral glycoproteins on their surface, they need to be activated by "latency reversing agents" to produce HIV-1 and express Env and hence will be recognizable by the targeted liposomes. These liposomes do not have to be administered for prolonged periods of time, since they will eliminate HIV reservoirs, unlike current treatment modalities with lifelong administration of antiviral agents. Thus, the inconvenience of subcutaneous, intravenous, intraperitoneal, or spinal delivery of liposomes is likely to be tolerable by patients who are likely to be cured of their HIV infection, perhaps after a series of injections.

The activated, previously latently infected cells are thus expected to express the HIV-1 Env protein on their surface, be recognized by the targeted cytotoxic liposomes, and be killed as a result of the intracellular delivery of the cytotoxic drug.

The fact that doxorubicin encapsulated in sterically stabilized liposomes is already approved for clinical use in the treatment of various cancers supports the feasibility of our approach [65,77]. An additional route of liposome administration for lymph node accumulation is intraperitoneal injection [78]. Anti-HLA-DR-bearing sterically stabilized liposomes accumulate in the lymph node cortex following subcutaneous injection [79]. Liposomes can also be injected into the spinal cord, as demonstrated in an animal model [80], enabling them to reach HIV-1-infected macrophages/microglia in the central nervous system [81]. Although this appears to be a difficult procedure, it is considerably more applicable than complete eradication of the immune system for bone marrow transplantation of HIV-1-resistant CCR5Δ32/Δ32 hematopoietic stem cells, a method that was applied in curing the "Berlin patient" and the "London patient" [82,83]. Therefore, after we demonstrate that targeted cytotoxic liposomes can specifically eliminate HIV-1-infected cells in culture, it will be possible to apply this method in vivo in HIV-1 infection models and eventually in patients.

7. Concluding Remarks

HIV-1 latency, the ability of the HIV-1 genome to remain in the chromosomes of resting CD4+ T cells and macrophages without being expressed, has been an important challenge in attaining HIV-1 remission and an eventual cure. It is astounding that a virus with just a few genes has evolved a way to reverse transcribe and integrate its genome into host cell chromosomes, but that virologists and molecular biologists throughout the world have not yet come up with an effective solution to excise or inactivate the viral genome or to specifically kill the infected cells. One possible reason for this is that the prevailing dogma in the scientific community soon after the identification of HIV-1 and HIV-2 as the etiologic agents of acquired immune deficiency syndrome (AIDS) was that it was impossible to cure HIV/AIDS and that our efforts should be focused on preventing viral replication. Nevertheless, in 1993, we proposed to use oligonucleotide-conjugated endonucleases [84,85] to cleave the chromosome-integrated HIV-1 provirus. In 2004, we also proposed to use triple-helix forming oligonucleotides [86,87] with an intervening spacer that would hybridize with the viral LTRs at the beginning and the end of the provirus, thereby connecting the two LTRs via the spacer and potentially inducing DNA repair mechanisms that would remove the looped DNA. We expect that the approaches we reviewed here (suicide gene therapy to kill infected cells, excision of chromosome-integrated HIV-1 DNA, and cytotoxic liposomes targeted to latency-reversed HIV-1-infected cells) will be developed further to be able to treat infected patients.

Author Contributions: Conceptualization, N.D. and K.K.; writing—original draft preparation, N.D.; writing—review and editing, N.D. and K.K.

Acknowledgments: We thank Matt Milnes, Senait Gebremedhin and Amy Au for their work on the LTR mutants described here.

References

1. Sundquist, W.I.; Kräusslich, H.-G. HIV-1 assembly, budding, and maturation. *Cold Spring Harb. Perspect. Med.* **2012**, 2, a006924. [CrossRef] [PubMed]

2. Baumgärtel, V.; Müller, B.; Lamb, D.C. Quantitative live-cell imaging of human immunodeficiency virus (HIV-1) assembly. *Viruses* **2012**, *4*, 777–799. [CrossRef]
3. Perelson, A.S.; Essunger, P.; Cao, Y.; Vesanen, M.; Hurley, A.; Saksela, K.; Markowitz, M.; Ho, D.D. Decay characteristics of HIV-1-infected compartments during combination therapy. *Nat. Cell Boil.* **1997**, *387*, 188–191. [CrossRef]
4. Kulkosky, J.; Sullivan, J.; Xu, Y.; Souder, E.; Hamer, D.H.; Pomerantz, R.J. Expression of latent HAART-persistent HIV Type 1 induced by novel cellular activating agents. *AIDS Hum. Retrovir.* **2004**, *20*, 497–505. [CrossRef] [PubMed]
5. Shehu-Xhilaga, M.; Tachedjian, G.; Crowe, S.; Kedzierska, K. Antiretroviral compounds: Mechanisms underlying failure of HAART to eradicate HIV-1. *Med. Chem.* **2005**, *12*, 1705–1719. [CrossRef]
6. Chun, T.W.; Engel, D.; Berrey, M.M.; Shea, T.; Corey, L.; Fauci, A.S. Early establishment of a pool of latently infected, resting CD4+ T cells during primary HIV-1 infection. *Proc. Natl. Acad. Sci. USA* **1998**, *95*, 8869–8873. [CrossRef]
7. Blankson, J.N.; Persaud, D.; Siliciano, R.F. The challenge of viral reservoirs in HIV-1 infection. *Annu. Med.* **2002**, *53*, 557–593. [CrossRef]
8. Siliciano, J.D.; Siliciano, R.F. A long-term latent reservoir for HIV-1: Discovery and clinical implications. *J. Antimicrob. Chemother.* **2004**, *54*, 6–9. [CrossRef] [PubMed]
9. Richman, D.D.; Margolis, D.M.; Delaney, M.; Greene, W.C.; Hazuda, D.; Pomerantz, R.J. The challenge of finding a cure for HIV infection. *Science* **2009**, *323*, 1304–1307. [CrossRef]
10. Murray, A.J.; Kwon, K.J.; Farber, D.L.; Siliciano, R.F. The latent reservoir for HIV-1: How immunologic memory and clonal expansion contribute to HIV-1 persistence. *J. Immunol.* **2016**, *197*, 407–417. [CrossRef]
11. Siliciano, R.F.; Greene, W.C. HIV latency. *Cold Spring Harb. Perspect. Med.* **2011**, *1*, a007096. [CrossRef]
12. Siliciano, R.F. Scientific rationale for antiretroviral therapy in 2005: Viral reservoirs and resistance evolution. *Top. HIV Med. Publ. Int. AIDS Soc. USA* **2005**, *13*, 96–100.
13. Ruelas, D.S.; Greene, W.C. An integrated overview of HIV-1 latency. *Cell* **2013**, *155*, 519–529. [CrossRef]
14. Lehrman, G.; Ylisastigui, L.; Bosch, R.J.; Margolis, D.M. Interleukin-7 induces HIV type 1 outgrowth from peripheral resting CD4+ T cells. *JAIDS J. Acquir. Immune Defic. Syndr.* **2004**, *36*, 1103–1104. [CrossRef] [PubMed]
15. Archin, N.M.; Cheema, M.; Parker, D.; Wiegand, A.; Bosch, R.J.; Coffin, J.M.; Eron, J.; Cohen, M.; Margolis, D.M. Antiretroviral intensification and valproic acid lack sustained effect on residual HIV-1 viremia or resting CD4+ cell infection. *PLoS ONE* **2010**, *5*, e9390. [CrossRef] [PubMed]
16. Margolis, D.M.; Garcia, J.V.; Hazuda, D.J.; Haynes, B.F. Latency reversal and viral clearance to cure HIV-1. *Science* **2016**, *353*, aaf6517. [CrossRef]
17. Sengupta, S.; Siliciano, R.F. Targeting the latent reservoir for HIV-1. *Immunity* **2018**, *48*, 872–895. [CrossRef] [PubMed]
18. Archin, N.M.; Bateson, R.; Tripathy, M.K.; Crooks, A.M.; Yang, K.H.; Dahl, N.P.; Kearney, M.F.; Anderson, E.M.; Coffin, J.M.; Strain, M.C.; et al. HIV-1 expression within resting CD4+ T cells after multiple doses of vorinostat. *J. Infect. Dis.* **2014**, *210*, 728–735. [CrossRef] [PubMed]
19. Chen, H.C.; Martinez, J.P.; Zorita, E.; Meyerhans, A.; Filion, G.J. Position effects influence HIV latency reversal. *Nat. Struct. Mol. Biol.* **2017**, *24*, 47–54. [CrossRef]
20. Lehrman, G.; Hogue, I.B.; Palmer, S.; Jennings, C.; A Spina, C.; Wiegand, A.; Landay, A.L.; Coombs, R.W.; Richman, D.D.; Mellors, J.W.; et al. Depletion of latent HIV-1 infection in vivo: A proof-of-concept study. *Lancet* **2005**, *366*, 549–555. [CrossRef]
21. Hamer, D.H.; Bocklandt, S.; McHugh, L.; Chun, T.-W.; Blumberg, P.M.; Sigano, D.M.; Marquez, V.E. Rational design of drugs that induce Human Immunodeficiency Virus replication. *J. Virol.* **2003**, *77*, 10227–10236. [CrossRef] [PubMed]
22. Bocklandt, S.; Blumberg, P.M.; Hamer, D.H. Activation of latent HIV-1 expression by the potent anti-tumor promoter 12-deoxyphorbol 13-phenylacetate. *Antivir. Res.* **2003**, *59*, 89–98. [CrossRef]
23. Demonte, D.; Quivy, V.; Colette, Y.; Van Lint, C. Administration of HDAC inhibitors to reactivate HIV-1 expression in latent cellular reservoirs: Implications for the development of therapeutic strategies. *Biochem. Pharmacol.* **2004**, *68*, 1231–1238. [CrossRef]

24. Macedo, A.B.; Novis, C.L.; De Assis, C.M.; Sorensen, E.S.; Moszczynski, P.; Huang, S.-H.; Ren, Y.; Spivak, A.M.; Jones, R.B.; Planelles, V.; et al. Dual TLR2 and TLR7 agonists as HIV latency-reversing agents. *JCI Insight* **2018**, *3*. [CrossRef] [PubMed]
25. Marsden, M.D.; Wu, X.; Navab, S.M.; Loy, B.A.; Schrier, A.J.; DeChristopher, B.A.; Shimizu, A.J.; Hardman, C.T.; Ho, S.; Ramirez, C.M.; et al. Characterization of designed, synthetically accessible bryostatin analog HIV latency reversing agents. *Virology* **2018**, *520*, 83–93. [CrossRef]
26. Spina, C.A.; Anderson, J.; Archin, N.M.; Bosque, A.; Chan, J.; Famiglietti, M.; Greene, W.C.; Kashuba, A.; Lewin, S.R.; Margolis, D.M.; et al. An in-depth comparison of latent HIV-1 reactivation in multiple cell model systems and resting CD4+ T cells from aviremic patients. *PLoS Pathog.* **2013**, *9*, e1003834. [CrossRef] [PubMed]
27. Beliakova-Bethell, N.; Hezareh, M.; Wong, J.K.; Strain, M.C.; Lewinski, M.K.; Richman, D.D.; Spina, C.A. Relative efficacy of T cell stimuli as inducers of productive HIV-1 replication in latently infected CD4 lymphocytes from patients on suppressive cART. *Virology* **2017**, *508*, 127–133. [CrossRef] [PubMed]
28. Richard, K.; Williams, D.E.; De Silva, E.D.; Brockman, M.A.; Brumme, Z.L.; Andersen, R.J.; Tietjen, I. Identification of novel HIV-1 latency-reversing agents from a Library of Marine Natural Products. *Viruses* **2018**, *10*, 348. [CrossRef] [PubMed]
29. Ukah, O.B.; Puray-Chavez, M.; Tedbury, P.R.; Herschhorn, A.; Sodroski, J.G.; Sarafianos, S.G. Visualization of HIV-1 RNA Transcription from Integrated HIV-1 DNA in Reactivated Latently Infected Cells. *Viruses* **2018**, *10*, 534. [CrossRef]
30. Bialek, J.K.; Dunay, G.A.; Voges, M.; Schäfer, C.; Spohn, M.; Stucka, R.; Hauber, J.; Lange, U.C. Targeted HIV-1 latency reversal using CRISPR/Cas9-derived transcriptional activator systems. *PLoS ONE* **2016**, *11*, e0158294. [CrossRef]
31. Saayman, S.M.; Lazar, D.C.; Scott, T.A.; Hart, J.R.; Takahashi, M.; Burnett, J.C.; Planelles, V.; Morris, K.V.; Weinberg, M.S. Potent and targeted activation of latent HIV-1 using the CRISPR/dCas9 activator complex. *Mol. Ther.* **2016**, *24*, 488–498. [CrossRef] [PubMed]
32. Walker-Sperling, V.E.; Pohlmeyer, C.W.; Tarwater, P.M.; Blankson, J.N. The effect of latency reversal agents on primary CD8+ T cells: Implications for shock and kill strategies for human immunodeficiency virus eradication. *EBioMedicine* **2016**, *8*, 217–229. [CrossRef] [PubMed]
33. Clutton, G.T.; Jones, R.B. Diverse impacts of HIV latency-reversing agents on CD8+ T-cell function: Implications for HIV cure. *Front. Immunol.* **2018**, *9*, 1452. [CrossRef]
34. Huang, S.H.; Ren, Y.; Thomas, A.S.; Chan, D.; Mueller, S.; Ward, A.R.; Patel, S.; Bollard, C.M.; Cruz, C.R.; Karandish, S.; et al. Latent HIV reservoirs exhibit inherent resistance to elimination by CD8+ T cells. *J. Clin. Investig.* **2018**, *128*, 876–889. [CrossRef] [PubMed]
35. Harrison, G.S.; Maxwell, F.; Long, C.J.; Rosen, C.A.; Glode, L.M.; Maxwell, I.H. Activation of a Diphtheria Toxin A gene by expression of human immunodeficiency virus-1 Tat and Rev proteins in transfected cells. *Hum. Gene Ther.* **1991**, *2*, 53–60. [CrossRef] [PubMed]
36. Harrison, G.S.; Long, C.J.; Curiel, T.J.; Maxwell, F.; Maxwell, I.H. Inhibition of Human Immunodeficiency Virus-1 production resulting from transduction with a retrovirus containing an HIV-regulated diphtheria toxin A chain gene. *Hum. Gene Ther.* **1992**, *3*, 461–469. [CrossRef] [PubMed]
37. Curiel, T.J.; Cook, D.R.; Wang, Y.; Hahn, B.H.; Ghosh, S.K.; Harrison, G.S. Long-Term inhibition of clinical and laboratory human immunodeficiency virus strains in human T-cell lines containing an HIV-regulated diphtheria toxin A chain gene. *Hum. Gene Ther.* **1993**, *4*, 741–747. [CrossRef] [PubMed]
38. Konopka, K.; Harrison, G.S.; Felgner, P.L.; Düzgüneş, N. Cationic liposome-mediated expression of HIV-regulated luciferase and diphtheria toxin genes in HeLa cells infected with or expressing HIV. *Biochim. Biophys. Acta (BBA) Mol. Cell Res.* **1997**, *1356*, 185–197. [CrossRef]
39. Gebremedhin, S.; Au, A.; Konopka, K.; Milnes, M.; Düzgüneş, N. A gene therapy approach to eliminate HIV-1-infected cells. *J. Calif. Dent. Assoc.* **2012**, *40*, 402–406.
40. Young, M.; Overlid, N.; Konopka, K.; Düzgüneş, N. Gene therapy for oral cancer: Efficient delivery of a 'suicide gene' to murine oral cancer cells in physiological milieu. *J. Calif. Dent. Assoc.* **2005**, *33*, 967–971.
41. Gebremedhin, S.; Singh, A.; Koons, S.; Bernt, W.; Konopka, K.; Düzgüneş, N. Gene delivery to carcinoma cells via novel non-viral vectors: Nanoparticle tracking analysis and suicide gene therapy. *Eur. J. Pharm. Sci.* **2014**, *60*, 72–79. [CrossRef]

42. Düzgüneş, N.; Cheung, J.; Konopka, K. Non-viral suicide gene therapy in cervical, oral and pharyngeal carcinoma cells with CMV- and EEV-plasmids. *J. Gene Med.* **2018**, *20*, e3054. [CrossRef] [PubMed]
43. Düzgüneş, N.; Cheung, J.; Konopka, K. Suicide gene therapy of oral squamous cell carcinoma and cervical carcinoma in vitro. *Methods Mol. Biol.* **2019**, *1895*, 177–184.
44. Neves, S.; Faneca, H.; Bertin, S.; Konopka, K.; Düzgüneş, N.; Pierrefite-Carle, V.; Simoes, S.; De Lima, M.P. Transferrin lipoplex-mediated suicide gene therapy of oral squamous cell carcinoma in an immunocompetent murine model and mechanisms involved in the antitumoral response. *Cancer Gene Ther.* **2009**, *16*, 91–101. [CrossRef]
45. Faneca, H.; Düzgüneş, N.; Pedroso de Lima, M.C. Suicide gene therapy for oral squamous cell carcinoma. *Suicide Gene Ther.* **2019**, *1895*, 43–55.
46. Garg, H.; Joshi, A. Conditional cytotoxic anti-HIV gene therapy for selectable cell modification. *Hum. Gene Ther.* **2016**, *27*, 400–415. [CrossRef] [PubMed]
47. Mali, P.; Esvelt, K.M.; Church, G.M. Cas9 as a versatile tool for engineering biology. *Nat. Methods* **2013**, *10*, 957–963. [CrossRef] [PubMed]
48. Doudna, J.A.; Charpentier, E. The new frontier of genome engineering with CRISPR-Cas9. *Science* **2014**, *346*, 1258096. [CrossRef] [PubMed]
49. Ebina, H.; Misawa, N.; Kanemura, Y.; Koyanagi, Y. Harnessing the CRISPR/Cas9 system to disrupt latent HIV-1 provirus. *Sci. Rep.* **2013**, *3*, 2510. [CrossRef] [PubMed]
50. Wang, Z.; Pan, Q.; Gendron, P.; Zhu, W.; Guo, F.; Cen, S.; Wainberg, M.A.; Liang, C. CRISPR/Cas9-Derived mutations both inhibit HIV-1 replication and accelerate viral escape. *Cell Rep.* **2016**, *15*, 481–489. [CrossRef]
51. Wang, G.; Zhao, N.; Berkhout, B.; Das, A.T. CRISPR-Cas based antiviral strategies against HIV-1. *Virus Res.* **2018**, *244*, 321–332. [CrossRef] [PubMed]
52. Christian, M.; Cermak, T.; Doyle, E.L.; Schmidt, C.; Zhang, F.; Hummel, A.; Bogdanove, A.J.; Voytas, D.F. Targeting DNA double-strand breaks with TAL effector nucleases. *Genetics* **2010**, *186*, 757–761. [CrossRef] [PubMed]
53. Ebina, H.; Kanemura, Y.; Misawa, N.; Sakuma, T.; Kobayashi, T.; Yamamoto, T.; Koyanagi, Y. A high excision potential of TALENs for integrated DNA of HIV-based lentiviral vector. *PLoS ONE* **2015**, *10*, e0120047. [CrossRef] [PubMed]
54. Hu, W.; Kaminski, R.; Yang, F.; Zhang, Y.; Cosentino, L.; Li, F.; Luo, B.; Alvarez-Carbonell, D.; Garcia-Mesa, Y.; Karn, J.; et al. RNA-directed gene editing specifically eradicates latent and prevents new HIV-1 infection. *Proc. Natl. Acad. Sci. USA* **2014**, *111*, 11461–11466. [CrossRef] [PubMed]
55. Kaminski, R.; Chen, Y.; Fischer, T.; Tedaldi, E.; Napoli, A.; Zhang, Y.; Karn, J.; Hu, W.; Khalili, K. Elimination of HIV-1 genomes from human T-lymphoid cells by CRISPR/Cas9 gene editing. *Sci. Rep.* **2016**, *6*, 22555. [CrossRef] [PubMed]
56. Kaminski, R.; Bella, R.; Yin, C.; Otte, J.; Ferrante, P.; Gendelman, H.E.; Li, H.; Booze, R.; Gordon, J.; Hu, W.; et al. Excision of HIV-1 DNA by gene editing: A proof-of-concept in vivo study. *Gene Ther.* **2016**, *23*, 690–695. [CrossRef] [PubMed]
57. Walker, L.M.; Phogat, S.K.; Chan-Hui, P.-Y.; Wagner, D.; Phung, P.; Goss, J.L.; Wrin, T.; Simek, M.D.; Fling, S.; Mitcham, J.L.; et al. Broad and potent neutralizing antibodies from an African donor reveal a new HIV-1 vaccine target. *Science* **2009**, *326*, 285–289. [CrossRef]
58. Yee, M.; Konopka, K.; Balzarini, J.; Düzgüneş, N. Inhibition of HIV-1 Env-mediated cell-cell fusion by lectins, peptide T-20, and neutralizing antibodies. *Open Virol. J.* **2011**, *5*, 44–51. [CrossRef]
59. Stephenson, K.E.; Barouch, D.H. Broadly neutralizing antibodies for HIV eradication. *HIV/AIDS Rep.* **2016**, *13*, 31–37. [CrossRef]
60. Flasher, D.; Konopka, K.; Chamow, S.M.; Dazin, P.; Ashkenazi, A.; Pretzer, E.; Düzgüneş, N. Liposome targeting to human immunodeficiency virus type 1-infected cells via recombinant soluble CD4 and CD4 immunoadhesin (CD4-IgG). *Biochim. et Biophys. Acta (BBA) Biomembr.* **1994**, *1194*, 185–196. [CrossRef]
61. Slepushkin, V.A.; Salem, I.I.; Andreev, S.M.; Dazin, P.; Düzgüneş, N. Targeting of liposomes to HIV-1-infected cells by peptides derived from the CD4 receptor. *Biochem. Biophys. Commun.* **1996**, *227*, 827–833. [CrossRef] [PubMed]
62. Park, J.; Kirpotin, D.; Hong, K.; Shalaby, R.; Shao, Y.; Nielsen, U.; Marks, J.; Papahadjopoulos, D.; Benz, C. Tumor targeting using anti-her2 immunoliposomes. *J. Control. Release* **2001**, *74*, 95–113. [CrossRef]

63. Eliaz, R.E.; Nir, S.; Marty, C.; Szoka, F.C., Jr. Determination and modeling of kinetics of cancer cell killing by doxorubicin and doxorubicin encapsulated in targeted liposomes. *Cancer Res.* **2004**, *64*, 711–718. [CrossRef] [PubMed]
64. Li, R.; Hu, S.; Chang, Y.; Zhang, Z.; Zha, Z.; Huang, H.; Shen, G.; Liu, J.; Song, L.; Wei, W.; et al. Development and characterization of a humanized anti-HER2 antibody HuA21 with potent anti-tumor properties in breast cancer cells. *Int. J. Mol. Sci.* **2016**, *17*, 563. [CrossRef] [PubMed]
65. Gabizon, A.A.; Patil, Y.; La-Beck, N.M. New insights and evolving role of pegylated liposomal doxorubicin in cancer therapy. *Drug Resist. Updat.* **2016**, *29*, 90–106. [CrossRef] [PubMed]
66. Oussoren, C.; Storm, G. Liposomes to target the lymphatics by subcutaneous administration. *Adv. Drug Deliv. Rev.* **2001**, *50*, 143–156. [CrossRef]
67. Allen, T.M.; Hansen, C.B.; Guo, L.S.S. Subcutaneous administration of liposomes: A comparison with the intravenous and intraperitoneal routes of injection. *Biochim. Biophys. Acta (BBA) Biomembr.* **1993**, *1150*, 9–16. [CrossRef]
68. Pantaleo, G.; Graziosi, C.; Butini, L.; Pizzo, P.A.; Schnittman, S.M.; Kotler, D.P.; Fauci, A.S. Lymphoid organs function as major reservoirs for human immunodeficiency virus. *Proc. Natl. Acad. Sci. USA* **1991**, *88*, 9838–9842. [CrossRef] [PubMed]
69. Pantaleo, G.; Graziosi, C.; Demarest, J.F.; Butini, L.; Montroni, M.; Fox, C.H.; Orenstein, J.M.; Kotler, D.P.; Fauci, A.S. HIV infection is active and progressive in lymphoid tissue during the clinically latent stage of disease. *Nat. Cell Boil.* **1993**, *362*, 355–358. [CrossRef]
70. Embretson, J.; Zupancic, M.; Ribas, J.L.; Burke, A.; Racz, P.; Tenner-Racz, K.; Haase, A.T. Massive covert infection of helper T lymphocytes and macrophages by HIV during the incubation period of AIDS. *Nat. Cell Boil.* **1993**, *362*, 359–362. [CrossRef]
71. Désormeaux, A.; Bergeron, M.G. Lymphoid tissue targeting of anti-HIV drugs using liposomes. *Methods Enzymol.* **2005**, *391*, 330–351. [PubMed]
72. Kinman, L.; Brodie, S.J.; Tsai, C.C.; Bui, T.; Larsen, K.; Schmidt, A.; Anderson, D.; Morton, W.R.; Hu, S.-L.; Ho, R.J.Y. Lipid–drug association enhanced HIV-1 protease inhibitor Indinavir localization in lymphoid tissues and viral load reduction: A proof of concept study in HIV-2287-infected macaques. *JAIDS J. Acquir. Immune Defic. Syndr.* **2003**, *34*, 387–397. [CrossRef]
73. Pretzer, E.; Flasher, D.; Düzgüneş, N. Inhibition of human immunodeficiency virus type-1 replication in macrophages and H9 cells by free or liposome-encapsulated L-689,502, an inhibitor of the viral protease. *Antivir. Res.* **1997**, *34*, 1–15. [CrossRef]
74. Clayton, R.; Öhagen, Å.; Nicol, F.; Del Vecchio, A.M.; Jonckers, T.H.; Goethals, O.; Van Loock, M.; Michiels, L.; Grigsby, J.; Xu, Z.; et al. Sustained and specific in vitro inhibition of HIV-1 replication by a protease inhibitor encapsulated in gp120-targeted liposomes. *Antivir. Res.* **2009**, *84*, 142–149. [CrossRef] [PubMed]
75. Slepushkin, V.A.; Simões, S.; Dazin, P.; Newman, M.S.; Guo, L.S.; de Lima, M.C.P.; Düzgüneş, N. Sterically stabilized pH-sensitive liposomes. Intracellular delivery of aqueous contents and prolonged circulation in vivo. *J. Biol. Chem.* **1997**, *272*, 2382–2388. [CrossRef] [PubMed]
76. Slepushkin, V.; Simões, S.; de Lima, M.C.; Düzgüneş, N. Sterically stabilized pH-sensitive liposomes. *Methods Enzymol.* **2004**, *387*, 134–147. [PubMed]
77. Gabizon, A.; Shmeeda, H.; Grenader, T. Pharmacological basis of pegylated liposomal doxorubicin: Impact on cancer therapy. *Eur. J. Pharm. Sci.* **2012**, *45*, 388–398. [CrossRef]
78. Phillips, W.T.; Medina, L.A.; Klipper, R.; Goins, B. A novel approach for the increased delivery of pharmaceutical agents to peritoneum and associated lymph nodes. *J. Pharmacol. Exp. Ther.* **2002**, *303*, 11–16. [CrossRef] [PubMed]
79. Bestman-Smith, J.; Gourde, P.; Désormeaux, A.; Tremblay, M.J.; Bergeron, M.G. Sterically stabilized liposomes bearing anti-HLA-DR antibodies for targeting the primary cellular reservoirs of HIV-1. *Biochim. Biophys. Acta (BBA) Biomembr.* **2000**, *1468*, 161–174. [CrossRef]
80. Kim, S.; Scheerer, S.; Geyer, M.A.; Howell, S.B. Direct cerebrospinal fluid delivery of an antiretroviral agent using multivesicular liposomes. *J. Infect. Dis.* **1990**, *162*, 750–752. [CrossRef]
81. Bissel, S.J.; Wiley, C.A. Human immunodeficiency virus infection of the brain: Pitfalls in evaluating infected/affected cell populations. *Brain Pathol.* **2004**, *14*, 97–108. [CrossRef] [PubMed]

82. Hütter, G.; Nowak, D.; Mossner, M.; Ganepola, S.; Müßig, A.; Allers, K.; Schneider, T.; Hofmann, J.; Kücherer, C.; Blau, O.; et al. Long-term control of HIV by CCR5Delta32/Delta32 stem-cell transplantation. *N. Engl. J. Med.* **2009**, *360*, 692–698. [CrossRef] [PubMed]
83. Gupta, R.K.; Abdul-Jawad, S.; McCoy, L.E.; Mok, H.P.; Peppa, D.; Salgado, M.; Martinez-Picado, J.; Nijhuis, M.; Wensing, A.M.J.; Lee, H.; et al. HIV-1 remission following CCR5Δ32/Δ32 haematopoietic stem-cell transplantation. *Nat. Cell Boil.* **2019**, *568*, 1. [CrossRef] [PubMed]
84. Corey, D.; Schultz, P. Generation of a hybrid sequence-specific single-stranded deoxyribonuclease. *Science* **1987**, *238*, 1401–1403. [CrossRef] [PubMed]
85. Pei, D.; Corey, D.R.; Schultz, P.G. Site-specific cleavage of duplex DNA by a semisynthetic nuclease via triple-helix formation. *Proc. Natl. Acad. Sci. USA* **1990**, *87*, 9858–9862. [CrossRef]
86. Guieysse, A.; Praseuth, D.; François, J.; Helene, C. Inhibition of replication initiation by triple helix-forming oligonucleotides. *Biochem. Biophys. Commun.* **1995**, *217*, 186–194. [CrossRef]
87. Faria, M.; Wood, C.; Perrouault, L.; Nelson, J.S.; Winter, A.; White, M.R.H.; Helene, C.; Giovannangeli, C. Targeted inhibition of transcription elongation in cells mediated by triplex-forming oligonucleotides. *Proc. Natl. Acad. Sci. USA* **2000**, *97*, 3862–3867. [CrossRef]

4

Antiproliferative Aspidosperma-Type Monoterpenoid Indole Alkaloids from *Bousigonia mekongensis* Inhibit Tubulin Polymerization

Yu Zhang [1,2], Masuo Goto [2,*], Akifumi Oda [3], Pei-Ling Hsu [2], Ling-Li Guo [1], Yan-Hui Fu [1], Susan L. Morris-Natschke [2], Ernest Hamel [4], Kuo-Hsiung Lee [2,5,*] and Xiao-Jiang Hao [1,*]

1 Key Laboratory of Phytochemistry and Plant Resources in West China, Kunming Institute of Botany, Chinese Academy of Sciences, Kunming 650201, China; zhangyu@mail.kib.ac.cn (Y.Z.); guolingli@mail.kib.ac.cn (L.-L.G.); fuyanhui80@163.com (Y.-H.F.)

2 Natural Product Research Laboratories, UNC Eshelman School of Pharmacy, University of North Carolina, Chapel Hill, NC 27599, USA; peiling96@livemail.tw (P.-L.H.); susan_natschke@unc.edu (S.L.M.-N.)

3 Graduate School of Pharmacy, Meijo University, 150 Yagotoyama, Tempaku-ku, Nagoya, Aichi 468-8503, Japan; oda@meijo-u.ac.jp

4 Screening Technologies Branch, Developmental Therapeutics Program, Division of Cancer Treatment and Diagnosis, Frederick National Laboratory for Cancer Research, National Cancer Institute, Frederick, MD 21702, USA; hamele@dc37a.nci.nih.gov

5 Chinese Medicine Research and Development Center, China Medical University and Hospital, 2 Yuh-Der Road, Taichung 40447, Taiwan

* Correspondence: goto@med.unc.edu (M.G.); khlee@unc.edu (K.-H.L.); haoxj@mail.kib.ac.cn (X-J.H.)

Abstract: Monoterpenoid indole alkaloids are structurally diverse natural products found in plants of the family Apocynaceae. Among them, vincristine and its derivatives are well known for their anticancer activity. *Bousigonia mekongensis*, a species in this family, contains various monoterpenoid indole alkaloids. In the current study, fourteen known aspidosperma-type monoterpenoid indole alkaloids (**1–14**) were isolated and identified from a methanol extract of the twigs and leaves of *B. mekongensis* for the first time. Among them, compounds **3**, **6**, **9**, and **13** exhibited similar antiproliferative activity spectra against A549, KB, and multidrug-resistant (MDR) KB subline KB-VIN cells with IC_{50} values ranging from 0.5–0.9 μM. The above alkaloids efficiently induced cell cycle arrest at the G2/M phase by inhibiting tubulin polymerization as well as mitotic bipolar spindle formation. Computer modeling studies indicated that compound **7** likely forms a hydrogen bond (H-bond) with α- or β-tubulin at the colchicine site. Evaluation of the antiproliferative effects and SAR analysis suggested that a 14,15-double bond or 3α-acetonyl group is critical for enhanced antiproliferative activity. Mechanism of action studies demonstrated for the first time that compounds **3**, **4**, **6**, **7**, and **13** efficiently induce cell cycle arrest at G2/M by inhibiting tubulin polymerization by binding to the colchicine site.

Keywords: aspidosperma-type; monoterpenoid indole alkaloids; antiproliferative activity; tubulin inhibitor; *Bousigonia mekongensis*

---

1. Introduction

Microtubule-binding agents have been developed as an effective therapy in cancer treatment due to the key roles of microtubules in cell proliferation, signal transduction, and cell migration [1]. Currently, many microtubule-binding agents, including taxanes, vinca alkaloids, epothilones, halichondrins, maytansinoids, colchicine-site binding agents, and others, have been discovered from natural products and later progressed to clinical studies and clinical use [2]. However, innate and acquired drug resistance, especially multidrug resistance (MDR), are major obstacles in cancer chemotherapy [3]. Overexpression of P-glycoprotein (P-gp) encoded by the ABCB1 gene leads to poor disease prognosis, and most clinical antimicrotubule drugs, including paclitaxel (PXL), vincristine (VIN), halichondrin B, and their analogs, are P-gp substrates [4]. A recent study indicated that antimitotic agents that target the colchicine site (CS) on the α/β-tubulin dimer were generally active in cells overexpressing βIII-tubulin, which is important in tumor aggressiveness and resistance to chemotherapy [5]. Hence, the discovery of other antimitotic CS-targeting agents might be a valuable approach for effective cancer chemotherapy, especially agents with enhanced tumor specificity and insensitivity to chemoresistance mechanisms.

Monoterpenoid indole alkaloids (MIAs) are secondary metabolites characteristic of plants in the family Apocynaceae [6]. Among them, the vinca alkaloids exhibit significant anticancer activity and vincristine, vinblastine, vinorelbine, vindesine, and vinflunine have been approved for clinical use in the treatment of hematological and lymphatic neoplasms [7]. Previous chemical studies on MIAs mostly focused on the dimeric compounds (vindoline-catharanthine), which generally exhibit superior anticancer activities compared with the corresponding monomeric units. Aspidosperma-type MIAs contain only the vindoline structural unit found in vincristine and are widely distributed in the genera *Tabernaemontana*, *Melodinus*, and *Bousigonia* (family Apocynaceae) [6]. In prior biological activity studies, several aspidosperma-type MIAs, such as jerantinines A, B, and E from *T. corymbose*, displayed significant antiproliferative activity against cancer cells [8]. Further mechanistic studies demonstrated that these alkaloids significantly arrested cells at the G2/M phase by inhibiting tubulin polymerization and, thus, they merit development as potential chemotherapeutic agents [9–11].

The genus *Bousigonia* (family Apocynaceae) contains only two species (*B. mekongensis* and *B. angustifolia*), distributed mainly in Southern China, Laos, and Vietnam [12]. Previous chemical investigation on this genus conducted in our group resulted in a series of new eburnamine-aspidospermine-type bisindole alkaloids and aspidosperma-type MIAs [13–15]. As part of our ongoing work, the present study investigated the antiproliferative activity of aspidosperma-type MIAs (**1–14**) against five cancer cell lines, A549, MDA-MB-231, KB, P-gp-overexpressing KB subline KB-VIN, and MCF-7, as well as a primary structure activity relationship (SAR) analysis including computer modeling. The detailed mechanisms of action of these alkaloids (Figure 1) were also further investigated and are described herein.

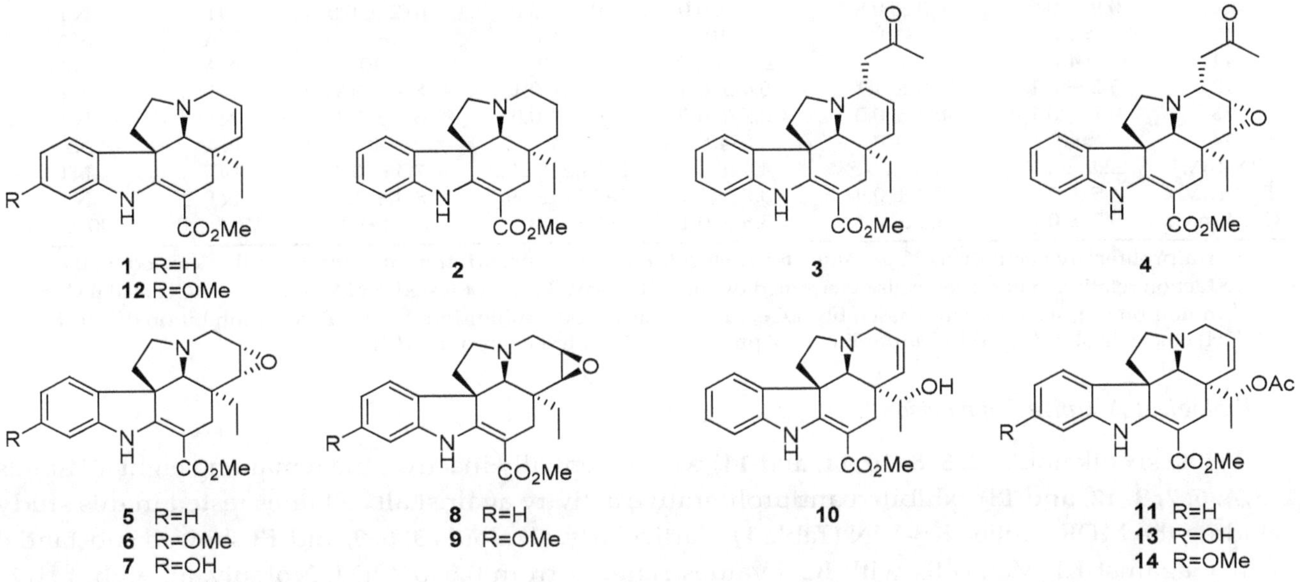

Figure 1. Structures of aspidosperma-type MIAs (**1–14**) from *B. mekongensis*.

2. Results and Discussion

2.1. Chemistry

Fourteen aspidosperma-type monoterpenoid indole alkaloids, tabersonine (**1**) [16], vincadifformine (**2**) [16], 3α-acetonyl-tabersonine (**3**) [17], melodinine S (**4**) [18], lochnericine (**5**) [19], 14,15-α-epoxy-11-methoxytabersonine (**6**) [20], 11-hydroxylochnericine (**7**) [20], pachysiphine (**8**) [21], lochnerinine (**9**) [22], 19-(*R*)-hydroxytabersonine (**10**) [23], 19-(*R*)-acetoxytabersonine (**11**) [24], 11-methoxytabersonine (**12**) [16], 19-(*R*)-acetoxy-11-hydroxytabersonine (**13**) [24], 19-(*R*)-acetoxy-11-methoxytabersonine (**14**) [24] were isolated and identified from the methanol extract of *B. mekongensis* for the first time by a combination of chromatographic and spectroscopic methods (Figure 1, Tables S1–S3). The effects of the substituents at positions C-3, C-11, C-14/C-15, and C-19 were evaluated by considering the hydrophilic or hydrophobic properties.

2.2. Antiproliferative Activity of Compounds 1–14

We tested the fourteen known aspidosperma-type alkaloids (**1–14**) against chemosensitive KB (originally isolated from epidermoid carcinoma of the nasopharynx) and P-gp over-expressing multidrug-resistant (MDR) KB subline KB-VIN, as well as three additional human cancer cell lines, A549 (lung carcinoma), MDA-MB-231 (triple negative breast cancer), and MCF-7 (estrogen receptor-positive breast cancer), using a sulforhodamine B (SRB) assay (Table 1). Vincristine (VIN), paclitaxel (PXL), and a CS agent combretastatin A-4 (CA-4) were also tested as positive controls.

Table 1. Antiproliferative activity and effect on tubulin assembly.

Compound	IC_{50} (μM) [a]					Tubulin Assay	
	A549	MDA-MB-231	KB	KB-VIN	MCF-7	ITA [d] (μM)	ICB [e] (%)
1	6.9 ± 0.1	5.9 ± 0.0	5.5 ± 0.0	7.4 ± 0.3	7.2 ± 0.4	NT [b]	NT
2	>40	>40	>40	>40	>40	NA [c]	NA
3	0.6 ± 0.0	0.9 ± 0.0	0.6 ± 0.0	0.6 ± 0.1	2.2 ± 0.2	NT	NT
4	5.6 ± 0.0	8.2 ± 0.8	5.8 ± 0.3	6.3 ± 0.2	10.0 ± 0.9	NT	NT
5	>40	>40	>40	>40	>40	NA	NA
6	0.5 ± 0.0	0.8 ± 0.0	0.5 ± 0.0	0.5 ± 0.0	0.8 ± 0.0	0.7 ± 0.0	54 ± 0.8
7	5.6 ± 0.1	9.8 ± 0.9	5.4 ± 0.3	6.1 ± 0.4	10.8 ± 0.8	4.6 ± 0.1	35 ± 1
8	27.7 ± 0.1	34.5 ± 0.2	>40	>40	>40	NA	NA
9	0.8 ± 0.0	6.0 ± 0.8	0.9 ± 0.0	0.7 ± 0.0	10.2 ± 0.5	NT	NT
10	>40	>40	>40	>40	>40	NA	NA
11	>40	>40	26.5 ± 2.5	>40	>40	NA	NA
12	5.2 ± 0.1	6.8 ± 1.1	5.4 ± 0.4	5.8 ± 0.1	8.2 ± 0.9	NT	NT
13	0.7 ± 0.1	0.9 ± 0.0	0.7 ± 0.0	0.7 ± 0.0	6.7 ± 0.1	NT	NT
14	>40	>40	>40	>40	>40	NA	NA
VIN (nM)	22.9 ± 2.4	32.0 ± 0.5	4.4 ± 0.1	2479.2 ± 28.2	7.3 ± 0.2	NT	NT
PXL (nM)	4.5 ± 0.9	7.0 ± 0.9	3.7 ± 1.1	2357.7 ± 59.5	8.8 ± 1.0	NT	NT
CA-4 (nM)	5.5 ± 0.1	8.2 ± 0.5	3.6 ± 0.1	3.8 ± 0.1	487.4 ± 11	0.7 ± 0.0	100 ± 0.4

[a] Antiproliferative activity as IC_{50} values for each cell line, the concentration of compound that caused a 50% reduction relative to untreated cells determined by the SRB assay. [b] NT, not tested. [c] NA, not active (IC_{50} > 40 μM). [d] Inhibition of purified tubulin assembly, EC_{50} (μM) values of 50% inhibition (ITA). [e] Percent inhibition of 5 μM [^{3}H] colchicine binding to 1 μM tubulin in the presence of 5 μM test compound (ICB).

2.3. Biological Activity Comparison

While six alkaloids (**2, 5, 8, 10, 11,** and **14**) were essentially inactive, the remaining eight alkaloids (**1, 3, 4, 6, 7, 9, 12,** and **13**) exhibited antiproliferative activity against all cell lines tested in this study, including the MDR subline KB-VIN (Table 1). Particularly, alkaloids **3, 6, 9,** and **13** showed substantial potency against KB-VIN cells with IC_{50} values ranging from 0.5–0.7 μM. Notably, all eight active alkaloids were effective against both chemosensitive and MDR cells, as compared with well-known P-gp substrates VIN and PXL, which required 600-fold higher concentration against KB-VIN cells.

The results indicate that the tested alkaloids are not substrates of P-gp and, thus, could be effective against tumors expressing the MDR phenotype.

Alkaloids **1–14** have the same carbon skeleton but differ in the substituents or oxidation state at various positions. Based on the antiproliferative activity data, a 14,15-double bond is critical for activity as alkaloids **2**, **5**, and **8** with a 14,15-single bond lost potency. Addition of a 3α-acetonyl group led to greatly increased potency (compare **3** versus **1**, **4** versus **5**). Potency was lost when the α-carbon of the ethyl group attached at C-19 of **1** was substituted with a hydroxyl (**10**) or acetoxy (**11**) moiety. The presence of a hydroxyl group at C-11 had a significant effect on potency (compare **7** versus **5**, **13** versus **11**), while a methoxy group at the same position led to both increased (~60-fold rise between **5** and **6**, **8** and **9**) and negligible (compare **1** versus **12**, **14** and **11**) potency.

Taken together, a 14,15-double bond or 3α-acetonyl group was required for antiproliferative activity against human cancer cell lines, including the MDR subline KB-VIN. A hydroxyl group at C-11 is necessary, while the effect of a methoxy group at C-11 was dependent on the parent skeleton. The compatibility of the synergistic groups will be considered in subsequent SAR studies.

2.4. Mechanisms of Action of 3, 4, 6, 7, and 13 in KB-VIN Cells

Bioactive analogs **6** and **7** were tested for inhibitory effects on tubulin assembly as well as inhibition of [^{3}H] colchicine binding to tubulin in a cell-free system, using highly purified bovine brain tubulin (Table 1). The results showed that alkaloid **6** strongly inhibited tubulin assembly with an EC_{50} (50% effective concentration for inhibiting tubulin assembly) value of 0.7 μM and inhibited the binding of colchicine to tubulin by 54%, while **7** showed moderate inhibition of tubulin assembly with an EC_{50} value of 4.6 μM. The data for **6** and **7** indicate that both alkaloids bind to tubulin and inhibit its assembly, and these effects are closely related to their antiproliferative activities against tumor cells. Thus, we further investigated whether the inhibition of tubulin polymerization was the major action of these alkaloids.

CA-4, a colchicine site (CS) agent, and other tubulin polymerization inhibitors induce cell cycle arrest at G2/M. Accordingly, we investigated whether the MIAs affected the cell cycle progression. KB-VIN cells were treated with compounds **3**, **4**, **6**, **7**, and **13** at their IC_{50} ($1 \times IC_{50}$) or three-fold IC_{50} ($3 \times IC_{50}$) concentration, and the cell cycle progression was analyzed by flow cytometer (Figure 2A). Expectedly, the accumulation of cells in the G2/M phase was observed in cells treated with alkaloids **3**, **4**, **6**, **7**, and **13**, as compared with CA-4 and vincristine (VIN).

To determine whether the cell cycle arrest was due to an antimicrotubule effect, cells treated with compounds were analyzed by immunocytochemistry using antibodies to α-tubulin for microtubules and mitotic spindles, Ser10-phosphorylated histone H3 (pH3) for the condensed chromatins and 4′,6-diamidino-2-phenylindole (DAPI) for DNA. In cells treated with alkaloids **3**, **4**, **6**, **7**, and **13**, dotted tubulin aggregations without spindles were seen in the pH3-positive mitotic cells, while microtubules were undetectable in pH3-negative interphase cells (Figure 2B). These observations demonstrated that the tested alkaloids inhibited tubulin polymerization in both interphase and mitosis for bipolar spindle formation, inducing cell cycle arrest at G2/M, probably at prometaphase. In addition, alkaloid **7** was less active than **6**, which corresponded to the inhibitory activity observed in cell-based proliferation and cell-free tubulin assembly assays. Thus, we concluded that these alkaloids are tubulin polymerization inhibitors. Furthermore, the immunocytochemical data suggest that alkaloids **3**, **4**, **6**, **7**, and **13** probably interact with tubulin in a biological manner similar to that of CA-4. These results agreed with those in a recent study on aspidosperma-type MIAs, such as jerantinine A, which potentially inhibit tubulin polymerization by binding to the CS on tubulin dimers [25].

Accordingly, we performed molecular docking studies to predict how alkaloid **7** binds to the tubulin dimer. An inactive alkaloid **5** was used as a comparison compound. In the tubulin binding assay described above (Table 1), CA-4 totally inhibited colchicine binding to tubulin, while **5** or **7** inhibited binding with 0 or 35% ICB value, respectively. Thus, compared with CA-4, alkaloid **5** and its hydroxyl analog **7** might bind differently to the CS. As expected, an overview of the predicted binding modes of **5** and **7** in the crystal structure of the α/β-tubulin dimer revealed considerable differences (Figures 3 and 4). The docked model of **5** showed an H-bond between the carbonyl oxygen and the side chain of Val181 on α-tubulin (αVal181), while that of **7** showed an H-bond between the C-11 hydroxyl group and the side chain of Val315 on β-tubulin (βVal315). Interestingly, in a cell-free tubulin assembly assay, compound **7** (EC_{50} 4.6 μM) was more potent than **5** (EC_{50} > 40 μM). These analyses suggested that the binding mode of **5** was insufficient to inhibit tubulin assembly. The docking model also predicted that active compound **13** (IC_{50} 0.6~6.7 μM) forms an H-bond with βAsn249, while less active compounds **4** (IC_{50} 5.6~10.0 μM) and **11** (IC_{50} > 26.5 μM) form H-bonds with αThr179 and αSer178, respectively (Supplementary Figure S2). However, H-bonding with αVal181 may also be important and depends on a steric hindrance due to the parent skeleton (compare **3** versus **5**). This docking model suggested that the force of the H-bond between βVal315 or βAsn249 and the C-11 hydroxyl group of **7** might be critical for greater inhibition of tubulin assembly, which is also reflected in greater antiproliferative activity.

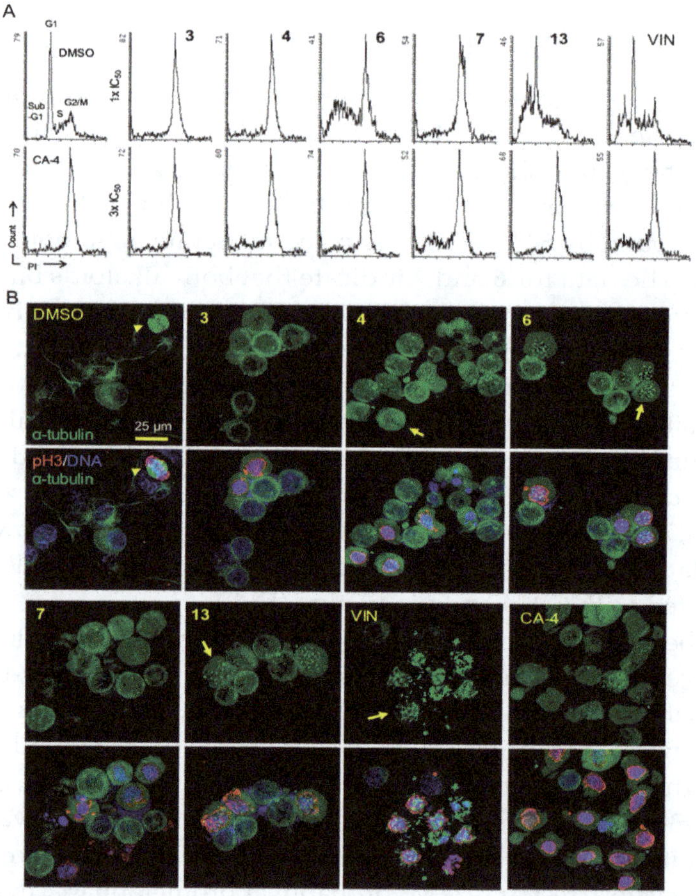

Figure 2. Mitotic defects in KB-VIN cells treated by compounds. (**A**) Vincristine-resistant subline KB-VIN cells were treated with compounds for 24 h at a concentration of one- or three-fold IC_{50} (1× IC_{50} or 3 × IC_{50}). CA-4 at 0.2 μM was used as a colchicine-type tubulin polymerization inhibitor. Cell cycle distributions (sub-G1, G1, S, G2/M) were analyzed using flow cytometry after staining cells with propidium iodide (PI). (**B**) KB-VIN cells were treated with compounds for 24 h at a concentration of 3 × IC_{50}. CA-4 was used at 0.2 μM. Fixed cells were stained with antibodies to α-tubulin (green) and phospho-histone H3 (pH3, red), and DAPI was used for DNA (blue). Stained cells were observed by confocal fluorescence microscope. The represented image is a projection of 15~20 optical sections acquired at 0.5~1 μm intervals. Normal mitotic spindle formation (arrow head) in control (DMSO) and dotted tubulin aggregations without spindles (**4, 6, 13**) or with multipolar spindles (VIN) were observed (arrows). Bar, 0.025 mm. Additional images are available in Supplementary Figure S1.

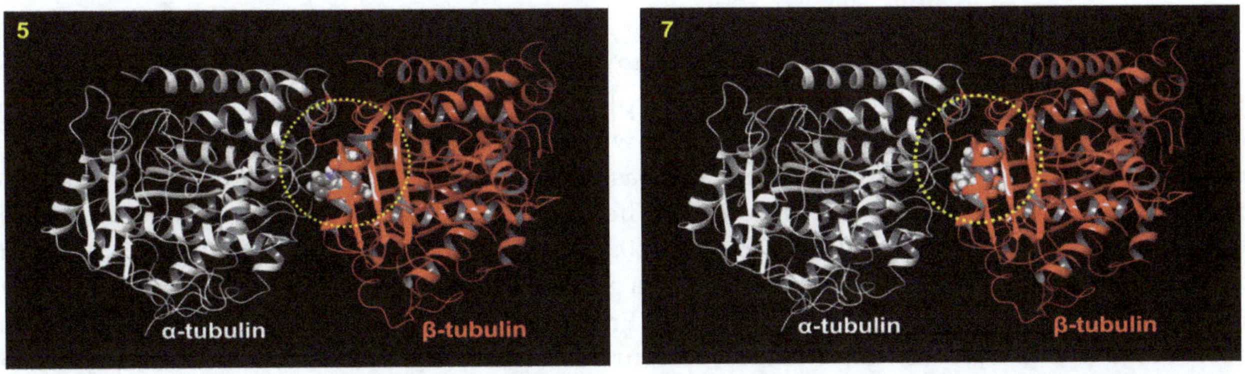

Figure 3. Predicted docking models for **5** and **7** binding to tubulin. Top 1 ranked docking models of **5** and **7** (sphere in 3D with gray in carbon, proton in white, oxygen in red, nitrogen in blue) in the colchicine site (CS, yellow circle) of the tubulin crystal structure (α and β tubulin heterodimer: α- (white) and β-tubulin (red)) (PDB: 1SA0) are shown as a ribbon diagram.

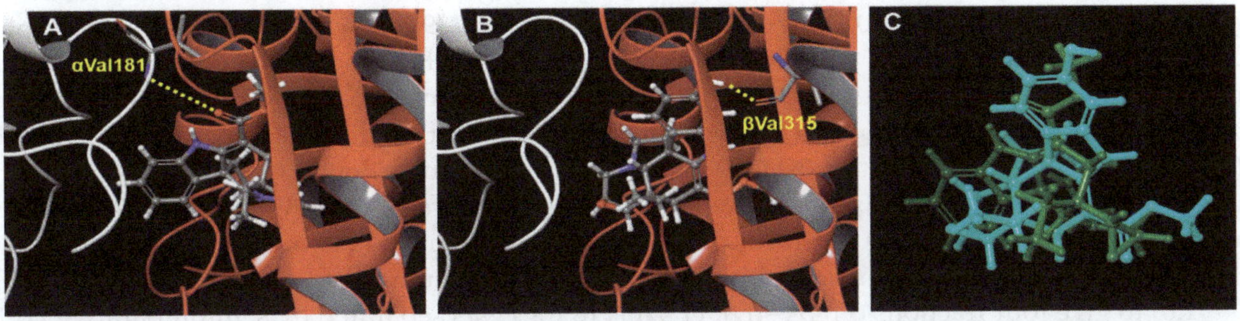

Figure 4. Predicted docking models for **5** and **7** binding in the CS. The crystal structures (PDB: 1SA0) of α- (white) and β-tubulin (red) are shown as ribbon diagrams. The distances calculated to be less than 5 Å between heavy atoms are represented by dashed lines. Docking models of compounds (gray skeleton with oxygen in red and nitrogen in blue) **5** (**A**) and **7** (**B**) in the CS are shown. Superimposition of docked compound **5** or **7** shows H-bonds with the side chain of αVal181 or βVal315, respectively. (**C**) Comparison of docking mode of **5** (green) with that of **7** (blue) in CS.

3. Materials and Methods

3.1. General Experimental Procedures

All chemicals and solvents were used as purchased. ESIMS data were obtained on a Finnigan MAT 90 spectrometer. NMR spectra were recorded on Bruker DRX-500 and Avance III -600 NMR spectrometers using TMS as an internal standard. All chemical shifts are reported in ppm, and apparent scalar coupling constants *J* are given in Hertz. Silica gel (300–400 mesh, Qingdao Marine Chemical Inc., Shandong, China), silica gel H (10–40 µm, Qingdao Marine Chemical Inc.), Lichroprep RP-18 gel (40–63 µm, Merck, Darmstadt, Germany), and Sephadex LH-20 (40–70 µm, Amersham Biosciences, Waltham, MA, USA) were used for column chromatography (CC). All target compounds were characterized and determined to be at least >95% pure by ^{1}H NMR and analytical HPLC.

3.2. Plant Material

The twigs and leaves of *B. mekongensis* were collected during April 2010 from Mengla County, Yunnan Province, PR China and identified by Mr. Jing-Yun Cui, Xishuangbanna Tropical Plant Garden. A voucher specimen (No. CUI20100419) has been deposited at the State Key Laboratory of Phytochemistry and Plant Resources in West China, Kunming Institute of Botany, Chinese Academy of Science (CAS).

3.3. Extraction and Isolation

The dried twigs and leaves of *B. mekongensis* (12 kg) were extracted with CH_3OH, the crude extract was dissolved in aqueous solution, and then the pH was adjusted to 2 by adding saturated tartaric acid with adequate stirring. The acidic mixture was defatted with petroleum ether (PE) and then extracted with $CHCl_3$. The aqueous phase was basified to pH~10 with saturated Na_2CO_3 and then extracted with $CHCl_3$ to obtain crude alkaloids. The crude alkaloids (60 g) were separated on a silica gel column (200–300 mesh; $CHCl_3/CH_3OH$, 1:0 $\rightarrow$ 0:1), yielding five major fractions (Fr 1–5). Fraction 1 (12.8 g) was chromatographed with a series of silica gel columns ($CHCl_3$/acetone and $CHCl_3/CH_3OH$) to afford compounds **3** (21 mg) and **4** (16 mg). Fraction 2 (11.2 g) was further chromatographed on a reversed-phase C_{18} silica gel medium-pressure column (CH_3OH/H_2O, 1:1 $\rightarrow$ 1:0) to give four fractions (Fr 2A–2D). Fraction 2C (3.2 g) was separated on a silica gel column (300–400 mesh; PE/acetone, 3:1), yielding three fractions (Fr 2C1–2C3). Compound **1** (16 mg) was separated from fraction 2C2 (760 mg) by semipreparative HPLC using a Waters XBridge C_{18} (10 $\times$ 250 mm, 5 μm) column with 70% CH_3CN/H_2O with added 0.1 *v*/*v* diethylamine. Compound **11** (36 mg) was obtained from fraction 2C3 (368 mg) by semipreparative HPLC using a Waters XBridge C_{18} (10 $\times$ 250 mm, 5 μm) column with 70% CH_3OH/H_2O with added 0.1 *v*/*v* diethylamine. Fraction 3 (9.8 g) was further chromatographed over a reversed-phase C_{18} silica gel medium-pressure column (CH_3OH/H_2O, 1:1 $\rightarrow$ 1:0) to give four fractions (Fr 3A–3D). Fraction 3A (480 mg) was separated by semipreparative HPLC using a Waters XBridge C_{18} (10 $\times$ 250 mm, 5 μm) column with 45% CH_3OH/H_2O to give compounds **5** (21 mg), **10** (4.0 mg) and **12** (28 mg). Fraction 3C (780 mg) was purified using a Sephadex LH-20 column eluted with CH_3OH, followed by semipreparative HPLC using a Waters XBridge C_{18} (19 $\times$ 250 mm, 5 μm) column with 70% CH_3OH/H_2O to afford compounds **8** (22 mg) and **14** (48 mg). Fraction 4 (9.8 g) was further chromatographed over a reversed-phase C_{18} silica gel medium-pressure column (CH_3OH/H_2O, 1:1 $\rightarrow$ 1:0) to give four fractions (Fr 4A–4D). Fr 4A (518 mg) was separated by semipreparative HPLC using a Waters XBridge C_{18} (10 $\times$ 250 mm, 5 μm) column with 40% CH_3OH/H_2O to afford compounds **2** (9 mg), **6** (28 mg), **7** (20 mg), and **9** (12 mg). Fr 4B (300 mg) was further purified using a Sephadex LH-20 column eluted with CH_3OH to afford **13** (35 mg).

3.4. Antiproliferative Activity Assay

Antiproliferative activity was determined by the sulforhodamine B (SRB) colorimetric assay as previously described [26]. In brief, human tumor cell lines were cultured in RPMI-1640 medium containing 2 mM l-glutamine and 25 mM HEPES (Gibco), supplemented with 10% fetal bovine serum (Speciality Media), 100 μg/mL streptomycin, 100 IU/mL penicillin, and 0.25 μg/mL amphotericin B (Corning). MDR stock cells (KB-VIN) were maintained in the presence of 100 nM vincristine (VIN) (Sigma-Aldrich, Saint Louis, MI, USA).

Freshly trypsinized cell suspensions were seeded in 96-well microtiter plates at densities of 4000–11,000 cells per well (based on the cell lines) with compounds. After 72 h in culture with test compounds, cells were fixed in 10% trichloroacetic acid followed by staining with 0.04% sulforhodamine B (Sigma-Aldrich). The bound SRB was solubilized in 10 mM Tris-base and the absorbance at 515 nm was measured using a Microplate Reader (ELx800, Bio-Tek Instruments, Winooski, VT, USA) operated by Gen5 software (BioTek) after solubilizing the protein-bound dye with 10 mM Tris base. The mean IC_{50} is the concentration of agent that reduced cell growth by 50% compared with vehicle (DMSO) control under the experimental conditions and is the average from at least three independent experiments with duplicate samples.

The following human tumor cell lines were used in the assay: A549 (lung carcinoma), MDA-MB-231 (triplen-egative breast cancer), KB (originally isolated from epidermoid carcinoma of the nasopharynx), KB-VIN (VIN-resistant KB subline showing MDR phenotype by overexpressing P-gp), MCF-7 (estrogen receptor (ER)-positive, HER2-negative breast cancer). It should be noted that we confirmed the KB and KB-VIN cell lines were identical to AV-3 (ATCC number, CCL-21) as a HeLa (cervical carcinoma) contaminant by short tandem repeat (STR) profiling. All cell lines were obtained from the Lineberger Comprehensive Cancer Center (UNC-CH) or from ATCC (Manassas, VA), except KB-VIN, which was a generous gift from Professor Y.-C. Cheng (Yale University). Paclitaxel was purchased from Sigma-Aldrich.

3.5. Tubulin Assays

Inhibitory effects of compounds on tubulin assembly were evaluated using electrophoretically homogeneous bovine brain tubulin as described previously [27,28] using 1.0 mg/mL (10 μM) tubulin. The turbidity development as tubulin assembly was initiated by adding 0.4 mM GTP and followed for 20 min at 30 °C following a rapid temperature jump. Compound concentrations as EC_{50} values that inhibited the increase in turbidity by 50% relative to a control sample were determined. In colchicine inhibition assays, tubulin (1.0 μM) was incubated with 5.0 μM [^{3}H] colchicine and 5.0 μM test compound at 37 °C for 10 min, when about 40–60% of maximum colchicine binding occurs in control samples.

3.6. Cell Cycle Analysis

KB-VIN cells were seeded in 12-well plates at a density of 1×10^5 per well and incubated overnight. After 24 h of treatment with tested compounds at a concentration of one- or three-fold IC_{50}, the cells were harvested and fixed in 70% EtOH at −20 °C overnight followed by staining with propidium iodide (PI) containing RNase (BD Pharmingen, Franklin Lakes, NJ, USA) for 30 min at 37 °C. The DNA contents of stained cells were analyzed by flow cytometer (LSRFortessa, BD Biosciences) controlled by FACSDiva software (BD Biosciences). Paclitaxel (PXL) was used at 3 or 6 μM. Combretastatin A-4 (CA-4) was purchased from Sigma-Aldrich and used at 0.2 μM. Experiments were repeated a minimum of two times.

3.7. Immunofluorescence Staining

Immunocytochemical analysis was performed as previously described [26]. KB-VIN cells were grown on an 8-well chamber slide (Lab-Tech) for 24 h prior to treatment with the compound at a concentration of three-fold IC_{50}. CA-4 was used at 0.2 μM (Figure 2A and Supporting Information, Supplementary Figure S1). After treatment of cells with the agent for 24 h, cells were fixed with 4% paraformaldehyde in PBS and permeabilized with 0.5% Triton X-100 in PBS. Fixed cells were labeled with mouse monoclonal antibody to α-tubulin (B5-1-2, Sigma) and rabbit IgG to Ser10-phosphorylated histone H3 (p-H3) (#06570, EMD Millipore), followed by FITC-conjugated antibody to mouse IgG (Sigma) and Alexa Fluor 549-conjugated antibody to rabbit IgG (Life Technologies). Nuclei were labeled with DAPI (Sigma). Fluorescently-labeled cells were observed using a confocal microscope (Zeiss, LSM700) with ZEN (black edition) software (Zeiss). The 15~20 optical sections acquired at 0.5~1 μm intervals were stacked and reconstructed using ZEN (black edition) software. Experiments were repeated at least twice for each compound. Final images were prepared using Adobe Photoshop CS3.

3.8. Computer Modeling

GOLD 5.1 software with default settings was used to predict the three-dimensional (3D) structures of tubulin-ligand complexes [29]. The human tubulin 3D structure (TUBA1A and TUBB2B) used in this study was built from a Protein Data Bank entry (PDB ID: 1SA0) [30]. Absent hydrogen atoms in the crystal structure were added computationally by Hermes software 5.1 version. The active site radius was set to 10.0 Å, and the active site center was defined as the ligand center in 1SA0. The docking calculations used the quantum chemically-optimized ligand structures as the initial structures. Structural optimizations of ligands were performed with B3LYP/6-311+G (df, p) using Gaussian 09, Revision B.01 [31].

4. Conclusions

Fourteen aspidosperma-type monoterpenoid indole alkaloids (**1–14**) were isolated from a methanol extract of the twigs and leaves of *Bousigonia mekongensis*. All isolates were evaluated for antiproliferative activity against five human tumor cell lines, including the MDR subline KB-VIN. Alkaloids **3**, **4**, **6**, **7**, and **13** showed significant antiproliferative effects against all five tumor cell lines. Because activity was retained against KB-VIN, the active alkaloids are not P-gp substrates and, thus, could be effective against tumors expressing the MDR phenotype. SAR studies suggested that the presence of a 14,15-double bond or 3α-acetonyl group is critical for antiproliferative activity. Furthermore, mechanistic studies revealed for the first time that the five active alkaloids cause significant arrest of the cell cycle progression at the G2/M cell cycle phase via inhibition of tubulin polymerization. In addition, the compounds interact with tubulin in a manner distinct from that of CA-4.

Author Contributions: Conceptualization, Y.Z. and M.G.; Methodology, M.G., P.-L.H. and E.H.; Software, A.O.; Formal Analysis, Y.Z. and M.G.; Resources, Y.-H.F. and L.-L.G.; Data Curation, Y.Z. and M.G.; Writing—Original Draft Preparation, Y.Z.; Writing—Review & Editing, M.G., S.L.M.-N. and K.-H.L.; Supervision, K.-H.L. and X.-J.H.; Project Administration, Y.Z. and X.-J.H.; Funding Acquisition, Y.Z.

Acknowledgments: We wish to thank the Microscopy Service Laboratory (UNC-CH) for its expertise in the confocal microscopy studies.

Disclaimer: The content of this paper is solely the responsibility of the authors and does not necessarily reflect the official views of the National Institutes of Health.

References

1. Dumontet, C.; Jordan, M.A. Microtubule-binding agents: A dynamic field of cancer therapeutics. *Nat. Rev. Drug Discov.* **2010**, *9*, 790–803. [CrossRef]
2. Perez, E.A. Microtubule inhibitors: Differentiating tubulin-inhibiting agents based on mechanisms of action, clinical activity, and resistance. *Mol. Cancer Ther.* **2009**, *8*, 2086–2095. [CrossRef]
3. Szakács, G.; Hall, M.D.; Gottesman, M.M.; Boumendjel, A.; Kachadourian, R.; Day, B.J.; Baubichon-Cortay, H.; Pietro, A.D. Targeting the Achilles heel of multidrug-resistant cancer by exploiting the fitness cost of resistance. *Chem. Rev.* **2014**, *114*, 5753–5774. [CrossRef]
4. Eckford, P.D.; Sharom, F.J. ABC efflux pump-based resistance to chemotherapy drugs. *Chem. Rev.* **2009**, *109*, 2989–3011. [CrossRef] [PubMed]
5. Kavellaris, M. Microtubules and resistance to tubulin-binding agents. *Nat. Rev. Cancer* **2010**, *10*, 194–204. [CrossRef] [PubMed]
6. Dewick, P.M. Alkaloids. In *Medicinal Natural Products: A Biosynthetic Approach*, 3rd ed.; John Wiley & Sons Ltd.: Chichester, UK, 2009; pp. 369–380. ISBN 978-0-470-74168-9.
7. Martino, E.; Casamassima, G.; Castiglione, S.; Cellupica, E.; Pantalone, S.; Papagni, F.; Rui, M.; Siciliano, A.M.; Collina, S. Vinca alkaloids and analogues as anti-cancer agents: Looking back, peering ahead. *Bioorg. Med. Chem. Lett.* **2018**, *28*, 2816–2826. [CrossRef] [PubMed]
8. Lim, K.H.; Hiraku, O.; Komiyama, K.; Kam, T.S. Jerantinines A–G, cytotoxic Aspidosperma alkaloids from *Tabernaemontana corymbosa*. *J. Nat. Prod.* **2008**, *71*, 1591–1594. [CrossRef] [PubMed]
9. Frei, R.; Staedler, D.; Raja, A.; Franke, R.; Sasse, F.; Gerber-Lemaire, S.; Waser, J. Total synthesis and biological evaluation of Jerantinine E. *Angew. Chem. Int. Ed.* **2013**, *52*, 13373–13376. [CrossRef]
10. Raja, V.J.; Lim, K.H.; Leong, C.O.; Kam, T.S.; Bradshaw, T.D. Novel antitumor indole alkaloid, Jerantinine A, evokes potent G2/M cell cycle arrest targeting microtubules. *Invest New Drugs* **2014**, *32*, 838–850. [CrossRef] [PubMed]
11. Qazzaz, M.E.; Raja, V.J.; Lim, K.H.; Kam, T.S.; Lee, J.B.; Gershkovich, P.; Bradshaw, T.D. In vitro anticancer properties and biological evaluation of novel natural alkaloid jerantinine B. *Cancer Lett.* **2016**, *370*, 185–197. [CrossRef] [PubMed]
12. Li, B.T.; Leeuwenberg, J.M.; Middleton, D.J. *Flora of China*; Science Press: Beijing, China, 1995; Volume 16, p. 150.
13. Fu, Y.H.; He, H.P.; Di, Y.T.; Li, S.L.; Zhang, Y.; Hao, X.J. Mekongenines A and B, two new alkaloids from *Bousigonia mekongensis*. *Tetrahedron Lett.* **2012**, *53*, 3642–3646. [CrossRef]

14. Fu, Y.H.; Di, Y.T.; He, H.P.; Li, S.L.; Zhang, Y.; Hao, X.J. Angustifonines A and B, cytotoxic bisindole alkaloids from *Bousigonia angustifolia*. *J. Nat. Prod.* **2014**, *77*, 56–62. [CrossRef]
15. Fu, Y.H.; Li, S.L.; Li, S.F.; He, H.P.; Di, Y.T.; Zhang, Y.; Hao, X.J. Cytotoxic eburnamine-aspidospermine type bisindole alkaloids from *Bousigonia mekongensis*. *Fitoterapia* **2014**, *98*, 45–52. [CrossRef]
16. Baassou, S.; Mehri, H.; Plat, M. Plants of New Caledonia. Part 49. Alkaloids of *Melodinus aeneus*. *Phytochemistry* **1978**, *17*, 1449–1450. [CrossRef]
17. Fahn, W.; Kaiser, V.; Schübel, H.; Stöckigt, J.; Danieli, B. *Catharanthus roseus* enzyme mediated synthesis of 3-hydroxyvoafrine A and B—A simple route to the voafrines. *Phytochemistry* **1990**, *29*, 129–133. [CrossRef]
18. Liu, Y.P.; Li, Y.; Cai, X.H.; Li, X.Y.; Kong, L.M.; Cheng, G.G.; Luo, X.D. Melodinines M-U, cytotoxic alkaloids from *Melodinus suaveolens*. *J. Nat. Prod.* **2012**, *75*, 220–224. [CrossRef]
19. Nair, C.P.N.; Pillay, P.P. Lochnericine. A new alkaloid from *Lochnera rosea*. *Tetrahedron* **1959**, *6*, 89–93. [CrossRef]
20. Guo, L.W.; Zhou, Y.L. Alkaloids from *Melodinus hemsleyanus*. *Phytochemistry* **1993**, *34*, 563–566. [CrossRef]
21. Men-Olivier, L.L.; Richard, B.; Men, J.L. Alcaloïdes des grains du *Pandaca retusa*. *Phytochemistry* **1993**, *34*, 563–566.
22. Feng, T.; Li, Y.; Cai, X.H.; Gong, X.; Liu, Y.P.; Zhang, R.T.; Zhang, X.Y.; Tan, Q.G.; Luo, X.D. Monoterpenoid indole alkaloids from *Alstonia yunnanensis*. *J. Nat. Prod.* **2009**, *72*, 1836–1841. [CrossRef]
23. Langlois, N.; Andriamialisoa, R.Z. Studies on vindolinine. 6. Partial synthesis of aspidospermane-type alkaloids. *J. Org. Chem.* **1979**, *44*, 2468–2471. [CrossRef]
24. Kutney J., P.; Choi, L.S.L.; Kolodziejczyk, P.; Sleigh, S.K.; Stuart, K.L.; Worth, B.R.; Kurz, W.G.W.; Chatson, K.B.; Constabel, F. Alkaloid production in *Catharanthus roseus* cell cultures: Isolation and characterization of alkaloids from one cell line. *Phytochemistry* **1980**, *19*, 2589–2595. [CrossRef]
25. Smedley, C.J.; Stanley, P.A.; Qazzaz, M.E.; Prota, A.E.; Olieric, N.; Collins, H.; Eastman, H.; Barrow, A.S.; Lim, K.H.; Kam, T.S.; et al. Sustainable syntheses of (-)-jerantinines A & E and structural characterisation of the jerantinine-tubulin complex at the colchicine binding Site. *Sci. Rep.* **2018**, *8*, 10617. [PubMed]
26. Nakagawa-Goto, K.; Oda, A.; Hamel, E.; Ohkoshi, E.; Lee, K.H.; Goto, M. Development of a novel class of tubulin inhibitor from desmosdumotin B with a hydroxylated bicyclic B-ring. *J. Med. Chem.* **2015**, *58*, 2378–2389. [CrossRef]
27. Hamel, E. Evaluation of antimitotic agents by quantitative comparisons of their effects on the polymerization of purified tubulin. *Cell Biochem. Biophys.* **2003**, *38*, 1–22. [CrossRef]
28. Verdier-Pinard, P.; Lai, J.Y.; Yoo, H.D.; Yu, J.; Marquez, B.; Nagle, D.G.; Nambu, M.; White, J.D.; Falck, J.R.; Gerwick, W.H.; et al. Structure−activity analysis of the interaction of curacin A, the potent colchicine site antimitotic agent, with tubulin and effects of analogs on the growth of MCF-7 breast cancer cells. *Mol. Pharmacol.* **1998**, *53*, 62–76. [CrossRef] [PubMed]
29. Jones, G.; Willett, P.; Glen, R.C. Molecular recognition of receptor sites using a genetic algorithm with a description of desolvation. *J. Mol. Biol.* **1995**, *245*, 43–53. [CrossRef]
30. Ravelli, R.B.; Gigant, B.; Curmi, P.A.; Jourdain, I.; Lachkar, S.; Sobel, A.; Knossow, M. Insight into tubulin regulation from a complex with colchicine and a stathmin-like domain. *Nature* **2004**, *428*, 198–202. [CrossRef]
31. Frisch, M.J.; Trucks, G.W.; Schlegel, H.B.; Scuseria, G.E.; Robb, M.A.; Cheeseman, J.R.; Scalmani, G.; Barone, V.; Mennucci, B.; Petersson, G.A.; et al. *Gaussian 09 (Revision B.01)*; Gaussian, Inc.: Wallingford, CT, USA, 2010.

5

Caffeic Acid Attenuates Multi-Drug Resistance in Cancer Cells by Inhibiting Efflux Function of Human P-Glycoprotein

Yu-Ning Teng [1], Charles C.N. Wang [2], Wei-Chieh Liao [3], Yu-Hsuan Lan [3,*] and Chin-Chuan Hung [3,4,*]

1 Department of Medicine, College of Medicine, I-Shou University, 8 Yida Road, Kaohsiung 82445, Taiwan; eunicegh520@gmail.com
2 Department of Bioinformatics and Medical Engineering, Asia University, 500 Lioufeng Rd., Wufeng, Taichung 41354, Taiwan; chaoneng.wang@gmail.com
3 Department of Pharmacy, College of Pharmacy, China Medical University, 91 Hsueh-Shih Road, Taichung 40402, Taiwan; u102003316@cmu.edu.tw
4 Department of Pharmacy, China Medical University Hospital, 2 Yude Road, Taichung 40447, Taiwan
* Correspondence: lanyh@mail.cmu.edu.tw (Y.-H.L.); cc0206hung@gmail.com (C.-C.H.)

Academic Editor: Kyoko Nakagawa-Goto

Abstract: Multidrug resistance (MDR) is a complicated ever-changing problem in cancer treatment, and P-glycoprotein (P-gp), a drug efflux pump, is regarded as the major cause. In the way of developing P-gp inhibitors, natural products such as phenolic acids have gotten a lot of attention recently. The aim of the present study was to investigate the modulating effects and mechanisms of caffeic acid on human P-gp, as well as the attenuating ability on cancer MDR. Calcein-AM, rhodamine123, and doxorubicin were used to analyze the interaction between caffeic acid and P-gp, and the ATPase activity of P-gp was evaluated as well. Resistance reversing effects were revealed by SRB and cell cycle assay. The results indicated that caffeic acid uncompetitively inhibited rhodamine123 efflux and competitively inhibited doxorubicin efflux. In terms of P-gp ATPase activity, caffeic acid exhibited stimulation in both basal and verapamil-stimulated activity. The combination of chemo drugs and caffeic acid resulted in decreased IC_{50} in *ABCB1*/Flp-In^{TM}-293 and KB/VIN, indicating that the resistance was reversed. Results of molecular docking suggested that caffeic acid bound to P-gp through GLU74 and TRY117 residues. The present study demonstrated that caffeic acid is a promising candidate for P-gp inhibition and cancer MDR attenuation.

Keywords: caffeic acid; cancer multidrug resistance; P-glycoprotein; phenolic acid

1. Introduction

As cancer is one of the leading causes of death worldwide, cancer treatment is always on the top of listed hot research topics [1]. With advanced scientific researches and abundant medical resources in recent decades, diverse options have been developed to conquer cancer and related diseases. Nevertheless, the multi-drug resistance (MDR) of cancer treatment is still an ever-changing problem and more in-depth studies have been conducted to unveil the complicated characteristics of cancer treatment. Cancer MDR manifests cross resistance to several structurally and mechanically different chemo-agents and could be contributed to the following reasons [2]. The change in tumor microenvironment [3–5], decreased drug uptake [6], adapted cell apoptotic pathways [7–9], drug inactivation through metabolism [10,11], the influence of epigenetic regulation [12,13], mutation of drug target site [14], and the increased drug efflux [15] have been reported to play important roles in causing cancer MDR. Among the above mechanisms, the increased drug efflux by ATP-binding cassette (ABC) transporters has been regarded as the most influential cause. ABC transporter superfamily consists of several subfamilies, and P-glycoprotein (P-gp) is one of the most comprehensively studied proteins [16]. P-gp is encoded by human *ABCB1* gene and can recognize various clinically used drugs, including antidepressants, HIV protease inhibitors, immunosuppressive agents, and chemotherapeutic drugs [17,18]. The diverse structures recognizing and effluxing the ability of P-gp, result in insufficient chemo-drug concentration inside cancer cells, therefore, causing cancer MDR.

There have been a series of P-gp inhibitor developments along the cancer MDR reversing agents discovering history, and the improvements have been based on previous failure experiences [19]. First generation P-gp inhibitors are potent but toxic as the required dose is high; examples of this are quinidine and verapamil [20]. Second generation inhibitors have exhibited better effects with lower IC_{50}, but the involvement of these inhibitors in CYP450 interaction has impeded their further application [21,22]. Third generation inhibitors, including tariquidar and zosuquidar, have demonstrated prominent MDR reversal effects. However, they have still faced failure in clinical studies [23,24]. Therefore, severe toxicity and interaction of the above chemical reagents have turned the research direction toward natural resources, aiming at discovering low toxic and potent structures from plants, fungi, or marine organisms.

Among various natural resources, phytochemicals such as flavonoids and phenolic acids get much attention due to their multiple pharmacological effects, including antioxidant and antitumor activity [25,26]. Several phytochemicals, such as cyanidin, catechin, quercetin, caffeic acid, and ellagic acid, have been related to the down-regulation of human LDL oxidation [27]. Ellagic acid and ursolic acid have been reported to exhibit preventive and therapeutic effects against breast cancer cells [28]. Caffeic acid (Figure 1), a phenolic acid that widely exists in vegetables, fruits, and tea extracts, is well-known as a natural antioxidant [29]. Besides, caffeic acid has also been identified to have anti-inflammatory, antibacterial, and antiviral effects [30,31]. With regards to cancer treatment, caffeic acid and its derivative, caffeic acid phenethyl ester (CAPE), exhibit some therapeutic effects toward lung cancer and breast cancer cells, as well as breast cancer pre-clinical models [32–34]. CAPE has been well studied in previous researches, including its *MDR1* gene down-regulating effects in MCF-7 and MDA-MB-231 breast cancer cells [34] and P-gp inhibitory effects in HeLa resistant cancer subline and human intestinal LS174T cell line [35,36]. Nevertheless, the P-gp inhibitory and MDR modulating information of the caffeic acid was insufficient and warrants further detailed investigation.

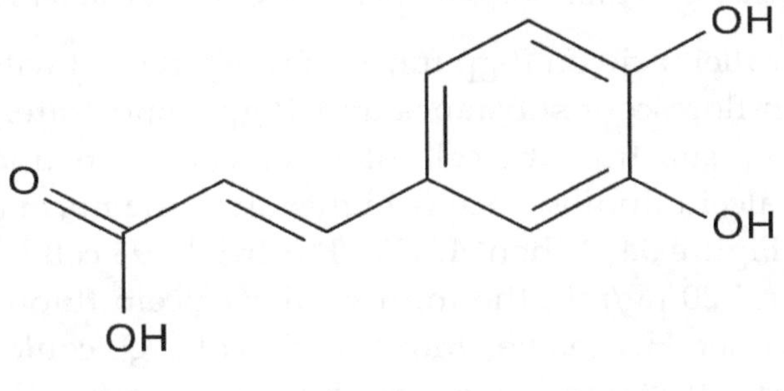

Figure 1. The chemical structure of caffeic acid.

Therefore, in the present study, comprehensive researches of caffeic acid were conducted. The interaction of caffeic acid with human P-gp, as well as the inhibitory effects and mechanisms were assessed in P-gp over-expressing cell line *ABCB1*/Flp-In^{TM}-293. The cancer MDR reversing ability of caffeic acid was then evaluated in both *ABCB1*/Flp-In^{TM}-293 and KB/VIN MDR cancer cell lines. The present study demonstrated that caffeic acid is a promising candidate for P-gp inhibition and cancer MDR attenuation.

2. Results

2.1. Caffeic Acid Is Non-Cytotoxic toward Experimental Cell Lines and Is Not a Substrate of P-gp

Before conducting further experiments, the cytotoxicity of caffeic acid was examined in HeLaS3, KB/VIN, Flp-In^{TM}-293, and *ABCB1*/Flp-In^{TM}-293 cell lines to select a rational concentration range. Caffeic acid exhibited higher than 80% cell viability in all tested cell lines under the treatment of 100 μg/mL for 72 h. Hence, the following assays were conducted with caffeic acid of not more than 100 μg/mL.

The first characteristic of caffeic acid on P-gp was demonstrated through MDR1 shift assay, which revealed whether a compound is a substrate of P-gp. P-gp's substrates activate a conformational change detected by the structure-sensitive UIC2 antibody. As Figure 2 showed, the fluorescent peaks of caffeic acid 20 and 25 μg/mL did not shift to the right as the positive control vinblastine did, indicating that the conformation of P-gp was not influenced by caffeic acid. Therefore, caffeic acid is not P-gp's substrate.

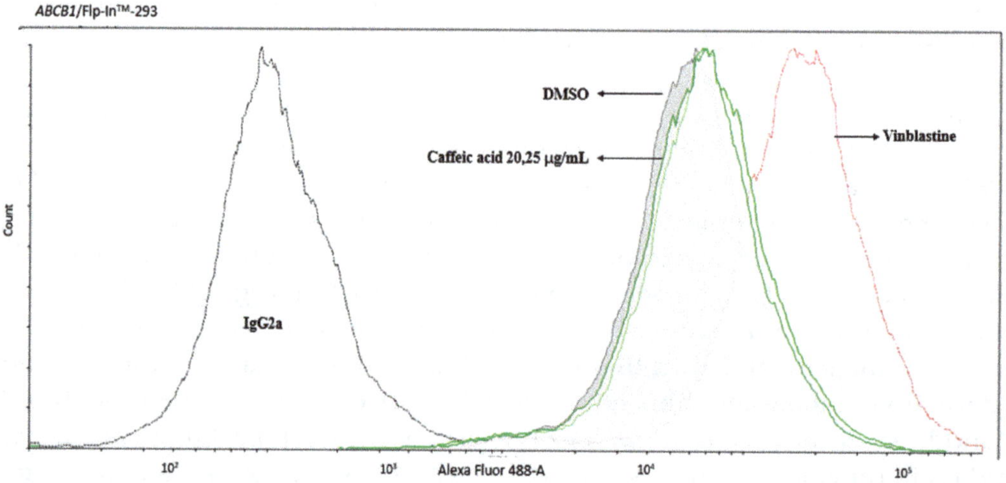

Figure 2. The result of MDR1 shift assay. The conformation of P-gp was not influenced under the treatment of 20 and 25 μg/mL caffeic acid. Vinblastine (a standard substrate of P-gp) was used as a positive control.

2.2. The Inhibitory Effects, Mechanisms and Binding Modes of Caffeic Acid on Human P-gp Function

The inhibitory effect of caffeic acid on P-gp function was screened with calcein-AM accumulation assay. Calcein-AM is a non-florescent substance and P-gp's substrate. It will be transformed to fluorescent calcein (not a P-gp substrate) by cell esterase. Therefore, under the treatment of P-gp's inhibitor, the intracellular calcein fluorescence is higher than the normal condition. The results of caffeic acid are revealed in Figure 3a. When *ABCB1*/Flp-In^{TM}-293 cell line was treated with caffeic acid in amounts of 5, 10, and 20 μg/mL, the intracellular calcein fluorescence was increased in a concentration-dependent manner. Hence, the efflux function of P-gp could be inhibited by caffeic acid.

Caffeic acid's inhibitory effects and mechanisms were further demonstrated via the other two substrates of P-gp, rhodamine123 and doxorubicin. As Figure 3b showed, the efflux of fluorescent substrate rhodamine123 was inhibited by caffeic acid 10 and 20 μg/mL treatment and followed Michaelis-Menten kinetics. The Lineweaver-Burk plot (Figure 3c) indicated that caffeic acid inhibited rhodamine123 efflux in an uncompetitive pattern, both V_{max} and K_m decreased when the *ABCB1*/Flp-In^{TM}-293 cell line was treated with increased caffeic acid concentrations (Table 1). Same as rhodamine123, the efflux of the chemotherapeutic drug doxorubicin was also inhibited by caffeic acid dose-dependently (Figure 3d). However, the inhibitory mechanism of caffeic acid on doxorubicin was competitive inhibition, different from rodamine123 (Figure 3e). When the *ABCB1*/Flp-In^{TM}-293 cell line was treated with an increased concentration of caffeic acid, the K_m (affinity) increased accordingly and the V_{max} remained constant (Table 1).

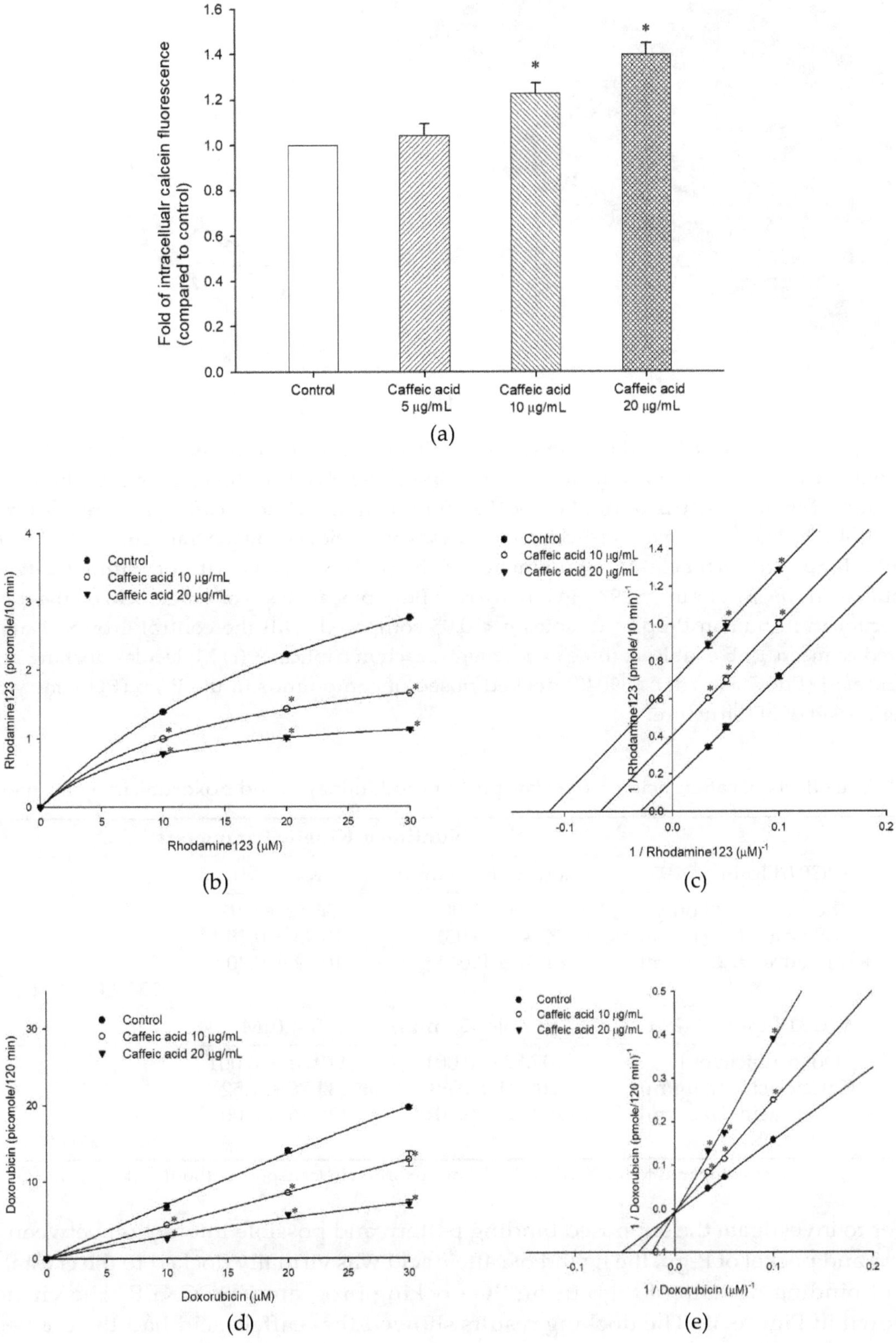

Figure 3. *Cont.*

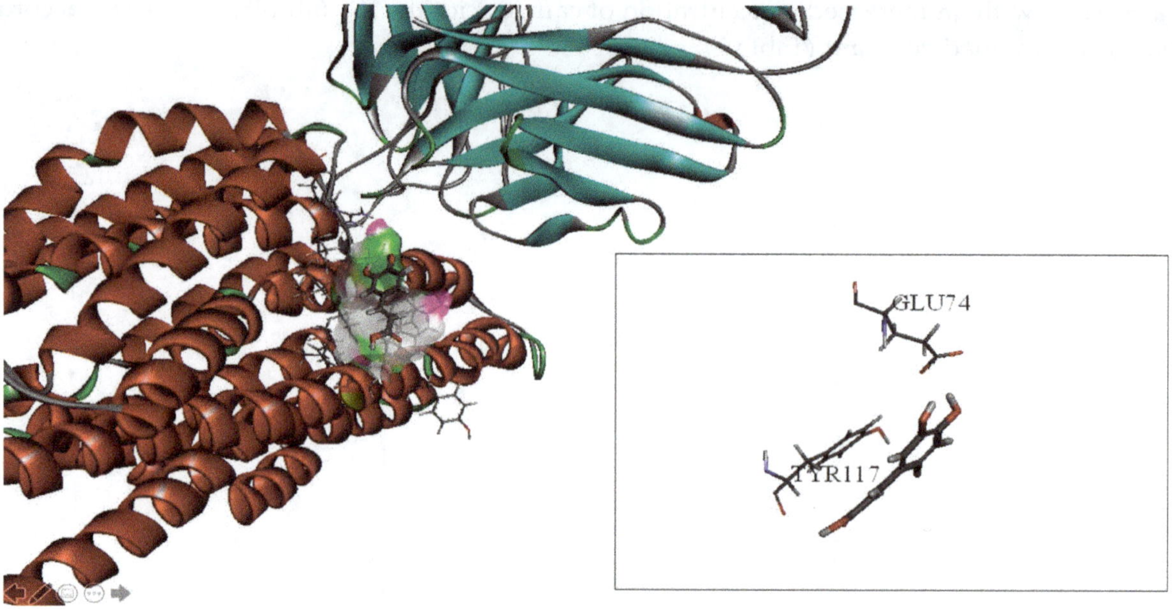

(f)

Figure 3. The effects of caffeic acid on human P-gp efflux function. (**a**) Intracellular calcein fluorescence with or without caffeic acid pretreatment in *ABCB1*/Flp-In^{TM}-293 cell line (over-expressing human P-gp). (**b**) Michaelis-Menten kinetics of rhodamine123 efflux with or without caffeic acid pretreatment in *ABCB1*/Flp-In^{TM}-293. (**c**) Lineweaver-Burk plot analyses of caffeic acid on the transport of rhodamine123 in human P-gp. (**d**) Michaelis-Menten kinetics of doxorubicin efflux with or without caffeic acid pretreatment in *ABCB1*/Flp-In^{TM}-293. (**e**) Lineweaver-Burk plot analyses of caffeic acid on the transport of doxorubicin in human P-gp. * denotes $p < 0.05$ compared with the control group. Data were presented as mean ± SE of at least three experiments, each in triplicate. (**f**) Molecular docking analysis of caffeic acid (PubChem CID: 689043) docked posed of compounds in the P-gp (PDB entry 6QEX) binding pocket of 3D structure.

Table 1. The effects of caffeic acid on the transport of rhodamine123 and doxorubicin by human P-gp.

	Nonlinear Kinetic Parameters		
ABCB1/Flp-In^{TM}-293	V_m (pmole/10 min)	K_m (μM)	
Rhodamine123 only	9.04 ± 1.00	56.52 ± 6.97	
+ Caffeic acid, 10 μg/mL	2.47 ± 0.03*	15.93 ± 0.18 *	
+ Caffeic acid, 20 μg/mL	1.57 ± 0.04 *	10.72 ± 0.30 *	
K_i			253.44 ± 2.64
ABCB1/Flp-In^{TM}-293	V_m (pmole/120 min)	K_m (μM)	
Doxorubicin only	107.52 ± 0.001	179.81 ± 0.001	
+ Caffeic acid, 10 μg/mL	108.31 ± 0.68	234.76 ± 1.52 *	
+ Caffeic acid, 20 μg/mL	107.52 ± 0.001	426.16 ± 0.00 *	
K_i			14.13 ± 0.005

* $p < 0.05$ as compared to the rhodamine123 or doxorubicin transport without caffeic acid.

In order to investigate the supposed binding pattern and possible interaction between the ligand of caffeic acid and pocket of P-gp, the ligand of caffeic acid was virtually docked to the crystal structures of the ligand-binding domain of P-gp using the docking program CDOCKER. The virtual binding result is shown in Figure 3f. The docking results showed that caffeic acid had the the best binding energies active site of P-gp with a -CDOCKER energy score of 20.1292, and binding energy was 44.4058 Kcal/mol. The binding model clearly indicated that the caffeic acid bound to P-gp with residues GLU74 and TRY117. Our docking results further demonstrated the binding behavior between P-gp and caffeic acid, providing insight into the design of novel P-gp modulators.

The interaction between caffeic acid and ATP binding site of P-gp was carried out with Pgp-Glo™ Assay System. As Figure 4a shows, when the P-gp membrane was treated with caffeic acid with amounts of 1, 10, and 50 μg/mL, the basal P-gp ATPase activity was inhibited. On the other hand, the ATPase activity was stimulated under the treatment of 100 μg/mL caffeic acid. Besides, when combining caffeic acid with 200 μM verapamil, the elevated ATPase activity produced by verapamil was further stimulated and especially high under 100 μg/mL concentration (Figure 4b).

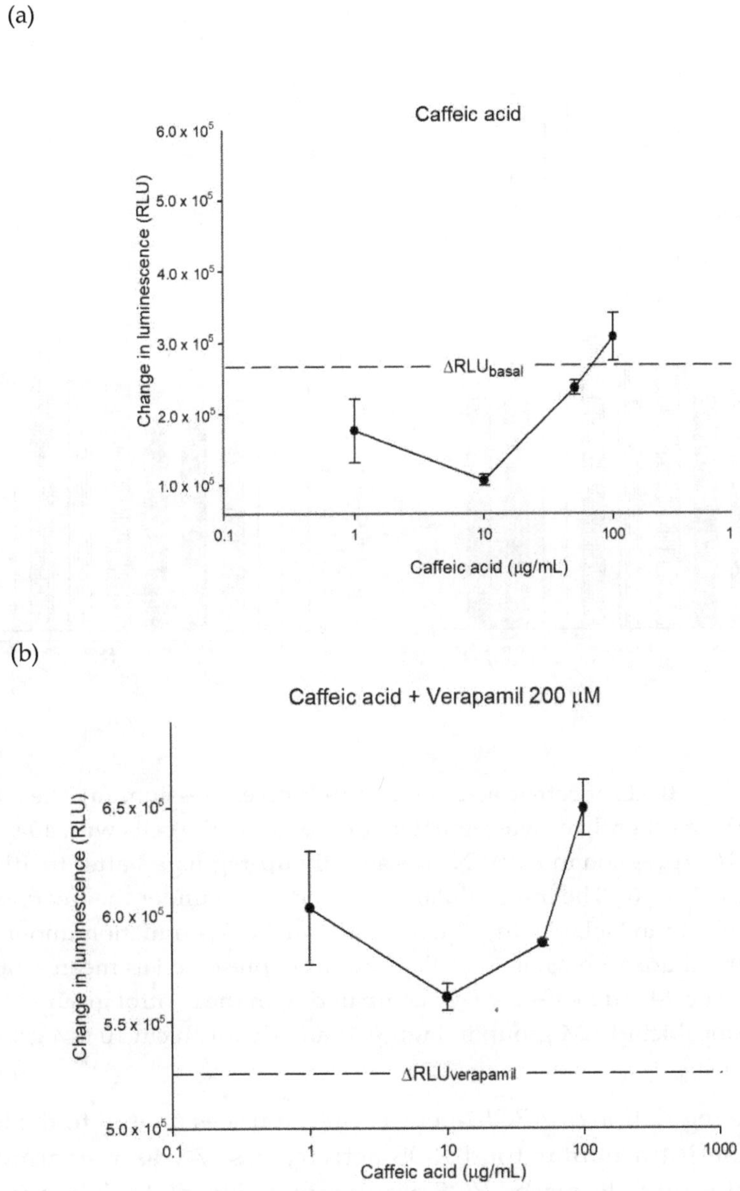

Figure 4. The P-gp ATPase modulating effects of caffeic acid. (**a**) Caffeic acid stimulated ATPase activity dose-dependently (10–100 μg/mL). (**b**) The verapamil-stimulated ATPase activity was further stimulated by caffeic acid. Data were analyzed in terms of the change of luminescence (ΔRLU). Data were presented as mean ± SE of at least three experiments, each in triplicate.

2.3. The Influences of Caffeic Acid on Human P-gp Expression

The modulatory ability of caffeic acid on *ABCB1* gene expression was performed in both *ABCB1*/Flp-In^{TM}-293 and KB/VIN cell lines. In *ABCB1* overexpressing cell line *ABCB1*/Flp-In^{TM}-293, caffeic acid after 72 h treatment slightly down-regulated the expression of P-gp (Figure 5a). Nevertheless, the same treatment for MDR cancer cell line KB/VIN exhibited the opposite phenomenon. Caffeic acid elevated *ABCB1* gene expression under 72 h treatment (Figure 5b).

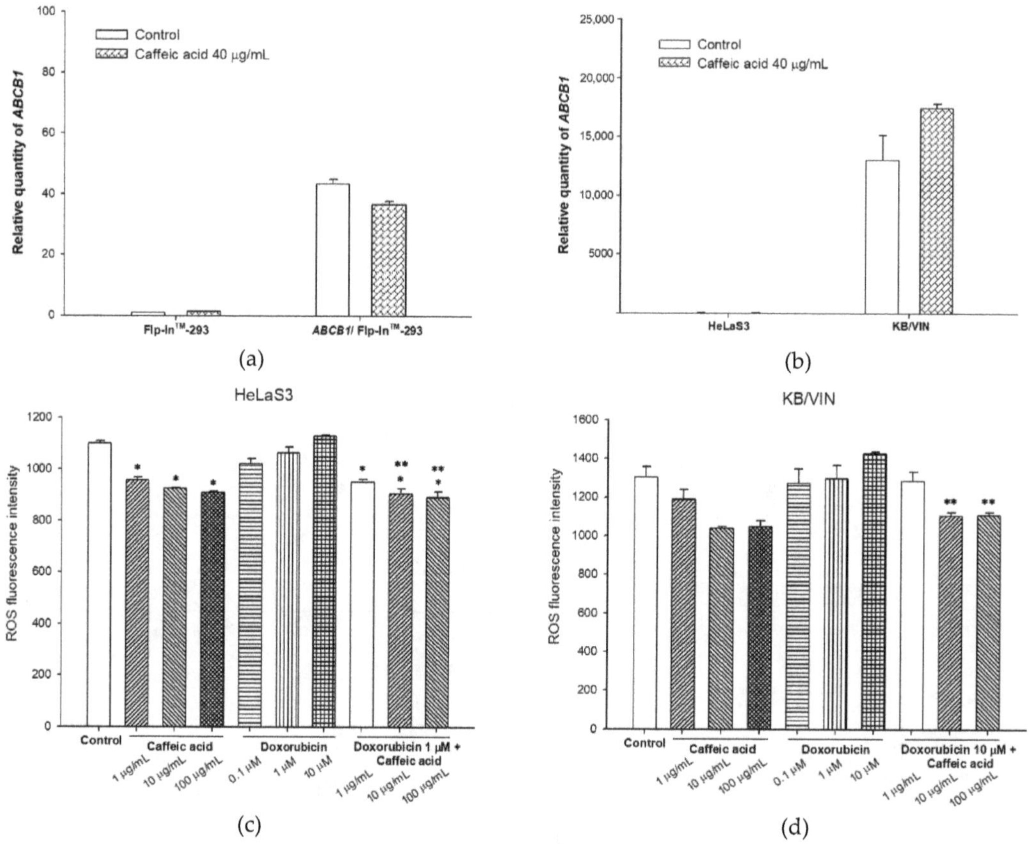

Figure 5. The modulating effects of caffeic acid on human P-gp expression. (**a**) The *ABCB1* expression in *ABCB1*/Flp-In^{TM}-293 was slightly down-regulated after treating the cells with 40 μg/mL caffeic acid for 72 h. (**b**) The *ABCB1* expression in KB/VIN was slightly up-regulated after treating the cells with 40 μg/mL caffeic acid for 72 h. (**c**) The intracellular ROS production under the treatment of caffeic acid with or without doxorubicin in HeLaS3. (**d**) The intracellular ROS production under the treatment of caffeic acid with or without doxorubicin in KB/VIN. Data were presented as mean ± SE of at least three experiments, each in triplicate. * denotes $p < 0.05$ compared with the control group. ** denotes $p < 0.05$ compared with the doxorubicin 1 μM group in Figure 5c and doxorubicin 10 μM group in Figure 5d.

To study whether the regulation of *ABCB1* gene expression was related to the intracellular reactive oxygen species status, the intracellular total ROS activity assay was performed. As Figure 5c,d indicates, caffeic acid significantly decreased ROS production in HeLaS3 cell line and slightly decreased ROS production in KB/VIN cell line. When both cell lines were treated with chemotherapeutic drug doxorubicin and caffeic acid, the ROS production exhibited no difference compared to caffeic acid treatment alone. However, the doxorubicin-induced oxidative challenge was significantly reversed by caffeic acid in amounts of 10 μg/mL and 100 μg/mL in both HeLaS3 and KB/VIN cell lines.

2.4. The Modulating Effects of Caffeic Acid on Cancer Multi-Drug Resistance

The MDR reversal ability of caffeic acid was examined in both P-gp over-expressing cell line *ABCB1*/Flp-In^{TM}-293 and MDR cancer cell line KB/VIN. As Table 2 shows, 30 μg/mL caffeic acid reversed vincristine, paclitaxel, and doxorubicin resistance by 3.90, 4.96, and 15.11-fold, respectively. The IC_{50} of doxorubicin decreased from 9023.61 nM to 569.90 nM with the treatment of caffeic acid 30 μg/mL in *ABCB1*/Flp-In^{TM}-293. The MDR reversal phenomenon was further approved and analyzed by cell cycle. Compared to paclitaxel alone treatment, the addition of caffeic acid 20 and 25 μg/mL significantly increased subG1 population (from 11.3% to 24.1% and 33.0%), indicating that the cell underwent obvious apoptosis under combinatorial treatment (Figure 6a and Table 3).

Table 2. The reversal effects of caffeic acid on chemotherapeutic drug resistance in P-gp over-expressing cell line *ABCB1*/Flp-In^{TM}293.

Cell Line	**Flp-In^{TM}293**		***ABCB1*/Flp-In^{TM}293**	
Compound	**IC_{50} ± S.E. (nM)**	**RF**	**IC_{50} ± S.E. (nM)**	**RF**
Vincristine	9.34 ± 0.43	1.00	778.11 ± 14.77	1.00
+ 30 μg/mL Caffeic acid	3.37 ± 4.30	2.77	198.04 ± 6.62	3.90
+ 20 μg/mL Caffeic acid	7.08 ± 0.09	1.31	557.46 ± 8.70	1.40
+ 10 μg/mL Caffeic acid	9.11 ± 0.32	1.02	615.03 ± 3.09	2.26
Paclitaxel	89.99 ± 0.50	1.00	604.09 ± 7.09	1.00
+ 30 μg/mL Caffeic acid	40.9 ± 0.50	2.20	121.55 ± 13.50	4.96 *
+ 20 μg/mL Caffeic acid	79.3 ± 0.67	1.13	313.06 ± 37.71	1.92
+ 10 μg/mL Caffeic acid	86.9 ± 0.12	1.03	597.87 ± 11.25	1.01
Doxorubicin	8.55 ± 0.19	1.00	9023.61 ± 272.90	1.00
+ 30 μg/mL Caffeic acid	4.07 ± 4.49	2.10	596.90 ± 24.18	15.11 *
+ 20 μg/mL Caffeic acid	7.34 ± 4.67	1.20	1299.7 ± 37.18	6.94 *
+ 10 μg/mL Caffeic acid	8.48 ± 2.58	1.00	2628.1 ± 24.49	3.43

* $p < 0.05$ as compared to the chemotherapeutic drug treatment (vincristine, paclitaxel, or doxorubicin) without caffeic acid. The reversal fold (RF) was calculated by dividing the individual IC_{50} of chemotherapeutic drugs by the IC_{50} of chemotherapeutic drugs in the presence of caffeic acid.

Table 3. The percentage of each cell cycle phase under various treatments in *ABCB1*/Flp-In^{TM}-293 cell line and KB/VIN cell line.

***ABCB1*/Flp-In^{TM}-293**	**Percentage of Phase ± SE (%)**			
	Sub G1	**G0/G1**	**S**	**G2/M**
Control	0.4 ± 0.17	35.7 ± 1.5	46.2 ± 2.9	17.6 ± 4.3
Paclitaxel 250 nM	11.3 ± 0.2	27.4 ± 0.6	29.3 ± 1.6	31.8 ± 1.3
Caffeic acid 20 μg/mL	3.7 ± 0.6	27.4 ± 0.6	29.3 ± 1.6	31.8 ± 1.3
Caffeic acid 25 μg/mL	1.2 ± 0.1	41.7 ± 0.5	37.7 ± 0.2	19.2 ± 0.6
Paclitaxel 250 nM + Caffeic acid 20 μg/mL	24.1 ± 0.3	36.6 ± 1.4	24.1 ± 1.8	15.0 ± 0.5
Paclitaxel 250 nM + Caffeic acid 25 μg/mL	33.0 ± 9.0	27.5 ± 8.5	29.7 ± 4.8	14.8 ± 0.6
KB/VIN	**Percentage of Phase ± SE (%)**			
	Sub G1	**G0/G1**	**S**	**G2/M**
Control	0.6 ± 0.07	37.3 ± 4.0	39.2 ± 0.7	22.9 ± 3.3
Paclitaxel 250 nM	12.8 ± 1.5	44.6 ± 1.0	29.2 ± 0.4	13.3 ± 0.1
Caffeic acid 20 μg/mL	1.5 ± 0.04	40.3 ± 0.9	45.5 ± 1.3	12.8 ± 0.5
Caffeic acid 25 μg/mL	1.3 ± 0.1	37.2 ± 0.4	50.1 ± 0.5	11.4 ± 0.3
Paclitaxel 250 nM + Caffeic acid 20 μg/mL	13.2 ± 1.2	44.3 ± 0.5	31.6 ± 1.0	11.0 ± 0.2
Paclitaxel 250 nM + Caffeic acid 25 μg/mL	12.7 ± 1.3	46.9 ± 0.1	23.6 ± 1.5	16.8 ± 0.2

(**a**)

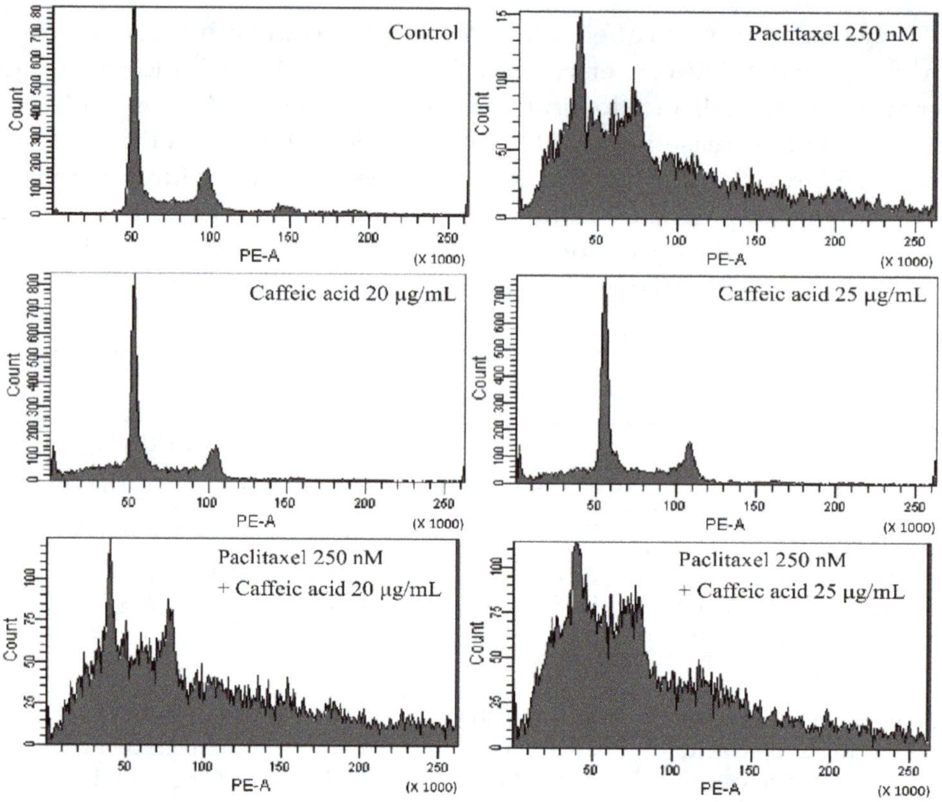

(**b**)

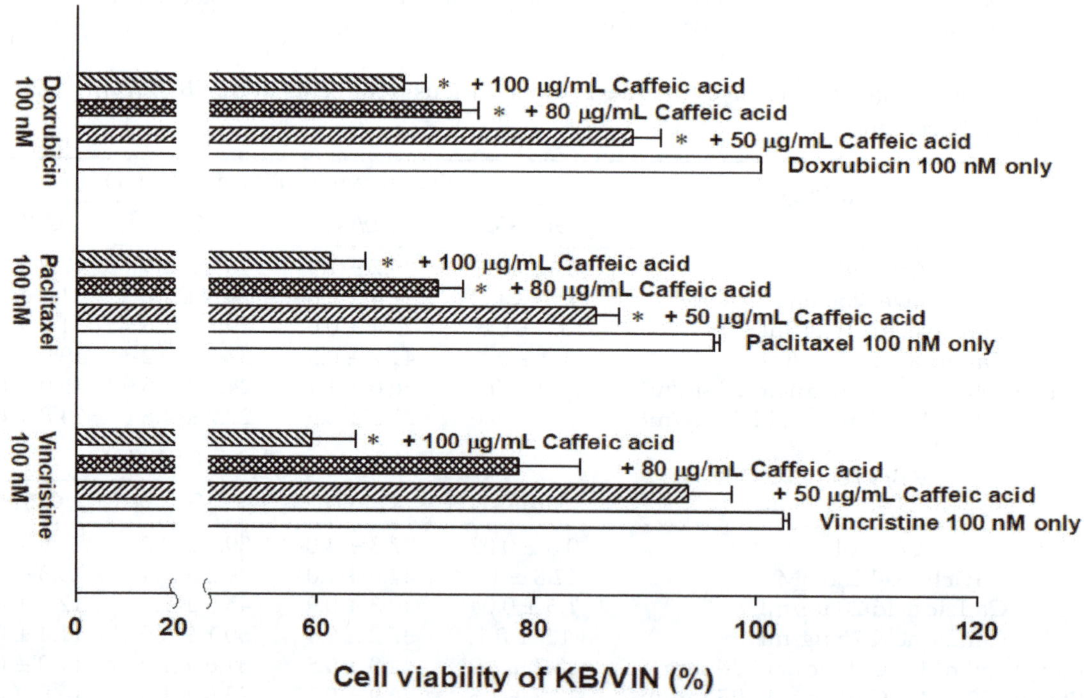

Figure 6. *Cont.*

(c)

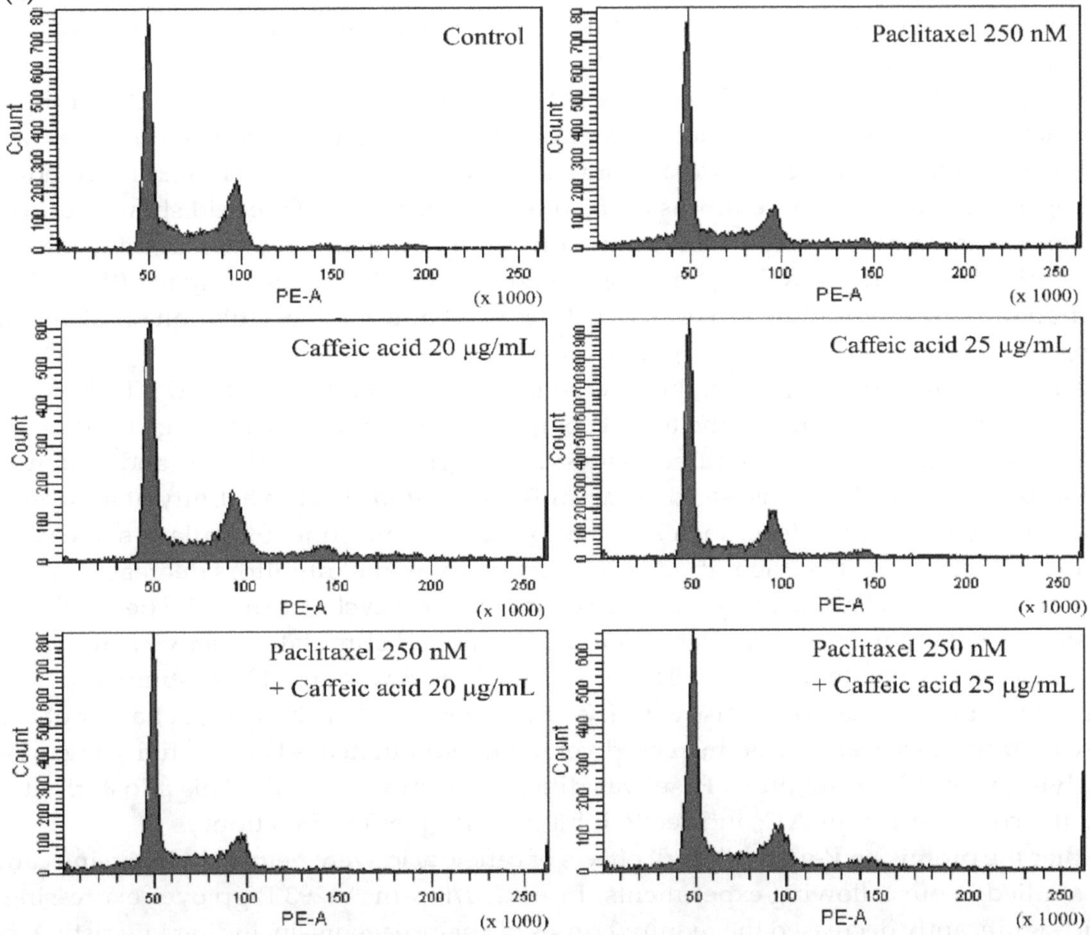

Figure 6. The cytotoxicity-enhancing effects of combinatorial treatment with caffeic acid. (**a**) The cell cycle distribution of 72 h treatment in *ABCB1*/Flp-In^{TM}-293 cell line. (**b**) The cell viability of KB/VIN under the treatment of chemotherapeutic drugs with or without caffeic acid. Data were presented as mean ± SE of at least three experiments, each in triplicate. * $p < 0.05$ as compared to the chemotherapeutic drug treatment (doxorubicin, paclitaxel, or vincristine) without caffeic acid. (**c**) The cell cycle distribution of 72 h treatment in KB/VIN cell line.

In MDR cancer cell line KB/VIN, with 100 µg/mL caffeic acid treatment, the cytotoxicity of 100 nM doxorubicin, paclitaxel, and vincristine significantly increased. The cell viability decreased from nearly 100% to 67.91%, 61.18%, and 59.50% for doxorubicin, paclitaxel, and vincristine, respectively. In addition, the cytotoxic-enhancing ability of caffeic acid on chemotherapeutic drugs was in a dose-dependent manner (Figure 6b). However, the further cell cycle analyses showed that the combination of caffeic acid and paclitaxel did not prominently increase the apoptosis of KB/VIN cells, revealing distinct cell effects among *ABCB1*/Flp-In^{TM}-293 and KB/VIN (Figure 6c and Table 3).

3. Discussion

Caffeic acid, a dietary non-flavonoid phenolic compound, has been a popular candidate among several research fields. The present study has demonstrated its usability in cancer MDR. Caffeic acid can attenuate this severe resistant problem by inhibiting the efflux function of human P-gp. Through diverse modulating mechanisms, caffeic acid helps resistant cancer cells retain chemotherapeutic drugs inside their cells, promoting further apoptosis and cell death.

Through investigating the history of P-gp inhibitor development, the ideal characteristics of potential candidates have been revealed. The inhibitor itself is not a substrate of P-gp, but is one of the favorable properties [19]. Our present research performed an experiment and the results indicated that caffeic acid was not P-gp's substrate. In this way, more caffeic acid could stay inside the cells to help P-gp inhibition, resulting in a higher intracellular chemotherapeutic drugs concentration.

The inhibitory effects of caffeic acid on P-gp efflux function were demonstrated on three P-gp fluorescent substrates, calcein-AM, rhodamine123, and doxorubicin. The different binding modes of each substrate revealed the inhibitory mechanisms of caffeic acid on P-gp drug binding sites. A previous investigation found that doxorubicin was a R-site substrate while rhodamine123 exhibited both M and R sites binding affinity [37–39]. Our efflux assay results indicated that caffeic acid showed uncompetitive inhibition on rhodamine123 transport and competitive inhibition on doxorubicin transport. Therefore, caffeic acid might compete the R drug binding site with doxorubicin, resulting in efflux inhibition. In terms of rhodamine123 inhibition, caffeic acid exhibited an allosteric modulation on M site, indirectly prohibiting the pump out behavior of P-gp.

In addition to drug binding sites, the interaction between caffeic acid and ATP binding sites of P-gp was also studied. According to the tested compound's behavior toward P-gp ATPase regulation, substances could be categorized into three classes: dual regulators, stimulators, and inhibitors [40,41]. Dual regulators stimulate both basal and verapamil-stimulated ATPase activity at a lower dose, but inhibit the activity at a higher dose, such as paclitaxel and vinblastine. Stimulators like valinomycin and bisantrene increase ATPase activity dose-dependently while inhibitors decrease both basal and verapamil-stimulated ATPase activity, such as rapamycin and cyclosporine A. The results of ATPase assay in the present study indicated that caffeic acid exhibited stimulatory activity from 10 μg/mL to 100 μg/mL in a dose-dependent manner. Therefore, caffeic acid was an ATPase stimulator. Besides, the results of verapamil-stimulated ATPase activity further revealed the binding behavior of caffeic acid on ATPase binding sites. Caffeic acid increased verapamil-stimulated ATPase activity regardless of the dose, implying its binding site on ATPase was different from verapamil. This allosteric stimulation advanced the consumption of ATP, indirectly inhibiting P-gp efflux function.

Whether the promising P-gp inhibitory effects of caffeic acid were helpful in reversing cancer MDR was than studied in our following experiments. In *ABCB1*/Flp-In^{TM}-293 P-gp over-expressing cell line, caffeic acid significantly decreased the required doses of chemo-agents, including vincristine, paclitaxel, and doxorubicin. Under the treatment of 30 μg/mL caffeic acid, the IC_{50} of paclitaxel largely decreased from 604.09 nM to 121.55 nM. This advanced cytotoxicity was related to the increased apoptotic effects revealed by cell cycle assay results. With caffeic acid as a combinatory agent, the percentage of subG1 apoptotic population induced by paclitaxel significantly increased in a dose-dependent manner. The above results were consistent with previous researches, which revealed that caffeic acid could sensitize ovarian carcinoma cells and lung cancer cells to cisplatin and paclitaxel, respectively [33,42]. Caffeic acid exhibited chemo-sensitizing effects in the combination group by cell cycle arresting in G2/M (caffeic acid 20 μg/mL with paclitaxel) and G1 (caffeic acid 25 μg/mL with paclitaxel). These effects were not only due to the modulation of P-gp, other cellular targets and multiple mechanistic possibilities may be involved and need further investigation. The MDR reversing ability of caffeic acid was also investigated in MDR cancer cell line KB/VIN. The results exhibited a trend on increasing the cytotoxicity of chemo-agents. With the treatment of 100 μg/mL caffeic acid, the cell viability decreased from nearly 100% to 67.91%, 61.18%, and 59.50% for doxorubicin, paclitaxel, and vincristine, respectively. However, compared to the promising results in *ABCB1*/Flp-In^{TM}-293 cell line, the MDR modulating effects of caffeic acid in KB/VIN seemed to be less potent and did not show increased apoptosis in the cell cycle analyses, exhibiting cell type-dependent effects. This phenomenon could be explained by the regulation of caffeic acid on P-gp expression. As Figure 5a,b shows, caffeic acid slightly decreased *ABCB1* gene expression in *ABCB1*/Flp-In^{TM}-293 but increased the expression level in KB/VIN cell line. This up-regulating trend in KB/VIN diminished the functional inhibitory potency of caffeic acid, resulting in weaker MDR reversing effects. Previous research has revealed that the oxidative stress might have a role in the regulation of P-gp expression [43]. As caffeic acid exhibited significant ROS-related anti-oxidant effects, the influence of caffeic acid on ROS production in KB/VIN cell line was performed. The results showed that caffeic acid significantly decreased ROS production in HeLaS3 cell line and slightly decreased ROS production in KB/VIN cell line. However, the doxorubicin-induced oxidative challenge was significantly reversed by caffeic acid in amounts of 10 μg/mL and 100 μg/mL in both HeLaS3 and KB/VIN cell lines. Therefore, the relationship between the reactive oxygen species levels and the up-regulation of *ABCB1* gene in KB/VIN might be related to the insufficient ROS regulation of caffeic acid. The above results indicated that the MDR reversal effects of caffeic acid might be cell line-dependent and warrant further detailed investigation.

The present study provided in-depth and comprehensive researches on the relationship between caffeic acid and human P-gp, and demonstrated the ability of caffeic acid on sensitizing MDR cancer cells toward chemotherapeutic drugs treatment. In order for caffeic acid to find a role in clinical application, some attempts could be applied to this phenolic prototype agent, including structural modification and pharmaceutical design.

4. Materials and Methods

4.1. Chemicals and Reagents

Acetic acid, β-Mercaptoethanol (β-ME), caffeic acid, dimethyl sulfoxide (DMSO), ethanol (Absolute; analytical grade), paclitaxel, rhodamine 123, sulforhodamine B (SRB), trichloroacetic acid (TCA), tris base, (±)-verapamil, and vincristine were obtained from Sigma-Aldrich Co. (St Louis, MO, USA). Calcein-AM was from AAT Bioquest (Sunnyvale, CA, USA), and doxorubicin was from US Biological (Woburn, MA, USA). Dulbecco's Modified Eagle Medium, RPMI 1640 medium, fetal bovine serum (FBS), phosphate buffered saline (PBS; pH 7.2), Trypsin-EDTA, and hygromycin B were purchased from Invitrogen (Carlsbad, CA, USA). Zeocin was from InvivoGen (San Diego, CA, USA).

4.2. Cell Lines

Human cervical epithelioid carcinoma HeLaS3 was purchased from Bioresource Collection and Research Center (Hsinchu, Taiwan), and the multi-drug resistant human cervical cancer cell line KB/VIN was kindly provided by Dr. Kuo-Hsiung Lee (University of North Carolina, Chapel Hill, NC, USA) and maintained with vincristine regularly. The human P-gp stable expression cells (*ABCB1*/Flp-In^{TM}-293) and parental cell line Flp-In^{TM}-293 were constructed as previously described [44]. All cells were cultured in DMEM or RPMI-1640 containing 10% FBS at 37 °C in a humidified atmosphere of 5% CO_2.

4.3. Cytotoxicity Determination Assay (SRB Assay)

The method has been described in our previous research [45]. Briefly, after 72 h of treatment of a series of concentrations of chemotherapeutic drugs with or without caffeic acid, 50% trichloroacetic acid (TCA) was added to fix cells for 30 min, and then the cells were washed with water and air-dried. After that, cells were stained with 0.04% sulforhodamine B (SRB) for 30 min, and then the unbound dye was removed by washing cells with 1% acetic acid and air-dried. The bound stain was solubilized in 10 mM Tris Base and the absorbance was measured using a BioTek Synergy HT Multi-Mode Microplate Reader (Winooski, VT, USA) at 515 nm.

4.4. MDR1 Shift Assay

The method has been described in our previous research [46]. The conformation change of P-gp after the addition of caffeic acid was examined by using a MDR1 Shift Assay kit (EMD Millipore Corp., Billerica, MA, USA) according to the manufacturer's protocol. UIC2 shift was shown in the presence of a P-gp substrate such as vinblastine. A total of 5×10^5–1×10^6 cells were prepared per reaction and resuspended with warm UIC2 binding buffer. Cells were incubated at 37 °C for 10 min and then treated with DMSO or vinblastine or test compounds. Cells were incubated at 37 °C for 30 min and then treated with IgG2a (negative control antibody) or UIC2 working solution (P-gp conformational sensitive antibody). Cells were incubated at 37 °C for 15 min and then washed with iced UIC2 binding buffer twice. A secondary antibody, goat anti-mouse IgG ALEXA 488, was added at 4 °C for 15 min, and then iced UIC2 binding buffer was added. The fluorescence was measured by FACS analysis (BD FACSCanto™ II System, South City-I, Haryana, India).

4.5. Intracellular Calcein Accumulation Assay

The method has been described in our previous research [46]. For the screening of an inhibitory effect on human P-gp efflux function, intracellular calcein accumulation assay was performed. Briefly, 1×10^5 cells/well were seeded in 96-well black plates for 24 h. Before the assay, cells were washed and pre-incubated with warm Hanks' balanced salt solution (HBSS) for 30 min and subsequently with caffeic acid for 30 min. After pre-incubation and three times washing with PBS, the calcein-AM was added (substrate of P-gp), and the calcein fluorescence generated within the cells was detected by BioTek Synergy HT Multi-Mode Microplate Reader using an excitation wavelength of 485 nm and emission wavelength of 528 nm at 37 °C temperature every 3 min for 30 min. Each experiment was performed at least three times, each in triplicate on different days.

4.6. Rhodamine123 and Doxorubicin Efflux Assay

The method has been described in our previous research [46]. 1×10^5 cells/well were placed on 96-well plates and incubated overnight. Before the efflux assay, cells were washed and pre-incubated with warm HBSS for 30 min, and subsequently with caffeic acid for 30 min. Then, the cells were treated with rhodamine123 for 30 min or doxorubicin for 3 h at 37 °C. After being washed with warm PBS, cells were allowed to efflux fluorescent rhodamin123 and doxorubicin for 10 min and 2 h, respectively. Supernatant samples (100 μL) were transferred to 96-well black plates. The fluorescence of rhodamine123 and doxorubicin was measured using a BioTek Synergy HT Multi-Mode Microplate Reader (excitation/emission: 485/528 nm for rhodamine123, 485/590 nm for doxorubicin). Each experiment was performed at least three times, each in triplicate on different days. Kinetic parameters were estimated by nonlinear regression using Scientist v2.01 (MicroMath Scientific Software, Salt Lake City, UT, USA) according to the following equation:

$$V = \frac{V_{max} \times C}{K_m + C}$$

where V denoted the efflux rate; V_{max}, the maximal efflux rate; K_m, the Michaelis-Menten constant; and C is the substrate concentration.

4.7. P-gp ATPase Activity Assay

The method has been described in our previous research [46]. For the evaluation of P-gp ATPase activity of caffeic acid, Pgp-Glo™ Assay System from Promega (Madison, WI, USA) was used. In a 96-well untreated white plate, 25 μg of recombinant human P-gp membranes were incubated with Pgp-Glo™ Assay Buffer (untreated control), 200 μM verapamil (positive control for drug induced P-gp ATPase activity), 100 μM sodium orthovanadate (selective inhibitor for P-gp ATPase activity), or a series of concentrations of caffeic acid. The reaction was initiated by adding 5 mM MgATP and incubated for 40 min at 37 °C, followed by stopping the reaction with 50 μL ATPase Detection Reagent for 20 min at room temperature. Luminescence was measured using a BioTek Synergy HT Multi-Mode Microplate Reader, and data were presented as Change in Luminescence (ΔRLU).

4.8. Real-Time Quantitative RT-PCR

The method has been described in our previous research [46]. *ABCB1* mRNA expression levels were quantified by real-time RT-PCR. Total RNA was extracted from HeLaS3, KB/VIN, Flp-In™-293, and *ABCB1*/Flp-In™-293 cells using Qiagen RNeasy kit (Valencia, CA, USA). Taqman Assay-On-Demand™ reagents of primers and probes for *ABCB1* (Hs00184500_m1) and *GAPDH* (Hs02758991_g1) genes were provided by Applied Biosystem (Foster City, CA, USA). The relative *ABCB1* mRNA expression levels were normalized to the amount of *GAPDH* in the same cDNA and evaluated by StepOnePlus™ Real-Time PCR System (Applied Biosystems®).

4.9. Intracellular Total ROS Activity Assay

The influence of caffeic acid on intracellular reactive oxygen species (ROS) was evaluated with Cell Meter™ Fluorimetric Intracellular Total ROS Activity Assay Kit (Catalog number: 22900) purchased from AAT Bioquest (Sunnyvale, CA, USA). Briefly, 4×10^4 cells/well were seeded in 96-well black plates for 24 h. Then the cells were stained with Amplite™ ROS Green working solution for 1 h; after that, caffeic acid with or without chemotherapeutic drugs were added to induce ROS production at room temperature for at least 15 min. The fluorescence was measured using a BioTek Synergy HT Multi-Mode Microplate Reader at 490/525 nm (same as FITC filter).

4.10. Cell Cycle Analysis

The method has been described in our previous research [45]. Cells were plated to 6-well plates with serum-free medium for starvation. Twenty-four hours later, cells were treated with chemotherapeutic drugs with or without caffeic acid for 72 h. After that, cells were harvested and washed in cold phosphate-buffered saline (PBS), followed by fixing in ice-cold 70% ethanol for at least 24 h. Then, cells were incubated with 50 µg/mL PI at 4 °C for 24 h in the dark. Cells were then analyzed by FACS analysis (BD FACSCanto™ II System with excitation laser 488 nm, measuring at emission 575 nm for PI).

4.11. Molecular Docking

Molecular docking helps us in predicting the intermolecular framework formed between a protein and a small molecule and suggests the binding modes responsible for inhibition of the protein. In this study, the existing structure of P-gp (PDB entry 6QEX) was used as a template for docking caffeic acid (PubChem CID: 689043) putative ligands using Discovery Studio 4.5. After removing all crystallized H_2O molecules from the former construction, hydrogen was added into the CDOCKER module. CDOCKER is a powerful CHARMm-based docking method that has been used to generate highly accurate docked poses. In this refinement application, the ligands were conceded to tilt around the rigid receptor [47].

4.12. Statistical Analysis

Statistical differences were evaluated by ANOVA followed by post hoc analysis (Tukey's test) or Student's t-test. The statistical significance was set at p value < 0.05.

Author Contributions: Conceptualization, Y.-N.T. and C.-C.H.; Data curation, Y.-N.T.; Formal analysis, Y.-N.T., C.C.N.W. and W.-C.L.; Funding acquisition, Y.-N.T. and C.-C.H.; Investigation, Y.-N.T., C.C.N.W., W.-C.L. and Y.-H.L.; Methodology, Y.-N.T., C.C.N.W., W.-C.L. and C.-C.H.; Project administration, C.-C.H.; Resources, Y.-H.L. and C.-C.H.; Software, Y.-N.T., C.C.N.W. and W.-C.L.; Supervision, Y.-H.L. and C.-C.H.; Validation, C.-C.H.; Visualization, C.-C.H.; Writing—original draft, Y.-N.T., C.C.N.W. and W.-C.L.; Writing—review & editing, Y.-H.L. and C.-C.H. All authors have read and agreed to the published version of the manuscript.

Acknowledgments: Flow cytometry analyses were performed at the Medical Research Core Facilities Center, Office of Research & Development at China Medical University, Taichung, Taiwan, R.O.C.

References

1. Silva, R.; Vilas-Boas, V.; Carmo, H.; Dinis-Oliveira, R.J.; Carvalho, F.; de Lourdes Bastos, M.; Remiao, F. Modulation of P-glycoprotein efflux pump: Induction and activation as a therapeutic strategy. *Pharmacol. Ther.* **2015**, *149*, 1–123. [CrossRef] [PubMed]
2. Kumar, A.; Jaitak, V. Natural products as multidrug resistance modulators in cancer. *Eur. J. Med. Chem.* **2019**, *176*, 268–291. [CrossRef] [PubMed]

3. Kathawala, R.J.; Wang, Y.J.; Ashby, C.R., Jr.; Chen, Z.S. Recent advances regarding the role of ABC subfamily C member 10 (ABCC10) in the efflux of antitumor drugs. *Chin. J. Cancer* **2014**, *33*, 223–230. [CrossRef] [PubMed]
4. Shi, R.; Wang, C.; Fu, N.; Liu, L.; Zhu, D.; Wei, Z.; Zhang, H.; Xing, J.; Wang, Y. Downregulation of cytokeratin 18 enhances BCRP-mediated multidrug resistance through induction of epithelial-mesenchymal transition and predicts poor prognosis in breast cancer. *Oncol. Rep.* **2019**, *41*, 3015–3026. [CrossRef]
5. Das, M.; Law, S. Role of tumor microenvironment in cancer stem cell chemoresistance and recurrence. *Int. J. Biochem. Cell Biol.* **2018**, *103*, 115–124. [CrossRef]
6. Giacomini, K.M.; Huang, S.M.; Tweedie, D.J.; Benet, L.Z.; Brouwer, K.L.; Chu, X.; Dahlin, A.; Evers, R.; Fischer, V.; Hillgren, K.M.; et al. Membrane transporters in drug development. *Nat. Rev. Drug Discov.* **2010**, *9*, 215–236.
7. Uddin, M.B.; Roy, K.R.; Hosain, S.B.; Khiste, S.K.; Hill, R.A.; Jois, S.D.; Zhao, Y.; Tackett, A.J.; Liu, Y.Y. An *N*(6)-methyladenosine at the transited codon 273 of p53 pre-mRNA promotes the expression of R273H mutant protein and drug resistance of cancer cells. *Biochem. Pharmacol.* **2019**, *160*, 134–145. [CrossRef]
8. Bedi, A.; Barber, J.P.; Bedi, G.C.; el-Deiry, W.S.; Sidransky, D.; Vala, M.S.; Akhtar, A.J.; Hilton, J.; Jones, R.J. BCR-ABL-mediated inhibition of apoptosis with delay of G2/M transition after DNA damage: A mechanism of resistance to multiple anticancer agents. *Blood* **1995**, *86*, 1148–1158. [CrossRef]
9. Wilson, C.S.; Medeiros, L.J.; Lai, R.; Butch, A.W.; McCourty, A.; Kelly, K.; Brynes, R.K. DNA topoisomerase IIalpha in multiple myeloma: A marker of cell proliferation and not drug resistance. *Mod. Pathol.* **2001**, *14*, 886–891. [CrossRef]
10. Filomeni, G.; Turella, P.; Dupuis, M.L.; Forini, O.; Ciriolo, M.R.; Cianfriglia, M.; Pezzola, S.; Federici, G.; Caccuri, A.M. 6-(7-Nitro-2,1,3-benzoxadiazol-4-ylthio)hexanol, a specific glutathione S-transferase inhibitor, overcomes the multidrug resistance (MDR)-associated protein 1-mediated MDR in small cell lung cancer. *Mol. Cancer Ther.* **2008**, *7*, 371–379. [CrossRef]
11. Rodriguez-Antona, C.; Ingelman-Sundberg, M. Cytochrome P450 pharmacogenetics and cancer. *Oncogene* **2006**, *25*, 1679–1691. [CrossRef] [PubMed]
12. Shoemaker, R.H. Genetic and epigenetic factors in anticancer drug resistance. *J. Natl. Cancer Inst.* **2000**, *92*, 4–5. [CrossRef] [PubMed]
13. Li, H.; Yang, B.B. Friend or foe: The role of microRNA in chemotherapy resistance. *Acta Pharm. Sin* **2013**, *34*, 870–879. [CrossRef] [PubMed]
14. Camidge, D.R.; Pao, W.; Sequist, L.V. Acquired resistance to TKIs in solid tumours: Learning from lung cancer. *Nat. Rev. Clin. Oncol.* **2014**, *11*, 473–481. [CrossRef] [PubMed]
15. Paskeviciute, M.; Petrikaite, V. Overcoming transporter-mediated multidrug resistance in cancer: Failures and achievements of the last decades. *Drug Deliv. Transl. Res.* **2019**, *9*, 379–393. [CrossRef] [PubMed]
16. Yakusheva, E.N.; Titov, D.S. Structure and Function of Multidrug Resistance Protein 1. *Biochem. Biokhimiia* **2018**, *83*, 907–929. [CrossRef]
17. Ling, V.; Thompson, L.H. Reduced permeability in CHO cells as a mechanism of resistance to colchicine. *J. Cell. Physiol.* **1974**, *83*, 103–116. [CrossRef]
18. Mollazadeh, S.; Sahebkar, A.; Hadizadeh, F.; Behravan, J.; Arabzadeh, S. Structural and functional aspects of P-glycoprotein and its inhibitors. *Life Sci.* **2018**, *214*, 118–123. [CrossRef]
19. Leopoldo, M.; Nardulli, P.; Contino, M.; Leonetti, F.; Luurtsema, G.; Colabufo, N.A. An updated patent review on P-glycoprotein inhibitors (2011-2018). *Expert Opin. Ther. Pat.* **2019**, *29*, 455–461. [CrossRef]
20. Joshi, P.; Vishwakarma, R.A.; Bharate, S.B. Natural alkaloids as P-gp inhibitors for multidrug resistance reversal in cancer. *Eur. J. Med. Chem.* **2017**, *138*, 273–292. [CrossRef]
21. O'Brien, M.M.; Lacayo, N.J.; Lum, B.L.; Kshirsagar, S.; Buck, S.; Ravindranath, Y.; Bernstein, M.; Weinstein, H.; Chang, M.N.; Arceci, R.J.; et al. Phase I study of valspodar (PSC-833) with mitoxantrone and etoposide in refractory and relapsed pediatric acute leukemia: A report from the Children's Oncology Group. *Pediatr. Blood Cancer* **2010**, *54*, 694–702. [CrossRef] [PubMed]
22. Li, W.; Zhang, H.; Assaraf, Y.G.; Zhao, K.; Xu, X.; Xie, J.; Yang, D.H.; Chen, Z.S. Overcoming ABC transporter-mediated multidrug resistance: Molecular mechanisms and novel therapeutic drug strategies. *Drug Resist. Updat.* **2016**, *27*, 14–29. [CrossRef] [PubMed]

23. Cripe, L.D.; Uno, H.; Paietta, E.M.; Litzow, M.R.; Ketterling, R.P.; Bennett, J.M.; Rowe, J.M.; Lazarus, H.M.; Luger, S.; Tallman, M.S. Zosuquidar, a novel modulator of P-glycoprotein, does not improve the outcome of older patients with newly diagnosed acute myeloid leukemia: A randomized, placebo-controlled trial of the Eastern Cooperative Oncology Group 3999. *Blood* **2010**, *116*, 4077–4085. [CrossRef] [PubMed]
24. Dash, R.P.; Jayachandra Babu, R.; Srinivas, N.R. Therapeutic Potential and Utility of Elacridar with Respect to P-glycoprotein Inhibition: An Insight from the Published In Vitro, Preclinical and Clinical Studies. *Eur. J. Drug Metab. Pharmacokinet.* **2017**, *42*, 915–933. [CrossRef]
25. Han, R.M.; Zhang, J.P.; Skibsted, L.H. Reaction dynamics of flavonoids and carotenoids as antioxidants. *Molecules* **2012**, *17*, 2140–2160. [CrossRef]
26. Kumar, S.; Pandey, A.K. Chemistry and biological activities of flavonoids: An overview. *Sci. World J.* **2013**, *2013*, 162750. [CrossRef]
27. Meyer, A.S.; Heinonen, M.; Frankel, E.N. Antioxidant interactions of catechin, cyanidin, caffeic acid, quercetin, and ellagic acid on human LDL oxidation. *Food Chem.* **1998**, *61*, 71–75. [CrossRef]
28. Jaman, M.S.; Sayeed, M.A. Ellagic acid, sulforaphane, and ursolic acid in the prevention and therapy of breast cancer: Current evidence and future perspectives. *Breast Cancer (TokyoJpn.)* **2018**, *25*, 517–528. [CrossRef]
29. Xing, Y.; Peng, H.Y.; Zhang, M.X.; Li, X.; Zeng, W.W.; Yang, X.E. Caffeic acid product from the highly copper-tolerant plant Elsholtzia splendens post-phytoremediation: Its extraction, purification, and identification. *J. Zhejiang Univ. Sci. B* **2012**, *13*, 487–493. [CrossRef]
30. Ahmed, N.; Escalona, R.; Leung, D.; Chan, E.; Kannourakis, G. Tumour microenvironment and metabolic plasticity in cancer and cancer stem cells: Perspectives on metabolic and immune regulatory signatures in chemoresistant ovarian cancer stem cells. *Semin. Cancer Biol.* **2018**, *53*, 265–281. [CrossRef]
31. Khan, F.A.; Maalik, A.; Murtaza, G. Inhibitory mechanism against oxidative stress of caffeic acid. *J. Food Drug Anal.* **2016**, *24*, 695–702. [CrossRef] [PubMed]
32. Ahn, C.H.; Choi, W.C.; Kong, J.Y. Chemosensitizing activity of caffeic acid in multidrug-resistant MCF-7/Dox human breast carcinoma cells. *Anticancer Res.* **1997**, *17*, 1913–1917. [PubMed]
33. Lin, C.L.; Chen, R.F.; Chen, J.Y.; Chu, Y.C.; Wang, H.M.; Chou, H.L.; Chang, W.C.; Fong, Y.; Chang, W.T.; Wu, C.Y.; et al. Protective effect of caffeic acid on paclitaxel induced anti-proliferation and apoptosis of lung cancer cells involves NF-kappaB pathway. *Int. J. Mol. Sci.* **2012**, *13*, 6236–6245. [CrossRef] [PubMed]
34. Wu, J.; Omene, C.; Karkoszka, J.; Bosland, M.; Eckard, J.; Klein, C.B.; Frenkel, K. Caffeic acid phenethyl ester (CAPE), derived from a honeybee product propolis, exhibits a diversity of anti-tumor effects in pre-clinical models of human breast cancer. *Cancer Lett.* **2011**, *308*, 43–53. [CrossRef]
35. Nabekura, T.; Kawasaki, T.; Furuta, M.; Kaneko, T.; Uwai, Y. Effects of Natural Polyphenols on the Expression of Drug Efflux Transporter P-Glycoprotein in Human Intestinal Cells. *Acs Omega* **2018**, *3*, 1621–1626. [CrossRef]
36. Takara, K.; Fujita, M.; Matsubara, M.; Minegaki, T.; Kitada, N.; Ohnishi, N.; Yokoyama, T. Effects of propolis extract on sensitivity to chemotherapeutic agents in HeLa and resistant sublines. *Phytother. Res. Ptr.* **2007**, *21*, 841–846. [CrossRef]
37. Montanari, F.; Ecker, G.F. Prediction of drug-ABC-transporter interaction–Recent advances and future challenges. *Adv. Drug Deliv. Rev.* **2015**, *86*, 17–26. [CrossRef]
38. Ferreira, R.J.; Ferreira, M.J.; dos Santos, D.J. Molecular docking characterizes substrate-binding sites and efflux modulation mechanisms within P-glycoprotein. *J. Chem. Inf. Model.* **2013**, *53*, 1747–1760. [CrossRef]
39. Martinez, L.; Arnaud, O.; Henin, E.; Tao, H.; Chaptal, V.; Doshi, R.; Andrieu, T.; Dussurgey, S.; Tod, M.; Di Pietro, A.; et al. Understanding polyspecificity within the substrate-binding cavity of the human multidrug resistance P-glycoprotein. *FEBS J.* **2014**, *281*, 673–682. [CrossRef]
40. Ambudkar, S.V.; Dey, S.; Hrycyna, C.A.; Ramachandra, M.; Pastan, I.; Gottesman, M.M. Biochemical, cellular, and pharmacological aspects of the multidrug transporter. *Ann. Rev. Pharmacol. Toxicol.* **1999**, *39*, 361–398. [CrossRef]
41. Dey, S.; Ramachandra, M.; Pastan, I.; Gottesman, M.M.; Ambudkar, S.V. Evidence for two nonidentical drug-interaction sites in the human P-glycoprotein. *Proc. Natl. Acad. Sci. USA* **1997**, *94*, 10594–10599. [CrossRef] [PubMed]

42. Sirota, R.; Gibson, D.; Kohen, R. The timing of caffeic acid treatment with cisplatin determines sensitization or resistance of ovarian carcinoma cell lines. *Redox Biol.* **2017**, *11*, 170–175. [CrossRef]
43. Huang, C.; Huang, S.; Li, H.; Li, X.; Li, B.; Zhong, L.; Wang, J.; Zou, M.; He, X.; Zheng, H.; et al. The effects of ultrasound exposure on P-glycoprotein-mediated multidrug resistance in vitro and in vivo. *J. Exp. Clin. Cancer Res.* **2018**, *37*, 232. [CrossRef] [PubMed]
44. Sheu, M.J.; Teng, Y.N.; Chen, Y.Y.; Hung, C.C. The functional influences of common ABCB1 genetic variants on the inhibition of P-glycoprotein by Antrodia cinnamomea extracts. *PLoS ONE* **2014**, *9*, e89622. [CrossRef]
45. Teng, Y.-N.; Wang, Y.-H.; Wu, T.-S.; Hung, H.-Y.; Hung, C.-C. Zhankuic Acids A, B and C from Taiwanofungus camphoratus Act as Cytotoxicity Enhancers by Regulating P-Glycoprotein in Multi-Drug Resistant Cancer Cells. *Biomolecules* **2019**, *9*, 759. [CrossRef] [PubMed]
46. Teng, Y.-N.; Hsieh, Y.-W.; Hung, C.-C.; Lin, H.-Y. Demethoxycurcumin Modulates Human P-Glycoprotein Function via Uncompetitive Inhibition of ATPase Hydrolysis Activity. *J. Agric. Food Chem.* **2015**, *63*, 847–855. [CrossRef] [PubMed]
47. Wu, G.; Robertson, D.H.; Brooks, C.L., 3rd; Vieth, M. Detailed analysis of grid-based molecular docking: A case study of CDOCKER-A CHARMm-based MD docking algorithm. *J. Comput. Chem.* **2003**, *24*, 1549–1562. [CrossRef]

6

Development of a Transdermal Delivery System for Tenofovir Alafenamide, a Prodrug of Tenofovir with Potent Antiviral Activity Against HIV and HBV

Ashana Puri [1], Sonalika A. Bhattacharjee [1], Wei Zhang [2], Meredith Clark [2], Onkar N. Singh [2], Gustavo F. Doncel [2] and Ajay K. Banga [1,*]

1 Center for Drug Delivery Research, Department of Pharmaceutical Sciences, College of Pharmacy, Mercer University, Atlanta, GA 30341, USA; ashana.puri@live.mercer.edu (A.P.); sonalika.arup.bhattacharjee@live.mercer.edu (S.A.B.)

2 CONRAD, Department of Obstetrics and Gynecology, Eastern Virginia Medical School, Arlington, VA 22209, USA; wzhang@conrad.org (W.Z.); mclark@conrad.org (M.C.); osingh@conrad.org (O.S.); gfdoncel@conrad.org (G.F.D.)

* Correspondence: banga_ak@mercer.edu

Abstract: Tenofovir alafenamide (TAF) is an effective nucleotide reverse transcriptase inhibitor that is used in the treatment of HIV-1 and HBV. Currently, it is being investigated for HIV prophylaxis. Oral TAF regimens require daily intake, which hampers adherence and increases the possibility of viral resistance. Long-acting formulations would significantly reduce this problem. Therefore, the aim of this study was to develop a transdermal patch containing TAF and investigate its performance in vitro through human epidermis. Two types of TAF patches were manufactured. Transparent patches were prepared using acrylate adhesive (DURO-TAK 87-2516), and suspension patches were prepared using silicone (BIO-PSA 7-4301) and polyisobutylene (DURO-TAK 87-6908) adhesives. In vitro permeation studies were performed while using vertical Franz diffusion cells for seven days. An optimized silicone-based patch was characterized for its adhesive properties and tested for skin irritation. The acrylate-based patches, comprising 2% w/w TAF and a combination of chemical enhancers, showed a maximum flux of 0.60 ± 0.09 μg/cm^2/h. However, the silicone-based patch comprising of 15% w/w TAF showed the highest permeation (7.24 ± 0.47 μg/cm^2/h). This study demonstrates the feasibility of developing silicone-based transdermal patches that can deliver a therapeutically relevant dose of TAF for the control of HIV and HBV infections.

Keywords: transdermal patch; tenofovir alafenamide; acrylate adhesive; in vitro permeation; silicone adhesive; suspension patch

---

1. Introduction

Tenofovir (TFV) represents the cornerstone of prophylactic and therapeutic approaches to control HIV infection [1]. Tenofovir alafenamide fumarate (TAF), a prodrug, is currently replacing TFV disoproxil fumarate, which shows better affinity for lymphoid tissue, yielding higher levels of TFV-diphosphate (active metabolite) and lower levels of plasma TFV, and displaying a better renal and bone safety profile [2]. Due to these advantages, TAF is also being considered in the treatment of chronic HBV infection [1]. For HIV, TAF is typically administered, in combination with other antiretrovirals (ARVs), in daily single tablet regimens (STRs). Although STRs represent a significant advantage over the need to take multiple tablets three times a day, which characterized the beginnings of highly active antiretroviral therapy, it still remains a high burden to the patient, leading to poor adherence, lower efficacy, and increased risk of viral resistance. Therefore, sustained release of ARVs, which can reduce these problems, is needed. The development of sustained release delivery technologies in this space would be of high clinical relevance.

A variety of delivery systems, such as tablets (oral), tablet-like inserts (vaginal/rectal), gels (rectal/vaginal), vaginal films, ointments, rings, diaphragm based devices and electrospun fibers, oral/parenteral liposomes and nanoparticles, injectables, and subdermal implants for prophylactic or therapeutic anti-HIV agents have been explored [3–9]. Drug delivery systems, such as daily oral tablets and coitally-dependent vaginal gels, are typically short-acting and they have been associated with poorer user adherence. Long-acting coitally-independent systems, such as implants and injectables, do not present these problems, but are riskier if safety or idiosyncratic issues arise [7,10–13]. An intermediate duration drug delivery system, such as a transdermal patch, exerting its pharmacological effect for a few days to a week, would thus be beneficial to the users, providing a more sophisticated and convenient therapy option.

Transdermal drug delivery offers an attractive alternative to oral and other systemic routes of delivery, allowing for the drug substances to reach the systemic circulation across the skin barrier. Transdermal drug delivery systems can be beneficial in preventing the hepatic first pass effect of drugs, eliminating peak and valley plasma drug concentrations, which are usually associated with the oral and injectable drug delivery, avoiding the degradation of drugs in GI tract, and, in general, being non-invasive and convenient to administer [14]. ARV drug substances may potentially be delivered through the transdermal route in a consistent and sustained manner (e.g., zero order release kinetics), which would provide several advantages over the other delivery systems that have been explored so far [15]. Being non-invasive and much easier to apply, without the intervention of a health care provider, transdermal patches may provide more user adherence than the injectable or implantable delivery systems that are currently under investigation. Additionally, transdermal patches can be easily discontinued if the need arises, making them safer to use. The aim of this study was to develop and characterize transdermal patches for the delivery of ARV agents, in particular TAF, and investigate its permeation through human epidermis.

There are generally two types of passive transdermal patches, namely, matrix (drug-in-adhesive) and reservoir. The matrix-based transdermal patch, which was the system of choice in this study, consists of a release liner, an adhesive matrix, and an impermeable backing membrane. In addition to the ease of use and manufacturability, as well as the acceptable cost of goods, one of the significant advantages of matrix type transdermal patches when compared to reservoir patches is the absence of dose dumping [16]. The matrix transdermal patches are usually prepared using organic solvent based pressure sensitive adhesives (PSAs), such as acrylate copolymer, silicone, polyisobutylene (PIB), either alone or in combination with each other [17]. Drug substance can be either dissolved or dispersed in the adhesive matrix, resulting in clear/transparent/translucent or suspension patches, respectively.

From a transdermal patch development perspective, drugs with low molecular weight (<500 Da), suitable melting point (<250 °C), and moderate log P (1–3) are ideal for passive permeation through skin. With a molecular weight of 476.47 g/mol, melting point of 279 °C, and having a logP =1.8, as calculated using chemicalize software (MarvinSketch: version 6.2.2, ChemAxon, Hungary, Europe), TAF, the newest prodrug of TFV in the market, is a promising ARV candidate for the development of transdermal patch formulation. TAF is commercially available with oral daily doses of 10 mg and 25 mg [18]. When considering the higher dose of 25 mg and low bioavailability of orally administered TAF (25%) vs transdermal, 6 mg of it would be needed in the systemic circulation [19,20]. However, 8 mg/day was established as the target dose to be on the safer side and keeping a window of deviations.

The aim of this study was to develop a transdermal patch for sustained release of TAF for approximately one-week duration. To our knowledge, transdermal patches comprising of ARV agents for HIV therapy or prophylaxis have not yet been developed. Thus, this is the first study to report such a system. In the present study, transparent acrylate based patches, as well as silicone and PIB based suspension patches of various compositions, were prepared and evaluated for in vitro permeation across human epidermis for seven days. In order to release a TAF dose of 8 mg/day from a 50 cm^2 transdermal patch, the targeted permeation flux was about 7 $\mu g/cm^2/h$. Different chemical enhancers, plasticizers, as well as crystallization inhibiting agents, were included in the patch formulations. Patches were evaluated for stability, skin irritation, and physical characteristics, such as tack, peel, and shear adhesion.

2. Materials and Methods

2.1. Materials

TAF (free base, CAS number: 379270-37-8) was purchased from Pharmacodia Co., LTD (Beijing, China). Backing membranes (Scotchpak™ 9733-2.05 mil polyester film; CoTran™ 9702, 9706, 9728- ethylene vinyl acetate copolymer (EVAC); CoTran™ 9718, 9720 – polyethylene film); and, release liner (Scotchpak™ 1022- 3 mil fluoropolymer coated polyester film) were gifted by 3M (St. Paul, MN, USA). Silicone coated poly-ethylene terephthalate (PET) films (1 mil): 48101-4400B/000, 44916-7300AM/000, and 40987-U4162/000 were procured from Loparex (Cary, NC, USA). Acrylate PSA (DURO-TAK 87-2516) as well as PIB adhesive (DURO-TAK 87-6908) were obtained as gift samples from Henkel Corporation (Dusseldorf, Germany). The Dow Corning Corporation provided Silicone adhesive (BIO-PSA 7-4301) provided as a gift sample (Washington, DC, USA). Mineral oil, oleyl alcohol, polyethylene glycol (PEG), and polyvinyl pyrrolidone (PVP 360) were obtained from Sigma–Aldrich (St. Louis, MO, USA). Propylene glycol (PG) and oleic acid (OA) were purchased from Ekichem (Joliet, IL, USA) and Croda Inc. (Edison, NJ, USA), respectively. Triacetin, octisalate, gentamycin sulfate, tetra hydrogen furan (THF), sodium dihydrogen phosphate, sodium hydroxide, and phosphate buffered saline, pH 7.4 (PBS) were obtained from Fisher Scientific (Pittsburgh, PA, USA). Kollidon® VA64, Kollidon® 90F, and Kollidon® 30LP were purchased from BASF (Florham Park, NJ, USA). Methanol, ethanol, acetonitrile, and trifluoroacetic acid were purchased from Pharmco-aaper (Brookfield, CT, USA). Dermatomed human cadaver skin was obtained from New York Fire Fighters (New York, NY, USA).

2.2. Methods

2.2.1. Slide Crystallization Studies

TAF was dissolved in methanol (10 mg/mL) and a drop of this solution was placed on a glass slide. Methanol was allowed to evaporate at room temperature (RT) under a fume hood. The drug crystals that were obtained were then observed under Leica DM 750 optical microscope (Leica Microsystems Inc., Buffalo Grove, IL, USA). The DFC-295 camera, which was attached to the microscope, was used to capture images at magnifications of 10× or 20× (as specified). Similar procedure was used to determine the saturation solubility of TAF in different adhesives (DURO-TAK 87-2516, DURO-TAK 87-6908, and BIO-PSA 7-4301), solution of 5% (*w*/*w*) OA in DURO-TAK 87-2516, as well as in the additives: PVP 360, Kollidon® VA64, Kollidon® 90F, and Kollidon® 30LP. For solubility studies in adhesives, blends of different concentrations of TAF in adhesives, ranging from 1–12% *w*/*w* (dry weight) were prepared and a drop of the transparent blends (with completely dissolved drug) was individually placed on glass slides and kept in a flameproof oven at 100 °C for 30 min. for the evaporation of the solvents in the adhesives. Similarly, different blends with TAF concentration, ranging from 3–5% (*w*/*w*) in a mixture of 5% (*w*/*w*) OA in DURO-TAK 87-2516 (dry weight basis), were prepared and a drop of each of the solutions was placed on the glass slides and then exposed to the same drying conditions, as mentioned above. In order to determine the solubility of TAF in different additives, the two components were weighed in the following ratios (% *w*/*w*): 1:9, 2:8, 3:7, 4:6, 5:5, 6:4, 7:3, 8:2, 9:1, and then dissolved in methanol.

A drop of each of these solutions was individually mounted on glass slides and observed for crystals after allowing for the evaporation of methanol at RT. The appearance of crystals in all of the test samples was observed for a week before concluding the saturation solubility of TAF in different components. The latter was indicated by the highest concentration at which no crystals were observed [21,22]. The percentages of solid content that were used to calculate the wet weight of adhesives were 41.5% for DURO-TAK 87-2516, 38% for DURO-TAK 87-6908, and 60% for BIO-PSA 7-4301.

2.2.2. Preparation of Drug in Adhesive Patches of TAF

Formulation of Acrylate-Based Patches

Pre-determined amounts of TAF, adhesives, and additives (OA, oleyl alcohol, PG, octisalate, triacetin, as specified in Table 1) were weighed into glass jars with airtight lids to minimize the loss of organic solvents. For the patch formulations AP4 to AP11, excipients, such as PVP 360, Kollidon® VA64, Kollidon® 90F, and Kollidon® 30LP were separately dissolved in methanol and the solutions were then added to the mixture of adhesive and other excipients. The blends were kept overnight on the rotary mixer (Preiser Scientific Inc., St. Albans, WV, USA). Table 1 shows the compositions of the different acrylate based TAF patches. Solid content % of 41.5 was used for the calculation of the wet weight of DURO-TAK 87-2516 for the formulations. The homogenous mixtures were then casted on the release liner (fluoropolymer coated side of Scotchpak™ 1022) using a Gardner film casting knife (BYK-AG-4300 series, Columbia, MD, USA). The target coat weight of different patches varied from 100–400 gsm (grams per square meter). The casted sheets were dried in a flameproof oven at 95 °C for 40 min. After drying, they were laminated using Scotchpak™ 9733 (backing membrane) with the help of a roller, ensuring that no air pockets were formed. The 200 gsm and 400 gsm patches were made by preparing one 100 gsm patch and then stacking 1 and 3, 100 gsm cast films (coated on release liner), respectively, on that one by one, after removing the liner of the previous laminate.

Table 1. Composition of acrylate based Tenofovir alafenamide fumarate (TAF) transdermal patches.

Properties	Patch Formulation Codes														
	AP1	AP2	AP3	AP4	AP5	AP6	AP7	AP8	AP9	AP10	AP11	AP12	AP13	AP14	AP15
Coat weight (gsm)	200	200	200	100	100	100	100	100	100	100	100	400	400	400	400
Composition	**Components (% Dry Weight, *w/w*)**														
TAF	2	3	4	5	10	15	10	10	10	7.5	7.5	2	2	2	2
OA	5	5	5	5	5	5	5	5	5	5	5	5	5	5	-
DURO-TAK 87-2516	93	92	91	87.86	80.71	73.57	83.89	83.89	83.89	77.50	79.29	83	83	79.5	83
PVP 360	-	-	-	2.14	4.29	6.43	-	-	-	5	-	-	-	-	-
Kollidon® VA64	-	-	-	-	-	-	1.11	-	-	-	-	-	-	-	-
Kollidon® 90 F	-	-	-	-	-	-	-	1.11	-	-	-	-	-	-	-
Kollidon® 30 LP	-	-	-	-	-	-	-	-	1.11	-	3.21	-	-	-	-
Oleyl alcohol	-	-	-	-	-	-	-	-	-	-	-	5	-	-	10
PG	-	-	-	-	-	-	-	-	-	5	5	5	5	5	5
Triacetin	-	-	-	-	-	-	-	-	-	-	-	-	5	-	-
Octisalate	-	-	-	-	-	-	-	-	-	-	-	-	-	8.5	-

Table 2. Composition and manufacturing parameters of the silicone based TAF suspension transdermal patches.

Properties	Patch Formulation Codes													
	SP1	SP2	SP3	SP4	SP5	SP6	SP7	SP8	SP9	SP10	SP11	SP12	SP13	SP14
Composition of matrix	Components (% Dry Weight, *w/w*)													
TAF	15	15	15	15	15	15	15	15	15	5	10	20	25	15
OA	5	5	5	5	5	5	5	5	5	5	5	5	5	5
Oleyl alcohol	-	10	10	10	10	10	10	10	10	10	10	10	10	-
Mineral oil	14	14	14	14	14	14	14	14	14	14	14	14	14	14
BIO-PSA 7-4301	66	56	56	56	56	56	56	56	56	66	61	51	46	-
DURO-TAK 87-6908	-	-	-	-	-	-	-	-	-	-	-	-	-	66
Coat weight (gsm)	~100	~250	~250	~250	~250	~250	~300	~300	~300	~350	~350	~200	~200	~50
Release liner	Fluoro-polymer coated side of Scotchpak™ 1022	Uncoated side of Scotchpak™ 1022												Fluoro-polymer coated side of Scotchpak™ 1022
Backing membrane	Scotchpak™ 9733 (polyester)	Scotchpak™ 9733 (polyester)	CoTran™ 9702, 9706, 9728 (EVAC)	CoTran™ 9720 (poly-ethylene)	CoTran™ 9718 (poly-ethylene)	CoTran™ 9718 (poly-ethylene)	Silicone coated PET film (48101)	Silicone coated PET film (44916)	Silicone coated PET film (40987)	Silicone coated PET film (48101)				Scotchpak™ 9733 (polyester)
Homogenization speed (rpm) and time (min) before addition of adhesive	5000; 3	30,000; 20				32,000; 30	32,000; 5							5000; 3
Homogenization speed (rpm) and time (min) after addition of adhesive	5000; 1	30,000; 1				32,000; 1	15,000; 1							5000; 1
Drying conditions	78 °C for 10 min	Air drying for 5 min. followed by drying at 78 °C for 15 min					Air drying, 15 min							78 °C for 10 min

Microscopy of Acrylate-Based Patches

The prepared acrylate patches were punched and stored at 40 °C, RT, and −20 °C, and then observed for the occurrence of crystallization under an optical microscope (Leica DM 750) at predetermined time points for up to six months [23]. In case of patches that showed the appearance of crystals in the first week of storage at RT or 40 °C, microscopic observations after storage at −20 °C were not performed.

Formulation of TAF Suspension Patches

The suspension patches of TAF were prepared using silicone (BIO-PSA 7-4301) and PIB (DURO-TAK 87-6908) adhesive. TAF was first levigated with mineral oil and other additives (OA and oleyl alcohol) were then added and mixed using Benchmixer™ (Benchmark Scientific Inc., Edison, NJ, USA). Heptane was then added to the blend and the drug suspension was homogenized using a high-speed homogenizer (OmniTHQ, Omni International, NW, GA, USA). Heptane was then allowed to evaporate at 90 °C for 5 min. and the adhesive was added to the remaining mixture. The final blend was allowed to mix overnight, then homogenized for 1 min, and then casted on the release liner. It was dried in a flameproof oven and the casted film was then laminated with the backing membrane. Table 2 elaborates on the compositions, homogenization conditions, release liners, backing membranes, and drying conditions employed for the formulation of different TAF suspension patches.

Visual Observations of the TAF Suspension Patches

The suspension patches with varying composition and material components were prepared and observed for the following visual changes for about two weeks: phase separation, contraction/shrinkage of the film, residue on release liner after peeling, ease of peeling off the patches applied on human skin, as well as any residue on skin after removal of the patches.

Effect of Homogenization on Particle Size of TAF

The particle size of TAF, before and after homogenization, was determined using optical microscopy. For the former, pure TAF was dispersed in heptane and a drop of the same was placed on a glass slide and observed under optical microscope. For the size of TAF particles after homogenization, a drop of the suspension, before the addition of the adhesive, was mounted on glass slide and observed under the optical microscope. Size of particles (n = 50) was measured using ImageJ 1.41o software (National Institutes of Health, USA) and it has been reported as average ± SD.

2.2.3. Coat Weight and TAF Content of the Patches

Punching and weighing 4.91 cm^2 or 1 cm^2 laminates (from different areas of the patch, n = 3) using analytical balance (Mettler Toledo, Columbus, OH, USA) and subtracting the weight of equal sized respective release liner and backing membrane from the same determined the coat weight of the prepared patches. For the determination of drug content in the patches, the punched patches were placed in 10 mL of THF after removal of the release liner and allowed to shake overnight. The solutions were then diluted ten times with methanol and centrifuged at 13,400 rpm for 10 min. The supernatants were then analyzed while using high performance liquid chromatography (HPLC) to quantitate the amount of TAF in the same. Comparing the experimental and theoretical drug content values used for processing indicated the stability of TAF after exposure to high temperature conditions. The latter were calculated based on the targeted coat weight for each laminate and the percentage of drug loaded (dry weight% when considering the solvent loss upon drying) in the formulation blend. Results have been reported as average ± SD.

2.2.4. In Vitro Skin Permeation Studies

In vitro permeation studies of TAF from transdermal patches through human epidermis were performed for seven days using in vitro vertical Franz diffusion cells (PermeGear, Inc., Hellertown, PA, USA), providing an effective diffusion area of 0.64 cm^2 ($n = 6$).

Separation of Epidermis

For each permeation study, human epidermis was freshly isolated from dermatomed human skin by the heat-separation method. Skin was immersed in 10 mM PBS, pH 7.4 for 2 min. at 60 °C. Epidermis was then carefully manually peeled off, with the help of forceps and spatula, and thereafter cut into pieces of suitable size for mounting on the Franz cells [24].

Epidermal Integrity and Thickness Assessment

Resistance of human epidermis was measured in order to select the pieces with acceptable initial barrier integrity for the in vitro permeation study [25]. This was carried out with the use of silver-silver chloride electrodes that were attached to a digital multimeter: 34410A 6 $\frac{1}{2}$ (Agilent Technologies, CA, USA) as well as an arbitrary waveform generator (Agilent 33220A, 20 MHz Function). Epidermis was mounted on the Franz diffusion cells and left for equilibration for 15 min. Phosphate buffer, pH 6.0, was then added in the donor (300 µL) and receptor (5 mL), respectively. Following equilibration, silver and silver chloride electrodes were placed in the receptor and donor compartment, respectively. Load resistor (R_L) attachment was in series with skin, and the voltage drop across the entire circuit and skin (V_S) was displayed on the multimeter (V_O). The following formula was used to measure the skin resistance (R_S):

$$Rs = Vs\, R_L / \ (Vo \ - \ Vs)$$

where, V_O and R_L were 100 mV and 100 kΩ, respectively. Epidermis pieces with electrical resistance of more than 10 kΩ were selected for the permeation study. A thickness gauge measured the thickness of the selected epidermis pieces (Cedarhurst, NY, USA).

Selection of the Receptor Solution

The stability of TAF in different solvent systems (10 mM PBS, pH 7.4; phosphate buffer, pH 6.0; 10 mM PBS, pH 7.4: PEG 400 - 1:1; PEG 400) at 37 °C was assessed in order to select a suitable receptor solution for the seven day permeation studies. For this study, different concentrations of TAF were prepared (0.5, 5, 50 µg/mL) in the above specified solvents and kept at 37 °C. The solutions were analyzed for drug content at 0, and after 24 h using HPLC. The solubility of TAF in the selected receptor media (phosphate buffer, pH 6.0) was determined to ensure the maintenance of sink conditions. For this purpose, excess drug was added to 1.0 mL of the buffer and it was allowed to shake for 24 h at RT. Thereafter, the solution was filtered using 0.22 µm syringe filters (Cell treat Scientific Products, Shirley, MA, USA) and analyzed using HPLC after suitable dilution.

In Vitro Skin Permeation Set Up

The permeation of TAF from different transdermal patch formulations (donor), through human epidermis was investigated using the Franz diffusion cell set up as mentioned in Table 3. While taking the stability of TAF, as well as the maintenance of sink conditions, into consideration, phosphate buffer, pH 6.0 having gentamycin sulfate (80 mg/L) as an anti-microbial agent for the seven day permeation study [22], was selected as the receptor compartment. The temperature of the receptor phase was maintained at 37 °C and it was constantly stirred at 600 rpm. The freshly isolated epidermis pieces were clamped between the donor and receptor compartments. After measuring the skin resistance through the procedure described above, phosphate buffer from the donor was pipetted out, epidermis was removed, placed flat on a glass plate, and then dried with the help of Kimwipes. The release liners of the patches (of size enough to cover the diffusion area) were removed and the latter were applied carefully on the dried epidermis, such that the adhesive layer of the patch was adhered to the stratum corneum side of the skin. The glass rod was rolled on the patches to ensure their adherence to the skin. The epidermis pieces with the applied patches were then mounted between the donor and receptor compartment and the entire set up was secured in place using a clamp. Receptor (0.3 mL) was sampled at 0, 2, 4, 6, and 8 h with replacement with fresh receptor solution and entire receptor (5 mL) was removed and replaced with fresh buffer at 24, 48, 72, 96, 120, 144, and 168 h. All of the samples were analyzed for TAF content using HPLC. As human skin from different donors was employed for the different permeation studies, the in vitro permeation data was normalized using the flux that was obtained by repeating permeation of a previously evaluated patch, within every new permeation study. Permeation flux was calculated from the slope of the linear profile of amount of TAF permeated/ cm^2 and time. The average of all the replicates ± SE has been reported. The calculated flux was extrapolated to patch size of 50 cm^2 and time duration of 24 h, in order to calculate the dose administered/day.

Table 3. Coat weight and drug content of TAF patches.

Patch Formulation Code	COAT WEIGHT (mg/cm^2), mean ± SD		DRUG CONTENT (mg/0.64 cm^2), mean ± SD	
	Targeted	Experimental	Theoretical	Experimental
AP1	20	18.20 ± 1.88	0.256	0.25 ± 0.02
AP5	10	7.10 ± 0.14	0.640	0.53 ± 0.05
AP12	40	37.37 ± 6.94	0.512	0.478 ± 0.09
AP13	40	40.80 ± 1.47	0.512	0.522 ± 0.02
AP14	40	44.17 ± 4.96	0.512	0.565 ± 0.06
AP15	40	40.43 ± 2.35	0.512	0.643 ± 0.106
SP1	10	12.30 ± 3.15	0.96	1.35 ± 0.28
SP5	25	24.23 ± 2.88	2.40	2.52 ± 0.19
SP6	25	20.99 ± 5.80	2.40	2.17 ± 0.55
SP7	30	29.60 ± 1.94	2.88	2.94 ± 0.65
SP10	35	34.15 ± 3.75	1.12	1.11 ± 0.06
SP11	35	36.05 ± 1.29	2.24	2.53 ± 0.11
SP12	20	16.43 ± 0.39	2.56	2.31 ± 0.16
SP13	20	18.29 ± 1.82	3.20	3.02 ± 0.14
SP14	5	4.54 ± 0.55	0.48	0.80 ± 0.06

2.2.5. In Vitro Drug Release Studies

The release profile of TAF from the optimized patch (SP7) was evaluated using Paddle over Disk, USP V dissolution bath apparatus (Sotax AT7 Smart, Sotax AG, Switzerland) [26,27]. This study was performed during week 1 and after 1.5 and 3 months of patch preparation and storage at RT and 40 °C. The patches (0.712 cm^2) were applied on the teflon mesh and then placed on the glass discs, such that the release surface was facing upwards (n = 3). The distance between the paddle and the surface of the disk was about 25 mm. The disks were placed at the bottom of the vessels containing 500 mL of phosphate buffer (pH 6) as the receptor media. Temperature of the media was set at 32 ± 0.5 °C and the paddle speed was 100 rpm. The samples (1 mL) were drawn at 0, 2, 4, 6, 8 h with replacement with fresh media and the entire receptor (500 mL) was removed and replaced with fresh buffer at 24, 48, 72, 96, 120, 144, 168 h. All the samples were analyzed for TAF content using HPLC. Results have been presented as average cumulative amount of TAF released ± SE. The average percentage of TAF released after 7 days from the tested patches has been reported as well and was calculated for each replicate using the following equation:

$$\%TAF\ released = \left(\frac{Cumulative\ amount\ of\ TAF\ released\ over\ 7\ days}{Total\ amount\ of\ TAF\ in\ patch\ tested}\right) \times 100\%$$

2.2.6. Coat Thickness, Coat Weight, and Drug Content of Optimized Patch

Coat thickness of the 1 cm^2 laminates of SP7 (from different areas of the patch) was determined by measuring the patch thickness using a thickness gauge (Cedarhurst, NY, USA), and then subtracting the thickness of the release liner and backing membrane from the former. The coat weight and drug content of the optimized patch were determined using the procedure described in Section 2.2.3. These parameters were determined at day 1 and after 1.5 and 3 months of storage of patch at RT and 40 °C (n = 4–6).

2.2.7. Quantitative Analysis

A UV detection based reverse phase HPLC method was used for quantitative analysis of TAF. Waters Alliance 2695 separation module (Milford, MA, USA) that was attached to a 2996 photodiode array detector was used. Isocratic elution was performed on Phenomenex Luna 5μ C8 (2) 100A, 250 × 4.6 mm (Phenomenex, CA, USA), at a flow rate of 1.0 mL/min. and column temperature of 35 °C, after injecting 50 μL of sample. The mobile phase consisted of acetonitrile (phase A) and 0.1% v/v trifluoroacetic acid in DI water (phase B) in the ratio of 30:70. The run time was 12 min. and the retention time of TAF was around 7.4 min. The drug standards were prepared in the receptor solution and were detected at wavelength of 262 nm. The precision limit of detection and quantification were 0.01 μg/mL and 0.03 μg/mL, respectively, and linearity was observed in the concentration range of 0.1–50 μg/mL (R^2 = 0.9999).

2.2.8. Physical Characterizations of Optimized Patch

Peel Adhesion

The 180° peel adhesion tester (ChemInstruments, Fairfield, OH, USA) was used to evaluate the peel adhesion force (force that is required to peel away the transdermal patch from dermatomed human cadaver skin) [28]. The instrument was calibrated for experimental parameters, such as tension, speed, and peel length with a load cell weighing 50 g prior to running the test patches. Transdermal patches with the length and width of 3.0 inches and 1.0 inch, respectively, were cut. One end of the adhesive coated backing membrane was adhered to the human skin affixed on the stainless steel plate and the other end was attached to load cell grip. The average force that is required to peel off the adhesive film was measured and recorded during the first week after patch preparation at RT and after three months of its storage at RT and 40 °C (n = 3) as well. The results have been shown as average ± SD.

Tack Properties

A texture analyzer (Texture Technologies Corp, Marietta, GA, USA) consisting of a 7 mm probe was used to determine the adhesion efficiency of the TAF suspension patch [29]. Prior to running the test samples, the instrument was calibrated and parameters, such as target force, approach speed, return speed, as well as distance and hold time, were optimized. A transdermal patch (width and length of about 1.0 inch × 1.0 inch, respectively) was cut and adhered on to the sample holder after removal of release liner. As the test run was initiated, the probe was allowed to touch the adhesive film with a target force and hold time of 50 g and 10 s, respectively. This resulted in the creation of a bond between the probe surface and transdermal patch. Further, as the probe was pulled off, it resulted in debonding between the two surfaces. Parameters, such as work of adhesion, positive area, and separation distance were hence recorded during the first week after patch preparation at RT and after three months of storage at RT and 40 °C (n = 3). The results have been shown as average ± SD.

2.2.9. Evaluation of Skin Irritation Potential of Optimized Patch

An in vitro EpiDerm™ skin irritation test (EPI-200-SIT) with a three-dimensional (3D) in vitro reconstructed epidermis (RhE) model (MatTek Corporation 200 Homer Ave, Ashland, MA 01721) was employed to assess the cell viability of skin while using a methyl thiazolyl tetrazolium viability assay [30] after the application of patch SP7. Three replicates of each of the patches were tested and compared to a negative control (Dulbecco's phosphate buffered saline) and positive control (5% aqueous sodium dodecyl sulfate solution). After the removal of the release liners, patches were adhered to the tissues and kept in an incubator for 1 h at 37 °C. Afterwards, the patches were removed from the surface of tissue inserts, the inserts were washed using PBS, and then transferred to a fresh assay medium for 24 h incubation. The media for the inserts was exchanged and incubated again for 18 h. This was followed by transferring the inserts into yellow methyl thiazolyl tetrazolium solution and incubation for 3 h. During the 3 h incubation, mitochondrial metabolism was expected to occur and it was detected by the formation of a purple-blue formazan salt. The plate with the inserts was filled with isopropyl alcohol (2 mL) and kept on a shaker at 120 rpm for 2 -3 h. The aliquots were then transferred to a 96 well enzyme linked immunosorbent assay (ELISA) plate and the optical density of the extracted formazan salt was measured at 560 nm while using a Synergy HT plate reader (BioTek Instruments, Inc, Winooski, VT, USA).

2.2.10. Data Analysis

Microsoft Excel and SPSS software package version 21.0 (IBM, USA) were used for analyzing data. Single factor analysis of variance (ANOVA) and Student's *t*-test were used for statistical analysis and a p value of less than 0.05 was considered for concluding significant difference between the test groups.

3. Results and Discussion

3.1. Slide Crystallization Studies

Adhesiveness is a fundamental property of transdermal patches that is essentially required to ensure the complete contact between the entire surface area of the patch and skin during the wear period, for the efficient delivery of drugs. PSAs deform upon the application of slight pressure, provide intimate contact with surfaces by establishing inter-atomic and molecular forces at the interface, and are thus used for the preparation of transdermal patches [31]. A good adhesive is one that does not leave any residue upon removal, is easy to use, stable to environmental changes, non-irritant and non-sensitive to skin, compatible with other formulation components, allows sufficient drug solubility, and possesses the necessary adhesive properties, such as tack, shear, and skin adhesion [22,32]. Acrylic, silicone, and PIB-based adhesives are most commonly used in the design of transdermal patches [33]. Therefore, all three types of adhesives (acrylate: DURO-TAK 87-2516, silicone: BIO-PSA 7-4301, and PIB: DURO-TAK 87-6908) were explored for formulation development of TAF transdermal patches.

The determination of saturation solubility of TAF in different adhesives was required to determine the maximum amount of dissolvable drug that could be incorporated in the adhesives. Slide crystallization is a preliminary and relatively fast method that is employed as an alternate to preparing complete patches for estimating the solubility of drugs in adhesives [21]. Images of pure TAF, as observed under the microscope at a magnification of 10×, are shown in Figure 1A. TAF, at a concentration of 1% *w*/*w* (dry weight), was not soluble in silicone (BIO-PSA 7-4301) as well as PIB (DURO-TAK 87-6908) adhesive, even before the evaporation of solvents. Therefore, due to poor solubility in these adhesives, further slide crystallization studies were not performed with them. However, TAF blends at a concentration of 1–12% *w*/*w* (dry weight) in DURO-TAK 87-2516 were successfully prepared and drops of these were allowed to dry on glass slides and images of dried drug-adhesive blends, as observed under the microscope, are shown in Figure 1B–F. TAF at concentrations of 3–12% *w*/*w* was observed to immediately crystallize after drying (Figure 1B–D). However, 2% *w*/*w* TAF blend crystallized after three days (Figure 1E) and 1% *w*/*w* blend did not crystallize, even after seven days at RT (Figure 1F). Therefore, the saturation solubility of TAF in DURO-TAK 87-2516 was observed to be between 1–2% *w*/*w* (dry weight). Moreover, the addition of 5% *w*/*w* OA to DURO-TAK 87-2516 adhesive enhanced the solubility of TAF to about 4% *w*/*w*.

The blend containing 5% *w*/*w* TAF in adhesive-OA blend showed crystals after seven days, whereas the 4% *w*/*w* TAF solution did not, as shown in Figure 1H,G, respectively. Further, in order to select the composition ratios of different crystallization inhibitors and TAF for patch formulations with 5%, 10%, and 15% *w*/*w* TAF (higher than its solubility in adhesive alone), different ratios of the two components were tested in slide crystallization studies. The mixtures of TAF and PVP 360 in the ratios of 9:1 and 8:2 showed the appearance of crystals after seven days, but the compositions with TAF:PVP ratios from 7:3 to 1:9 did not show any crystals (Figure 1I–K). All of the other crystallization inhibitors (Kollidon® VA64, Kollidon® 90F, and Kollidon® 30LP) with TAF, each in the ratio of 1:9, did not show appearance of any crystals after seven days. Therefore, ratios of 7:3 (TAF:PVP 360) and 9:1 (TAF: Kollidon® VA64 or Kollidon® 90F or Kollidon® 30LP), comprising of the lowest amount of PVP with the potential to inhibit crystallization, were selected for the preparation of patches containing 5% *w*/*w* or higher concentrations of TAF.

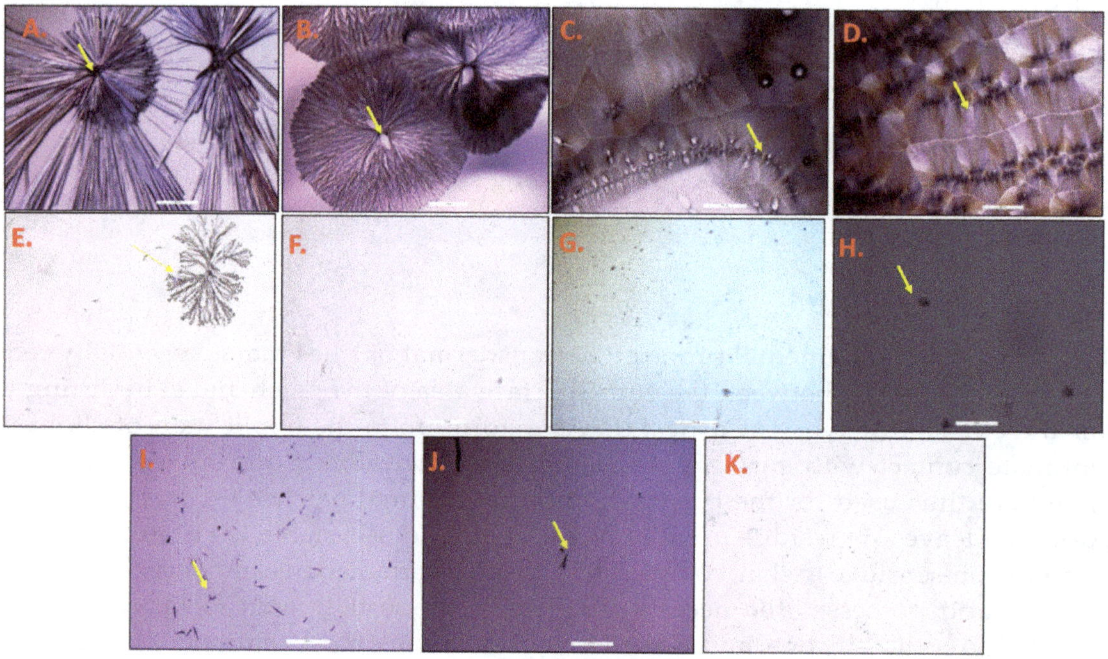

Figure 1. Images of slide crystallization studies, under optical microscope. (**A**). Pure TAF (at 10×). (**B–D**). TAF crystals in DURO-TAK 87-2516 immediately after evaporation of organic solvent at 10×: (**B**) 3% *w*/*w* TAF (**C**). 5% *w*/*w* TAF (**D**). 12% *w*/*w* TAF. (**E**). 2% *w*/*w* TAF in DURO-TAK 87-2516, 3 days after evaporation of organic solvent (10×). (**F**). 1% *w*/*w* TAF in DURO-TAK 87-2516, 7 days after evaporation of organic solvent (20×). (**G**). 4% *w*/*w* TAF in 5% *w*/*w* OA in DURO-TAK 87-2516 (10×). (**H**). 5% *w*/*w* TAF in 5% *w*/*w* OA in DURO-TAK 87-2516 (20×). (**I**). TAF:PVP 360 (9:1) under 20×. (**J**). TAF:PVP 360 (8:2) under 10×. (**K**).TAF:PVP 360 (7:3) under 20× (arrows depicting TAF crystals).

3.2. *Formulation of TAF Acrylate Patches*

Slide crystallization is a faster means for estimating the saturation solubility of drugs in adhesives. However, the thickness of the actual patches, as well as processing conditions and scale up procedures, may affect the phenomenon of crystallization. Therefore, based on the observations of slide crystallization studies, different transparent TAF patches were prepared in DURO-TAK 87-2516 adhesive, as shown in Table 1 and observed for crystallization for six months under the microscope. The solubility of TAF in 5% *w*/*w* OA in DURO-TAK 87-2516 blend (dry weight basis), as determined by slide crystallization studies, was found to be about 4%. Therefore, 2%, 3%, and 4% TAF patches (200 gsm) were prepared in this matrix (AP1, AP2, AP3, as specified in Table 1). Due to the solubility limitations of TAF in the adhesive, it was not possible to prepare patches with higher drug concentrations in the absence of crystallization inhibiting agents that act as solubilizers and anti-nucleants. The use of different grades of PVP as crystallization inhibitors has been well-reported in literature and some of them were, hence, investigated in the current study [22,34,35]. In order to prepare 100 gsm patches containing higher percentage of TAF (5%, 10%, and 15% *w*/*w*—AP4, AP5, AP6, respectively), PVP 360 was added as a solubilizer and crystallization inhibitor, with drug and PVP in the ratio of 7:3, in addition to OA. Patch 'AP10' was prepared to investigate the effect of enhancing the percentage of PVP 360, as well as the addition of 5% *w*/*w* PG in the 7.5% TAF patch on drug crystallization (100 gsm). Drug and PVP were in the ratio of 6:4 (*w*/*w*) in this formulation. Formulations AP7 to AP9 included the addition of other grades of PVP (Kollidon® VA64, Kollidon® 90F, and Kollidon® 30LP) as solubilizers and crystallization inhibitors with TAF (10% *w*/*w*), in the ratio of 1:9 (PVP: TAF) in OA and DURO-TAK 87-2516 blend. Patch AP11 (100 gsm) was prepared to investigate the effect of enhancing the percentage of Kollidon® 30LP as well as the addition of 5% *w*/*w* PG in the 7.5% TAF patch on drug crystallization. Drug and Kollidon® 30LP were in the ratio of 7:3 (*w*/*w*) in this formulation. Further, patches AP12 to AP14 (400 gsm) containing 2% *w*/*w* TAF were prepared to evaluate the effect of combination of permeation enhancers (5% *w*/*w* OA+ 5% *w*/*w* PG + 5% *w*/*w* oleyl alcohol, 5% *w*/*w* OA+ 5% *w*/*w* PG + 5% *w*/*w* triacetin, 5% *w*/*w* OA+ 5% *w*/*w* PG + 8.5% *w*/*w* octisalate, respectively), as well as increasing the coat weight on the skin permeation of TAF and comparing it with that of AP1. Further, the AP15 (400 gsm) patch was prepared by replacing 5% *w*/*w* OA in AP12 with 5% oleyl alcohol, such that the total oleyl alcohol content was 10% *w*/*w* in this formulation. The transdermal permeation enhancing effects of OA [36–38], oleyl alcohol [39,40], triacetin [41–43], and octisalate [44,45] are well-known and they have been reported in literature, and thus these chemical enhancers were selected for the formulation development of TAF patches.

Microscopy and Stability Assessment of TAF Acrylate Patches

During the storage period, changes in temperature can alter the thermodynamic activity of the transdermal patch formulation, and they result in precipitation or crystallization or changes in the crystal habit of the active ingredient. Therefore, during stability testing, patches are exposed to stress and real world storage conditions that are representative of the product's proposed marketing conditions [46]. The stability of the acrylate based TAF patches was assessed in terms of the occurrence of crystallization over a period of time at different temperature conditions. Table 4 shows the microscopic observations of the same after six months. Figure 2 shows the representative images of TAF crystals in transdermal patches.

Table 4. Microscopy observations of acrylate based TAF transdermal patch formulations up to 6 months.

Patch Codes	Temperature		
	−20 °C	RT	40 °C
AP1	NO	NO	NO
AP2	NO	Crystals after three weeks	Crystals after three weeks
AP3	NO	Crystals after two weeks	Crystals after two weeks
AP4	NO	Crystals after three weeks	Crystals after three weeks
AP5	NO	Crystals after two weeks	Crystals after two weeks
AP6	Crystals after 2 months	Crystals after 9 days	Crystals after one week
AP7	Not observed	Crystals in first week	Crystals in first week
AP8	Not observed	Crystals in first week	Crystals in first week
AP9	Not observed	Smaller crystals than AP7 and AP8 after 12 days	Crystals in first week (2–3 crystals)
AP10	NO	Crystals after three weeks	Crystals after two weeks
AP11	NO	Crystals after three weeks	Crystals after two weeks
AP12	NO	NO	NO
AP13	NO	NO	NO
AP14	NO	NO	NO
AP15	NO	NO	NO

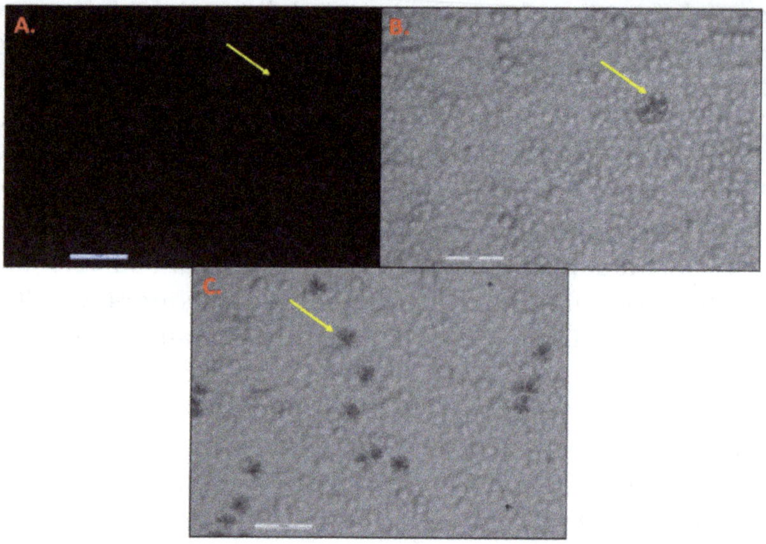

Figure 2. TAF crystals in acrylate based transdermal patches (at 10×). (**A**) Patch AP5 (crystals at 40 °C after 2 weeks). (**B**) Patch AP9 (crystals at RT in 12 days). (**C**) Patch AP8 (crystals at RT in first week). Arrows depict TAF crystals

Patches with 2% *w/w* TAF were found to be stable and they did not show crystals at all of the tested temperature conditions, even after six months, as the drug concentrations were within the saturation solubility limits in these matrices. However, in order to incorporate drugs in amounts that are higher than its saturation solubility in the adhesive alone, crystallization inhibitors were included in the patches. Mechanistically, these additives stabilize the systems against crystallization, either due to enhancing the solubility of the drug or by aiding adsorption of drug crystals in the adhesive matrix. PVP has been previously demonstrated as one of the most effective additives in inhibiting drug crystallization in patch formulations acting by the formation of amorphous co-precipitates with the drugs [35,47–49]. Additionally, it has been previously shown that PVP inhibits the crystallization of drugs by being adsorbed on the growing crystal surfaces [35,50]. Therefore, different grades of PVP were incorporated in patches containing higher concentrations of TAF. However, patches with 15% *w/w* TAF (AP6) and PVP 360, crystallized in less than ten days at RT and 40 °C, depicting the inability of PVP 360 to inhibit crystallization at high drug levels. At lower drug concentrations (5% and 10% *w/w* TAF, AP4, and AP5, respectively), the addition of PVP 360 in the same ratio with TAF (3:7, *w/w*), as in AP6, slowed down the process of crystallization, where it was observed after three and two weeks, respectively, at RT as well as 40 °C. Further, increasing the PVP:TAF ratio to 4:6 (*w/w*) and adding PG as additional solubilizer in patch AP10 formulation did not delay the process of crystallization further and crystals were still observed in less than a month as well at RT and 40 °C. Interestingly, these patches did not show the presence of any crystals, even after six months at −20 ° C. Further, other crystallization inhibitors (Kollidon® VA64, Kollidon® 90F) were found to be ineffective, as crystals were visible during the first week after storage of all these patches at RT as well as 40 °C. However, the crystals that were observed in patch AP9 (containing Kollidon® 30LP) were smaller than AP7 and AP8 and they were observed after about two weeks at RT and after first week at 40 °C. Therefore, patch AP11 was formulated with reduced drug concentration (7.5% *w/w* TAF), a higher amount of Kollidon® 30LP than AP9, and the addition of PG, and showed a slower appearance of crystals (observed after three weeks at RT). However, the inability of PVP to prevent the appearance of TAF crystals in the transdermal patch formulation for longer time duration may be attributed to the difficulty in the molecular interactions between PVP and growing TAF crystals, because of the higher viscosity of the patch formulation as compared to a single drop of blend on the slides [35]. Overall, although most of the studies showed PVP to be an effective drug crystallization inhibitor, there are a few findings regarding ineffectiveness of some grades of PVP. For example, Weng et al. reported that PVP K30 was found to be ineffective in inhibiting the crystallization of risperidone in drug-in-acrylate adhesive transdermal patches. However, in the same study, OA was found to be an effective crystallization inhibitor [34]. In this study, all the compositions of 2% *w/w* TAF transdermal patches were found to be stable at all of the temperature conditions for more than six months, which may be attributed to drug solubility in the adhesive matrix being lower than the saturation level, as well as the crystallization inhibiting effect that is conferred by OA. Additionally, the transdermal patches formulated with higher drug concentrations (AP2, AP3, AP4, AP5, AP10, AP11) were only stable at −20 °C.

3.3. Formulation of TAF Suspension Patches

Due to low solubility of TAF in silicone and PIB adhesives, the drug was suspended in the blends of these adhesives with different additives, as elaborated in Table 2. Mineral oil was added as a plasticizer that increases diffusivity of the drug by decreasing the resistance that is offered by the patch matrix [22]. In addition to the plasticizing effect, mineral oil has also been reported as a transdermal permeation enhancer [51]. OA and oleyl alcohol are also well-known chemical penetration enhancers [36–40] that were included in the TAF suspension patches. A number of different silicone based TAF patches were prepared in order to select the optimal type of the release liner and the backing membrane. Homogenization speed and time were also optimized to reduce the particle size of the drug.

Patch SP1 (~100 gsm) was prepared while using the fluoropolymer coated side of Scotchpak™ 1022 and Scotchpak™ 9733 (polyester backing). For TAF suspension patch formulations, SP2-SP13, a higher coat weight (~200–350 gsm) was applied and oleyl alcohol was included as an additional enhancer. For the preparation of SP2 patch, the same release liner and backing membrane as SP1 were initially selected. However, in terms of the TAF suspension patch formulation with oleyl alcohol, it was found that, when the formulation was coated on the fluoropolymer coated side of the liner, it could not come off the release liner, depicting the affinity of the formulation binding to the fluoropolymer coated release liner was more than the polyester backing membrane. Therefore, the formulation was casted on the uncoated side of the release liner (polyester only) and then laminated while using the polyester (Scotchpak™ 9733) backing film. This was an interesting experimental observation, as silicone based transdermal patches are usually casted on the fluoropolymer coated side of release liner in order to have easy release/transfer of the formulation from the liner to backing. Further, when the patch formulation SP2 was peeled off, it was observed that the adhesive layer transiently formed a film on the skin, depicting less affinity of the formulation for polyester backing material.

Therefore, other materials, such as EVAC based (Corona-treated - CoTran™ 9702, 9706, 9728) and polyethylene based (CoTran™ 9720 and CoTran™ 9718), were tried for the optimization of the backing membrane, while the uncoated side of Scotchpak™ 1022 was used as the release liner for the patch formulations, SP3-SP6. The formulation SP5 and SP6, using CoTran™ 9718 as the backing membrane, showed comparatively better peeling characteristics than the SP4 patch. The SP3 patch could not be successfully prepared, as the formulation film did not come off from the liner onto the EVAC backing membranes. Higher speed and duration of homogenization was employed for formulation SP6 when compared to that SP5 in an attempt to investigate the effect of homogenization with different parameters on the drug particle size and skin permeation. However, the issue of the residual film of the formulation on skin was not completely resolved in SP5 and SP6, indicating the requirement of a more compatible backing membrane material to facilitate the peeling off process of the patch formulation. In addition, upon long term storage (after a month), patches SP5 and SP6 showed the contraction of the film and the appearance of streaks.

As was evident from patches SP2-SP6, the silicone-based TAF suspension patch formulation did not have sufficient affinity to the backing membrane materials, including polyester and polyethylene. Therefore, silicone coated PET films (48101-4400B/000, 44916-7300AM/000, and or 40987-U4162/000) were explored as the backing membrane for SP7, SP8, and SP9, respectively. Patch SP7 (containing 15% *w/w* TAF) showed the best efficiency in terms of least resistance and minimal formulation residue, while peeling the patch formulation off from the skin. Hence, patches SP10-13 were prepared while using the same material components and processing parameters as SP7, except that different concentrations of TAF (5, 10, 20, 25% *w*/*w*) were included in these patches. For the preparation of PIB-based TAF suspension patch formulation (SP14), Scotchpak^{TM} 1022 (Fluoropolymer coated side) and Scotchpak^{TM} 9733 were used as the release liner and the backing membrane, respectively.

3.3.1. Visual Observation of TAF Suspension Patches

Table 5 summarizes the details of the visual observations of the different TAF suspension patches. Patches SP1, SP7, SP10-13, and SP14 were observed to be acceptable in terms of the properties that are specified in the table. The visual observations depicted that the addition of oleyl alcohol in the silicone suspension formulation rendered it more lipophilic, and thus provided more affinity or binding with skin. Using a silicone-coated film as a backing membrane resolved the issue of the residual film after peeling off. The PIB patch formulation (SP14) did not have any issues during the peeling off process as compared to the silicone patch formulations.

Table 5. Visual observations of TAF suspension patches.

Formulation Code	Properties				
	Phase Separation	Contraction/Shrinkage of Films	Residue on Release Liner after Peeling	Ease of Peeling Patches off the Skin	Residue on the Glove after Patch Removal
SP1	No	No	No	Yes	No
SP2	No	No	No	Yes	Yes
SP4	No	No	No	Yes	Yes
SP5	No	Yes (after a month)	No	Yes	Not when applied afresh, but if applied after storing for few days
SP6	No	Yes (after a month)	No	Yes	Not when applied afresh, but if applied after storing for few days
SP7	No	No	No	Yes	No
SP8	No	No	No	No	No
SP9	No	No	No	No	No
SP10	No	No	No	Yes	No
SP11	No	No	No	Yes	No
SP12	No	No	No	Yes	No
SP13	No	No	No	Yes	No
SP14	No	No	No	Yes	No

3.3.2. Effect of Homogenization on the Particle Size of TAF

The effect of homogenization parameters on the particle size of TAF was also investigated, in order to eventually evaluate the effect of the particle size of API in the adhesive matrix on the skin permeation. Homogenization is a process that consists of micronizing or reducing the particle size of dispersions by the application of high sheer, pressure, turbulence, as well as acceleration and impact [52]. Decreased particle size would aid in enhancing the solubility of the drug in the adhesive formulation, and therefore improving its permeation rate [53]. The effect of homogenization speed and duration on the particle size of API has been previously reported, and thus similar parameters were selected to reduce the particle size of TAF [54,55]. As reported, homogenization speed is an indicator of the amount of energy that is applied to the system, as determined by the velocity of the rotating mixing heads. Further, the mechanical impingement of the particles against the wall, due to the high acceleration of the fluid and shear stress in the gap between the rotor and stator, leads to the reduction in the particle size of the drug substance [54].

The average particle size of the pure TAF was observed to be 53.39 $\pm$ 16.15 μm under the optical microscope (Figure 3A). After homogenization at 30,000 rpm for 20 min, the particle size of TAF was reduced to 11.51 $\pm$ 2.89 μm ($p < 0.05$) (Figure 3B). Further increasing the speed to 32,000 rpm and the homogenization time to 30 min. significantly reduced the particle size of TAF to 6.0 $\pm$ 1.8 μm as compared to that of homogenization at 30,000 rpm for 20 min. ($p < 0.05$) (Figure 3C). The observation of the reduction in the particle size of API after the increase in the speed and time of homogenization was in concordance with those that were reported previously [54]. As shown in Figure 3C, some of the particles were smaller and were not visible under the microscope, and thus could not be measured using the software. However, it was found that homogenization at 32,000 rpm over 5 min. resulted in a similar reduction in drug particle size (5.28 ± 2.71 μm, Figure 3D) to that of homogenization at 32,000 rpm for 30 min. Collectively, the speed of homogenization had relatively more impact on the reduction in particle size as compared to the duration of the homogenization. Thus, 32,000 rpm and 5 min. were the homogenization parameters that were employed for the formulation of SP7-SP13.

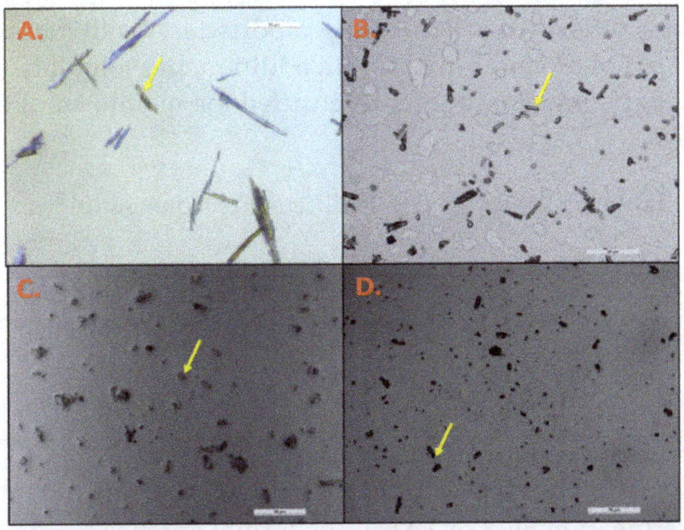

Figure 3. (**A**) Microscopic images of pure TAF particles suspended in heptane; TAF particles in suspension formulation, before addition of adhesive (at 20×) after homogenization at: (**B**) 30,000 rpm for 20 min; (**C**) 32,000 rpm for 30 min; (**D**) 32,000 rpm for 5 min.

3.4. Coat Weight and Drug Content

Coat weight and drug content of the patches evaluated for the in vitro permeation studies were measured and are reported in Table 3. These measured properties are influenced by various factors, such as percentage of non-volatile components in the adhesive blend, scale set-up, surface level of the casting knife, textural properties, of release liner and backing membrane, and they are reflective of the coating efficiency of the patches. The results showed that all of the patches (acrylate, silicone, PIB) had uniformity in both coat weight and drug assay. Additionally, the values of theoretical and experimental drug content were close for all of the patches that confirmed the stability of the drug after exposure to the temperature conditions used for the processing of respective patches.

3.5. In Vitro Permeation Studies

3.5.1. Epidermal Integrity and Thickness Assessment

The integrity of human epidermis samples must be evaluated prior to permeation studies, as the procedures that are employed for procurement of human skin, such as surgical removal, dermatoming, and storage, as well as technical procedure for the separation of epidermis from dermatomed skin, can damage the skin, and thus ultimately influence drug permeation. The physical integrity of stratum corneum has been reported to be indicated by its electrical properties. Therefore, the measurement of electrical conductivity is used as a means of assessing the barrier integrity for full thickness skin as well as epidermal membranes [27,56]. Hence, for the selection of epidermal pieces with optimum barrier integrity, electrical resistance of skin was measured and considered to be the main selection criterion.

Epidermal pieces with the resistance above 10 kΩ, were selected for the study. Further, the thickness of human epidermis used for the permeation studies ranged from 50–150 μm.

3.5.2. Selection of Receptor Solution

Table 6 shows the percentage degradation of TAF in different receptor solutions at 37 °C. It was evident that TAF degrades in PBS, pH 7.4, with or without PEG 400. Lowering the pH to 6.0 and using non-aqueous media, such as pure PEG 400, reduced the degradation of TAF. However, due to limitations, such as high viscosity as well as low drug sensitivity in HPLC, PEG 400 was not selected as the receptor media. Phosphate buffer, pH 6.0 was thus selected as the receptor solution, and it was completely replaced every 24 h during the seven-day skin permeation studies. The degradation of TAF at both acidic and basic pH has been previously reported in the literature. Additionally, TAF has been found to be stable at pH of around 5–6.8 [57]. In addition, the solubility of TAF in PBS was found to be 4.95 ± 0.07 mg/mL. Experimental conditions ensured the maintenance of sink conditions for our in vitro permeation studies.

Table 6. Stability of TAF in different receptor solutions.

TAF Concentration (μg/mL)	% Degradation of TAF in 24 h at 37 °C			
	PBS, pH 7.4	**Phosphate Buffer, pH 6.0**	**PEG 400: PBS, pH 7.4 (1:1)**	**PEG 400**
0.5	22.28	3.65	41.85	Not detected due to low LOD
5	28.29	1.61	32.40	0.00
50	30.54	2.27	33.84	0.85

3.5.3. Determination of Permeation Flux of TAF Transdermal Patches

Table 3 describes the different patches that were evaluated in seven day in vitro permeation studies.

Permeation of TAF from Acrylate-Based Clear Patches: Effect of Drug Concentration

The amount of TAF that permeated from patch AP1 (simplest matrix comprising of 2% *w*/*w* TAF dissolved in mixture of OA in acrylate adhesive) after seven days was found to be 19.20 ± 2.92 μg/cm^2. The average permeation flux over duration of seven days was calculated to be 0.12 ± 0.01 μg/cm^2/h. To evaluate the effect of drug concentration in the patch on its skin permeation, patch AP5 with 10% *w*/*w* TAF, which was found to be stable for about two weeks at RT, was selected for an in vitro permeation study. As shown in Figure 4, increasing the concentration of TAF to 10% *w*/*w* (AP5) significantly enhanced the drug permeation to 137.76 ± 10.42 μg/cm^2 after seven days and flux rate was calculated to be 0.88 ± 0.07 μg/cm^2/h as compared to that of AP1 ($p < 0.05$). Thus, increasing the drug concentration significantly enhanced its permeation across human epidermis. However, since AP5, as well as other acrylate adhesive-based patches with a TAF concentration of more than 2% (*w*/*w*), crystallized at RT over a period of time, transdermal patches with 2% *w*/*w* TAF, and consisting of combination of chemical penetration enhancers as well as higher coat weight, were prepared and evaluated for skin permeation testing (AP12 to AP15).

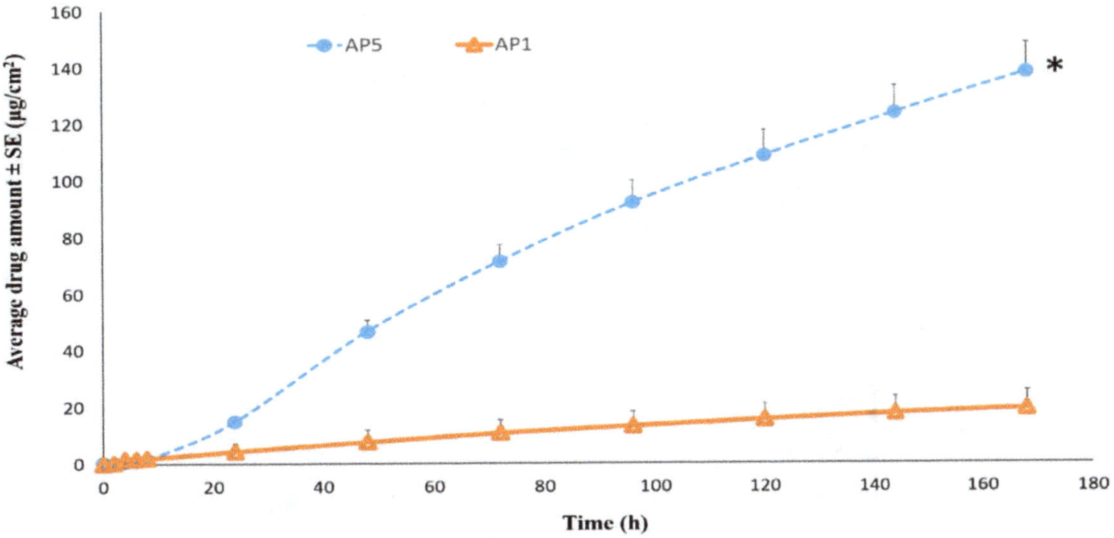

Figure 4. Permeation profiles of TAF from acrylate based patches across human epidermis. * Represents statistical significant difference, Student's t test ($p < 0.05$). AP1: Acrylate patch containing 2% TAF, AP5: Acrylate patch containing 10% TAF.

Permeation of TAF from Acrylate-Based Clear Patches: Effect of Coat Weight and Chemical Penetration Enhancers

As shown in Figure 5A, the cumulative amount of TAF permeation after seven days in the patches AP12 (96.40 ± 14.83 µg/cm^2), AP13 (87.15 ± 8.60 µg/cm^2), and AP14 (89.56 ± 17.28 µg/cm^2) was found to be significantly higher than that of AP1 (19.20 ± 2.92 µg/cm^2, $p < 0.05$). Additionally, the permeation flux that was observed from the three aforementioned groups was 0.60 ± 0.10 µg/cm^2/h, 0.54 ± 0.05 µg/cm^2/h, and 0.56 ± 0.12 µg/cm^2/h, respectively, which was about five-fold greater than that observed from AP1 (0.12 ± 0.01 µg/cm^2/h). Thus, increasing the patch coat weight to 400 gsm from 200 gsm along with the incorporation of a combination of chemical enhancers (OA+ PG+ oleyl alcohol, OA+ PG+ triacetin, or OA+ PG+ octisalate) resulted in the significant enhancement in drug permeation. However, no significant difference in TAF permeation between AP12, AP13, and AP14 was observed. As shown in Figure 5B, the amount of drug permeation over 6 h was significantly higher in patch AP12 (6.15 ± 0.41 µg/cm^2) than AP13 (3.38 ± 1.40 µg/cm^2), as well as AP14 (3.17 ± 1.30 µg/cm^2, $p < 0.05$). Patch AP15 was formulated by replacing 5% *w*/*w* OA in AP12 with oleyl alcohol, thus having total of 10% *w*/*w* oleyl alcohol and a coat weight of 400 gsm. However, as shown in Figure 6, there was no significant difference between the amount of TAF permeation after seven days between the two groups (AP12: 96.40 ± 14.83 µg/cm^2 and AP15: 122.69±28.34 µg/cm^2, $p > 0.05$).

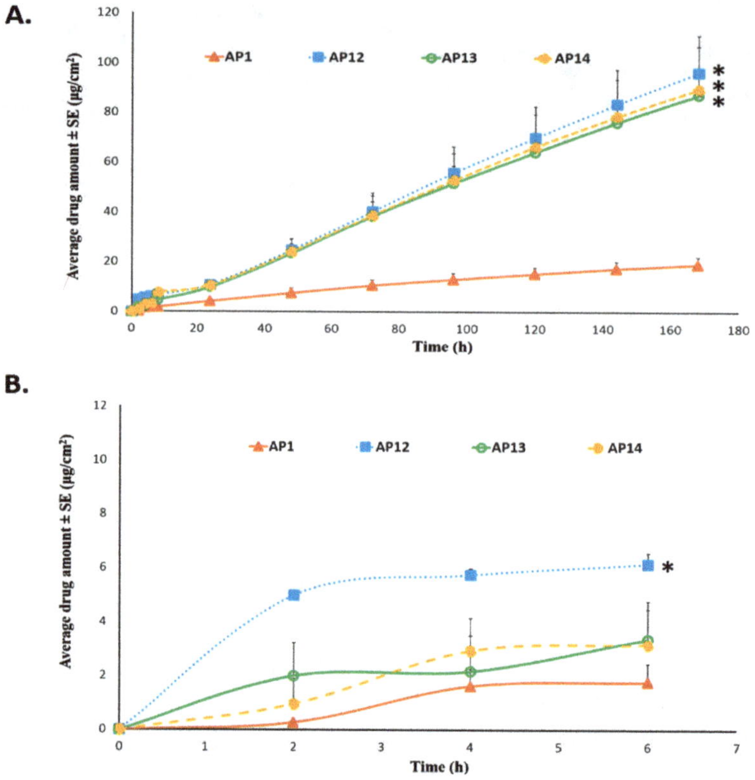

Figure 5. Effect of combination of enhancers and higher patch coat weight on permeation of TAF across human epidermis from acrylate patches: (**A**) Seven day permeation profile (**B**) Six hours permeation profile. * Represents statistically significant difference, ANOVA one way test ($p < 0.05$). AP1: Acrylate based patch containing 2% TAF and 5% oleic acid. AP12: Acrylate based patch containing 2% TAF, 5% oleic acid, 5% PG, and 5% oleyl alcohol. AP13: Acrylate based patch containing 2% TAF, 5% oleic acid, 5% PG, and 5% triacetin. AP14: Acrylate based patch containing 2% TAF, 5% oleic acid, 5% PG, and 8.5% octisalate.

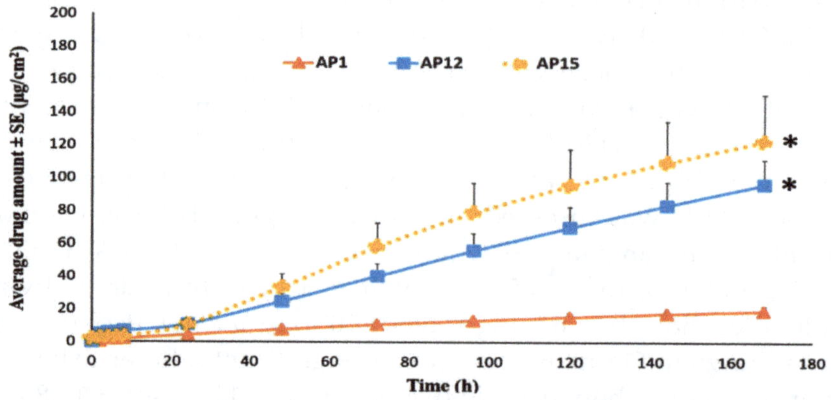

Figure 6. Permeation profile of acrylate based TAF patches comprising of oleyl alcohol and comparison with the control patch through human epidermis. * Represents statistically significant difference, ANOVA one way test ($p < 0.05$). AP1: Acrylate based patch containing 2% TAF and 5% oleic acid. AP12: Acrylate based patch containing 2% TAF, 5% oleic acid, 5% PG, and 5% oleyl alcohol. AP15: Acrylate based patch containing 2% TAF, 5% PG, and 10% oleyl alcohol.

The effects of various chemical enhancers that were used in the patches, such as OA [36–38], oleyl alcohol [39,40], triacetin [41–43], and octisalate [44,45] on skin permeation enhancement are well-known. Synergistic permeation enhancing effect of the combination of PG and OA has also been reported earlier [25,39,58]. In our study, PG is expected to act as a cosolvent, and thus enhance the concentrations of the drug substance as well as the enhancer in the stratum corneum. OA, on the other hand, has the potential to delipidize the stratum corneum, and therefore facilitate the partitioning of the drug molecules and PG into skin [38,59]. Additionally, the synergistic effect of PG and oleyl alcohol was found to markedly increase the skin permeation of tenoxicam across hairless mouse skin [60]. Furthermore, a combination use of PG and oleyl alcohol, under occlusive conditions, has been reported to result in considerable enhancement in the permeation of testosterone across full thickness neonatal porcine skin. The mechanism of penetration enhancement by octisalate is not fully understood. However, due to the structural similarity, as well as similar observations in differential scanning calorimetry and attenuated total reflectance spectroscopy, in terms of the effect of delipidization on stratum corneum, octisalate is assumed to mechanistically work in the similar way to azone [44]. Additionally, octisalate has been incorporated as a penetration enhancer in sunscreens, cosmetic products, as well as in metered spray transdermal systems [45]. Further, triacetin has been incorporated as a penetration enhancer in the commercially available Oxytrol® patch for overactive bladder [43,61]. Patel et al. also reported an enhancement in diclofenac permeation through human cadaver skin while using 10% triacetin [41].

Permeation of TAF from Suspension-Type Patches: PIB vs Silicone-Based

The PIB based TAF suspension patch (SP14) showed a permeation of 90.40 ± 10.18 μg/cm^2 after seven days through human epidermis. A TAF permeation flux rate of 0.60 ± 0.07 μg/cm^2/h and a lag time of about 19 h was observed with this patch. The results showed that the flux rate from SP14 was significantly higher than AP1 ($p < 0.05$), but was similar to that of AP12, AP13, AP14, and AP15 ($p > 0.05$). Further, silicone patch (SP1) with the same composition as PIB (SP14) was prepared. The cumulative amount of TAF that permeated from SP1 across human epidermis in seven days was observed to be 432.21 ± 41.25 μg/cm^2 and it was significantly higher than all of the other patches evaluated previously ($p < 0.05$). Figure 7 shows the skin permeation profiles of PIB (SP14) and silicone (SP1) based patch. The resultant permeation flux from SP1 for seven days was found to be 3.39 ± 0.03 μg/cm^2/h and the lag time was observed to be only 1.2 h. Further, with the addition of 10% w/w oleyl alcohol, as well as increased coat weight of ~250 gsm in patch SP5, the permeation flux of TAF was observed to significantly increase to 5.97 ± 0.47 μg/cm^2 /h ($p < 0.05$). The total amount of TAF observed in the receptor after seven days was 958.07 ± 82.81 μg/cm^2 and the lag time was about 1 h.

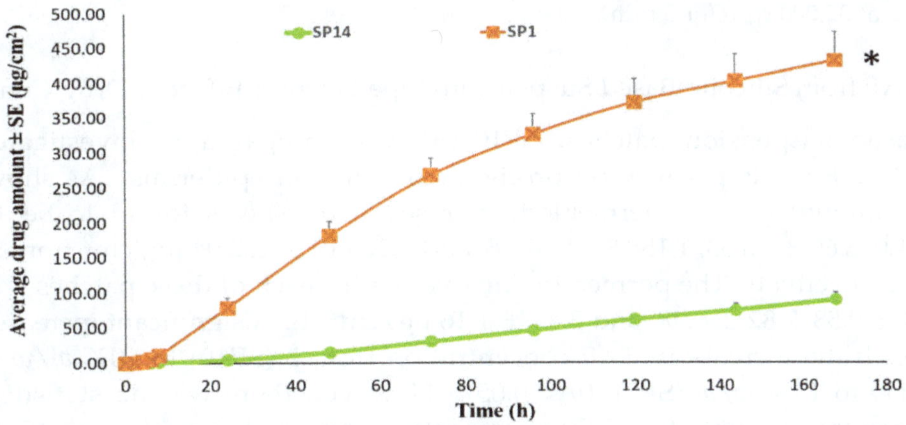

Figure 7. Comparison of permeation profile of silicone and PIB based TAF patches through human epidermis. * Represents statistical significant difference, Student's t test ($p < 0.05$). SP1: Silicone based 15% TAF patch. SP14: Poly isobutylene based 15% TAF patch.

Permeation of TAF from Silicone-Based Suspension-Type Patches: Effect of Homogenization

Briefly, the suspension blend for patch SP5 was homogenized at 30,000 rpm for 20 min, while homogenization at 32,000 rpm for 30 min. was performed for the preparation of SP6, to investigate the effect of homogenization parameters on the skin permeation. However, the amount of TAF permeation after seven days was not found to be significantly different between the two patch formulations (SP5: 958.07 ± 82.81 μg/cm^2 and SP6: 1,054.38 ± 214.40 μg/cm^2). It was found that a permeation flux rate of TAF from patch SP6 was 6.60 ± 1.48 μg/cm^2/h and lag time of about 1 h was observed. Furthermore, the patch SP7 blend was prepared by homogenization at 32,000 rpm for only 5 min., and it did not show any significant difference in the amount of TAF permeation as well as the lag time when compared to those of SP5 and SP6 ($p > 0.05$), as shown in Figure 8. The permeation flux of TAF observed from patch SP7 was 7.24 ± 0.47 μg/cm^2/h. Additionally, it can be inferred that the use of different backing materials in patches SP5/6 and SP7 did not impact the drug permeation across human epidermis.

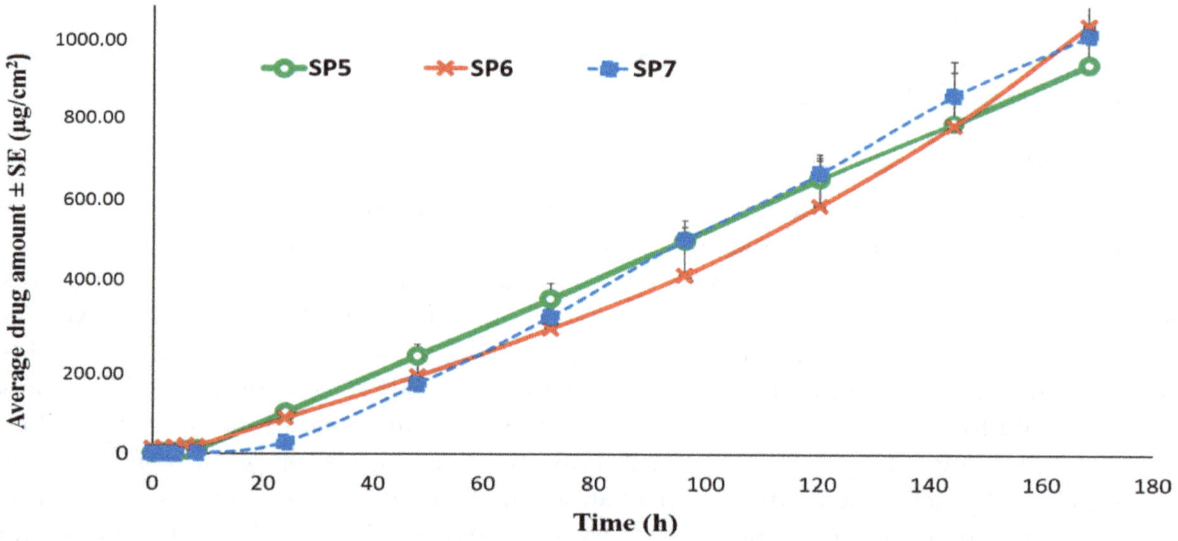

Figure 8. Comparison of permeation profile of silicone based TAF patches through human epidermis. SP5: Silicone-based 15% TAF patch prepared from formulation blend homogenized at 30,000 rpm for 20 min. SP6: Silicone-based 15% TAF patch prepared from formulation blend homogenized at 32,000 rpm for 30 min. SP7: Silicone-based 15% TAF patch prepared from formulation blend homogenized at 32,000 rpm for 5 min.

Permeation of TAF from Silicone-Based Suspension-Type Patches: Effect of Drug Concentration

Silicone based suspension patches, SP10-13, were prepared to investigate the effect of concentration of TAF on its permeation profile across human epidermis. As shown in Figure 9, the cumulative amount of TAF permeated after seven days was found to be 191.51 ± 23.26, 695.09 ± 68.85, 1,028.69 ± 78.63, 1,158.86 ± 57.96, and 1,266.19 ± 162.04 μg/cm^2 from SP10, SP11, SP7, SP12, and SP13, respectively. The permeation flux values for each of these patches were: 1.24 ± 0.13, 4.32 ± 0.47, 7.23 ± 0.58, 7.82 ± 0.48, and 8.44 ± 1.16 μg/cm^2/h. A significant increase in permeation was observed with the increase in TAF concentration from 5 (SP10) to 10% *w/w* (SP11), as well as from 10 (SP11) to 15% *w/w* (SP7), ($p < 0.05$). However, there was no statistically significant difference between the amount of TAF that permeated from patches containing 15 (SP7), 20 (SP12), and 25% *w/w* (SP13) drug ($p > 0.05$). Thus, increasing the TAF concentration from 5 to 15% *w/w* resulted in a higher amount of undissolved drug as a reservoir in the latter that probably provided an additional and constant driving force, eventually aiding in considerably enhancing the permeation of TAF. However, increasing the drug concentration from 15 to 25% *w/w* did not result in any further enhancement in permeation. Therefore, 15% drug concentration (SP7) was found to be optimum in order to achieve the targeted permeation flux.

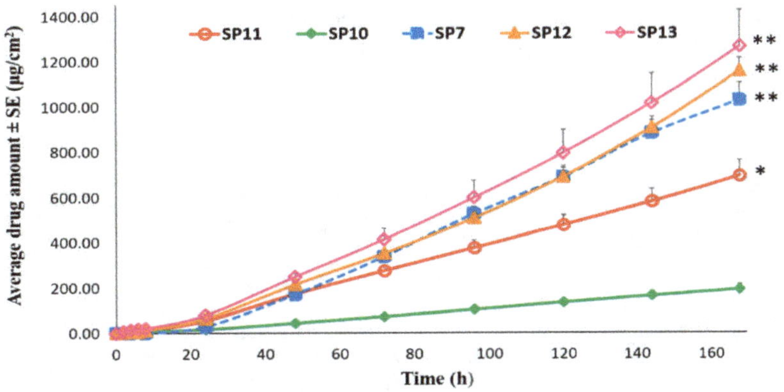

Figure 9. Effect of concentration of TAF in the silicone-based suspension patches on its permeation through human epidermis. * represents significant difference between 5 and 10% patch. ** represents significant difference as compared to 5 and 10% patch, ANOVA one-way test ($p < 0.05$). SP7: Silicone-based 15% TAF patch. SP10: Silicone-based 5% TAF patch. SP11: Silicone-based 10% TAF patch. SP12: Silicone-based 20% TAF patch. SP13: Silicone-based 25% TAF patch.

Permeation of TAF from Acrylate-Based Clear vs Silicone-Based Suspension-Type Patches

The aim of this study was to demonstrate a proof of concept for feasibility of developing a transdermal patch of TAF and achieve a clinically relevant flux of about 7 µg/cm^2/h across human epidermis. From an in vivo perspective, as blood vessels are present in the dermis layer, once the drug crosses the stratum corneum and the viable epidermis, it reaches the systemic circulation. Hence, human epidermis was used in this study for the in vitro permeation testing. Owing to the desirable physicochemical properties (molecular weight= 476.47 g/mol, log P= 1.8), TAF showed permeation from the simplest transdermal patch formulation (AP1), across the human epidermis, depicting its potential to passively permeate through human skin. However, for the acrylate-based TAF patch formulations, it was only possible to achieve a flux rate of 0.6 µg/cm^2/h, with a combination of different chemical penetration enhancers at a low drug concentration (2% *w*/*w*), with no issues regarding drug crystallization. However, the silicone based TAF suspension patch formulations containing 15–25% *w*/*w* drug showed higher permeation flux of about 7 µg/cm^2/h, as well as a lower lag time (about 1h), which may be attributed to the release characteristics of TAF from the silicone adhesive matrix, and a higher drug loading in a suspension form, which can provide constant concentration gradient/driving force for the drug release and continuous permeation through epidermis. In addition, all of the excipients that were included in the TAF suspension patch—mineral oil, OA, and oleyl alcohol—have been previously reported for transdermal permeation enhancing effects, which may contribute to higher flux.

In our study, it was possible to achieve a relatively high flux rate of 7 µg/cm^2/h, from silicone based TAF suspensions, and the optimized patch "SP7" was characterized for drug release, coat weight and thickness, and drug content after storage at RT and 40 °C for three months. This prototype patch was further characterized for physical properties, such as tack, shear, and peel adhesion.

3.6. In Vitro Drug Release Studies

Figure 10 presents the seven-day in vitro release profiles of TAF from the optimized patch "SP7". The average percentage of TAF released after 7 days was observed to be 64.27 ± 5.47, in the study performed during week 1 after the preparation of the patch. The release profile of TAF from the same batch of suspension patch was also studied after 1.5 and 3 months of storage at RT and 40 °C. Table 7 shows the results. No significant difference in the total percentage of TAF released from the patches that are exposed to different test conditions was observed (p>0.05). This depicted uniformity in the release profile and percentage of drug released after exposure to higher temperature for three months, further indicating the stability of TAF in the suspension-based patches.

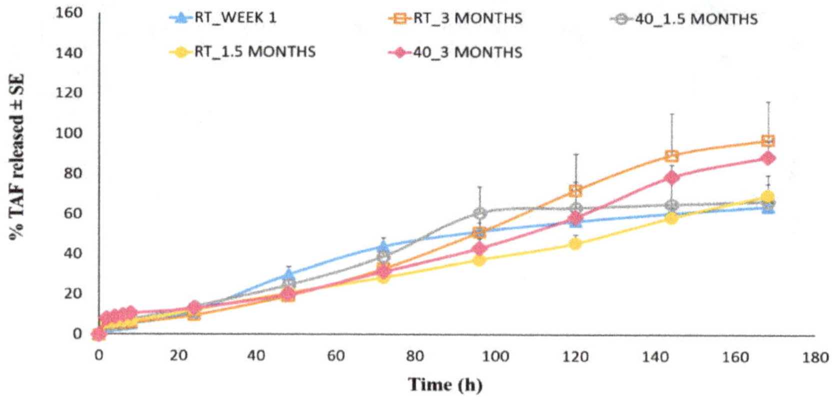

Figure 10. In vitro release profiles of TAF from the optimized suspension patch.

Table 7. Characterization parameters of optimized patch "SP7" up to three months at ambient and accelerated storage conditions.

Parameters	Week 1 (RT)	After 1.5 months (RT)	After 1.5 months (40 °C)	After 3 months (RT)	After 3 months (40 °C)
% TAF released after 7 days ± SE	64.27 ± 5.47	69.71 ± 5.63	66.82 ± 12.83	97.43 ± 19.03	88.86 ± 7.88
Coat weight (mg/cm2) ± SD	29.60 ± 1.94	30.38 ± 0.95	32.73 ± 3.06	29.39 ± 4.57	33.55 ± 3.14
Coat thickness (μm) ± SD	182.66 ± 1.15	186.67 ± 3.06	188.00 ± 3.46	186.00 ± 4.00	189.33 ± 3.06
Drug content (mg/cm2) ± SD	4.60 ± 1.01	4.95 ± 0.31	4.92 ± 0.39	5.25 ± 0.32	5.36 ± 0.43

3.7. *Coat Thickness, Coat Weight, and Drug Content of Optimized Patch*

Table 7 presents the average patch thickness, coat weight, and drug content of patch SP7, as measured after exposure to different temperature conditions for different durations. No significant difference in the measured parameters was observed after exposure of the patches to different test conditions ($p > 0.05$), signifying the stability and integrity of the suspension-based patches over time. Furthermore, as depicted by the results of drug content analysis, no degradation of TAF was observed after 1.5 and 3 months of patch storage at RT as well as 40 °C, further indicating the stability of TAF in the silicone-based suspension patches.

3.8. *Physical Characterization of the Optimized Patch*

3.8.1. Peel Adhesion

An ideal transdermal patch should peel off after application on skin, without causing delamination. Peel adhesion is not only affected by the intrinsic adhesiveness of the PSA, but it also involves the stretching and the bending of the patch matrix, and also the backing layer prior to the separation. The force that is required to peel the patch should be consistent for different batches and the value of peel adhesion obtained in the test varies the width of the test material [62]. No significant difference ($p > 0.05$) in the average force that is required to peel the patch from human dermatomed skin was observed when tested during week 1 (202.78 ± 43.07 g) and three months after patch storage at RT (149.35 ± 30.76 g) and 40 °C (171.17 ± 13.56 g). No delamination was observed for the tested patches.

3.8.2. Tack Properties

The adhesion efficiency of a transdermal patch can be tested by evaluating its tack, which is a measure of the force of debonding upon the application of a light pressure for a short time. A probe tack test was employed in this study, where the force that is required to separate a probe from the adhesive surface of a transdermal patch was measured. Tack was then expressed as the maximum value of the force that is required to break the bond between the probe and transdermal patch after a brief period of contact [62]. The average absolute positive force (adhesive or sticky property), average positive area (work of adhesion), and average separation distance (degree of legging), recorded for three replicates during the first week after patch preparation, was found to be 1,116.88 ± 167.79 g/cm^2, 34.30 ± 10.98 g.s, and 1.27 ± 0.50 mm, respectively. Storage at RT (1,012.03 ± 220.59 g/cm^2, 24.77 ± 8.50 g.s, and 0.8 ± 0.1 mm, respectively) and 40 °C (983.72 ± 201.56 g/cm^2, 23.33 ± 6.20 g.s, and 1.0 ± 0.17 mm, respectively) for three months did not impact the tack properties of the optimized patch formulation ($p > 0.05$). Additionally, the average absolute positive force that was observed in our study was comparable to that observed for the 9.5% fentanyl containing silicone-based suspension patch laminate (1,499 g/cm^2) reported in literature [63].

3.9. *Evaluation of Skin Irritation Potential of Optimized Patch*

The principle of irritation assay using the in vitro skin model is based on the premise that irritant chemicals can penetrate the stratum corneum by diffusion and they are cytotoxic to the cells in the underlying layers. In a transdermal patch, the drug by itself or in combination with other additives can be irritant to skin [30]. Hence, the entire patch was tested for its irritation potential, and not just the drug by itself. The tested transdermal patch (SP7) resulted in a mean relative cell viability of 104.64 ± 7.42%, which was comparable to the negative control (100.00 ± 6.09) and significantly higher than the positive control (14.27 ± 8.09). Hence, it can be concluded that the final optimized silicone suspension patch (SP7) is non-irritant to human skin.

4. Conclusions

Several solution and suspension-type patch formulations were developed for the transdermal delivery of TAF. Ultimately, the optimized silicone-based suspension patch design successfully achieved the target release and duration profile for TAF and it was found to be suitable for weekly drug dosing. Drug permeation flux of 7 μg/cm^2/h, as observed from the optimized patch, when extrapolated to 50 cm^2 patch size, indicates the delivery of 8.4 mg TAF/day, surpassing the target dose of 8 mg/day. Further studies are underway to characterize its safety and pharmacokinetic profiles in vivo.

Author Contributions: Conceptualization, A.P., W.Z. and A.K.B.; Methodology, A.P., S.A.B., W.Z. and A.K.B.; Formal Analysis, A.P. and S.A.B.; Investigation, A.P. and S.A.B.; Writing-Original Draft Preparation, A.P. and S.A.B.; Writing-Review & Editing, G.F.D., M.C. and O.N.S.; Visualization, A.P.; Supervision, A.K.B., O.N.S. and W.Z.; Project Administration, M.C., O.N.S. and W.Z.; Funding Acquisition, G.F.D. and M.C.

Abbreviations

ANOVA	Analysis of variance
EPI-200-SIT	EpiDerm™ skin irritation test
ELISA	Enzyme linked immunosorbent assay
EVAC	Ethylene vinyl acetate copolymer
HPLC	High performance liquid chromatography
PBS	Phosphate buffered saline
PDMS	Polydimethyl-siloxane
PEG	Polyethylene glycol
PET	poly-ethylene terephthalate
PIB	Polyisobutylene
PSA	Pressure sensitive adhesives
RhE	Reconstructed human epidermis
RT	Room temperature
STRs	Single tablet regimens
TFV	Tenofovir
TAF	Tenofovir alafenamide
THF	Tetrahydrofuran

References

1. De Clercq, E. Role of tenofovir alafenamide (TAF) in the treatment and prophylaxis of HIV and HBV infections. *Biochem. Pharmacol.* **2018**, *153*, 2–11. [CrossRef]
2. DeJesus, E.; Haas, B.; Segal-Maurer, S.; Ramgopal, M.N.; Mills, A.; Margot, N.; Liu, Y.-P.; Makadzange, T.; McCallister, S. Superior Efficacy and Improved Renal and Bone Safety After Switching from a Tenofovir Disoproxil Fumarate- to a Tenofovir Alafenamide-Based Regimen Through 96 Weeks of Treatment. *AIDS Res. Hum. Retrovir.* **2018**, *34*, 337–342. [CrossRef] [PubMed]
3. Kahn, P. AIDS Vaccine Handbook: Global Perspectives. Available online: http://www.avac.org/ (accessed on 2 November 2019).
4. Nelson, K.; Varadarajan, P.; Rajappan, M.; Chikkanna, N. Advances in Drug Delivery of Anti-HIV Drugs—An Overview. *Am. J. PharmTech Res.* **2012**, *2*, 231–244.
5. Vedha Hari, B.N.; Devendharan, K.; Narayanan, N. Approaches of novel drug delivery systems for Anti-HIV agents. *Int. J. Drug Dev. Res.* **2013**, *5*, 16–24.
6. Dou, H.; Destache, C.J.; Morehead, J.R.; Mosley, R.L.; Boska, M.D.; Kingsley, J.; Gorantla, S.; Poluektova, L.; Nelson, J.A.; Chaubal, M.; et al. Development of a macrophage-based nanoparticle platform for antiretroviral drug delivery. *Blood* **2006**, *108*, 2827–2835. [CrossRef] [PubMed]
7. Gunawardana, M.; Remedios-Chan, M.; Miller, C.S.; Fanter, R.; Yang, F.; Marzinke, M.A.; Hendrix, C.W.; Beliveau, M.; Moss, J.A.; Smith, T.J.; et al. Pharmacokinetics of long-acting tenofovir alafenamide (GS-7340) subdermal implant for HIV prophylaxis. *Antimicrob. Agents Chemother.* **2015**, *59*, 3913–3919. [CrossRef]
8. Ball, C.; Krogstad, E.; Chaowanachan, T.; Woodrow, K.A. Drug-Eluting Fibers for HIV-1 Inhibition and Contraception. *PLoS ONE* **2012**, *7*, e49792. [CrossRef] [PubMed]
9. Rohan, L.C.; Devlin, B.; Yang, H. Microbicide Dosage Forms. In *Microbicides for Prevention of HIV Infection*; Springer: Berlin/Heidelberg, Germany, 2013; pp. 27–54. ISBN 978-3-662-44596-9.
10. Nelson, A.G.; Zhang, X.; Ganapathi, U.; Szekely, Z.; Flexner, C.W.; Owen, A.; Sinko, P.J. Drug delivery strategies and systems for HIV/AIDS pre-exposure prophylaxis and treatment. *J. Control. Release* **2015**, *219*, 669–680. [CrossRef]
11. Karim, Q.A.; Karim, S.S.A.; Frohlich, J.A.; Grobler, A.C.; Baxter, C.; Mansoor, L.E.; Kharsany, A.B.M.; Sibeko, S.; Mlisana, K.P.; Omar, Z.; et al. Effectiveness and safety of tenofovir gel, an antiretroviral microbicide, for the prevention of HIV infection in women. *Science* **2010**, *329*, 1168–1174. [CrossRef]
12. Puri, A.; Sivaraman, A.; Zhang, W.; Clark, M.R.; Banga, A.K. Expanding the domain of drug delivery for HIV prevention: Exploration of the transdermal route. *Crit. Rev. Ther. Drug Carrier Syst.* **2017**, *34*, 551–587. [CrossRef] [PubMed]
13. Karim, S.S.A.; Kashuba, A.D.; Werner, L.; Karim, Q.A. Drug concentrations after topical and oral antiretroviral pre-exposure prophylaxis: Implications for HIV prevention in women. *Lancet* **2011**, *378*, 279–281. [CrossRef]
14. Banga, A.K. *Transdermal and Intradermal Delivery of Therapeutic Agents: Application of Physical Technologies*; CRC Press: Boca Raton, FL, USA, 2011; ISBN 9781439805107.
15. Ham, A.S.; Buckheit, R.W. Current and emerging formulation strategies for the effective transdermal delivery of HIV inhibitors. *Ther. Deliv.* **2015**, *6*, 217–229. [CrossRef]
16. Alexander, A.; Dwivedi, S.; Giri, T.K.; Saraf, S.; Saraf, S.; Tripathi, D.K. Approaches for breaking the barriers of drug permeation through transdermal drug delivery. *J. Control. Release* **2012**, *164*, 26–40. [CrossRef]
17. Pastore, M.; Kalia, Y.; Hortsmann, M.; Roberts, M. Transdermal patches: history, development and pharmacology. *Br. J. Phamacol.* **2015**, *172*, 2179–2209. [CrossRef]
18. De Clercq, E. Tenofovir alafenamide (TAF) as the successor of tenofovir disoproxil fumarate (TDF). *Biochem. Pharmacol.* **2016**, *119*, 1–7. [CrossRef]
19. Murphy, R.A.; Valentovic, M.A. Factors Contributing to the Antiviral Effectiveness of Tenofovir. *J. Pharmacol. Exp. Ther.* **2017**, *363*, 156–163. [CrossRef]
20. Babusis, D.; Phan, T.K.; Lee, W.A.; Watkins, W.J.; Ray, A.S. Mechanism for effective lymphoid cell and tissue loading following oral administration of nucleotide prodrug GS-7340. *Mol. Pharm.* **2013**, *10*, 459–466. [CrossRef]
21. Foreman, P.; Hansen, A.; Silverberg, E.; Manegold, T.; Yang, H.; Li, J.; Jacobson, S. Predicting Drug Solubility in Transdermal Adhesives. American Association of Pharmaceutical Scientists. In Proceedings of the 37th AAPS Annual Pharmaceutical Technologies Conference, New York, NY, USA, 13–18 January 2002.

22. Sachdeva, V.; Bai, Y.; Kydonieus, A.; Banga, A.K. Formulation and optimization of desogestrel transdermal contraceptive patch using crystallization studies. *Int. J. Pharm.* **2013**, *441*, 9–18. [CrossRef]
23. Banerjee, S.; Chattopadhyay, P.; Ghosh, A.; Bhattacharya, S.; Kundu, A.; Veer, V. Accelerated stability testing of a transdermal patch composed of eserine and pralidoxime chloride for prophylaxis against (±)-anatoxin A poisoning. *J. Food Drug Anal.* **2014**, *22*, 264–270. [CrossRef]
24. Kassis, V.; Søndergaard, J. Heat-separation of normal human skin for epidermal and dermal prostaglandin analysis. *Arch. Dermatol. Res.* **1982**, *273*, 301–306. [CrossRef]
25. Puri, A.; Murnane, K.S.; Blough, B.E.; Banga, A.K. Effects of chemical and physical enhancement techniques on transdermal delivery of 3-fluoroamphetamine hydrochloride. *Int. J. Pharm.* **2017**, *528*, 452–462. [CrossRef]
26. Lakhani, P.; Bahl, R.; Bafna, P. Transdermal Patches: Physiochemical and in-vitro Evaluation Methods. *Int. J. Pharm. Sci. Res.* **2015**, *6*, 1826–1836.
27. Cai, B.; Söderkvist, K.; Engqvist, H.; Bredenberg, S. A new drug release method in early development of transdermal drug delivery systems. *Pain Res. Treat.* **2012**, *2012*, 953140. [CrossRef]
28. Wokovich, A.M.; Prodduturi, S.; Doub, W.H.; Hussain, A.S.; Buhse, L.F. Transdermal drug delivery system (TDDS) adhesion as a critical safety, efficacy and quality attribute. *Eur. J. Pharm. Biopharm.* **2006**, *64*, 1–8.
29. Lu, Z.; Fassihi, R. Influence of colloidal silicon dioxide on gel strength, robustness, and adhesive properties of diclofenac gel formulation for topical application. *AAPS PharmSciTech* **2015**, *16*, 636–644. [CrossRef]
30. Kandárová, H.; Hayden, P.; Klausner, M.; Kubilus, J.; Sheasgreen, J. An in vitro skin irritation test (SIT) using the EpiDerm reconstructed human epidermal (RHE) model. *J. Vis. Exp. JoVE* **2009**, *29*, e1336.
31. Banerjee, S.; Chattopadhyay, P.; Ghosh, A.; Datta, P.; Veer, V. Aspect of adhesives in transdermal drug delivery systems. *Int. J. Adhes. Adhes.* **2014**, *50*, 70–84.
32. Pocius, A. Adhesives. In *Kirk-Othmer Encyclopedia of Chemical Technology*; Howe-Grants, M., Ed.; Wiley-Interscience: New York, NY, USA, 1991; pp. 445–466.
33. Lobo, S.; Sachdeva, S.; Goswami, T. Role of pressure-sensitive adhesives in transdermal drug delivery systems. *Ther. Deliv.* **2016**, *7*, 33–48. [CrossRef]
34. Weng, W.; Quan, P.; Liu, C.; Zhao, H.; Fang, L. Design of a Drug-in-Adhesive Transdermal Patch for Risperidone: Effect of Drug-Additive Interactions on the Crystallization Inhibition and In Vitro/In Vivo Correlation Study. *J. Pharm. Sci.* **2016**, *10*, 3153–3161. [CrossRef]
35. Jain, P.; Banga, A.K. Induction and inhibition of crystallization in drug-in-adhesive-type transdermal patches. *Pharm. Res.* **2013**, *30*, 562–571. [CrossRef]
36. Saini, S.; Shikha, B.; Chauhan, S.S. Recent development in penetration enhancers and techniques in transdermal drug delivery system. *J. Adv. Pharm. Educ. Res.* **2014**, *4*, 31–40.
37. Pathan, I.B.; Setty, C.M. Chemical penetration enhancers for transdermal drug delivery systems. *Trop. J. Pharm. Res.* **2009**, *8*, 173–179. [CrossRef]
38. Mitragotri, S. Synergistic effect of enhancers for transdermal drug delivery. *Pharm. Res.* **2000**, *17*, 1354–1359. [CrossRef]
39. Santoyo, S.; Arellano, A.; Ygartua, P.; Martin, C. Penetration enhancer effects on the in vitro percutaneous absorption of piroxicam through rat skin. *Int. J. Pharm.* **1995**, *117*, 219–224. [CrossRef]
40. Andega, S.; Kanikkannan, N.; Singh, M. Comparison of the effect of fatty alcohols on the permeation of melatonin between porcine and human skin. *J. Control. Release* **2001**, *77*, 17–25. [CrossRef]
41. Patel, K.N.; Patel, H.K.; Patel, V.A. Formulation and characterization of drug in adhesive transdermal patches of diclofenac acid. *Int. J. Pharm. Pharm. Sci.* **2012**, *4*, 296–299.
42. Moghimipour, E.; Rezaee, S.; Omidi, A. The effect of formulation factors on the release of oxybutynin hydrochloride from transdermal polymeric patches. *J. Appl. Pharm. Sci.* **2011**, *1*, 73–76.
43. Nicoli, S.; Penna, E.; Padula, C.; Colombo, P.; Santi, P. New transdermal bioadhesive film containing oxybutynin: In vitro permeation across rabbit ear skin. *Int. J. Pharm.* **2006**, *325*, 2–7. [CrossRef]
44. Nicolazzo, J.A.; Morgan, T.M.; Reed, B.L.; Finnin, B.C. Synergistic enhancement of testosterone transdermal delivery. *J. Control. Release* **2005**, *103*, 577–585. [CrossRef]
45. Fraser, I.S.; Weisberg, E.; Kumar, N.; Kumar, S.; Humberstone, A.J.; McCrossin, L.; Shaw, D.; Tsong, Y.Y.; Sitruk-Ware, R. An initial pharmacokinetic study with a Metered Dose Transdermal System® for delivery of the progestogen Nestorone® as a possible future contraceptive. *Contraception* **2007**, *76*, 432–438. [CrossRef]

46. European Meedicines Agency. Guideline on quality of transdermal patches Guideline on quality of transdermal patches Table of contents. *Eur. Med. Agency* **2014**, *44*, 1–28.
47. Sekikawa, H.; Nakano, M.; Arita, T. Inhibitory effect of polyvinylpyrrolidone on the crystallization of drugs. *Chem. Pharm. Bull.* **1978**, *26*, 118–126. [CrossRef]
48. Gong, K.; Viboonkiat, R.; Rehman, I.U.; Buckton, G.; Darr, J.A. Formation and characterization of porous indomethacin-PVP coprecipitates prepared using solvent-free supercritical fluid processing. *J. Pharm. Sci.* **2005**, *94*, 2583–2590. [CrossRef]
49. Ohm, A. Interaction of Bay t 3839 coprecipitates with insoluble excipients. *Eur. J. Pharm. Biopharm.* **2000**, *49*, 183–189. [CrossRef]
50. Ma, X.; Taw, J.; Chiang, C.M. Control of drug crystallization in transdermal matrix system. *Int. J. Pharm.* **1996**, *142*, 115–119. [CrossRef]
51. Karande, P.; Mitragotri, S. Enhancement of transdermal drug delivery via synergistic action of chemicals. *Biochim. Biophys. Acta-Biomembr.* **2009**, *1788*, 2362–2373. [CrossRef]
52. Dhankhar, P. Homogenization Fundamentals. *IOSR J. Eng.* **2014**, *4*, 1–8. [CrossRef]
53. Chu, K.R.; Lee, E.; Jeong, S.H.; Park, E.-S. Effect of particle size on the dissolution behaviors of poorly water-soluble drugs. *Arch. Pharm. Res.* **2012**, *35*, 1187–1195. [CrossRef]
54. Anarjan, N.; Jafarizadeh-Malmiri, H.; Nehdi, I.A.; Sbihi, H.M.; Al-Resayes, S.I.; Tan, C.P. Effects of homogenization process parameters on physicochemical properties of astaxanthin nanodispersions prepared using a solvent-diffusion technique. *Int. J. Nanomed.* **2015**, *10*, 1109–1118.
55. Sharma, N.; Madan, P.; Lin, S. Effect of process and formulation variables on the preparation of parenteral paclitaxel-loaded biodegradable polymeric nanoparticles: A co-surfactant study. *Asian J. Pharm. Sci.* **2016**, *11*, 404–416. [CrossRef]
56. Lawrence, J.N. Electrical resistance and tritiated water permeability as indicators of barrier integrity of in vitro human skin. *Toxicol. Vitr.* **1997**, *11*, 241–249. [CrossRef]
57. Golla, V.M.; Kurmi, M.; Shaik, K.; Singh, S. Stability behaviour of antiretroviral drugs and their combinations. 4: Characterization of degradation products of tenofovir alafenamide fumarate and comparison of its degradation and stability behaviour with tenofovir disoproxil fumarate. *J. Pharm. Biomed. Anal.* **2016**, *131*, 146–155. [CrossRef]
58. Larrucea, E.; Arellano, A.; Santoyo, S.; Ygartua, P. Combined effect of oleic acid and propylene glycol on the percutaneous penetration of tenoxicam and its retention in the skin. *Eur. J. Pharm. Biopharm.* **2001**, *2*, 113–119. [CrossRef]
59. Benson, H.A.E. Transdermal drug delivery: Penetration enhancement techniques. *Curr. Drug Deliv.* **2005**, *2*, 23–33. [CrossRef]
60. Chatterjee, D.J.; Li, W.Y.; Koda, R.T. Effect of vehicles and penetration enhancers on the in vitro and in vivo percutaneous absorption of methotrexate and edatrexate through hairless mouse skin. *Pharm. Res.* **1997**, *14*, 1058–1065. [CrossRef]
61. Quan, D.; Deshpanday, N.; Venkateshwaran, S.; Ebert, C. Triacetin as a Penetration Enhancer for Transdermal Delivery of a Basic Drug. U.S. Patent No 5,834,010, 10 November 1998.
62. Cilurzo, F.; Gennari, C.G.M.; Minghetti, P. Adhesive properties: A critical issue in transdermal patch development. *Expert Opin. Drug Deliv.* **2012**, *9*, 33–45. [CrossRef]
63. Miller, K.; Govil, S.; Bhatia, K. Fentanyl Suspension-Based Silicone Adhesive Formulations and Devices for Transdermal Delivery of Fentanyl. U.S. Patent 7556823B2, 28 October 2008.

7

Design of Poly(lactic-*co*-glycolic Acid) (PLGA) Nanoparticles for Vaginal Co-Delivery of Griffithsin and Dapivirine and their Synergistic Effect for HIV Prophylaxis

Haitao Yang [1,2], Jing Li [1,2], Sravan Kumar Patel [1,2], Kenneth E. Palmer [3], Brid Devlin [4] and Lisa C. Rohan [1,2,5,*]

1 Department of Pharmaceutical Sciences, School of Pharmacy, University of Pittsburgh, Pittsburgh, PA 15261, USA; hyang96@its.jnj.com (H.Y.); jil132@pitt.edu (J.L.); patels10@mwri.magee.edu (S.K.P.)
2 Magee-Womens Research Institute, Pittsburgh, PA 15213, USA
3 Center for Predictive Medicine and Department of Pharmacology and Toxicology, University of Louisville School of Medicine, Louisville, KY 40202, USA; kenneth.palmer@louisville.edu
4 International Partnership for Microbicides, Silver Spring, MD 20910, USA; bdevlin@ipmglobal.org
5 Department of Obstetrics, Gynecology and Reproductive Sciences, University of Pittsburgh, Pittsburgh, PA 15261, USA
* Correspondence: rohanlc@upmc.com

Abstract: Long-acting topical products for pre-exposure prophylaxis (PrEP) that combine antiretrovirals (ARVs) inhibiting initial stages of infection are highly promising for prevention of HIV sexual transmission. We fabricated core-shell poly(lactide-*co*-glycolide) (PLGA) nanoparticles, loaded with two potent ARVs, griffithsin (GRFT) and dapivirine (DPV), having different physicochemical properties and specifically targeting the fusion and reverse transcription steps of HIV replication, as a potential long-acting microbicide product. The nanoparticles were evaluated for particle size and zeta potential, drug release, cytotoxicity, cellular uptake and in vitro bioactivity. PLGA nanoparticles, with diameter around 180–200 nm, successfully encapsulated GRFT (45% of initially added) and DPV (70%). Both drugs showed a biphasic release with initial burst phase followed by a sustained release phase. GRFT and DPV nanoparticles were non-toxic and maintained bioactivity (IC_{50} values of 0.5 nM and 4.7 nM, respectively) in a cell-based assay. The combination of drugs in both unformulated and encapsulated in nanoparticles showed strong synergistic drug activity at 1:1 ratio of IC_{50} values. This is the first study to co-deliver a protein (GRFT) and a hydrophobic small molecule (DPV) in PLGA nanoparticles as microbicides. Our findings demonstrate that the combination of GRFT and DPV in nanoparticles is highly potent and possess properties critical to the design of a sustained release microbicide.

Keywords: microbicides; HIV; combination ARVs; sustained release; synergism; PLGA nanoparticles; co-delivery

---

1. Introduction

Human immunodeficiency virus (HIV) infection is one of the world's most serious health challenges, and the development of means to prevent its spread is urgently needed. By the end of 2017, approximately 36.9 million people were living with HIV, with 1.8 million more becoming newly infected globally [1]. Women, especially young (15–24 years) and adolescent (10–19 years), are disproportionately affected by HIV due to social, cultural, economic, and biological vulnerabilities [2,3]. Sexual transmission is the principal cause of new HIV-1 infections in women in the U.S. and worldwide [2].

To protect women from this global epidemic, it is critical to develop effective biomedical interventions for HIV/AIDS prevention and treatment. However, there is no effective vaccine available. In addition, the low instance of condom use by men and other social factors could significantly increase HIV-1 infection in women [4,5]. With these considerations in mind, oral or topical pre-exposure prophylaxis (PrEP) with antiretroviral (ARV) drugs could be the most promising avenue for preventing sexually transmitted HIV infection. Topical PrEP products could be applied by women in the vaginal or rectal tract before sexual intercourse to inactivate pathogens, including HIV, thus providing a female-controlled strategy against HIV-1 infection [6–8]. Rectal-specific topical PrEP products are equally applicable to men who have sex with men (MSM).

HIV-specific ARV drugs that can target specific steps in HIV's life cycle and then effectively inhibit its replication have been selected in the development of current microbicides [9]. To reach maximum protection effect of microbicides, ARVs inhibiting early stage of HIV replication can be beneficial. A combination strategy that includes multiple ARVs targeting different steps of HIV infection lifecycle could potentially improve the antiretroviral activity of each product with synergistic effect as a viable PrEP product for preventing acquisition of HIV-1. It has been proven that combination ARV (cARV) therapy can increase the efficacy of each drug in clinic, reduce resistance, decrease the risk of both HIV disease progression and death, reduce doses and cost, and improve patient adherence and compliance [10].

Dapivirine (DPV) is a diarylaminopyrimidine compound with high activity against HIV-1, and it belongs to the family of non-nucleoside reverse transcriptase inhibitors (NNRTIs). It is extremely potent in inhibiting both wild-type and mutant HIV-1 in vitro [11]. No vaginal or systemic toxicity of DPV was observed in sheep, indicating a desirable safety profile of DPV as a microbicide candidate [12]. In an intravaginal ring dosage form, DPV has shown great promise in Phase III clinical trials, ASPIRE and The Ring study [13,14]. Another promising molecule is Griffithsin (GRFT), a 121–amino acid and13-kDa-molecular-mass lectin that was originally isolated from the red alga *Griffithsia* sp. [15]. Binding to the mannose-rich glycans gp120 and gp41, GRFT inhibits HIV-1 gp120 and exposes the CD4 binding site [16,17]. GRFT is shown to exhibit high potency in inhibition of both X4- and R5-tropic HIV-1 virus at subnanomolar concentration, with high stability in cervical/vaginal lavage fluid [18]. It has been shown to be safe and tolerable in subcutaneous treatment in both guinea pigs and mice at 10 mg/kg and in rabbit vaginal irritation studies [19,20]. Furthermore, our previous investigation of the effect of GRFT rectal gel formulations on proteome and microbiome in non-human primates was supportive of their safety [21]. Importantly, GRFT has shown strong synergistic activity when combined with nucleoside reverse transcriptase inhibitor (NRTI), NNRTI and fusion inhibitor compounds, such as tenofovir, maraviroc, and enfuvirtide in vitro [22]. Furthermore, the broad-spectrum anti-HIV activity and unique safety profile of GRFT and DPV support their development as combined topical microbicides. Therefore, we hypothesized that GRFT will display strong synergistic activity with DPV when combined in application as a microbicide product.

The extreme opposite properties of these two molecules greatly hinder the development of a formulation for the simultaneous delivery of both drugs. The proteinaceous nature of GRFT and quick tissue elimination and low water solubility of DPV, pose limitations to their topical microbicide potential [23]. Additionally, developing a long-acting drug delivery system, which is more favorable for patient adherence of the PrEP product [24,25], will meet with additional challenges. Therefore, our goal was to develop a novel drug delivery system that overcomes formulation limitations and co-delivers GRFT and DPV with a sustained release profile to solve the clinical need in microbicides.

Nanoparticle drug delivery systems not only provide the sustained or controlled delivery of APIs, but also improve drug solubility, protect drug payloads, and enhance mucosal drug permeability [26]. With these advantages, nanoparticle delivery systems have been explored in the design of vaginal microbicides [27–31]. Polymeric nanoparticles can provide controlled or sustained release profiles for the payloads. Poly(ethylene oxide) (PEO) modified poly(caprolactone) (PCL) nanoparticles have been developed for the delivery of DPV as an alternative vaginal microbicide [31] and showed enhanced mucosal penetration and improved local pharmacokinetic profiles of DPV [29]. Nanoparticles made from PEO modified poly(lactic-*co*-glycolic acid) (PLGA) were applied to deliver rilpivirine and demonstrated improved vaginal tissue concentration [32]. Previous studies have utilized nanoparticles for delivery of DPV [33]. Here, we used a PLGA-based nanoparticle delivery system to deliver GRFT/DPV simultaneously in a sustained release pattern. Furthermore, encapsulation of GRFT and DPV in PLGA nanoparticles overcomes the limitations of poor tissue permeability and low aqueous solubility respectively. PLGA is one of the most widely used biodegradable polymers for drug delivery applications due to its superior biocompatibility and biodegradability [34]. It is an FDA-approved polymer that has been widely used for the delivery of proteins/peptides and small molecules [35–38]. Importantly, PLGA nanoparticles were found to have no immunogenicity in vivo, which is critical for the safety of an anti-HIV drug delivery system [39–42]. Additionally, PLGA nanoparticles have been studied in the delivery of several ARV drugs for HIV/AIDS treatment and prevention [38,43–46]. However, to our knowledge, no studies have yet been reported to deliver both a macromolecule and a small hydrophobic molecule simultaneously in one nanoparticle system for PrEP. This attempt on the co-delivery of a macromolecule and a small hydrophobic molecule with PLGA nanoparticles will have implications for the development of future microbicides.

In this study, we investigated the ability of PLGA nanoparticles to deliver both GRFT and DPV simultaneously and their anti-HIV efficacy in combined application as ARVs. We show that GRFT and DPV can be individually and simultaneously fabricated into biodegradable PLGA nanoparticles with a high encapsulation efficiency. The ARV-containing nanoparticles were nontoxic in cell culture. We also observed synergistic effects in the combined application of GRFT and DPV. Collectively, our data show that core-shell type PLGA nanoparticles are a promising strategy for delivering multiple ARV drugs with extreme physicochemical diversity. Our results support a viable nanoparticle platform for the delivery of multi-ARV combinations for sustained HIV-1 prevention.

2. Materials and Methods

2.1. Materials

PLGA with lactic acid to glycolic acid ratios of 50:50 was purchased from Sigma-Aldrich (Resomer® RG 502 H, MW, 30 kDa; St. Louis, MO, USA). Cell culture reagents were obtained from GIBCO, Invitrogen by Life Sciences, Inc. (Lenexa, KS, USA). DPV was obtained from International Partnership for Microbicides (Silver Spring, MD, USA). Recombinant GRFT (~13 kDa) was kindly provided by Kentucky Bioprocessing, LLC (Owensboro, KY, USA). The protein was supplied in a solution of phosphate buffered saline. Phosphate buffered saline 10× molecular biology grade was purchased from Mediatech, Inc. (Manassas, VA, USA). All other reagents used for nanoparticle formulation were purchased from Thermo Fisher Scientific (Pittsburgh, PA, USA).

2.2. Methods

2.2.1. Fabrication of ARV-Loaded Nanoparticles

The ARV loaded nanoparticles were prepared by using double emulsion-solvent evaporation technique as shown in Figure 1. Blank nanoparticles (vehicle control) were prepared using this technique at ambient temperature, as previously described, with some modifications [38]. Briefly, 100 μL Milli-Q water as inner water phase was added into a solution of PLGA (20 mg) in ethylacetate (EA) (1 mL). Then, the primary water-in-oil (W/O) emulsion was obtained by homogenization using a 6-mm diameter Vibra-Cell probe sonicator (Sonics and Materials, Newton, CT, USA) for 40 s at 50 W. The primary W/O emulsion was then added into 2 mL of 2% *w*/*v* aqueous solution of polyvinyl alcohol (PVA) with sonication for 50 s at 50 W to form the secondary water-in-oil-in-water (W/O/W) emulsion.

The W/O/W nanoparticle solution was then diluted with 10 mL of Milli-Q water under magnetic stirring for 4 h in an ice water bath to allow EA to evaporate. The hardened nanoparticles were washed with deionized water three times by centrifugation for 15 min at 15,000× *g* (Sorvall Ultra 80, Waltham, MA, USA). Nanoparticles were then re-suspended in 1 mL of Milli-Q water after removing the PVA supernatant and were then lyophilized overnight (approximately 12 h) under vacuum at 0.120 mbar and at −50 °C using a FreeZone 6 lyophilizer (Labconco, Kansas City, MO, USA). Nanoparticles loaded with GRFT, GRFT/DPV, and DPV were fabricated similar to the blank nanoparticles. GRFT (50 µL, 10 mg/mL) was dissolved in the inner water phase for GRFT nanoparticle preparation. DPV was dissolved in EA (0.033 mg/mL) with PLGA polymer in DPV nanoparticles. GRFT/DPV nanoparticles were prepared by dissolving GRFT in inner water phase and DPV in EA. GRFT and DPV loading levels were kept the same in each preparation unless noted otherwise. The lyophilized nanoparticles were stored in aliquots in glass vials at 4 °C until use. To prepare fluorescent nanoparticles, fluorescein isothiocyanate–dextran 70 (FITC-dextran, MW 70,000; Sigma LLC, St. Louis, MO, USA) and Nile red (Sigma LLC) were added to inner phase and EA respectively during the manufacture of blank NPs.

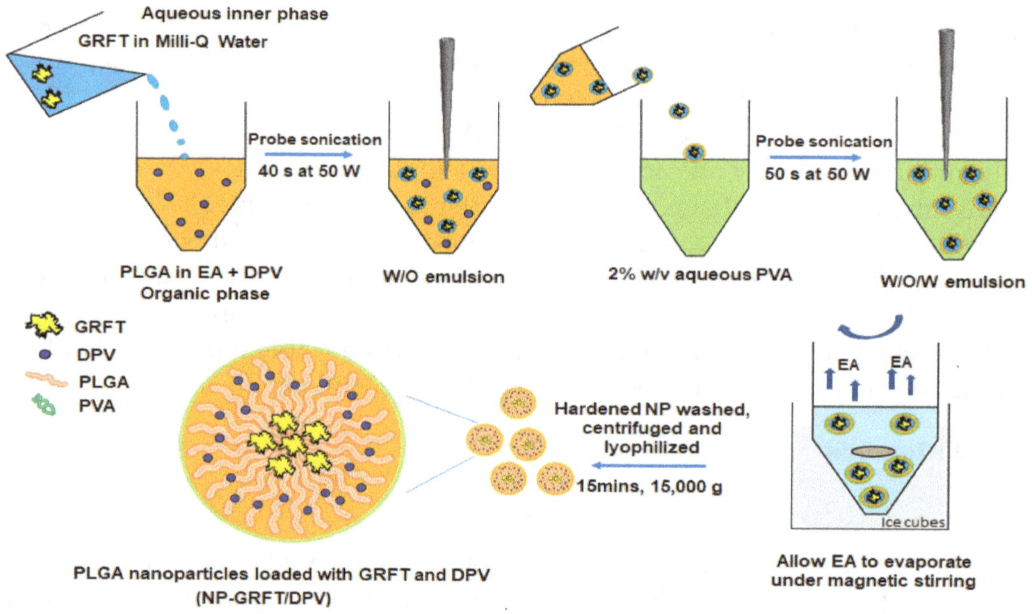

Figure 1. Schematic representation of DPV and GRFT-loaded PLGA nanoparticle preparation by double emulsion-solvent evaporation method.

2.2.2. Characterization of Nanoparticles

Size and zeta potential of the fabricated nanoparticles were determined using a Zetasizer Nano ZS90 (Malvern Instruments, Malvern, UK). Size and morphology of the nanoparticles were also confirmed by Transmission Electron Microscope (TEM), visualized with a JEM 1011 (JEOL, Sheboygan, WI, USA) scanning electron microscope. Samples of nanoparticles were negatively stained with ammonium phosphomolybdate and imaged using an 80 kV electron beam at the Center for Biologic Imaging of the University of Pittsburgh. The zeta potential of the PLGA nanoparticles, both drug-free and drug-loaded, in Milli-Q water, was measured using the zeta potential analysis mode in the Zetasizer.

2.2.3. Drug Loading

The amount of GRFT and DPV encapsulated in the nanoparticles was determined by analyzing the GRFT and DPV content in the supernatant after centrifugation by high-performance liquid chromatography (HPLC) to quantify encapsulation efficiency (Equation (1)). For GRFT analysis, an HPLC system (Waters Corporation, Milford, MA, USA) equipped with an auto injector (model 717), a quaternary pump (model 600), an ultraviolet detector (model 2487) at 280 nm, and a multi λ fluorescence detector (model 2475) at 370 nm was used. Separation of GRFT was achieved by using a Jupiter 5 μ 300 Å (250 × 4.6 mm) column (Phenomenex, Torrance, CA, USA) protected by a guard cartridge Jupiter C18 (4.0 × 3 mm). A gradient consisting of mobile phase A (0.1% trifluoroacetic acid [TFA] in Milli-Q water), and mobile Phase B (0.1% TFA in acetonitrile), at a flow rate of 1.0 mL/min, was used. Retention time of GRFT was approximately 16 min, and the total run time was 30 min. Empower Pro 3 software (Waters Corp., Milford, MA) was used to control the HPLC system.

DPV was assayed by using an Acquity ultra-performance liquid chromatography (UPLC) system H-class (Waters Corp., Milford, MA). Separation of DPV was achieved by using an Acquity UPLC BEH C18 (1.7 μm, 2.1 × 50 mm) column (Waters Corp., Milford, MA). A gradient consisting of mobile phase A (0.1% TFA in Milli-Q water) and mobile Phase B (0.1% TFA in acetonitrile), at a flow rate of 0.25 mL/min, was used. Retention time of DPV was approximately 8.5 min, and the total run time was 15 min. Empower Pro 3 software was used to control the UPLC system. Drug encapsulation efficiency is calculated by following equation as described by Papadimitriou et al. [47]:

$$\begin{aligned}\text{Drug encapsulation efficiency (\%)} &= \frac{\text{weight of drug in nanoparticles}}{\text{weight of drug fed initially}} \\ &= \frac{\text{weight of drug fed initially weight of drug in supernantant}}{\text{weight of drug fed initially}}\end{aligned} \quad (1)$$

2.2.4. In Vitro Release of ARVs from PLGA Nanoparticles

To determine the extent and rate of GRFT and DPV released from the nanoparticles, an in vitro release study was conducted over a 7-day period. In this study, vaginal fluid simulant (VFS, pH 4.5) was selected as dissolution medium to evaluate drug release from the fabricated nanoparticles because of its physiological relevance to the cervicovaginal fluid [48]. ARV-loaded nanoparticles were dispersed in 3 mL of VFS, with continuous shaking, at a temperature of 37 °C. At regular intervals, the nanoparticles were isolated via centrifugation (12,000× *g*, 4 °C, 30 min), and the entire VFS solution was decanted for analysis using chromatographic methods describe above. The nanoparticles were then re-suspended in fresh VFS and returned to the in vitro release set-up.

To determine the impact of medium and pH on drug release, in vitro release studies were also performed in 1 M phosphate-buffered saline (PBS) at pH 7.4 and 1 M PBS at pH 4.5 (1 M PBS adjusted to pH 4.5 with 10% hydrochloric acid). The amount of GRFT and DPV released into the release media was determined by HPLC or UPLC methodology as previously detailed.

2.2.5. Anti-HIV-1 Activity and Cellular Viability Assay of ARVs

The cytotoxicity and anti-HIV-1 activity of free and nanoparticle-formulated ARVs against HIV-1_{BaL} was determined in TZM-bl cells by luciferase quantification of cell lysates [49–51]. The HIV-1_{BaL} and TZM-bl indicator cell line were kindly provided by Dr. Charlene Dezzutti of Magee-Womens Research Institute. TZM-bl is a HeLa cell line derivation that stably expresses high levels (% positive cells) of CD4 (32%), CCR5 (82%) and CXCR4 (85%) [52]. The cells contain HIV-1 Tat-regulated reporter genes for firefly luciferase and β-galactosidase for quantitative analysis of HIV-1, simian immunodeficiency virus (SIV), and simian/human immunodeficiency virus (SHIV) infection [53]. The evaluation of cytotoxicity and anti-HIV-1 activity were conducted following methods previously described [54]. The cells were regularly cultured in Dulbecco's Modified Eagle Medium (DMEM) with 10% fetal bovine serum (FBS), 100 U/mL penicillin, 100 μg/mL streptomycin, and 1% 200 mM L-glutamine at 37 °C in 5% CO_2 atmosphere.

The TZM-bl cells were seeded into a 96-well clear-view plate, at a concentration of 5×10^4 cells per well, in 100 μL of DMEM medium (10% FBS) and allowed to adhere for 24 h at 37 °C [54]. Identical, but separate, plates were set up to measure efficacy and cellular toxicity. 100 μL of medium was removed and replaced with 100 μL of DMEM dilutions of test articles i.e., each drug and ARV-loaded nanoparticles (NP-ARVs). Cells exposed to media without test articles was used as a control. For toxicity testing, additional 100 μL of medium (without test articles) was added to each well to bring the total volume to 200 μL. The next day, 100 μL of medium was removed and replaced with 100 μL of CellTiter-Glo® (Promega, Madison, WI, USA) and the luminescence measured using SpectraMax M3 plate reader (Molecular Devices, Sunnyvale, CA, USA). Viability was determined on the basis of deviations from the cell-only control and presented as the percentage viability ± SD (standard deviation).

For efficacy testing, following addition of media with and without test articles, 100 μL of medium containing HIV-1 was added to each well to reach a total volume in each well of 200 μL. HIV-1_{BaL} was added at an approximate $TCID_{50}$ (50% tissue culture infectious dose) of 3000 per well in the presence of 40 μg/mL of Diethylaminoethyl cellulose- Dextran (DEAE-Dextran, Sigma, St. Louis, MO, USA). After 48 h, 100 μL of medium was removed and replaced with 100 μL of Bright-Glo™ (Promega, Madison, WI, USA) and the luminescence measured as mentioned above. Inhibition of HIV infection was determined on the basis of luminescence deviations from the HIV-1-only control and presented as the percentage inhibition ± SEM. Untreated wells with cells only served as the negative infectivity control (100% inhibition), while wells with cells and HIV-1 served as positive infectivity control (0% inhibition). The percent inhibition was calculated for all test and control cultures to determine the 50% inhibition concentration (IC_{50}) value of each drug. The IC_{50} values of NP-ARVs were calculated via GraphPad Prism (V 5.02) software, using drug concentrations that corresponded to the actual drug loading determined by HPLC.

2.2.6. Combination Effects

The combined anti-HIV-1 activity of the dual-drug combination was evaluated by using the median-effect analysis described by Chou and Talalay [55]. Briefly, median values (IC_{50}) of each drug were obtained using the TZM-bl antiviral activity assay as described in the previous section. The drugs were then mixed according to the ratio of their individual IC_{50} values (1:8, due to the molecular weight difference between DPV and GRFT). For NP-ARVs, amounts of the individual compounds used in combinations were determined by measured drug loading. The drug mixtures were then serially diluted, and IC_{50} values were determined with the TZM-bl assay. Combination effects of ARVs were evaluated by (1) comparing HIV-1 inhibition between the combination and each individual ARV; and (2) identifying combination indices (CI) to quantify drug synergy, using CompuSyn software (ComboSyn, Inc., Paramus, NJ, USA). The CI of drug combination was plotted as a function of the fractional inhibition (Fa), by computer simulation, from Fa = 0.10 to 0.95. In this analysis, the combined effect at the 50% fractional inhibition (CI_{50}) and 90% fractional inhibition (CI_{90}) were reported as synergistic, additive, or antagonistic when CI < 1, = 1, or >1, respectively.

2.2.7. Cellular Uptake Assay

The mouse macrophage cell line RAW264.7 (ATCC, Manassas, VA, USA) was maintained in DMEM culture medium with 10% FBS, 100 U/mL penicillin, 100 μg/mL streptomycin, and 1% 200 mM L-glutamine at 37 °C in 5% CO_2 atmosphere. RAW264.7 cells were cultured on a 1-cm diameter coverslip pre-coated with polylysine (BD BioCoat, BD Biosciences, Bedford, MA, USA) in DMEM culture medium for 48 h before uptake assay. Fluorescent dye-loaded NPs were added to the cells at 2.5% (*w/v*) of the total 200 μL of cell culture media for 4 h at 37 °C. NPs were then washed from cells with PBS for 4 times. The coverslips with cells grown on them were first stained with 4′,6-diamidino-2-phenylindole (DAPI, Molecular Probes, and Eugene) in PBS in order to visualize the nuclei and were then mounted on glass slides for fluorescent imaging. The fluorescent images were obtained by ApoTome Confocal Microscope Observer Z1 (Carl Zeiss Microscopy, Zaventem, Belgium). Cell images were taken at 358/461 nm for DAPI, 495/519 nm for FITC-dextran, and 552/636 nm for Nile red.

2.2.8. Statistical Analyses

All differences were evaluated by Student's t-test or ANOVA analysis. $p < 0.05$ was considered statistically significant. Drug release profiles were analyzed using DD Solver, an Excel add-in package [56]. All error bars represent standard deviations unless otherwise noted.

3. Results

3.1. PLGA Nanoparticle Characterization

In this study, PLGA core-shell nanoparticles were successfully developed that simultaneously encapsulate and deliver both a protein drug and a small-molecule hydrophobic drug without compromising the effectiveness of either. The manufactured PLGA nanoparticles are near-spherical in shape, possess high drug-loading capability, and are of a reproducible size. It has been reported that the duration and intensity of sonication can significantly affect the size of the nanoparticles produced using double-emulsion method [57,58]. The targeted particle size and distribution can be obtained by optimizing sonication intensity and time within a given system. With the sonication parameters described in the Methods section, the diameters of the fabricated nanoparticles were confined to a narrow range (Table 1): 182.8 ± 1.7 nm (placebo nanoparticles) to 188.8 ± 1.7 nm (GRFT, DPV, or GRFT/DPV nanoparticles) and had low polydispersity index (PDI < 0.1), indicating that nearly monodispersed nanoparticles were manufactured (Figure 2). Zeta potential measurements showed minimal change between unloaded and loaded nanoparticles, falling within a range of −23.4 ± 0.3 mV to −24.9 ± 1.3 mV, respectively, at a pH of 7.4. The high similarity in colloidal properties of all nanoparticles such as size, PDI, and zeta potential demonstrates that the formed nanoparticles are composed of PLGA-PVA system. It is highly unlikely that the particles are primarily composed of GRFT alone. Table 1 lists properties of placebo nanoparticles (vehicle) and ARV-loaded nanoparticles fabricated using double emulsion evaporation.

A GRFT encapsulation efficiency of 40.7 ± 5.9% and 45.9 ± 13.7% was obtained from the manufactured single (NP-GRFT) and combination nanoparticles (NP-GRFT/DPV), respectively. A DPV encapsulation efficiency of 70.1 ± 4.4% and 69.4 ± 5.1% was obtained from NP-DPV and NP-GRFT/DPV, respectively. Our results indicate that the encapsulation efficiency of DPV and GRFT are independent of each other in the combined NPs. Our findings are similar to those describing the manufacture of PLGA nanoparticles via double-emulsion or solvent displacement methods [30,38,43]. Our results suggest that the double-emulsion technique is suitable for encapsulating both hydrophilic macromolecules and hydrophobic small molecules in PLGA-based core-shell type nanoparticles simultaneously.

Table 1. Physicochemical properties of PLGA nanoparticles loaded with ARVs.

Drugs	Size (d.nm ± SD)	PDI	Zeta Potential (mV ± SD)	Encapsulation Efficiency (% ± SD)
Placebo	182.8 ± 1.7	0.066	−23.7 ± 0.6	-
GRFT	188.8 ± 1.7	0.069	−23.5 ± 0.3	40.7 ± 5.9
DPV	186.6 ± 1.6	0.079	−24.9 ±1.3	70.1 ± 4.4
GRFT/DPV	184.3 ± 1.0	0.063	−23.4 ± 0.3	45.9 ± 13.7 (GRFT) 69.4 ± 5.1 (DPV)

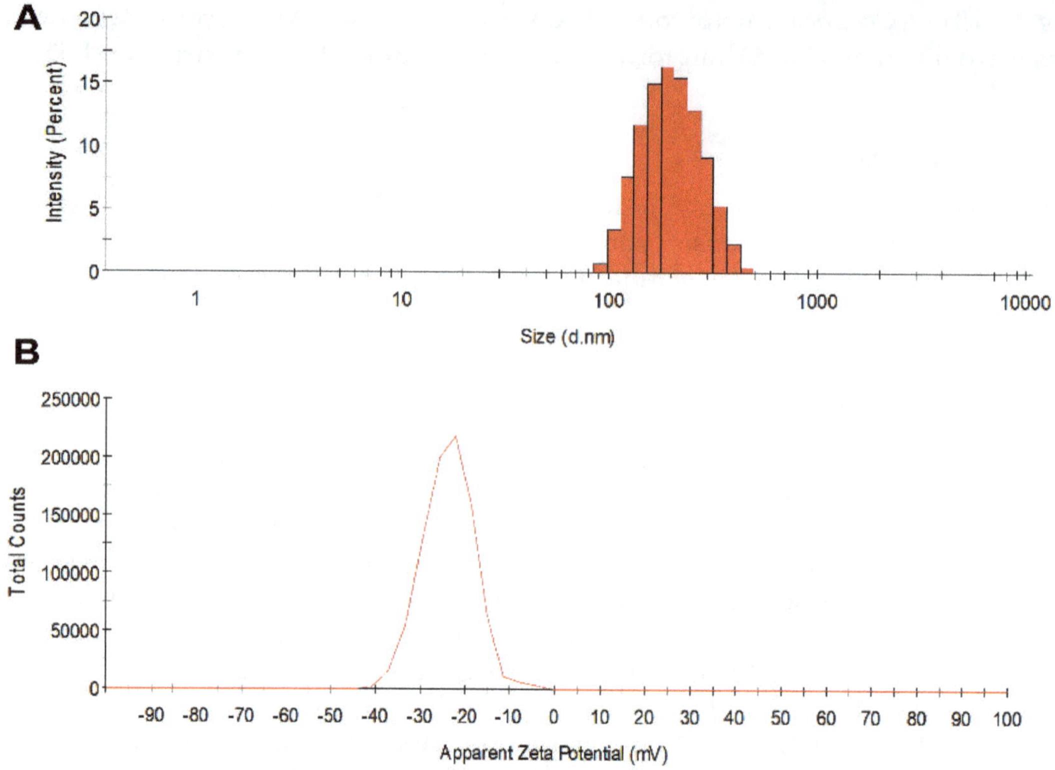

Figure 2. Characterization of PLGA nanoparticles loaded with GRFT and DPV. (**A**) Size and (**B**) zeta potential distribution graphs of nanoparticles encapsulated with anti-HIV drugs GRFT and DPV (NP-DPV/GRFT).

3.2. *In Vitro Release Studies of ARVs from PLGA Nanoparticles Resulting in Sustained Drug Release*

The in vitro drug release profile of GRFT and DPV from NP-ARVs was measured over 7 days in VFS at pH 4.5 that mimics the composition, pH, and viscoelastic properties of vaginal fluid produced by healthy, adult, nonpregnant women [48,59,60], as well as in buffers at pH 7.4 and pH 4.5. Our findings indicate that the combination of ARVs and media pH/composition affect the release profile of individual ARVs from core-shell PLGA nanoparticles as shown in Figure 3.

The in vitro release of GRFT and DPV from both single-entity and combination nanoparticles followed a biphasic release profile (Figure 3A,B). In VFS, the combination nanoparticles showed an initial burst release within first 24 h, where 15.1 ± 2.6% of the GRFT had been released. A sustained release of GRFT was obtained over the remaining 7 days. The total amount of drug released over the 7-day period was 16.7 ± 2.8%. Although not statistically significant, less GRFT was released from NP-GRFT, in both burst phase (11.1 ± 2.2%) and total amount of GRFT released (12.1 ± 2.8%) than that from combination nanoparticles.

The in vitro release of DPV showed a different and more prolonged initial burst release profiles (Figure 3C,D). In VFS, after 1 day, 51.7 ± 7.8% of DPV was released from the combination nanoparticles (NP-DPV/GRFT). DPV was released continuously over the next 7 days. The total amount of drug released over the 7-day period was 76.9 ± 13.1%. Similar to GRFT release, DPV release was lower from single entity nanoparticles in both burst phase (45.9 ± 10.0%), as well as the total amount of DPV released in 7 days (69.0 ± 12.8%) compared to combination nanoparticles in VFS and pH 7.4 media.

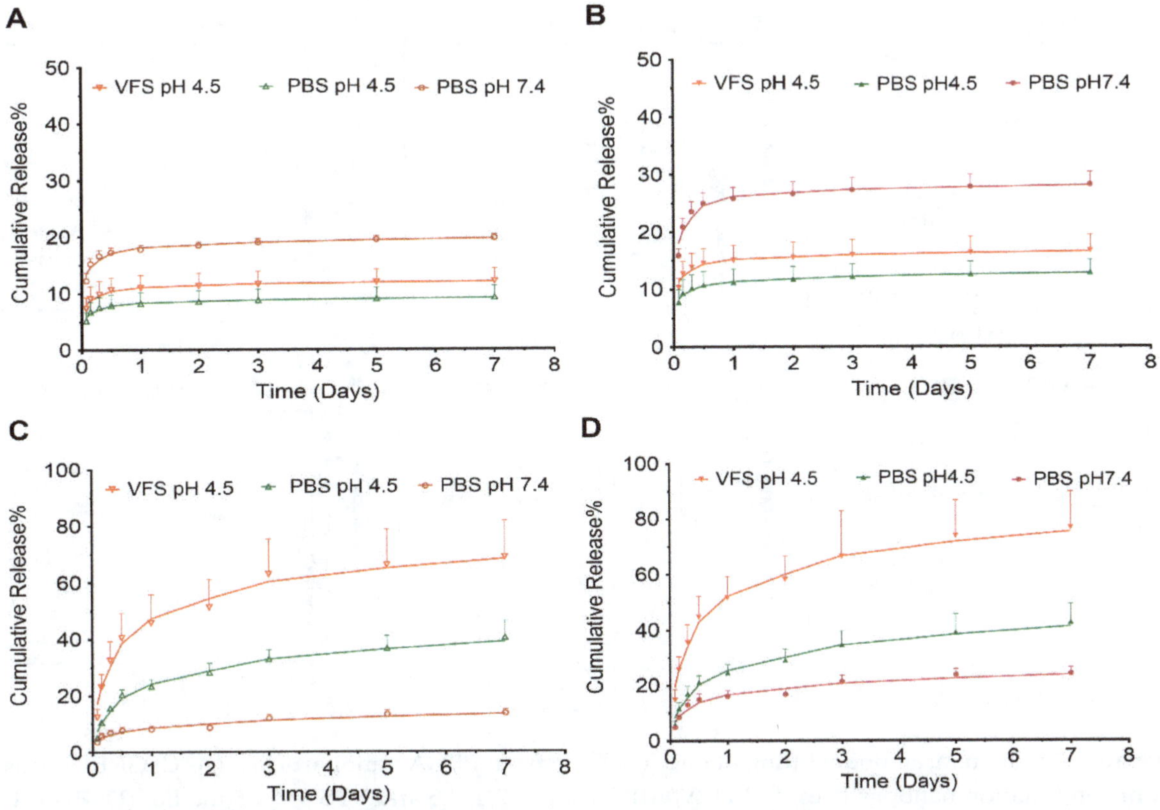

Figure 3. In vitro release of ARVs from PLGA nanoparticles in VFS at pH 4.5, and buffers at pH 4.5 and pH 7.4. (**A**) GRFT release from NP-GRFT and (**B**) NP-DPV/GRFT. (**C**) DPV release from NP-DPV and (**D**) NP-DPV/GRFT. NP-nanoparticles.

We also investigated the effect of pH and release media on the in vitro release of the PLGA nanoparticles. Total release of DPV from NP-DPV/GRFT was significantly higher in pH 4.5 media than that in pH 7.4 media (42.7 ± 6.7% vs. 24.3 ± 2.2%, $p < 0.05$). Even more DPV was released in VFS (pH 4.5) (76.9 ± 13.1%, $p < 0.05$) than in pH 4.5 media. However, pH showed an opposite effect on GRFT's release from nanoparticles. The total release of GRFT from NP-DPV/GRFT was significantly less in pH 4.5 media than that in pH 7.4 (12.9 ± 2.2% vs. 28.2 ± 2.2%, $p < 0.05$), while the total release of GRFT in VFS (16.7 ± 2.8%) was only slightly higher than that in pH 4.5 media. The order of release in the media remained similar for the single entity nanoparticles (NP-DPV and NP-GRFT) compared to combination nanoparticles; however, stronger statistical differences were noted. The order of release rate of NP-ARVs is pH 7.4 > VFS > pH 4.5 for GRFT and VFS > pH 4.5 > pH 7.4 for DPV. These results suggest that co-encapsulation could lead to enhanced release of each ARV from PLGA nanoparticles in all the media investigated.

To reveal the mechanism of drug release from fabricated nanoparticles, we used mathematical modeling to analyze the in vitro release profiles of GRFT and DPV by various kinetic models. Three empirical and semi-empirical models used were the Higuchi model, the Peppas–Sahlin model, and the Weibull model [56]. Higher correlation was observed in the Peppas model and Weibull model (Figures 4 and 5). Therefore, our results indicate that release of ARVs from PLGA nanoparticles is not predominantly driven by a solo mechanism, but a combined mechanism of Fickian (pure diffusion phenomenon) and non-Fickian release (due to the relaxation of the polymer chains between the networks).

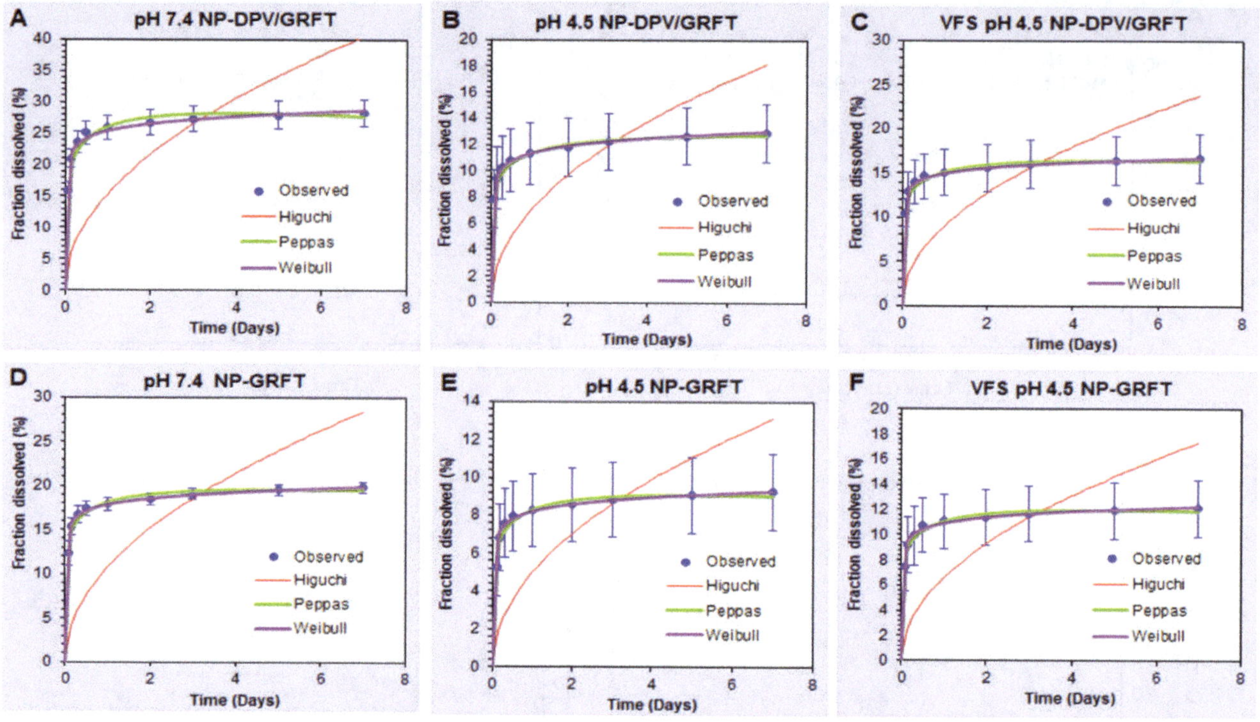

Figure 4. Mathematical model fitting of GRFT release from PLGA nanoparticles. (**A–C**) GRFT release from combination nanoparticles (NP-DPV/GRFT) at pH 7.4, 4.5 and VFS pH 4.5 media. (**D–F**) GRFT release from single entity nanoparticles (NP-GRFT) at pH 7.4, 4.5 and VFS pH 4.5 media. Dissolution profiles were fitted to Higuchi, Peppas, and Weibull models.

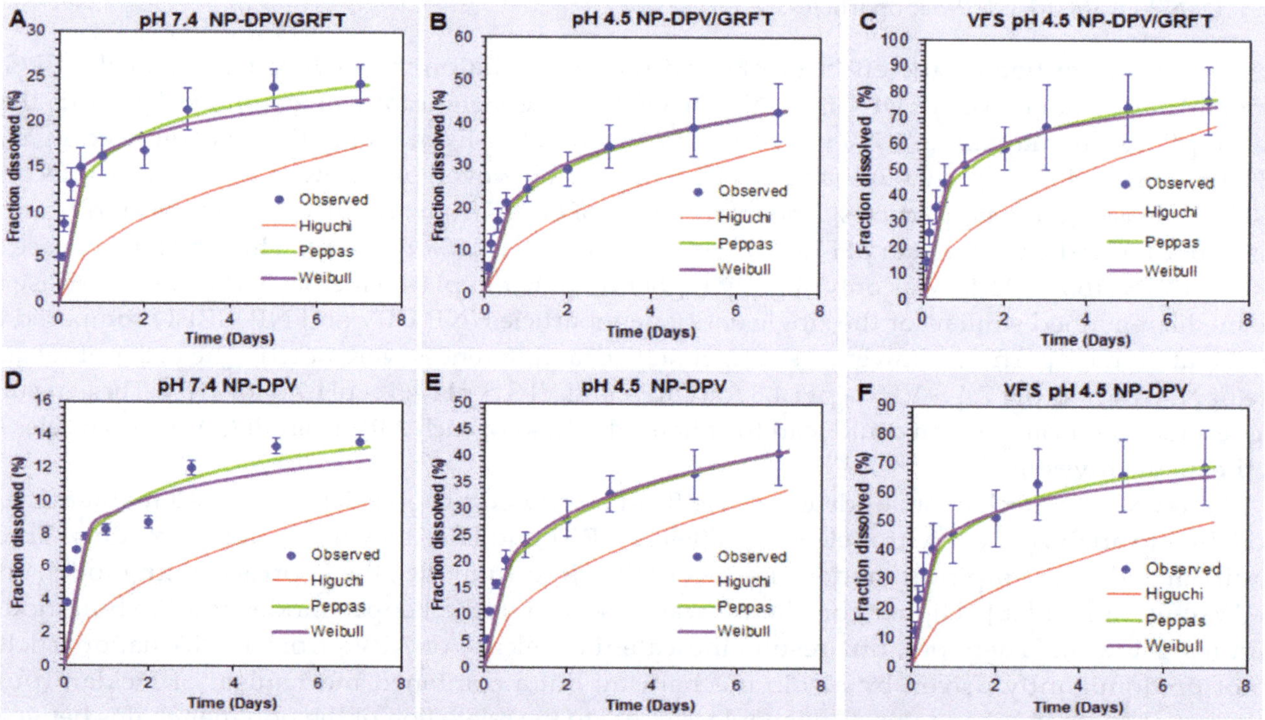

Figure 5. Mathematical model fitting of DPV release from PLGA nanoparticles. (**A–C**) DPV release from combination nanoparticles (NP-DPV/GRFT) at pH 7.4, 4.5 and VFS pH 4.5 media. (**D–F**) DPV release from single entity nanoparticles (NP-DPV) at pH 7.4, 4.5 and VFS pH 4.5 media. Dissolution profiles were fitted to Higuchi, Peppas, and Weibull models.

3.3. PLGA NP-ARVs Potently Inhibit HIV-1_{BaL} Infection In Vitro

To ensure that the anti-HIV-1 activity of the ARVs was retained after being loaded into nanoparticles, we tested the protection of NP-ARVs and unformulated ARVs against HIV-1_{BaL} infection, using the TZM-bl assay. Anti-HIV-1 efficacy of NP-ARVs and unformulated ARVs was measured as percent of HIV inhibition, which is calculated using percent relative luminescence units of TZM-bl cells treated with ARVs or NP-ARVs compared to untreated (media only) TZM-bl cells after exposure to HIV-1_{BaL} as noted in the Methods section.

The anti-HIV-1 activity of blank PLGA nanoparticles was not observed in the TZM-bl assay, which was comparable to the negative media control. After exposure of TZM-bl cells to NP-ARVs or free ARVs; however, we observed potent antiviral activity against HIV-1_{BaL}, with estimated IC_{50} values in the nanomolar ranges for GRFT and DPV, respectively (Table 2). Compared with free DPV, NP-DPV showed slightly enhanced HIV inhibitory activity, with an IC_{50} of 4.7 nM for the unformulated DPV to 3.6 nM for NP-DPV (Figure 6). The encapsulation of GRFT in PLGA nanoparticles slightly shifted the IC_{50} from 0.5 nM for the unformulated GRFT to 0.8 nM for the NP-GRFT. However, no statistically significant difference was observed between NP-GRFT and unformulated GRFT.

Table 2. IC_{50} of ARVs and NP-ARVs estimated by TZM-bl assay.

Drug	**Alone (nM)**	
	Unformulated	**NP-GRFT/NP-DPV**
DPV	4.7 ± 2.9	3.6 ± 2.9
GRFT	0.5 ± 0.3	0.8 ± 0.7

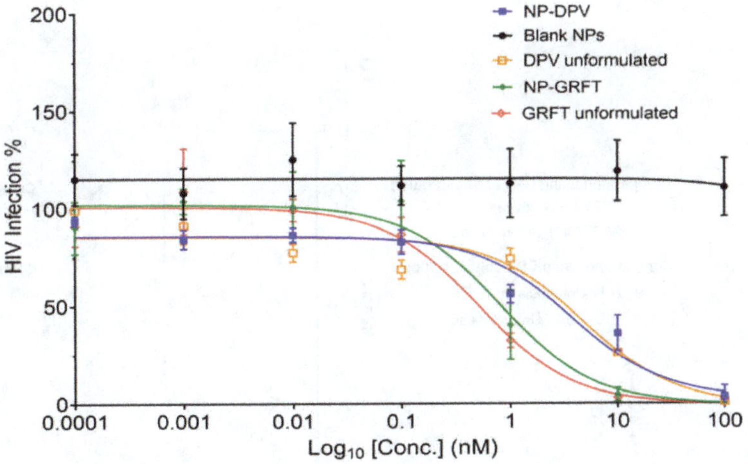

Figure 6. Anti-HIV activity of GRFT or DPV in PLGA nanoparticles. Anti-HIV activity of unformulated ARVs and fabricated NP-ARVs were evaluated in TZM-bl cells exposed to HIV-1. Luciferase luminescent readings of treated TZM-bl cells were compared against untreated cells infected with HIV-1 to obtain % HIV infection. Results are reported on a log scale of ARVs dosing levels versus percent of infection.

We hypothesized that NP-DPV can increase the intracellular concentration of DPV, resulting in greater potency due to enhanced internalization and intracellular uptake of PLGA nanoparticles [46,61]. For GRFT, whose target is on the cell membrane, the internalization and intracellular uptake of nanoparticles may cause the loss of bioactivity as we observed in the experiment, which is consistent with other reports on protein fusion inhibitors, such as RANTES [38]. However, no significant loss of GRFT's bioactivity was observed. Together, our results suggest that both GRFT and DPV can be loaded into nanoparticles without compromising their potent bioactivity.

3.4. NP-ARV Combination Exhibits Strong Synergistic Bioactivity

To identify the interactive effects on our ARVs' bioactivity, we evaluated the activity of their combination in nanoparticle and unformulated drugs, using the TZM-bl assay. The equipotency ratio of GRFT and DPV (i.e., 1:1 ratios of IC_{50} values), were used to assess the effect of the drug combination, when drugs were combined as unformulated or as distinct nanoparticles. This equipotency translated to a 1:8 molar ratio for GRFT:DPV. Notably, this exact ratio cannot be maintained in the manufactured combination nanoparticles (NP-DPV/GRFT), therefore these nanoparticles were tested at the loaded ARV levels.

The efficacy of GRFT and DPV was significantly improved when tested in combination compared with when tested alone, either as unformulated GRFT and DPV or combined as distinct nanoparticles (NP-GRFT and NP-DPV) or when co-encapsulated into combination nanoparticles. Figure 7 shows the dose-response relationships of unformulated GRFT or DPV alone versus unformulated GRFT/DPV combination (Figure 7A), NP-GRFT or NP-DPV alone vs NP-GRFT and NP-DPV combination (Figure 7B). The results demonstrate that GRFT and DPV combined as unformulated or distinct nanoparticles or in a combination nanoparticle system display similar reduction in HIV infection. Interestingly, although the combination system does not include GRFT and DPV at equipotency ratio, a similar reduction in HIV infection was observed. IC_{50} values for combinations were not calculated, because even at the lowest tested concentration, high potency was observed, i.e., <50% HIV infection. Overall, the combination of GRFT and DPV showed significant leftward shift in the dose-response curve compared to single ARVs, indicating a strong synergy. The results also suggest that the efficacy is comparable between combination in unformulated, NP-GRFT and NP-DPV combination, and NP-GRFT/DPV, as shown in Figure 8.

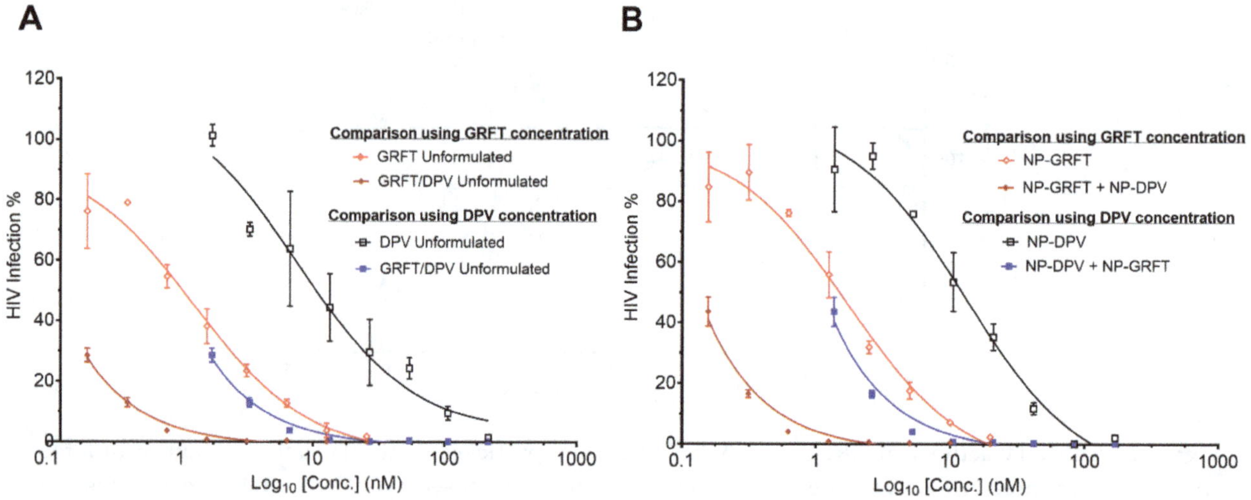

Figure 7. Strong synergistic effect of GRFT and DPV in free drug combination, in NP-GRFT and NP-DPV combination. The dose-response curve shows antiviral activity of (**A**) free GRFT, free DPV or combination of free GRFT and free DPV. (**B**) GRFT-loaded nanoparticles (NP-GRFT), DPV-loaded nanoparticles (NP-DPV) alone or in combination (NP-GRFT + NP-DPV). At a 1:8 molar ratio (GRFT and DPV), the antiviral activity of each drug in combination showed a significant reduction in %HIV infection (IC_{50} cannot be computed) compared to single ARV drug in unformulated or encapsulated forms. No difference in anti-HIV activity of GRFT or DPV were found in unformulated or nanoparticle combinations.

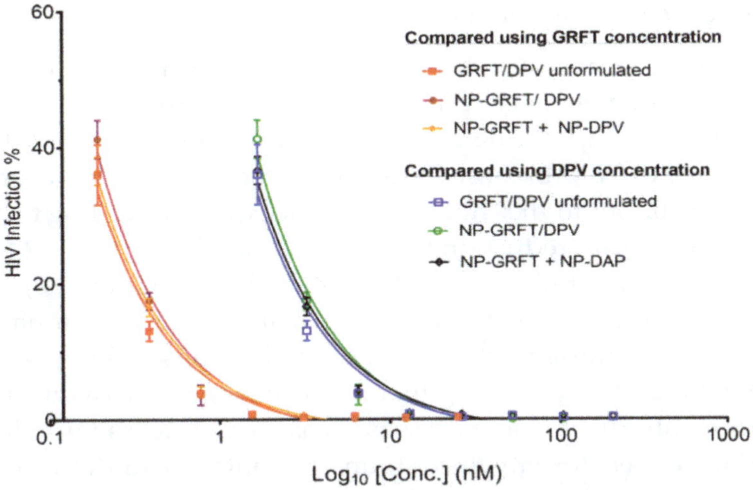

Figure 8. Potent and comparable anti-HIV effect of GRFT and DPV combinations. The dose-response curve shows potent antiviral activity of the combination of free drugs (GRFT/DPV unformulated), combination of single ARV nanoparticles (NP-GRFT + NP-DPV), and nanoparticles encapsulating both GRFT and DPV (NP-GRFT/DPV). Comparable inhibition of HIV infection was achieved with combination nanoparticles although the ARV ratio is not maintained at equipotency values (1:1 IC_{50} or 1:8 molar ratio for GRFT:DPV).

The CI was determined for the ARV drugs combined at molar ratios to achieve anti-HIV equipotency (1:1 ratios of IC_{50} values), leading to a 1:8 (GRFT: DPV) molar ratio in concentration. The CI of each unformulated ARV or NP-ARV combination was plotted as a function of the fractional inhibition (Fa) from 0.10 to 0.95 (Figure 9). The CI values were very low over the range from 0.10 to 0.95 of Fa. We interpreted the combination effects, at the CI_{50} and CI_{90} values, of unformulated GRFT/DPV and NP-GRFT/NP-DPV in combination ($CI_{50/90} < 0.1$) as demonstrating an extremely strong synergistic effect of anti-HIV infection.

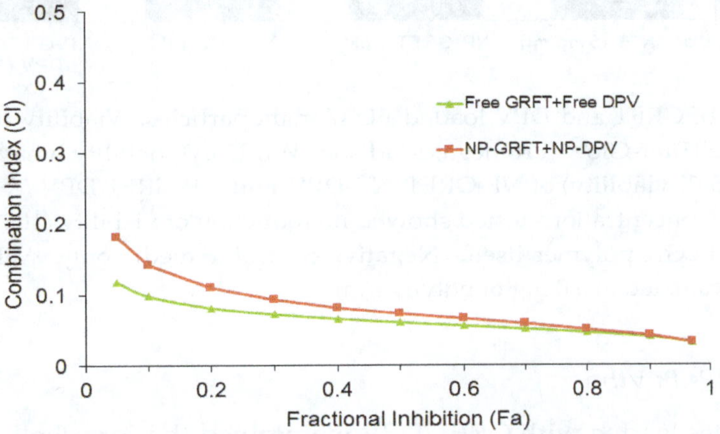

Figure 9. Combination index (CI) of free GRFT with free DPV or GRFT nanoparticles (NP-GRFT) with DPV nanoparticles (NP-DPV) were quantified using the TZM-bl infectivity assay. CI < 1, = 1, and >1 indicate synergistic, additive, and antagonistic effects, respectively. Combination of GRFT and DPV at a 1:8 molar ratio (GRFT:DPV) demonstrated very strong synergism, with CI at 50% inhibition (CI_{50}) of 0.086 and 0.066 for unformulated and nanoparticle combinations respectively. CI 0.90–1.10: nearly additive; CI 0.85–0.95: slight synergism; CI 0.7–0.85: moderate synergism; CI 0.3–0.7: synergism; CI 0.1–0.3 strong synergism; CI < 0.1: Very strong synergism.

3.5. NP-ARVs Are Nontoxic to In Vitro Cell Lines

Neither blank PLGA nanoparticles nor ARV-loaded PLGA nanoparticles were observed to be cytotoxic to cells over the range of concentrations evaluated in the TZM-bl assay. The cytotoxicity of NP-ARVs was evaluated during testing of their bioactivity in order to exclude any effects of the nanoparticles on the viability of TZM-bl cells. Cytotoxicity of our NP-ARVs was measured over a range of ARV concentrations, from 0.0001 to 1000 nM, after 24 h of exposure, leading to polymer concentration less than 0.1 mg/mL. No significant reduction ($p < 0.05$) in viability of the TZM-bl cells was observed in NP-ARV-treated cells as compared to untreated TZM-bl cells (Figure 10). In addition, we tried to evaluate the upper limit of cytotoxicity of nanoparticle vehicles. Compared with the negative control (media only), vehicle-control/blank NPs, at concentrations of 5 mg polymer/mL, showed no reduction of viability (100% ± 8%), suggesting that PLGA nanoparticles alone are not cytotoxic below this concentration. Since anti-HIV bioactivity was measured at doses far below 5 mg/mL polymer concentrations, we did not expect toxicity to confound the outcome of the antiviral activity assays.

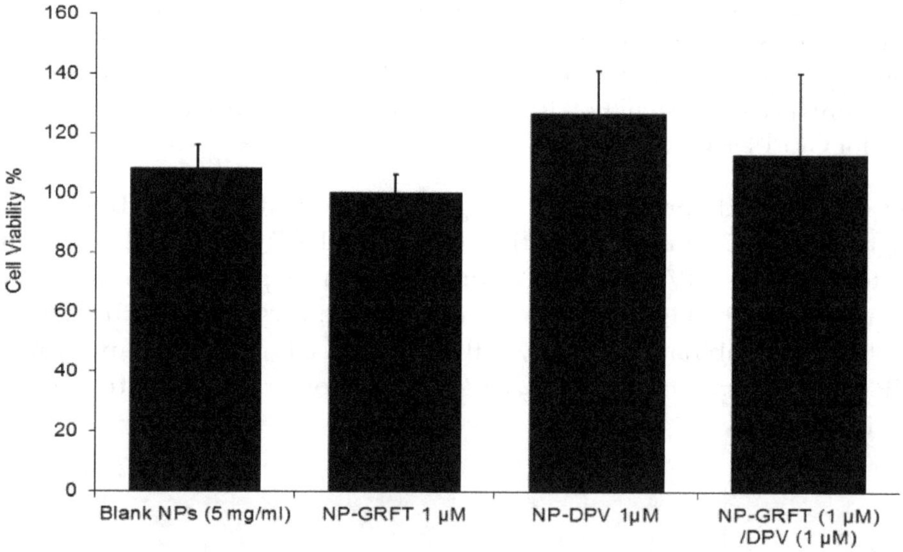

Figure 10. Toxicity of GRFT and DPV loaded PLGA nanoparticles. Viability of TZM-bl cells was measured by the CellTiter-Glo® (Promega, Madison, WI, USA) viability assay kit demonstrating non-toxic nature (≥80% viability) of NP-GRFT, NP-DPV, and NP-GRFT/DPV. Vehicle control (blank nanoparticles) at the concentrations tested showed no reduction of viability (108% ± 7%), indicating non-cytotoxicity of PLGA polymer itself. Negative control = media only. Vehicle control for all nanoparticles was evaluated at 5.0 mg of polymer/mL.

3.6. Cellular Uptake of NPs In Vitro

PLGA nanoparticles loaded with GRFT/DPV maintained the core-shell structure after cellular uptake. FITC-dextran and Nile red were incorporated into NPs as to evaluate the cellular uptake of NP-ARVs using fluorescence imaging as shown in Figure 11. FITC-dextran (Green) was used to mimic GRFT due to its water solubility and its molecular weight of 70 kDa. Nile red (Red) was used to mimic DPV due to its hydrophobicity. Coincident red and green fluorescence signals could be observed in the cytoplasm of RAW264.7 after 4 h incubation. The results demonstrate that the nanoparticles were taken up intact. Therefore, they could be delivered simultaneously in vivo with their synergistic anti-HIV effect.

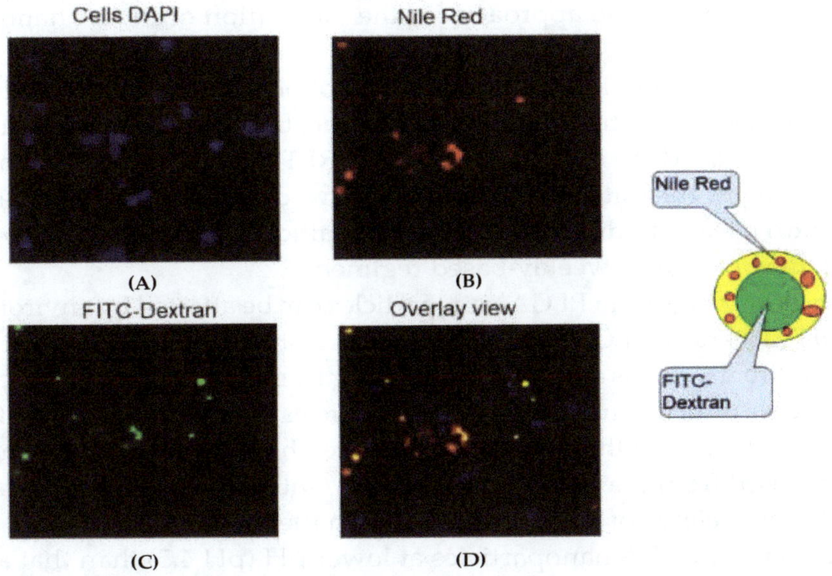

Figure 11. The cellular uptake of nanoparticles loaded with both FITC-Dextran (green, GRFT mimic) and Nile Red (red, DPV mimic) was investigated in RAW264.7 cells. Representative fluorescent microscopy images of RAW264.7 cells post nanoparticle exposure at 40× magnification. (**A**) Fluorescence images show RAW264.7 cells nuclei stained with DAPI (blue) for positioning purpose, (**B**) images of Nile red (red) and (**C**) FITC-dextran (green) of same field were taken through different channels to illustrate the position of FITC-dextran (green)/Nile red (red) encapsulated nanoparticles in cells. (**D**) Overlay image showing coincident green and red signals as yellow color indicating uptake of intact nanoparticles.

4. Discussion

Combination and long-acting drug products are emerging approaches for the prevention of HIV-1 infection, due to the clinical need for effectiveness, safety, and patient adherence. To date, no combination PrEP is available, either as a vaginal or a rectal product, although efforts are underway. The only oral PrEP currently approved by the FDA (in 2004) is Truvada, which is a combination of emtricitabine and tenofovir disoproxil fumarate. Patient adherence plays a key role in the effectiveness of PrEP products [62], a lesson to be learned from several HIV prevention trials, which found that higher adherence resulted in lower HIV incidence [13,14,63]. Long-acting formulations offer a promising paradigm to overcome the adherence challenge in the development of PrEP products [64,65].

Two PrEP candidates have been intensively studied, individually, as potential microbicides in pre-clinical evaluations. GRFT, a fusion inhibitor, has demonstrated high efficacy against HIV-1 infection at nanomolar concentrations, with enhanced anti-HIV-1 activity and extended contact time with HIV-1 [18,20]. However, cervicovaginal secretions tend to inhibit GRFT-gp120 binding, as well as oxidize its methionine at position 78, resulting in compromise of GRFT in vivo [66]. DPV is an NNRTI with extreme potency against HIV-1 infection. Yet, its quick elimination from tissue may lower its anti-HIV-1 activity as a microbicide [23]. We hypothesized that core-shell polymeric nanocarriers could enhance the anti-HIV-1 effect of these two candidate ARVs via simultaneous co-delivery and sustained release for long-acting prevention of HIV-1 infection via vaginal route.

In this study, we demonstrated that a protein drug and a small hydrophobic drug can be encapsulated within polymeric nanoparticles to provide prophylaxis in combination. Anti-HIV-1 drugs were encapsulated into fabricated PLGA nanoparticles without compromising their anti-HIV-1 bioactivity. The nanoparticles were near-monodispersed, mostly spherical in shape. The constant negative zeta potential of the nanoparticles from the unloaded to the loaded state suggests that the hydrophilic microbicide is encapsulated in the core structure of nanoparticles rather than adsorbed onto the surface. High encapsulation efficiency of both GRFT and DPV suggests that the double emulsion method would be a viable approach for the fabrication of PLGA nanoparticles for other microbicide candidates.

We were able to demonstrate the sustained release of both GRFT and DPV, one of the defining characteristics of fabricated PLGA nanoparticles and indicating a potential long-acting nanoparticle delivery system. The in vitro drug release profiles of GRFT and DPV from the nanoparticles were characterized by two stages: the initial burst release followed by a sustained release over the time of the experiment. In vitro release studies showed that a significant amount of drug was released over a 7-day period, which may provide a weekly-based regimen.

The in vitro release of drugs from PLGA nanoparticles can be affected by environmental conditions such as changes in pH. Generally, PLGA polymer degrades faster at lower pH than at neutral pH [67,68]. The normal vaginal environment has an acidic pH, ranging from 3.8 to 4.5, as a protective barrier [69,70]. Therefore, in vitro release of drugs from PLGA nanoparticles was evaluated in buffers and VFS. Our studies showed that pH changes in the environment affected both the release rate and the total amount of GRFT and DPV released from the PLGA nanoparticles. Interestingly, we observed that pH change has opposite effects on the release of DPV and GRFT from the nanoparticles. More DPV was released into dissolution media from PLGA nanoparticles at lower pH (pH 4.5) than that at pH 7.4, which is expected due to the increased hydrolysis or erosion of PLGA polymers at lower pH [71]. Furthermore, DPV is likely to be in the protonated form at low pH, leading to increased solubility and release. Although both media possess similar pH, DPV release in VFS was much higher compared to the pH 4.5 buffer, possibly due to increased solubility of hydrophobic DPV in VFS, which contains bovine serum albumin. On the contrary, less GRFT was released from PLGA nanoparticles at lower pH (pH 4.5) than that at neutral pH (pH 7.4). One possible explanation for this phenomenon is that GRFT is positively charged at pH 4.5 due to its low isoelectric point (pI) of 5.39. Thus, the electrostatic interaction between positively charged GRFT and negatively charged PLGA nanoparticles may suppress the release of GRFT from PLGA nanoparticles. PSC-RANTES, for instance, has a much higher pI (around 9.0), retaining positive charge at both pH 7.4 and pH 4.5 [72]. Therefore, the release of PSC-RANTES is only determined by environmental pH [38]. Further studies are needed to confirm our hypothesis.

This compensatory release profile of our nanoparticles could prove beneficial for HIV-1 prevention. In a regular vaginal environment, more DPV will be released from the nanoparticles at lower pH (pH 4.5); when the presence of semen results in a higher pH environment (pH 7.4), more GRFT will be released. Our nanoparticle system could provide protection against HIV-1 infection in both scenarios. Therefore, it could be used in either a coitally dependent or coitally independent manner and provide protection over a wide range of environmental pH values.

Mathematical models were applied to evaluate the drug release from the nanoparticles. The results suggest that the release may be governed by a mixed mechanism of diffusion and polymer degradation, which is different from the polymer degradation–only mechanism of PSC-RANTES release from PLGA nanoparticles reported by Ham et al. [38]. However, the polymer chain relaxation may be the rate-limiting step for the drug release from the PLGA nanoparticle system. Further detailed studies are needed to elucidate the mechanisms involved, which is beyond the scope of this work.

Since the combination of GRFT and DPV is extremely potent, the HIV infection could not reach 50% in CI study, even at extremely low concentration of GRFT and DPV in combination, which made the estimation of IC_{50} for GRFT and DPV combination not very reliable. However, that also confirmed the potency of our combination strategy using GRFT and DPV. We found that the combination of free GRFT with free DPV at a 1:1 ratio of IC_{50} values demonstrated a strong synergistic effect (Figure 7). Importantly, the same synergistic effect was also demonstrated when the combination of drugs was released from nanoparticles, indicating that our PLGA nanoparticle system is suitable for delivering highly potent anti-HIV-1 drugs in combination. We quantified the synergistic effects of free GRFT and free DPV and NP-GRFT/NP-DPV using the median effect analysis developed by Chou and Talalay [73]. We believe that this synergy suggests a promising combination of ARVs as candidates for HIV-1 PrEP. Importantly, our studies demonstrated that GRFT and DPV possess a strong synergistic effect in vitro and that this synergistic effect can be maintained in PLGA nanoparticle delivery system. It had been reported that GRFT can have synergistic effects when used in combination with other anti-HIV-1 drugs, such as tenofovir [22]. However, it has never been studied in combination with DPV either as free drugs or in a nanoparticle system. Our findings indicate that the antiviral activity against HIV-1_{BaL} of our NP-ARVs was maintained similar to unformulated ARVs. The IC_{50} of DPV and GRFT did not change significantly in nanoparticles compared to unformulated form. Our results, however, show enhanced anti-HIV activity of NP-DPV (but $p > 0.05$), which may be caused by more uptake of nanoparticles [61]. The uptake of nanoparticles was visually confirmed in the RAW267.4 cell model. The combination NP-DPV/GRFT system also showed high anti-HIV-1 activity comparable to combination of unformulated ARVs and distinct NP-ARVs. Even without accomplishing 1:8 molar ratio of ARVs, our developed system displayed high potency and suitable for long-term application.

Interestingly, the potency of a drug may play an important role in the extent of combination effect with other drugs. Chaowanachan et al. reported that only additive effects were identified in a study of tenofovir and efavirenz delivery in combination in PLGA nanoparticles; this may be due to the limited drug release from the nanoparticles within the first hour [43]. Here, both tenofovir and efavirenz have an IC_{50} at a micromolar level, resulting in higher drug concentration needed for efficacy. Therefore, a faster drug release rate is required to achieve effective concentration against HIV infection. On the contrary, in our studies, both GRFT and DPV have an IC_{50} at a nanomolar level, indicating that only a small amount of the released drugs would be sufficient for complete HIV-1 inhibition. The difference between these studies using PLGA nanoparticles shows that the drug release rate needs to be optimized according to the drug potency by altering manufacturing and formulation conditions of the nanoparticles.

5. Conclusions

Although nanoparticles have been intensively investigated in numerous biomedical applications, not many studies have been conducted on nanoparticles as a drug delivery system for PrEP products, especially the combination delivery of a protein drug with a water-insoluble drug. In this study, successful encapsulation of both GRFT and DPV into core-shell nanoparticles resulted in monodispersed, near-spherical particles with low PDI that maintained their anti-HIV-1bioactivity. Furthermore, we have shown that our NP-ARVs act synergistically in preventing HIV-1 infection in vitro, and that the formulated PLGA nanoparticles provide sustained release of the drugs. To our knowledge, this is the first quantitative measure of synergistic effect of GRFT and DPV combination in a nanoparticle system. Additionally, the sustained release property of manufactured NPs provides a delivery system that could potentially reduce the dosing frequency to a weekly based regimen, which could significantly increase the compliance and acceptability in women.

However, additional research is required to further develop PLGA nanoparticles as PrEP products for delivery of combined GRFT and DPV. In particular, the relationship between protein pI and protein release in different media e.g., VFS. The model for drug release study in this paper only provides an empirical explanation on the mechanism of protein drug release from nanoparticles. Further investigation will help to reveal the mechanism of drug release from PLGA-based nanoparticles, particularly for protein drugs. In addition, the distribution of nanoparticles in the reproductive tract may affect the efficacy in vivo and needs to be investigated. These studies are beyond the scope of this paper and will be investigated in our future work.

Author Contributions: Conceptualization, L.C.R. and H.Y.; methodology, L.C.R., H.Y., and J.L.; formal analysis, H.Y., S.K.P., J.L., and L.C.R.; investigation, L.C.R., H.Y., J.L., and S.K.P.; resources, L.C.R., H.Y., K.E.P., and B.D.; data curation, H.Y., L.C.R., J.L., and S.K.P.; writing—H.Y., L.C.R., S.K.P., J.L., D.P., K.E.P.; review and editing, H.Y., L.C.R., J.L., S.K.P.; funding acquisition, L.C.R., H.Y., and K.E.P."

Acknowledgments: We would like to thank Charlene Dezzutti (deceased) for her help with anti-HIV testing. We greatly acknowledge Hima Bindu Ruttala for designing the schematic showing nanoparticle preparation and critical review of the manuscript. We greatly acknowledge Won-Bin Young for his help with uptake study. We would like to thank the Center for Biologic Imaging (CBI) of the University of Pittsburgh for access to the electron microscopy instrumentation and for assistance with the execution of this part of the study.

References

1. UNAIDS. Global HIV & AIDS Statistics—2018 Fact Sheet. Available online: http://www.unaids.org/en/resources/fact-sheet (accessed on 19 February 2019).
2. AVERT. Women and Girls, HIV and AIDS. Available online: https://www.avert.org/professionals/hiv-social-issues/key-affected-populations/women (accessed on 19 February 2019).
3. Centers for Disease Control and Prevention. HIV Among Women. Available online: https://www.cdc.gov/hiv/group/gender/women/index.html (accessed on 14 April 2019).
4. Bedimo, A.L.; Bennett, M.; Kissinger, P.; Clark, R.A. Understanding barriers to condom usage among HIV-infected African American women. *J. Assoc. Nurses AIDS Care* **1998**, *9*, 48–58. [CrossRef]
5. Santelli, J.S.; Kouzis, A.C.; Hoover, D.R.; Polacsek, M.; Burwell, L.G.; Celentano, D.D. Stage of behavior change for condom use: the influence of partner type, relationship and pregnancy factors. *Fam. Plan. Perspect.* **1996**, *28*, 101–107. [CrossRef]
6. Moench, T.R.; Chipato, T.; Padian, N.S. Preventing disease by protecting the cervix: the unexplored promise of internal vaginal barrier devices. *AIDS* **2001**, *15*, 1595–1602. [CrossRef]
7. Minnis, A.M.; Padian, N.S. Effectiveness of female controlled barrier methods in preventing sexually transmitted infections and HIV: current evidence and future research directions. *Sex. Transm. Infect.* **2005**, *81*, 193–200. [CrossRef]
8. Matthews, J.; Harrison, T. An update on female-controlled methods for HIV prevention: Female condom, microbicides and cervical barriers. *S. Afr. J. HIV Med.* **2006**, *7*, 7–11.
9. Padian, N.S.; Buve, A.; Balkus, J.; Serwadda, D.; Cates, W., Jr. Biomedical interventions to prevent HIV infection: evidence, challenges, and way forward. *Lancet* **2008**, *372*, 585–599. [CrossRef]
10. Maenza, J.; Flexner, C. Combination antiretroviral therapy for HIV infection. *Am. Fam. Physician* **1998**, *57*, 2789–2798. [PubMed]
11. Ludovici, D.W.; De Corte, B.L.; Kukla, M.J.; Ye, H.; Ho, C.Y.; Lichtenstein, M.A.; Kavash, R.W.; Andries, K.; de Bethune, M.P.; Azijn, H.; et al. Evolution of anti-HIV drug candidates. Part 3: Diarylpyrimidine (DAPY) analogues. *Bioorg. Med. Chem. Lett.* **2001**, *11*, 2235–2239. [CrossRef]
12. Holt, J.D.; Cameron, D.; Dias, N.; Holding, J.; Muntendam, A.; Oostebring, F.; Dreier, P.; Rohan, L.; Nuttall, J. The Sheep as a Model for Preclinical Safety and Pharmacokinetic Evaluations of Candidate Microbicides. *Antimicrob. Agents Chemother.* **2015**, *59*, 3761–3770. [CrossRef] [PubMed]
13. Baeten, J.M.; Palanee-Phillips, T.; Brown, E.R.; Schwartz, K.; Soto-Torres, L.E.; Govender, V.; Mgodi, N.M.; Matovu Kiweewa, F.; Nair, G.; Mhlanga, F.; et al. Use of a Vaginal Ring Containing Dapivirine for HIV-1 Prevention in Women. *N. Engl. J. Med.* **2016**, *375*, 2121–2132. [CrossRef] [PubMed]
14. Nel, A.; van Niekerk, N.; Kapiga, S.; Bekker, L.G.; Gama, C.; Gill, K.; Kamali, A.; Kotze, P.; Louw, C.; Mabude, Z.; et al. Safety and Efficacy of a Dapivirine Vaginal Ring for HIV Prevention in Women. *N. Engl. J. Med.* **2016**, *375*, 2133–2143. [CrossRef] [PubMed]
15. Mori, T.; O'Keefe, B.R.; Sowder, R.C., 2nd; Bringans, S.; Gardella, R.; Berg, S.; Cochran, P.; Turpin, J.A.; Buckheit, R.W., Jr.; McMahon, J.B.; et al. Isolation and characterization of griffithsin, a novel HIV-inactivating protein, from the red alga Griffithsia sp. *J. Biol. Chem.* **2005**, *280*, 9345–9353. [CrossRef]
16. Kagiampakis, I.; Gharibi, A.; Mankowski, M.K.; Snyder, B.A.; Ptak, R.G.; Alatas, K.; LiWang, P.J. Potent strategy to inhibit HIV-1 by binding both gp120 and gp41. *Antimicrob. Agents Chemother.* **2011**, *55*, 264–275. [CrossRef]
17. Alexandre, K.B.; Gray, E.S.; Pantophlet, R.; Moore, P.L.; McMahon, J.B.; Chakauya, E.; O'Keefe, B.R.; Chikwamba, R.; Morris, L. Binding of the mannose-specific lectin, griffithsin, to HIV-1 gp120 exposes the CD4-binding site. *J. Virol.* **2011**, *85*, 9039–9050. [CrossRef] [PubMed]

18. Emau, P.; Tian, B.; O'Keefe, B.R.; Mori, T.; McMahon, J.B.; Palmer, K.E.; Jiang, Y.; Bekele, G.; Tsai, C.C. Griffithsin, a potent HIV entry inhibitor, is an excellent candidate for anti-HIV microbicide. *J. Med. Primatol.* **2007**, *36*, 244–253. [CrossRef]
19. Barton, C.L. Evaluation of the Safety and Pharmacokinetic Profile of the Broad Spectrum Antiviral Lectin Griffithsin. Ph.D. Thesis, University of Louisville, Louisville, KY, USA, 2014.
20. O'Keefe, B.R.; Vojdani, F.; Buffa, V.; Shattock, R.J.; Montefiori, D.C.; Bakke, J.; Mirsalis, J.; d'Andrea, A.L.; Hume, S.D.; Bratcher, B.; et al. Scaleable manufacture of HIV-1 entry inhibitor griffithsin and validation of its safety and efficacy as a topical microbicide component. *Proc. Natl. Acad. Sci. USA* **2009**, *106*, 6099–6104. [CrossRef]
21. Girard, L.; Birse, K.; Holm, J.B.; Gajer, P.; Humphrys, M.S.; Garber, D.; Guenthner, P.; Noel-Romas, L.; Abou, M.; McCorrister, S.; et al. Impact of the griffithsin anti-HIV microbicide and placebo gels on the rectal mucosal proteome and microbiome in non-human primates. *Sci. Rep.* **2018**, *8*, 8059. [CrossRef]
22. Ferir, G.; Palmer, K.E.; Schols, D. Synergistic activity profile of griffithsin in combination with tenofovir, maraviroc and enfuvirtide against HIV-1 clade C. *Virology* **2011**, *417*, 253–258. [CrossRef]
23. Kiser, P.F.; Mesquita, P.M.; Herold, B.C. A perspective on progress and gaps in HIV prevention science. *AIDS Res. Hum. Retroviruses* **2012**, *28*, 1373–1378. [CrossRef] [PubMed]
24. Gupta, S.K.; Nutan. Clinical use of vaginal or rectally applied microbicides in patients suffering from HIV/AIDS. *HIV AIDS (Auckl)* **2013**, *5*, 295–307. [CrossRef]
25. Thurman, A.R.; Clark, M.R.; Hurlburt, J.A.; Doncel, G.F. Intravaginal rings as delivery systems for microbicides and multipurpose prevention technologies. *Int. J. Womens Health* **2013**, *5*, 695–708. [CrossRef]
26. das Neves, J.; Nunes, R.; Rodrigues, F.; Sarmento, B. Nanomedicine in the development of anti-HIV microbicides. *Adv. Drug Deliv. Rev.* **2016**, *103*, 57–75. [CrossRef]
27. Cunha-Reis, C.; Machado, A.; Barreiros, L.; Araujo, F.; Nunes, R.; Seabra, V.; Ferreira, D.; Segundo, M.A.; Sarmento, B.; das Neves, J. Nanoparticles-in-film for the combined vaginal delivery of anti-HIV microbicide drugs. *J. Control. Release* **2016**, *243*, 43–53. [CrossRef]
28. Malik, T.; Chauhan, G.; Rath, G.; Kesarkar, R.N.; Chowdhary, A.S.; Goyal, A.K. Efaverinz and nano-gold-loaded mannosylated niosomes: a host cell-targeted topical HIV-1 prophylaxis via thermogel system. *Artif. Cells Nanomed. Biotechnol.* **2017**. [CrossRef]
29. das Neves, J.; Araujo, F.; Andrade, F.; Amiji, M.; Bahia, M.F.; Sarmento, B. Biodistribution and pharmacokinetics of dapivirine-loaded nanoparticles after vaginal delivery in mice. *Pharm. Res.* **2014**, *31*, 1834–1845. [CrossRef]
30. das Neves, J.; Araujo, F.; Andrade, F.; Michiels, J.; Arien, K.K.; Vanham, G.; Amiji, M.; Bahia, M.F.; Sarmento, B. In vitro and ex vivo evaluation of polymeric nanoparticles for vaginal and rectal delivery of the anti-HIV drug dapivirine. *Mol. Pharm.* **2013**, *10*, 2793–2807. [CrossRef]
31. das Neves, J.; Michiels, J.; Arien, K.K.; Vanham, G.; Amiji, M.; Bahia, M.F.; Sarmento, B. Polymeric nanoparticles affect the intracellular delivery, antiretroviral activity and cytotoxicity of the microbicide drug candidate dapivirine. *Pharm. Res.* **2012**, *29*, 1468–1484. [CrossRef]
32. Kovarova, M.; Council, O.D.; Date, A.A.; Long, J.M.; Nochi, T.; Belshan, M.; Shibata, A.; Vincent, H.; Baker, C.E.; Thayer, W.O.; et al. Correction: Nanoformulations of Rilpivirine for Topical Pericoital and Systemic Coitus-Independent Administration Efficiently Prevent HIV Transmission. *PLoS Pathog.* **2015**, *11*, e1005170. [CrossRef]
33. das Neves, J.; Sarmento, B. Precise engineering of dapivirine-loaded nanoparticles for the development of anti-HIV vaginal microbicides. *Acta Biomater.* **2015**, *18*, 77–87. [CrossRef]
34. Bala, I.; Hariharan, S.; Kumar, M.N. PLGA nanoparticles in drug delivery: The state of the art. *Crit. Rev. Ther. Drug Carrier Syst.* **2004**, *21*, 387–422. [CrossRef]
35. Makadia, H.K.; Siegel, S.J. Poly Lactic-co-Glycolic Acid (PLGA) as Biodegradable Controlled Drug Delivery Carrier. *Polymers* **2011**, *3*, 1377–1397. [CrossRef] [PubMed]
36. Bouissou, C.; Rouse, J.J.; Price, R.; van der Walle, C.F. The influence of surfactant on PLGA microsphere glass transition and water sorption: remodeling the surface morphology to attenuate the burst release. *Pharm. Res.* **2006**, *23*, 1295–1305. [CrossRef] [PubMed]
37. Jain, R.A. The manufacturing techniques of various drug loaded biodegradable poly(lactide-co-glycolide) (PLGA) devices. *Biomaterials* **2000**, *21*, 2475–2490. [CrossRef]

38. Ham, A.S.; Cost, M.R.; Sassi, A.B.; Dezzutti, C.S.; Rohan, L.C. Targeted delivery of PSC-RANTES for HIV-1 prevention using biodegradable nanoparticles. *Pharm. Res.* **2009**, *26*, 502–511. [CrossRef]
39. Menei, P.; Daniel, V.; Montero-Menei, C.; Brouillard, M.; Pouplard-Barthelaix, A.; Benoit, J.P. Biodegradation and brain tissue reaction to poly(D,L-lactide-co-glycolide) microspheres. *Biomaterials* **1993**, *14*, 470–478. [CrossRef]
40. Shive, M.S.; Anderson, J.M. Biodegradation and biocompatibility of PLA and PLGA microspheres. *Adv. Drug Deliv. Rev.* **1997**, *28*, 5–24.
41. McRae, A.; Ling, E.A.; Hjorth, S.; Dahlstrom, A.; Mason, D.; Tice, T. Catecholamine-containing biodegradable microsphere implants as a novel approach in the treatment of CNS neurodegenerative disease. A review of experimental studies in DA-lesioned rats. *Mol. Neurobiol.* **1994**, *9*, 191–205. [CrossRef]
42. Engman, C.; Wen, Y.; Meng, W.S.; Bottino, R.; Trucco, M.; Giannoukakis, N. Generation of antigen-specific Foxp3+ regulatory T-cells in vivo following administration of diabetes-reversing tolerogenic microspheres does not require provision of antigen in the formulation. *Clin. Immunol.* **2015**, *160*, 103–123. [CrossRef]
43. Chaowanachan, T.; Krogstad, E.; Ball, C.; Woodrow, K.A. Drug synergy of tenofovir and nanoparticle-based antiretrovirals for HIV prophylaxis. *PLoS ONE* **2013**, *8*, e61416. [CrossRef]
44. Mallipeddi, R.; Rohan, L.C. Progress in antiretroviral drug delivery using nanotechnology. *Int. J. Nanomed.* **2010**, *5*, 533–547.
45. das Neves, J.; Amiji, M.M.; Bahia, M.F.; Sarmento, B. Nanotechnology-based systems for the treatment and prevention of HIV/AIDS. *Adv. Drug Deliv. Rev.* **2010**, *62*, 458–477. [CrossRef]
46. Destache, C.J.; Belgum, T.; Christensen, K.; Shibata, A.; Sharma, A.; Dash, A. Combination antiretroviral drugs in PLGA nanoparticle for HIV-1. *BMC Infect. Dis.* **2009**, *9*, 198. [CrossRef]
47. Papadimitriou, S.; Bikiaris, D. Novel self-assembled core-shell nanoparticles based on crystalline amorphous moieties of aliphatic copolyesters for efficient controlled drug release. *J. Control. Release* **2009**, *138*, 177–184. [CrossRef]
48. Owen, D.H.; Katz, D.F. A vaginal fluid simulant. *Contraception* **1999**, *59*, 91–95. [CrossRef]
49. Dezzutti, C.S.; Brown, E.R.; Moncla, B.; Russo, J.; Cost, M.; Wang, L.; Uranker, K.; Kunjara Na Ayudhya, R.P.; Pryke, K.; Pickett, J.; et al. Is wetter better? An evaluation of over-the-counter personal lubricants for safety and anti-HIV-1 activity. *PLoS ONE* **2012**, *7*, e48328. [CrossRef]
50. Montefiori, D.C. Measuring HIV neutralization in a luciferase reporter gene assay. *Methods Mol. Biol.* **2009**, *485*, 395–405. [CrossRef]
51. Dezzutti, C.S.; Shetler, C.; Mahalingam, A.; Ugaonkar, S.R.; Gwozdz, G.; Buckheit, K.W.; Buckheit, R.W., Jr. Safety and efficacy of tenofovir/IQP-0528 combination gels - a dual compartment microbicide for HIV-1 prevention. *Antiviral Res.* **2012**, *96*, 221–225. [CrossRef]
52. Kohli, A.; Islam, A.; Moyes, D.L.; Murciano, C.; Shen, C.; Challacombe, S.J.; Naglik, J.R. Oral and vaginal epithelial cell lines bind and transfer cell-free infectious HIV-1 to permissive cells but are not productively infected. *PLoS ONE* **2014**, *9*, e98077. [CrossRef] [PubMed]
53. Montefiori, D.C. Evaluating neutralizing antibodies against HIV, SIV, and SHIV in luciferase reporter gene assays. *Curr. Protoc. Immunol.* **2005**. [CrossRef]
54. Dezzutti, C.S.; Rohan, L.C.; Wang, L.; Uranker, K.; Shetler, C.; Cost, M.; Lynam, J.D.; Friend, D. Reformulated tenofovir gel for use as a dual compartment microbicide. *J. Antimicrob. Chemother.* **2012**, *67*, 2139–2142. [CrossRef]
55. Chou, T.C. Theoretical basis, experimental design, and computerized simulation of synergism and antagonism in drug combination studies. *Pharmacol. Rev.* **2006**, *58*, 621–681. [CrossRef]
56. Zhang, Y.; Huo, M.; Zhou, J.; Zou, A.; Li, W.; Yao, C.; Xie, S. DDSolver: An add-in program for modeling and comparison of drug dissolution profiles. *AAPS J.* **2010**, *12*, 263–271. [CrossRef]
57. Bilati, U.; Allemann, E.; Doelker, E. Poly(D,L-lactide-co-glycolide) protein-loaded nanoparticles prepared by the double emulsion method–processing and formulation issues for enhanced entrapment efficiency. *J. Microencapsul.* **2005**, *22*, 205–214. [CrossRef]
58. Xu, B.; Dou, H.; Tao, K.; Sun, K.; Lu, R.; Shi, W. Influence of experimental parameters and the copolymer structure on the size control of nanospheres in double emulsion method. *J. Polym. Res.* **2011**, *18*, 131–137. [CrossRef]

59. Liu, J.; Qiu, Z.; Wang, S.; Zhou, L.; Zhang, S. A modified double-emulsion method for the preparation of daunorubicin-loaded polymeric nanoparticle with enhanced in vitro anti-tumor activity. *Biomed. Mater.* **2010**, *5*, 065002. [CrossRef] [PubMed]
60. Marques, M.R.C.; Loebenberg, R.; Almukainzi, M. Simulated Biological Fluids with Possible Application in Dissolution Testing. *Dissolution Technol.* **2011**, *18*, 15–28. [CrossRef]
61. Destache, C.J.; Belgum, T.; Goede, M.; Shibata, A.; Belshan, M.A. Antiretroviral release from poly(DL-lactide-co-glycolide) nanoparticles in mice. *J. Antimicrob. Chemother.* **2010**, *65*, 2183–2187. [CrossRef] [PubMed]
62. Friend, D.R.; Kiser, P.F. Assessment of topical microbicides to prevent HIV-1 transmission: concepts, testing, lessons learned. *Antiviral. Res.* **2013**, *99*, 391–400. [CrossRef] [PubMed]
63. Abdool Karim, Q.; Abdool Karim, S.S.; Frohlich, J.A.; Grobler, A.C.; Baxter, C.; Mansoor, L.E.; Kharsany, A.B.; Sibeko, S.; Mlisana, K.P.; Omar, Z.; et al. Effectiveness and safety of tenofovir gel, an antiretroviral microbicide, for the prevention of HIV infection in women. *Science* **2010**, *329*, 1168–1174. [CrossRef] [PubMed]
64. Dolgin, E. Long-acting HIV drugs advanced to overcome adherence challenge. *Nat. Med.* **2014**, *20*, 323–324. [CrossRef]
65. Andrews, C.D.; Spreen, W.R.; Mohri, H.; Moss, L.; Ford, S.; Gettie, A.; Russell-Lodrigue, K.; Bohm, R.P.; Cheng-Mayer, C.; Hong, Z.; et al. Long-acting integrase inhibitor protects macaques from intrarectal simian/human immunodeficiency virus. *Science* **2014**, *343*, 1151–1154. [CrossRef] [PubMed]
66. Kramzer, L. Preformulation and Biological Evaluations for the Intravaginal Delivery of Griffithsin for HIV Prevention. Ph.D. Thesis, University of Pittsburgh, Pittsburgh, PA, USA, 2015.
67. Zolnik, B.S.; Burgess, D.J. Effect of acidic pH on PLGA microsphere degradation and release. *J. Control. Release* **2007**, *122*, 338–344. [CrossRef] [PubMed]
68. Ding, A.G.; Schwendeman, S.P. Acidic microclimate pH distribution in PLGA microspheres monitored by confocal laser scanning microscopy. *Pharm. Res.* **2008**, *25*, 2041–2052. [CrossRef] [PubMed]
69. Smith, P. Estrogens and the urogenital tract. Studies on steroid hormone receptors and a clinical study on a new estradiol-releasing vaginal ring. *Acta Obstet. Gynecol. Scand.* **1993**, *72*, 5–26. [CrossRef]
70. Boskey, E.R.; Cone, R.A.; Whaley, K.J.; Moench, T.R. Origins of vaginal acidity: high D/L lactate ratio is consistent with bacteria being the primary source. *Hum. Reprod.* **2001**, *16*, 1809–1813. [CrossRef]
71. Fredenberg, S.; Wahlgren, M.; Reslow, M.; Axelsson, A. The mechanisms of drug release in poly(lactic-co-glycolic acid)-based drug delivery systems—A review. *Int. J. Pharm.* **2011**, *415*, 34–52. [CrossRef]
72. Secchi, M.; Xu, Q.; Lusso, P.; Vangelista, L. The superior folding of a RANTES analogue expressed in lactobacilli as compared to mammalian cells reveals a promising system to screen new RANTES mutants. *Protein Expr. Purif.* **2009**, *68*, 34–41. [CrossRef]
73. Chou, T.C. Drug combination studies and their synergy quantification using the Chou-Talalay method. *Cancer Res.* **2010**, *70*, 440–446. [CrossRef]

8

Isolation, Structure Elucidation and Antiproliferative Activity of Butanolides and Lignan Glycosides from the Fruit of *Hernandia nymphaeifolia*

Simayijiang Aimaiti [1], Yohei Saito [1], Shuichi Fukuyoshi [1], Masuo Goto [2], Katsunori Miyake [3], David J. Newman [4], Barry R. O'Keefe [5,6], Kuo-Hsiung Lee [2,7] and Kyoko Nakagawa-Goto [1,2,*]

1 School of Pharmaceutical Sciences, College of Medical, Pharmaceutical and Health Sciences, Kanazawa University, Kanazawa 920-1192, Japan; ismayil507@stu.kanazawa-u.ac.jp (S.A.); saito-y@staff.kanazawa-u.ac.jp (Y.S.); fukuyosi@p.kanazawa-u.ac.jp (S.F.)
2 Natural Products Research Laboratories, UNC Eshelman School of Pharmacy, University of North Carolina at Chapel Hill, Chapel Hill, NC 27599-7568, USA; goto@med.unc.edu (M.G.); khlee@unc.edu (K.-H.L.)
3 Tokyo University of Pharmacy and Life Sciences, Hachioji, Tokyo 192-0392, Japan; miyake@toyaku.ac.jp
4 NIH Special Volunteer, Wayne, PA 19087, USA; newmand@mail.nih.gov
5 Natural Products Branch, Developmental Therapeutics Program, Division of Cancer Treatment and Diagnosis, National Cancer Institute, NCI at Frederick, Frederick, MD 21702-1201, USA; okeefeba@mail.nih.gov
6 Molecular Targets Program, Center for Cancer Research, National Cancer Institute, NCI at Frederick, Frederick, MD 21702-1201, USA
7 Chinese Medicine Research and Development Center, China Medical University and Hospital, Taichung 40447, Taiwan
* Correspondence: kngoto@p.kanazawa-u.ac.jp

Academic Editor: Maria Carla Marcotullio

Abstract: Seven new butanolides, peltanolides A–G (**1–7**), and two lignan glucosides, peltasides A (**8**) and B (**9**), along with eleven known compounds, **10–20**, were isolated from a crude CH_3OH/CH_2Cl_2 (1:1) extract of the fruit of *Hernandia nymphaeifolia* (Hernandiaceae). The structures of **1–9** were characterized by extensive 1D and 2D NMR spectroscopic and HRMS analysis. The absolute configurations of newly isolated compounds **1–9** were determined from data obtained by optical rotation and electronic circular dichroism (ECD) exciton chirality methods. Butanolides and lignan glucosides have not been isolated previously from this genus. Several isolated compounds were evaluated for antiproliferative activity against human tumor cell lines. Lignans **15** and **16** were slightly active against chemosensitive tumor cell lines A549 and MCF-7, respectively. Furthermore, both compounds displayed significant activity (IC_{50} = 5 μM) against a P-glycoprotein overexpressing multidrug-resistant tumor cell line (KB-VIN) but were less active against its parent chemosensitive cell line (KB).

Keywords: *Hernandia nymphaeifolia*; butanolides; lignan glycosides; antiproliferative activity

1. Introduction

Plants in the genus *Hernandia* (Hernandiaceae) are found in subtropical and tropical areas [1]. They contain diverse bioactive secondary metabolites, especially lignans, including podophyllotoxin analogues [2,3], and benzylisoquinolines [4], including aporphines [5–7]. These compounds exhibit various biological activities, including significant cytotoxic [8,9], antiplasmodial [9,10], and antibacterial activities [2]. *H. nymphaeifolia* (C.Presl) Kubitzki (synonym: *H. peltata* Meisn.) is a common coastal tree and grows to 12–20 m in height. This plant has been used for the treatment of abdominal pains, boils, cough, diarrhea, eye problems, and convulsions as a traditional medicine in western Samoa [11]. A CH_3OH/CH_2Cl_2 (1:1) extract of *H. nymphaeifolia* (N053499, originally described as *H. peltata*) provided by the U.S. National Cancer Institute Natural Products Branch (NCI, Frederick, MD, USA) exhibited broad cytotoxicity in the NCI-60 human tumor cell line (HTCL) assay, possibly due to the above or similar cytotoxic constituents. To supplement the reported phytochemical research on *H. nymphaeifolia* [2,4,9,12–14], we conducted a thorough study to identify new chemical compounds as part of our continuing investigation of rainforest plants. Accordingly, the extract of N053499 yielded seven new butanolides, peltanolides A–G (**1–7**), and two new lignan glycosides, peltasides A (**8**) and B (**9**), as well as eleven known compounds **10–20** (Figure 1). Herein, we report the details of isolation, structure elucidation, and cytotoxicity of isolated compounds from *H. nymphaeifolia*.

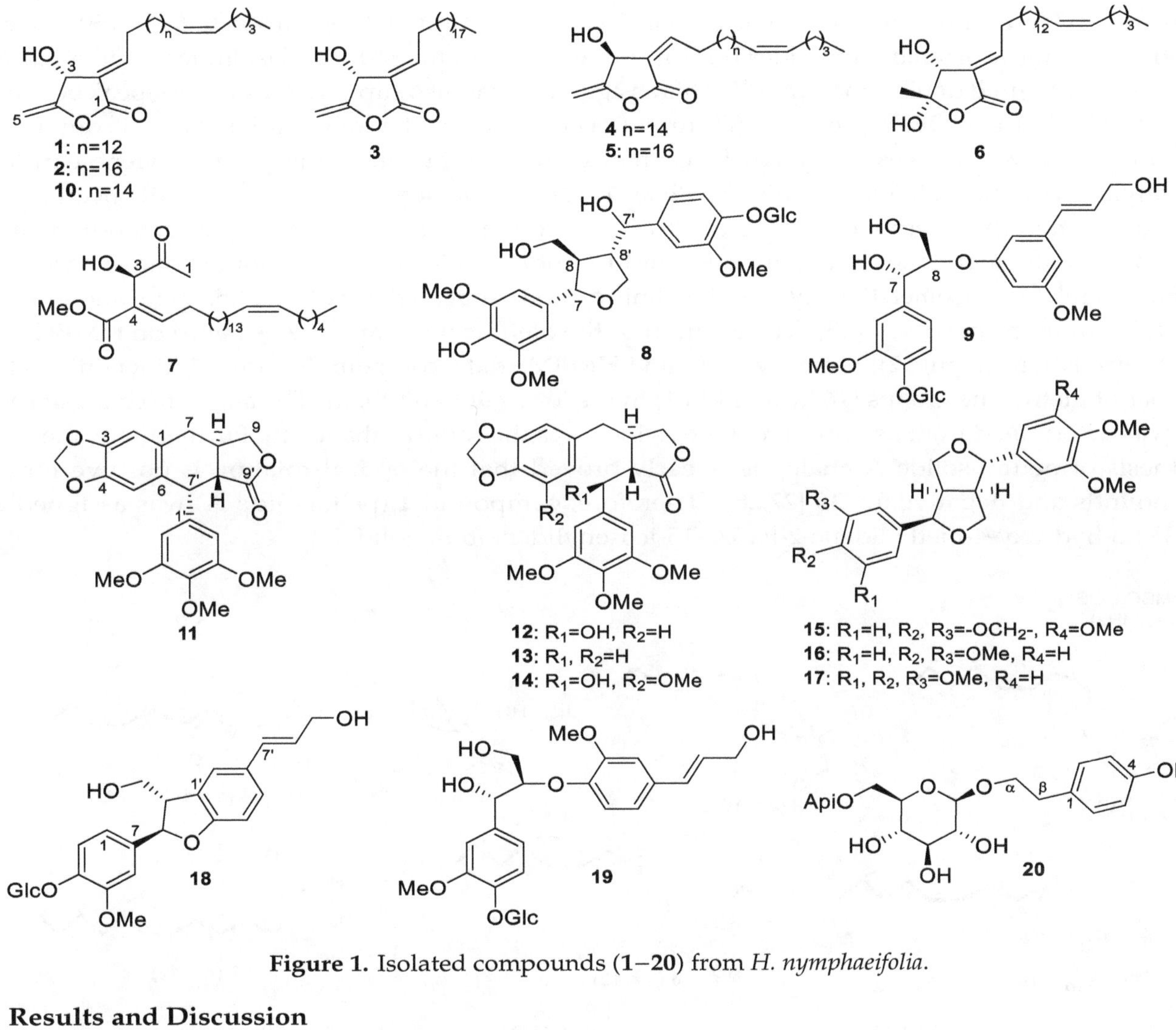

Figure 1. Isolated compounds (**1–20**) from *H. nymphaeifolia*.

2. Results and Discussion

2.1. Structure Elucidation of Isolated Compounds from H. nymphaeifolia

The CH_3OH/CH_2Cl_2 (1:1) extract of *H. nymphaeifolia* (fruit, N053499) was firstly partitioned with water and *n*-hexane. The water fraction was further partitioned with EtOAc and *n*-BuOH. All fractions were subjected to a combination of column chromatography, preparative HPLC, and preparative TLC using silica gel and octadecylsilyl (ODS) to give seven new butanolides, peltanolides A–G (**1–7**), and two new lignan glycosides, peltasides A (**8**) and B (**9**), as well as eleven known compounds, tambouranolide (**10**) [15], deoxypodophyllotoxin (**11**) [16], podorhizol (**12**) [17], bursehernin (**13**) [18], (2*S*,3*S*)-(+)-5′-methoxyyatein (**14**) [19], epiashantin (**15**) [20], epieudesmin (**16**) [21], (1*S*,3a*R*,4*R*,6a*R*)-

1-(3,4-dimethoxyphenyl)-4-(3′,4′,5′-trimethoxyphenyl)tetrahydro-1*H*,3*H*-furo-[3–*c*]furan (**17**) [20], (7*R*,8*S*)-dehydrodiconiferyl alcohol-4-*O*-β-D-glucoside (**18**) [22], alaschanioside A (**19**) [23], and osmanthuside H (**20**) [24]. The structures of all known compounds were identified by comparison of their spectroscopic data with reported values.

Compound **1** was obtained as a yellow amorphous solid: $[\alpha]^{25}_{D}$ + 27.3 (*c* 0.075, $CHCl_3$). It gave a $[M]^+$ peak at *m/z* 390.3137, appropriate for a molecular formula of $C_{25}H_{42}O_3$. The ^1H and ^{13}C NMR spectra (Tables 1 and 2) contained signals attributed to oxymethine [δ_H 5.26 (1H, brs); δ_C 66.5, C-3], methylidene [δ_H 4.96 (1H, dd, *J* = 2.8, 1.4 Hz), 4.72 (1H, dd, *J* = 2.8, 1.4 Hz); δ_C 91.4, 157.6, C-4,5], vinyl [δ_H 7.09 (1H, td, *J* = 7.8, 2.2 Hz); δ_C 127.3, 150.3, C-2,6], and carbonyl (δ_C 166.5, C-1) groups, consistent with a β-hydroxy-γ-methylene-α,β-unsaturated-γ-lactone. The chemical shifts of H-6 (δ_H 7.09) and H-7 (δ_H 2.48) as well as allylic carbon C-3 (δ_C 66.5) and olefinic carbon C-6 (δ_C 150.3) were identical with those of tambouranolide (**10**) [15] and related linderanolides and isolinderanolides [25,26] with an *E*-configured double bond [$\Delta^{2(6)}$]. This assignment was also supported by a cross-peak between H-3 and H-7 in the NOESY spectrum (Figure 3). The presence of a long aliphatic chain containing a double bond was suggested by NMR resonances for olefinic and multiple methylene carbons. The allylic (δ_C 27.0, 27.2) and olefinic (δ_C 129.8, 129.9) carbon signals in the ^{13}C NMR spectrum of **1** suggested that the internal olefin has the typical *Z*-configuration, comparable with those of **10** as well as the abovementioned linderanolides and isolinderanolides with *Z*-double bonds in the side chain. In a related *E*-isomer, the allylic and olefinic carbons appeared at 32.6 and 25.6 ppm and at 131.9 and 129.3 ppm, respectively [25]. The location of the olefinic bond at Δ^{20} was based on HMBC and COSY correlations (Figure 2). From the NMR and HREIMS data, compounds **10** and **1** differ only in the number of methylene groups (16 in **10**, 14 in **1**) in the long aliphatic chain. The absolute configuration of **1** was determined from its optical rotation, which was the same as that of **10**. Furthermore, the total synthesis of peumusolide A analogues clearly proved that the optical rotation is positive for 3*R* compounds and negative for 3*S* [27,28]. Therefore, compound **1** (peltanolide A) was assigned as (2*E*,3*R*)-3-hydroxy-4-methylidene-2-[(15*Z*)-15-icosenylidene]butanolide.

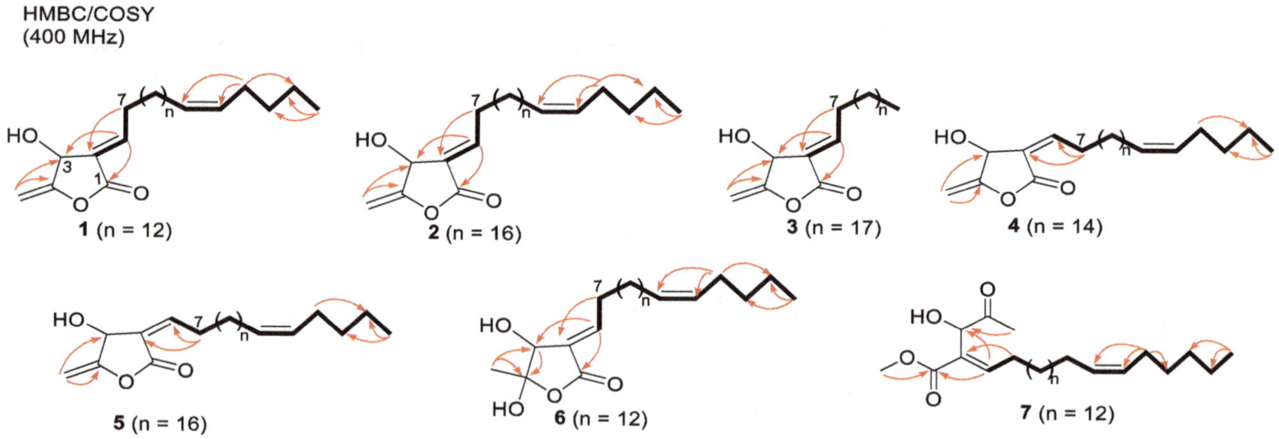

Figure 2. Selected HMBC correlations (arrows in red), COSY connectivities (bold lines) for compounds **1–7**.

Compound **2** was isolated as a yellow solid, $[\alpha]^{25}_{D}$ +26.1 (*c* 0.12, $CHCl_3$). The HREIMS data supported a molecular formula of $C_{29}H_{51}O_3$ from the peak at *m/z* 446.3743 $[M]^+$. The MS data and NMR spectra indicated four additional methylene units compared with **1**, and the optical rotation suggested the same configuration as that of **1**. Thus, compound **2** (peltanolide B) was defined as (2*E*,3*R*)-3-hydroxy-4-methylidene-2-[(19*Z*)-19-tetracosenylidene]butanolide.

Compound **3** was obtained as a colorless oil: $[\alpha]^{25}_{D}$ +26.0 (*c* 0.07, $CHCl_3$). The HREIMS data indicated a molecular formula of $C_{25}H_{44}O_3$ from the peak at *m/z* 392.3302 $[M]^+$, which was identical to that of miaolinolide [29]. One dimensional NMR spectra of **3** also displayed the similar signal pattern with one exception: the chemical shift of H-6 is δ_H 7.10 (1H, td, *J* = 7.8, 2.2 Hz) in **3** and δ_H 6.70 (1H, td, *J* = 8.0, 2.0 Hz) in miaolinolide. Thus, the $\Delta^{2(6)}$ double bond has an *E* configuration in **3**, rather than the *Z* configuration in miaolinolide [29]. This assignment was also proved that the chemical shift of H-6 in **3** was close to that of related butanolides with an *E* configuration of the $\Delta^{2(6)}$ double bond [15,25,26,30], including compounds **1** and **2**. A NOESY correlation between H-3 and H-7 (Figure 3) supported this conclusion. Based on their optical rotations, compound **3** and miaolinolide have the same absolute configuration. Hence, the structure of **3** (peltanolide C) was established as (2*E*,3*S*)-3-hydroxy-4-methylidene-2-icosylidenebutanolide.

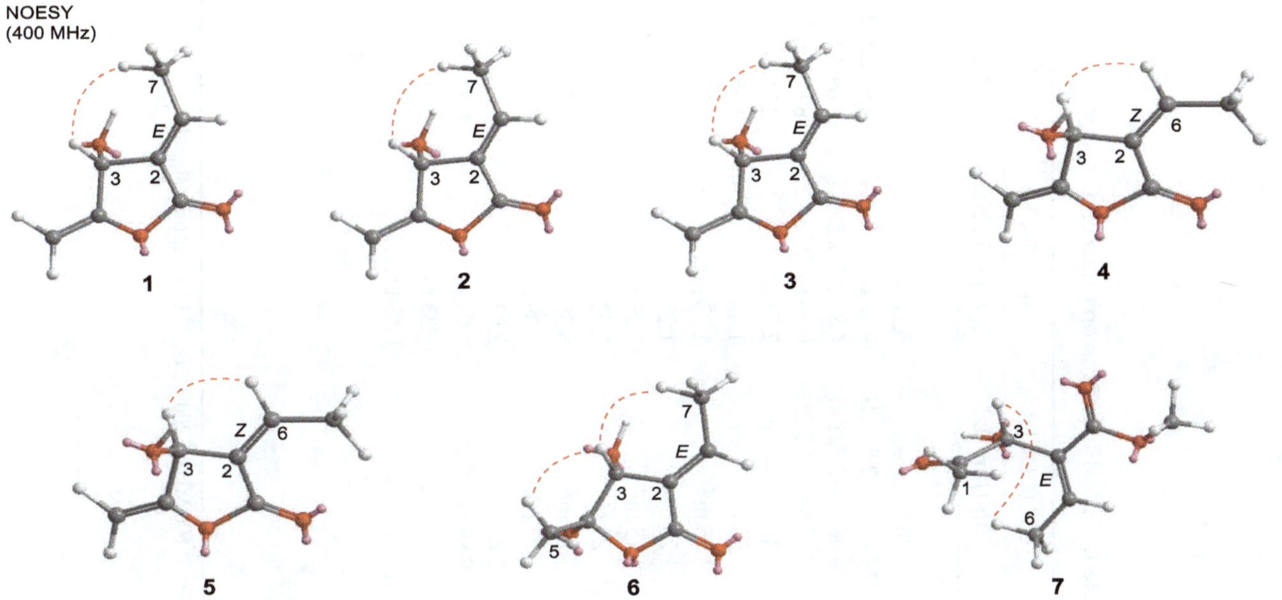

Figure 3. Key NOESY (red dashed lines) correlations for compounds **1–7**.

HRFABMS of compound **4** showed a molecular formula $C_{27}H_{46}O_3$ with a molecular ion at *m/z* 441.3357 $[M + Na]^+$. The ^1H and ^{13}C NMR spectra of **4** (Tables 1 and 2) were comparable to those of **10** but suggested different double bond [$\Delta^{2(6)}$] configurations and C-3 stereochemistries. For **4**, the $\Delta^{2(6)}$ configuration was determined as *Z* from a NOESY correlation between H-3 and H-6 (Figure 3) and the chemical shift of H-6 at 6.69 ppm rather than ca. 7.10 ppm for the *E* form. The C-3 stereochemistry was determined as *S* by comparison of optical rotations, $[\alpha]^{25}_{D}$ −29.7 (*c* 0.02, $CHCl_3$) for **4** and $[\alpha]^{25}_{D}$ + 18.0 (*c* 0.03, $CHCl_3$) for **10** with 3*R*. Thus, compound **4** (peltanolide D) was determined as (2*Z*,3*S*)-3-hydroxy-4-methylidene-2-[(17*Z*)-17-docosenylidene]butanolide.

Table 1. ^{1}H NMR Spectroscopic data of compounds **1–7**.

	1[a] ($CDCl_3$)	**2**[b] ($CDCl_3$)	**3**[b] ($CDCl_3$)	**4**[b] ($CDCl_3$)	**5**[b] ($CDCl_3$)	**6**[a] ($CDCl_3$)	**7**[b] ($CDCl_3$)
Position	δ_H (*J* in Hz)	δ_H (*J* in Hz)	δ_H (*J* in Hz)	δ_H (*J* in Hz)	δ_H (*J* in Hz)	δ_H (*J* in Hz)	δ_H (*J* in Hz)
1							2.15 s
3	5.26 brs	5.26 brs	5.26 brd (5.6)	5.11 m	5.10 brd (7.3)	4.82 brs	4.89 d (4.2)
5a	4.72 dd (2.8, 1.4)	4.72 dd (2.8, 1.4)	4.72 dd (2.8, 1.4)	4.67 dd (2.8, 1.4)	4.66 dd (2.8, 1.4)	1.62 s	7.07 t (8.0)
5b	4.96 dd (2.8, 1.4)	4.96 dd (2.8, 1.4)	4.96 dd (2.8, 1.4)	4.89 dd (2.8, 1.4)	4.89 dd (2.8, 1.4)		
6	7.09 td (7.8, 2.2)	7.09 td (7.8, 2.2)	7.10 td (7.8, 2.2)	6.69 td (7.8, 2.2)	6.67 td (7.8, 2.2)	7.04 td (7.8, 2.2)	2.34 td (14.8, 8.0)
7	2.48 m	2.48 m	2.48 m, 2.43 m	2.78 m	2.76 m	2.38 m	1.50 m
8	1.52 m	1.52 m	1.53 m	1.46 m	1.45 m	1.52 m	1.25 m[p]
9–18	1.26 m[c]	1.26 m[e]	1.25 m[g]	1.25 m[h]	1.25 m[j]	1.25 m[m]	1.25 m[p]
19	2.00 m	1.26 m[e]	1.25 m[g]	1.25 m[h]	1.25 m[j]	2.01 m[n]	2.00 m[q]
20	5.36 m[d]	1.26 m[e]	1.25 m[g]	1.25 m[h]	1.25 m[j]	5.34 t (4.8)[o]	5.34 t (4.8)[r]
21	5.36 m[d]	1.26 m[e]	1.25 m[g]	2.02 m	1.25 m[j]	5.34 t (4.8)[o]	5.34 t (4.8)[r]
22	2.02 m	1.26 m[e]	1.25 m[g]	5.35 m[i]	1.25 m[j]	2.01 m[n]	2.00 m[q]
23	1.26 m[c]	2.00 m	1.25 m[g]	5.35 m[i]	2.01 m[k]	1.25 m[m]	1.25 m[p]
24	1.32 m	5.36 m[f]	1.25 m[g]	2.02	5.33 m[l]	1.31	1.25 m[p]
25	0.89 t (6.9)	5.36 m[f]	0.89 br t (7.3)	1.25 m[h]	5.33 m[l]	0.89 t (6.0)	1.31 m
26		2.02 m		1.33 m	2.01 m[k]		0.89 t (6.0)
27		1.26 m[e]		0.88 t (6.9)	1.25 m[j]		
28		1.32 m			1.32 m		
29		0.89 t (7.3)			0.87 t (6.9)		
2-OH		2.26 m					
3-OH							4.00 brs
OCH_3							3.72 s

[a] 600 MHz, [b] 400 MHz, [c–r] Overlapping signals.

Table 2. ^{13}C NMR Spectroscopic data in $CDCl_3$ of compounds **1–7**.

	1[a]	**2**[b]	**3**[b]	**4**[b]	**5**[b]	**6**[a]	**7**[b]
Position	δ_c	δ_c	δ_c	δ_c	δ_c	δ_c	δ_c
1	166.5	166.5	166.3	163.1		166.4	24.8
2	127.3	127.3	127.2	127.4	127.3	125.2	206.3
3	66.5	66.5	66.6	68.9	68.9	70.9	73.4
4	157.6	157.6	157.5	160.1	160.2	100.1	129.8
5	91.4	91.4	91.5	90.3	90.4	26.8	149.0
6	150.3	150.3	150.3	151.4	151.4	151.9	28.7
7	29.8	29.8	29.8	29.8	29.8	30.1	29.3
8	28.4	28.4	28.4–29.6[d]	28.4	28.4	29.5–29.9[g]	29.4–30.0[h]
9–18	29.4–30.0	29.4–30.0[c]	28.4–29.6[d]	29.4–30.0[e]	29.4–30.0[f]	29.5–29.9[g]	29.4–30.0[h]
19	27.0	29.4–30.0[c]	28.4–29.6[d]	29.4–30.0[e]	29.4–30.0[f]	27.0	27.2
20	129.8	29.4–30.0[c]	28.4–29.6[d]	29.4–30.0[e]	29.4–30.0[f]	129.8	129.8
21	129.9	29.4–30.0[c]	28.4–29.6[d]	27.0	29.4–30.0[f]	129.9	129.9
22	27.2	29.4–30.0[c]	28.4–29.6[d]	129.8	29.4–30.0[f]	27.7	27.2
23	32.0	27.0	32.0	129.9	27.0	32.1	29.8
24	22.4	129.8	22.8	27.2	129.8	22.5	31.9
25	14.0	129.9	14.1	32.0	129.9	14.1	22.7
26		27.2		22.3	27.2		14.1
27		32.0		14.0	32.0		
28		22.4			22.4		
29		14.0			14.0		
COO							166.5
OCH_3							52.0

[a] 150 MHz, [b] 100 MHz, [c–h] Overlapping signals.

Compound **5** was obtained as a yellow solid and displayed a peak at *m/z* 446.3749 $[M]^+$ in the HREIMS spectrum, which agreed with a molecular formula of $C_{29}H_{50}O_3$ and two additional methylene units (C_2H_4) compared with **4**. This finding was also supported by the two NMR spectra. Both compounds also have the same absolute configurations based on their optical rotations, $[\alpha]^{25}{}_D$ −21.1 (*c* 0.015, $CHCl_3$) for **5** and $[\alpha]^{25}{}_D$ −29.7 (*c* 0.02, $CHCl_3$) for **4**. Thus, compound **5** (peltanolide E) was defined as (2*Z*,3*S*)-3-hydroxy-4-methylidene-2-[(15*Z*)-15-icosenylidene]butanolid.

Compound **6** was isolated as a colorless oil. The HREIMS data indicated a molecular formula of $C_{25}H_{44}O_4$ from the peak at *m/z* 408.3230 $[M]^+$. Compared with **1**, the ^{1}H and ^{13}C NMR spectra of **6** (Tables 1 and 2) showed the absence of signals for a methylidene group and the presence of signals for a methyl group [δ_H 1.62 (3H, s)/δ_C 26.8] and a doubly oxygenated carbon (δ_C 100.1). The doubly oxygenated carbon was assigned as C-4 with an attached methyl group; these assignments were confirmed by HMBC correlations (Figure 2). A NOESY correlation between H-7 and H-3 as well as the chemical shift of H-6 at 7.04 ppm were consistent with $\Delta^{2(6)}$ being the *E*-isomer. The stereochemistry of C-3 was determined as *R* based on the optical rotation $[\alpha]^{25}{}_D$ +116.0 (*c* 0.015, $CHCl_3$) by comparison with related 4-hydroxybutanolides [31–33]. The NOESY correlation between H-3 and H-5 supported the 4*S* stereochemistry (Figure 3). TDDFT-ECD calculation was also sorted the (3*R*,4*S*) absolute configuration (Figure 4). Therefore, compound **6** (peltanolide F) was assigned as (2*E*,3*R*,4*S*)-3,4-dihydroxy-5-methyl-2-[(15*Z*)-15-icosenylidene]butanolide.

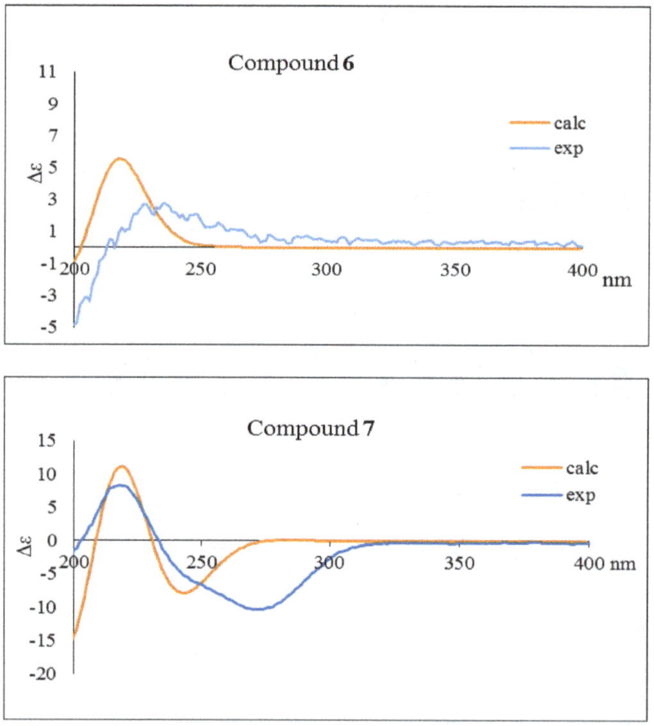

Figure 4. Experimental and calculated ECD spectra of compounds **6** and **7**.

Compound **7** has the molecular formula, $C_{28}H_{50}O_4$, based on the peak at *m/z* 450.3702 $[M]^+$ in the HREIMS. All NMR data and EIMS fragment peaks (Figure 5) of **7** were identical to those of illigerone A [34]. However, the ECD spectrum of **7** exhibited a different Cotton effect from that of illigerone A, and TDDFT-ECD calculation was indicated the 3*R* absolute configuration (Figure 4). In addition, the experimental optical rotation, $[\alpha]^{25}{}_D$ −78.5 (*c* 0.03, acetonitrile), of **7** had a negative (levorotary) rather than positive (dextrorotary) value, as found with illigerone A [34]. We concluded that compound **7** (peltanolide G) is (3*R*,4*E*,20*Z*)-3-hydroxy-4-(2-methoxy-2-oxo)hexacosa-4,20-dien-2-one, the enantiomer of illigerone A.

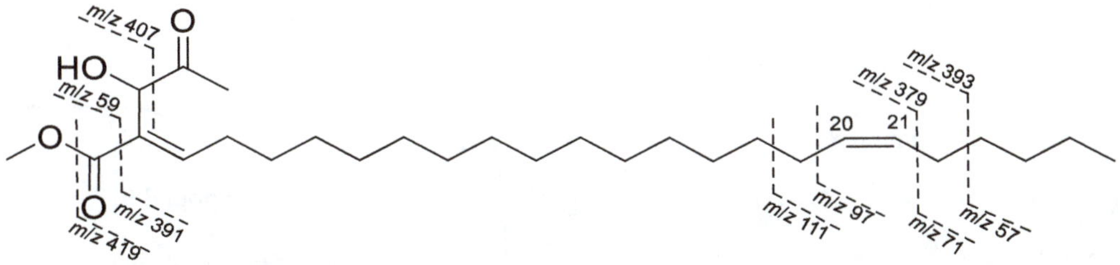

Figure 5. EIMS fragmentation of **7**.

Compound **8** was obtained as a yellow solid, and its molecular formula was determined to be $C_{27}H_{36}O_{13}$ on the HRFABMS ion at *m/z* 591.2022 [M + Na]$^+$. The ^{1}H NMR data displayed five aromatic [δ_H 7.11 (1H, d, J = 8.2 Hz), 6.92 (1H, d, J = 1.8 Hz), 6.82 (1H, dd, J = 8.2, 1.8 Hz), and 6.52 (2H, s, overlap)], two oxymethine [δ_H 4.63 (1H, d, J = 7.3 Hz), 4.52 (1H, d, J = 8.2 Hz)], four oxymethylene protons [δ_H 4.26 (1H, dd (J = 9.0, 4.6 Hz), 3.92 (1H, m), 3.87 (1H, m), and 3.63 (1H, m)], three methoxy groups [δ_H 3.84 (6H, s), and 3.83 (3H, s)], and two methine protons [δ_H 2.53 (1H, m), 1.89 (1H, m)]. In addition, a glucopyranosyl anomeric proton was observed at δ_H 4.84 (1H, m). The ^{13}C NMR spectrum showed 27 carbon signals, six from a glucose unit and three methoxy groups and the remaining 18 carbons from the lignan skeleton. The spectroscopic data of **8** resembled those of the known compound, (7*S*,8*R*,7′*S*,8′*S*)-4,9,7′-trihydroxy-3,3′-dimethoxy-7,9′-epoxylignan-4′-*O*-β-D-glucopyrano-side [35], except for the absence of the H-3 aromatic proton in the ^{1}H NMR spectrum and the presence of an additional methoxy group in **8**. The HMBC (Figure 6) and NOESY (Figure 7) spectra agreed with this structure, and the observed ROESY correlations between H-7/H-9, H-8/H-7′, and H-8′/H-9 (Figure 7) strongly suggested trans configurations of H-7/H-8 and H-8/H-8′. The CD spectrum of **8** showed positive Cotton effects at 237 nm and 274 nm (Figure 8), which were identical with those of the known compound [35]. Thus, the structure of **8** (peltaside A) was determined as (7*S*,8*R*,7′*S*,8′*S*)-4,9,7′-trihydroxy-3,5,3′-trimethoxy-7,9′-epoxylignan-4′-*O*-β-D-glucopyranoside.

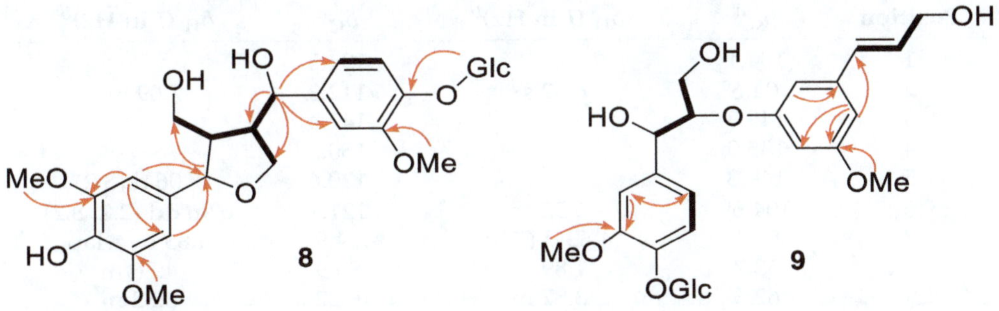

Figure 6. Selected HMBC correlations (arrows in red), COSY connectivities (bold lines) for **8** and **9**.

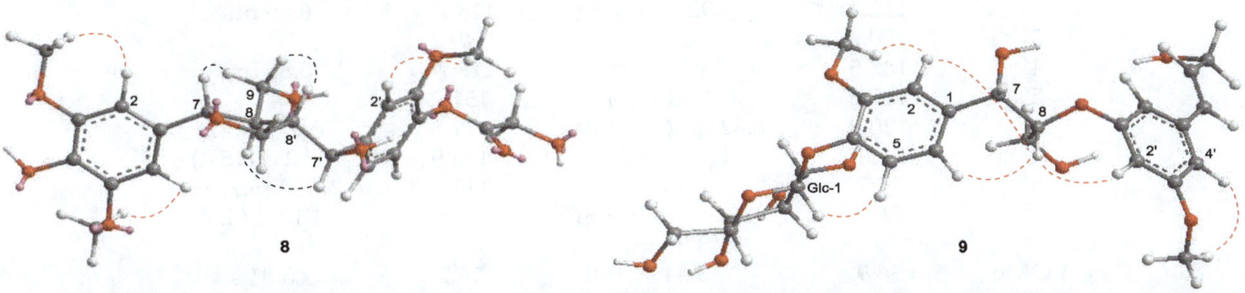

Figure 7. Key NOESY correlations (red lines) and Key ROESY correlations (blue lines) for **8** and **9**.

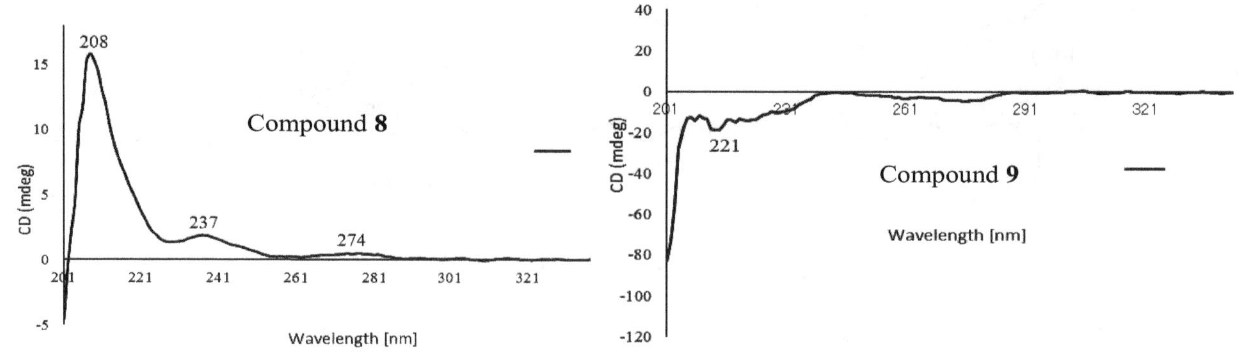

Figure 8. Experimental ECD spectra of compounds **8** and **9**.

Compound **9** was obtained as a yellow solid and its HRFABMS (*m/z* 561.1958 $[M + Na]^+$) indicated the molecular formula $C_{26}H_{34}O_{12}$. The 1H NMR spectrum of **9** displayed the signals for a trans-olefinic, two oxygenated methine, two oxygenated methylene, and six aromatic protons, as well as a β-glucose and two methoxy groups (Table 3). In addition, its ^{13}C-NMR spectrum showed the signals for 26 carbons, including 12 aromatic, two methoxy, two olefinic, and six glucopyranosyl carbons (Table 3). The COSY, HMQC, HMBC, and NOESY spectra suggested that the glucopyranosyl moiety was attached to C-4 (Figures 5 and 6). The relative configuration between C-7 and C-8 was assigned as erythro based on the small coupling constant (J = 4.8 Hz) in ^{1}H NMR (Figure S57). The absolute configuration of **9**, which showed a negative Cotton effect at 221 nm in the CD spectrum (Figure 8), was determined to be 7*S*,8*R* via a comparison with that of reported analogues [36–38]. Hence, compound **9** (peltaside B) is (7*S*,8*R*,7′*E*)-7,9,9′-trihydroxy-3,5′-dimethoxy-8-3′-oxyneolign-7′-ene-4-*O*-β-D-glucopyranoside.

Table 3. ^{1}H and ^{13}C NMR Spectroscopic Data of Compounds **8** and **9**.

	8 (CD_3OD)		9 (CD_3OD)	
Position	δ_C[a]	δ_H (J in Hz)[b]	δ_C[a]	δ_H (J in Hz)[b]
1	134.1		131.5	
2	104.6[c]	6.52 s[d]	112.3	7.09 brs
3	149.3		147.4	
4	135.9		150.5	
5	149.3		120.6	7.06 d (8.2)
6	104.6[c]	6.52 s[d]	121.1	6.96 dd (2.2, 8.2)
7	85.1	4.63 d (7.3)	74.9	4.85 overlap
8	53.7	1.89 m	85.9	4.36 m
9	62.3	3.87 m 3.63 m	62.2	3.82 m 3.47 m
1′	139.5		137.8	
2′	112.2	6.92 d (1.8)	118.7[g]	6.86 brs[g]
3′	150.7		149.2	
4′	147.5		118.7[g]	6.86 brs[g]
5′	117.5	7.11 d (8.2)	151.2	
6′	120.9	6.82 dd (8.2, 1.8)	111.3	6.97 d (2.2)
7′	74..8	4.52 d (8.2)	132.9	6.52 d (15.4)
8′	50.7	2.53 m	111.3	6.27 dd (5.7, 15.4)
9′	76.2	4.26 dd (9.0, 4.6) 3.92 m	63.8	4.19 d (5.9)
3-OMe	56.9	3.84 s[e]	56.7	3.81 s
5-OMe	56.8	3.84 s[e]	56.5	3.79 s
3′-OMe	56.7	3.83 s		

Table 3. *Cont.*

	8 (CD_3OD)		9 (CD_3OD)	
Position	δ_C [a]	δ_H (J in Hz) [b]	δ_C [a]	δ_H (J in Hz) [b]
Glc-1	102.7	4.84 m	103.1	4.81 d (6.9)
Glc-2	74.9	3.4–3.8 m[f]	73.9	3.4–3.8 m[h]
Glc-3	78.2	3.4–3.8 m[f]	78.2	3.4–3.8 m[h]
Glc-4	71.4	3.4–3.8 m[f]	71.4	3.4–3.8 m[h]
Glc-5	77.9	3.4–3.8 m[f]	77.9	3.4–3.8 m[h]
Glc-6	62.5	3.4–3.8 m[f]	62.5	3.4–3.8 m[h]

[a] 100 Hz, [b] 400 Hz, [c–h] Overlapping signals.

2.2. *Antiproliferative Activity of Isolated Compounds from H. nymphaeifolia*

Compounds **1**, **2**, **8**, **10**, and **13–18** were evaluated for antiproliferative effects against five human tumor cell lines, A549 (lung carcinoma), MCF-7 (estrogen receptor-positive and HER2-negative breast cancer), MDA-MB-231 (triple negative breast cancer), KB (cervical cancer cell line HeLa derivative), and P-glycoprotein (P-gp)-overexpressing multidrug-resistant (MDR) KB subline, KB-VIN (Table 4). The remaining compounds were not tested due to insufficient quantities. Butanolide **10** slightly inhibited MCF-7 and KB-VIN tumor cell growth with an IC_{50} value of **9** μM. Both lignans **15** and **16** showed antiproliferative activity against chemosensitive A549 and MCF-7 tumor cell lines, while **16** was also active against MDA-MB-231. Interestingly, compounds **15** and **16** also displayed moderate activity against the MDR cell line (KB-VIN) with an IC_{50} value of 5 μM but were less active against its parent chemosensitive cell line (KB). Compounds **1**, **2**, **8**, **14** and **18** exhibited no activity against all tested cell lines. These results demonstrated that the CH_3OH/CH_2Cl_2 (1:1) extract of *H. nymphaeifolia* contained antiproliferative natural products, which showed broad spectrum against HTCLs including MDR cells and could also work synergistically against MDR cells.

Table 4. Antiproliferative Activity of the Isolated Compounds.

Compounds	Cell Lines[a] (IC_{50} μM)[b]				
	A549	**MDA-MB-231**	**MCF-7**	**KB**	**KB-VIN**
1	>40	22.5	>40	25.7	31.7
2	21.9	24.6	24.6	22.6	21.4
8	35.1	35.3	35.7	32.7	21.7
10	12.5	10.8	8.8	18.6	8.8
13	32.8	37.7	33.5	>40	8.7
14	23.2	32.9	32.8	23.2	19.9
15	8.1	20.8	6.8	20.3	5.4
16	5.7	8.2	8.1	12.6	5.3
17	37.8	>40	38.0	>40	8.2
18	>40	>40	>40	>40	>40
Paclitaxel (nM)	6.5	8.4	12.1	7.1	2213

[a] A549 (lung carcinoma), MDA-MB-231 (triple-negative breast cancer), MCF-7 (estrogen receptor-positive & HER2-negative breast cancer), KB (cervical cancer cell line HeLa derivative), KB-VIN (P-gp-overexpressing multidrug-resistant (MDR) subline of KB). [b] Antiproliferative activity expressed as IC_{50} values for each cell line cultured with compound for 72 h, the concentration of compound that caused 50% reduction relative to untreated cells determined by the SRB assay. IC_{50} of all compounds were calculated.

3. Materials and Methods

3.1. *General Experimental Procedures*

Infrared spectra (IR) were obtained with a Thermo Fisher Scientific (Waltham, MA, USA) NICOLET iS5 FT-TR spectrometer from samples in $CHCl_3$ and MeOH. NMR spectra were measured on JEOL

(Akishima, Tokyo, Japan) JNM-ECA600 and JNM-ECS400 spectrometers with tetramethylsilane as an internal standard, and chemical shifts are stated as δ values. HRMS data were recorded on a JEOL JMS-700 Mstation (FAB or EI) mass spectrometer. Analytical and preparative TLC were carried out on precoated silica gel 60F254 and RP-18F254 plates (0.25 or 0.50 mm thickness; Merck, Darmstadt, Germany). MPLC was performed on a Combiflash R_f (Teledyne Isco, Lincoln, NE, USA) with silica gel and C18 cartridges (Biotage, Uppsala Sweden). Preparative HPLC was carried out with a GL Science (Shinjuku, Tokyo, Japan) recycling system (PU714 pump and UV702 UV-Vis detector) using an InertSustain C18 column (5 μM, 20 × 250 mm).

3.2. Plant Material

The crude CH_3OH/CH_2Cl_2 (1:1) extract (#N053499) from fruit of *H. nymphaeifolia* (Presl) Kubitzki (originally identified as *H. peltata*), collected in Java (Indonesia) was provided by NCI/NIH. The plant was collected on May 25, 1992 in a sandy habitat in the Ujung Kulon Reserve by A. McDonald. A voucher specimen for the plant collection was deposited at the Smithsonian Institution (Washington, WA, USA) and voucher extracts were deposited at the NCI (Frederick, MD, USA) and Kanazawa University (Kanazawa, Ishikawa, Japan).

3.3. Extraction and Isolation

The crude extract N053499 (25.0 g) was dissolved in CH_3OH/H_2O (9:1) then partitioned with n-hexane, EtOAc, and *n*-BuOH, yielding *n*-hexane (17.4 g), EtOAc (3.94 g), *n*-BuOH (1.72 g), and H_2O (0.997 g) fractions. The EtOAc-soluble fraction was subjected to silica gel column chromatography (CC) with a gradient system [*n*-hexane/EtOAc 100:0 (500 mL)→90:10 (500 mL)→70:30 (1000 mL)→50:50 (1000 mL)→30:70 (1000 mL)→10:90 (1000 mL)→0:100 (500 mL)→EtOAc/MeOH 50:50 (500 mL)→MeOH (1000 mL)] to yield nine fractions, F1–F9. F3 (123 mg) was subjected to silica gel MPLC (RediSep Rf GOLD High Performance 4 g) eluted with *n*-hexane/EtOAc (9:1 to 0:1) to afford five subfractions 3a–e. Subfraction 3b (21.6 mg) was purified by repeated recycling reversed-phase preparative HPLC with H_2O/MeOH (1:19) to provide compounds **2** (2.2 mg), **3** (1.4 mg), and **10** (1.2 mg). F4 (77.9 mg) was subjected to silica gel CC eluted with CH_2Cl_2 followed by MeOH to yield eight subfractions 4a–h. Subfraction 4d (1.0 mg) was further separated by preparative normal-phase TLC with CH_2Cl_2 to afford compound **5** (0.4 mg). Subfraction 4f (4.6 mg) was purified by repeated recycling preparative HPLC with H_2O/MeOH (1:2) to afford compound **7** (0.6 mg). Subfraction 4h (54.0 mg) was purified by preparative normal-phase TLC with CH_2Cl_2/EtOAc (19:1) to afford compounds 13 (13.2 mg) and 15 (2.1 mg). F6 was subjected to silica gel CC eluted with CH_2Cl_2/EtOAc (19:1 to 0:1) followed by MeOH to obtain six subfractions, 6a–f. Subfraction 6b (37.5 mg) was purified by repeated recycling preparative HPLC with H_2O/MeOH (1:2) to afford compounds **12** (7.1 mg) and **16** (20.3 mg). Subfraction 6c (15.9 mg) was purified by repeated recycling preparative HPLC with H_2O/MeOH (1:2), to provide compound **17** (4.1 mg). The *n*-hexane fraction (12.0 g) was subjected to silica gel MPLC (RediSep R_f GOLD High Performance 120 g) with a gradient system [*n*-hexane/CH_2Cl_2 1:1 (600 mL)→2:3 (1400 mL)→3:7 (1200 mL)→4:1 (1400 mL)→CH_2Cl_2 (1200 mL)→CH_2Cl_2/EtOAc 1:1 (1000 mL)→EtOAc (1000 mL)→MeOH (1400 mL)] to yield 15 fractions, F1–F15. F6 (695 mg) was applied to silica gel MPLC (RediSep Rf GOLD High Performance 24 g) eluted with *n*-hexane/EtOAc (9:1 to 0:1) followed by MeOH to yield ten subfractions 6a–j. Subfraction 6e (197 mg) was subjected to silica gel CC eluted with *n*-hexane/EtOAc (2:3 to 0:1) followed by MeOH to yield 11 subfractions 6e1–11. Subfraction 6e5 (4.9 mg) was purified by preparative normal-phase TLC with *n*-hexane/CH_2Cl_2 (3:1) to afford compound 6 (0.4 mg). F11 (1.12 g) was applied to silica gel MPLC (RediSep Rf GOLD High Performance 24 g) with *n*-hexane/EtOAc (9:1 to 0:1) followed by MeOH to yield seven subfractions 11a–g. Subfraction 11f (535 mg) was purified by MPLC on ODS-25 (YMC-DispoPack AT 12 g) with H_2O/CH_3OH (1:3), followed by recycling preparative HPLC with H_2O/MeOH (1:2) to afford compounds **13** (0.4 mg) and **14** (0.2 mg). F13 (1.35 g) was subjected to silica gel MPLC (RediSep Rf GOLD High Performance 24 g) with *n*-hexane/CH_2Cl_2/EtOAc (1:1:0 to 0:0:1) followed by MeOH to yield ten subfractions 13a–j.

Subfraction 13e (48.2 mg) was purified by ODS preparative TLC eluted three times using MeOH to afford compounds **1** (3.2 mg), **2** (1.1 mg), and **10** (1.0 mg). The *n*-BuOH-soluble fraction (1.72 g) was subjected to silica gel MPLC (RediSep R_f GOLD High Performance 120 g) with a gradient system [$CHCl_3$/MeOH 1:0 (1000 mL)→10:1 (1400 mL)→5:1 (1200 mL)→1:1 (1800 mL)→MeOH (1400 mL)] to yield nine fractions, F1–F9. F1 (147 mg) was subjected to silica gel CC eluted with CH_2Cl_2/EtOAc (1:0 to 0:1) followed by MeOH to obtain 14 subfractions, 1a–n. Compound **4** (0.3 mg) was obtained from subfraction 1e. Subfraction 1g (3.3 mg) was purified by preparative normal-phase TLC with CH_2Cl_2/EtOAc (95:5) to afford compound **10** (1.3 mg). Subfraction 1k was purified by recycling preparative HPLC with H_2O/MeOH (1:3) to afford compounds **11** (1.8 mg), **14** (0.3 mg), and **17** (0.4 mg). F2 (44.3 mg) was subjected to silica gel CC eluted with CH_2Cl_2/EtOAc (9:0 to 0:1) followed by MeOH to obtain nine subfractions, 2a–i. Subfraction 2b (1.1 mg) was purified by ODS preparative TLC eluted three times using H_2O/MeOH (1:8) to yield compound **13** (0.6 mg). F3 (33.8 mg) was purified by preparative normal-phase TLC with $CHCl_3$/MeOH (9:1) to afford compound **8** (1.0 mg). F5 (149 mg) was subjected to silica gel CC eluted with CH_2Cl_2/MeOH (10:1 to 1:1) followed by MeOH to obtain seven subfractions, 5a–g. Subfraction 5d (75.6 mg) was purified by MPLC on ODS-25 (YMC-DispoPack AT 12 g) with H_2O/MeOH (1:3), followed by recycling preparative HPLC with H_2O/MeOH (2:3) to afford compounds **9** (1.3 mg), **18** (2.3 mg), **19** (1.0 mg), and **20** (1.2 mg).

3.3.1. Peltanolide A (1)

Yellow amorphous solid; $[\alpha]^{25}_D$ +27.3 (*c* 0.075, $CHCl_3$); IR ν_{max} ($CHCl_3$) cm^{-1} 2923, 2853, 2017, 1733, 1457, 1278, 1219; ^1H and ^{13}C NMR, Tables 1 and 2; HREIMS *m/z* 390.3137 $[M]^+$ (calcd for $C_{25}H_{42}O_3$, 390.3134).

3.3.2. Peltanolide B (2)

Yellow amorphous solid; $[\alpha]^{25}_D$ +26.1 (*c* 0.12, $CHCl_3$); IR ν_{max} ($CHCl_3$) cm^{-1} 2923, 2852, 1731, 1464, 1265, 1074; ^1H and ^{13}C NMR, Tables 1 and 2; HREIMS *m/z* 446.3743 $[M]^+$ (calcd for $C_{29}H_{51}O_3$, 446.3760).

3.3.3. Peltanolide C (3)

Colorless oil; $[\alpha]^{25}_D$ +26.0 (*c* 0.07, $CHCl_3$); IR ν_{max} ($CHCl_3$) cm^{-1} 2916, 2849, 2016, 1750, 1678, 1470, 1278, 1184; ^1H and ^{13}C NMR, Tables 1 and 2; HREIMS *m/z* 392.3302 $[M]^+$ (calcd for $C_{25}H_{44}O_3$, 392.3290).

3.3.4. Peltanolide D (4)

Yellow amorphous solid; $[\alpha]^{25}_D$ −29.7 (*c* 0.02, $CHCl_3$); IR ν_{max} ($CHCl_3$) cm^{-1} 2923, 2852, 1783, 1733, 1465, 1373, 1287; ^1H and ^{13}C NMR, Tables 1 and 2; HRFABMS *m/z* 441.3357 $[M + Na]^+$ (calcd for $C_{27}H_{46}O_3Na$, 441.3345).

3.3.5. Peltanolide E (5)

Yellow amorphous solid; $[\alpha]^{25}_D$ −21.1 (*c* 0.015, $CHCl_3$); IR ν_{max} ($CHCl_3$) cm^{-1} 2922, 2852, 2017, 1770, 1731, 1557, 1458, 1375, 1287; ^1H and ^{13}C NMR, Tables 1 and 2; HREIMS *m/z* 446.3749 $[M]^+$ (calcd for $C_{29}H_{50}O_3$, 446.3760).

3.3.6. Peltanolide F (6)

Colorless oil; $[\alpha]^{25}_D$ +116.0 (*c* 0.015, $CHCl_3$); IR ν_{max} ($CHCl_3$) cm^{-1} 2923, 2852, 1733, 1558, 1540, 1456, 1287; ^1H and ^{13}C NMR, Tables 1 and 2; HREIMS *m/z* 408.3230 $[M]^+$ (calcd for $C_{25}H_{44}O_4$, 408.3240).

3.3.7. Peltanolide G (**7**)

Colorless oil; $[\alpha]^{25}{}_D$ −78.5 (*c* 0.03, acetonitrile); IR ν_{max} ($CHCl_3$) cm^{-1} 2922, 2852, 2016, 1717, 1669, 1558, 1456, 1436; ^1H and ^{13}C NMR, Tables 1 and 2; HREIMS *m/z* 450.3702 $[M]^+$ (calcd for $C_{28}H_{50}O_4$, 450.3709).

3.3.8. Peltaside A (**8**)

Yellow solid; $[\alpha]^{25}{}_D$ +5.6 (*c* 0.055, MeOH); IR ν_{max} ($CHCl_3$) cm^{-1} 3330, 2945, 2833, 1645, 1514, 1450, 1112; ^1H and ^{13}C NMR, Table 3; HRFABMS *m/z* 591.2022 $[M + Na]^+$ (calcd for $C_{27}H_{36}O_{13}Na$, 591.2054).

3.3.9. Peltaside B (**9**)

Yellow solid; $[\alpha]^{25}{}_D$ −71.8 (*c* 0.065, MeOH); IR ν_{max} ($CHCl_3$) cm^{-1} 3386, 3293, 1657, 1511, 1265; ^1H and ^{13}C NMR, Table 3; HRFABMS *m/z* 561.1958 $[M + Na]^+$ (calcd for $C_{26}H_{34}O_{12}Na$, 561.1948).

3.4. Calculation of ECD Spectra

Preliminary conformational analysis for each compound was carried out by using CONFLEX8 with the MMFF94 force field. The conformers were further optimized in MeCN by density functional theory (DFT) method with the B3LYP functional and 6–31(d) basis set. The ECD spectrum was calculated by the time-dependent DFT (TDDFT) method with the CAM-B3LYP functional and TZVP basis set. The calculation was completed by the use of conformers within 2 kcal/mol predicted in MeCN. The solvent effect was introduced by the conductor-like polarizable continuum model (CPCM). The DFT optimization and TDDFT-ECD calculation were performed using Gaussian09 (Gaussian, Inc., Wallingford, CT, USA). The calculated spectrum was displayed by GaussView 5.0.920 with the peak half-width at half height being 0.333 eV. The Boltzmann-averaged spectrum at 298.15K was calculated using Excel 2016 (Microsoft Co., Redmond, WA, USA). The calculations were re-optimized according to the literature [39].

3.5. Assay for Antiproliferative Activity

Antiproliferative activity of the compounds was determined by the sulforhodamine B (SRB) assay as described previously [40]. Briefly, cell suspensions were seeded on 96-well microtiter plates at a density of 4000–12,000 cells per well and cultured for 72 h with test compound. The cells were fixed in 10% trichloroacetic acid and then stained with 0.04% SRB. The absorbance at 515 nm of 10 mM Tris base-solubilized protein-bound dye was measured using a microplate reader (ELx800, BioTek, Winooski, VT, U.S) operated by Gen5 software (BioTek). IC_{50} data were calculated statistically (MS Excel) from at least three independent experiments performed with duplication ($n = 6$). All human tumor cell lines, except KB-VIN, were obtained from the Lineberger Comprehensive Cancer Center (UNC-CH, Chapel Hill, NC, USA) or from ATCC (Manassas, VA, USA). KB-VIN was a generous gift from Professor Y.-C. Cheng of Yale University (New Haven, CT, USA).

4. Conclusions

As part of our continuing investigation of rainforest plants, we conducted a thorough study to identify new chemical compounds to supplement the reported phytochemical research on *H. nymphaeifolia*. Consequently, a CH_3OH/CH_2Cl_2 (1:1) extract of *H. nymphaeifolia* (N053499) provided by NCI yielded seven new butanolides, peltanolides A–G (**1–7**), and two new lignan glycosides, peltasides A (**8**) and B (**9**), as well as eleven known compounds **10–20**. This is the first report to identify butanolides and lignan glucosides from this genus. The evaluation of antiproliferative activity against human tumor cell lines revealed that lignans **15** and **16** were slightly active against chemosensitive tumor cell lines A549 and MCF-7, respectively. Interestingly, both compounds displayed significant activity with IC_{50} valued of 5 μM against a P-glycoprotein overexpressing MDR tumor cell line (KB-VIN) although they were less active against its parent chemosensitive cell line (KB).

Author Contributions: S.A., Y.S; investigation, performed the chemical experiments and data collection, S.F.; ECD calculation and analysis, M.G.; investigation, performed cytotoxic experiments using SRB assay, M.G., K.M., D.J.N, B.R.O. K.-H.L.; editing and guidance, K.N.-G; writing, conceptualization, and supervision.

Acknowledgments: We appreciate critical comments, suggestions, and editing on the manuscript by Susan L. Morris-Natschke (UNC-CH).

References

1. Lakshmi, V.; Pandey, K.; Mishra, S.K.; Srivastava, S.; Mishra, M.; Agarwa, S.K. An overview of family *Hernandiaceae*. *Rec. Nat. Prod.* **2009**, *3*, 1–22.
2. Pettit, G.R.; Meng, Y.H.; Gearing, R.P.; Herald, D.L.; Pettit, R.K.; Doubek, D.L.; Chapuis, J.C.; Tackett, L.P. Antineoplastic Agents. 522. *Hernandia peltata* (Malaysia) and *Hernandia nymphaeifolia* (Republic of Maldives). *J. Nat. Prod.* **2004**, *67*, 214–220. [CrossRef] [PubMed]
3. Udino, L.; Abaul, J.; Bourgeois, P.; Corrichon, L.; Duran, H.; Zedde, C. Lignans from the seeds of *Hernandia sonora*. *Planta Med.* **1999**, *65*, 279–281. [CrossRef] [PubMed]
4. Chalandre, M.C.; Bruneton, J.; Cabalion, P.; Guinaudeau, H. Hernandiaceae. XII. Aporphine-benzylisoquinoline dimers isolated from *Hernandia peltata*. *Can. J. Chem.* **1986**, *64*, 123–126. [CrossRef]
5. Wei, C.Y.; Wang, S.W.; Ye, J.W.; Hwang, T.L.; Cheng, M.J.; Sung, P.J.; Chang, T.H.; Chen, J.J. New anti-inflammatory aporphine and lignan derivatives from the root wood of *Hernandia nymphaeifolia*. *Molecules* **2018**, *23*, 2286. [CrossRef]
6. Lavault, M.; Cabalion, P.; Bruneton, J. Study on Hernandiaceae. IV. Alkaloids of *Hernandia peltata*. *Planta Med.* **1982**, *46*, 119–121. [CrossRef]
7. Chen, J.J.; Tsai, I.L.; Chen, I.S. New Oxoaporphine Alkaloids from *Hernandia nymphaeifolia*. *J. Nat. Prod.* **1996**, *59*, 156–158. [CrossRef]
8. Chen, J.J.; Ishikawa, T.; Duh, C.Y.; Tsai, I.L.; Chen, I.S. New dimeric aporphine alkaloids and cytotoxic constituents of *Hernandia nymphaefolia*. *Planta Med.* **1996**, *62*, 528–533. [CrossRef]
9. Angerhofer, C.K.; Guinaudeau, H.; Wongpanich, V.; Pezzuto, J.M.; Cordell, G.A. Antiplasmodial and cytotoxic activity of natural bisbenzylisoquinoline alkaloids. *J. Nat. Prod.* **1999**, *62*, 59–66. [CrossRef]
10. Rasoanaivo, R.; Urverg, R.; Rafatro, H.; Ramanitrahasimbola, D.; Palazzino, G.; Galeffi, C.; Nicoletti, M. Alkaloids of *Hernandia voyronii*. Chloroquine-potentiating activity and structure elucidation of herveline D. *Planta Med.* **1998**, *64*, 58–62. [CrossRef]
11. Dittmar, A. The effectiveness of *Hernandia* spp. (Hernandiaceae) in traditional Samoan medicine and according to scientific analyses. *J. Ethnopharmacol.* **1991**, *33*, 243–251. [CrossRef]
12. Bruneton, J.; Shamma, M.; Minard, R.D.; Freyer, A.J.; Guinaudeau, H. Novel biogenetic pathways from (+)-reticuline. Three dimeric alkaloids: (+)-vanuatine, (+)-vateamine, and (+)-malekulatine. *J. Org. Chem.* **1983**, *48*, 3957–3960. [CrossRef]
13. Chen, I.S.; Chen, J.J.; Duh, C.Y.; Tsai, I.L. Cytotoxic lignans from Formosan *Hernandia nymphaeifolia*. *Phytochemistry* **1997**, *45*, 991–996. [CrossRef]
14. Chen, I.J.; Chang, Y.L.; Teng, C.M.; Chen, I.S. Anti-platelet aggregation alkaloids and lignans from *Hernandia nymphaefolia*. *Planta Med.* **2000**, *66*, 251–256. [CrossRef] [PubMed]
15. Yoder, B.J.; Cao, S.; Norris, A.; Miller, J.S.; Ratovoson, F.; Andriantsiferana, R.; Rasamison, V.E.; Kingston, D.G.I. Tambouranolide, a new cytotoxic hydroxybutanolide from a *Tambourissa* sp. (Monimiaceae). *Nat. Prod. Res.* **2007**, *21*, 37–41. [CrossRef] [PubMed]
16. Muto, N.; Tomokuni, T.; Haramoto, M.; Tatemoto, H.; Nakanishi, T.; Inatomi, Y.; Murata, H.; Inada, A. Isolation of apoptosis- and differentiation-inducing substances toward human promyelocytic leukemia HL-60 cells from leaves of *Juniperus taxifolia*. *Biosci. Biotechnol. Biochem.* **2008**, *72*, 477–484. [CrossRef] [PubMed]
17. Trazzi, G.; André, M.F.; Coelho, F.J. Diastereoselective synthesis of β-piperonyl-γ-butyrolactones from Morita-Baylis-Hillman adducts. Highly efficient synthesis of (±)-yatein, (±)-podorhizol and (±)-*epi*-podorhizol. *Braz. Chem. Soc.* **2010**, *21*, 2327–2339. [CrossRef]
18. Okunishi, T.; Umezawa, T.; Shimada, M. Enantiomeric compositions and biosynthesis of *Wikstroemia sikokiana* lignans. *J. Wood Sci.* **2000**, *46*, 234–242. [CrossRef]

19. Li, N.; Wu, J.L.; Sakai, J.I.; Ando, M. Dibenzylbutyrolactone and Dibenzylbutanediol Lignans from *Peperomia duclouxii*. *J. Nat. Prod.* **2003**, *66*, 1421–1426. [CrossRef]
20. Ahmed, A.A.; Mahmoud, A.A.; Ali, E.T.; Tzakou, O.; Couladis, M.; Mabry, T.J.; Gáti, T.; Tóth, G. Two highly oxygenated eudesmanes and ten lignans from *Achillea holosericea*. *Phytochemistry* **2002**, *59*, 851–856. [CrossRef]
21. Iida, T.; Nakano, M.; Ito, K. Hydroperoxysesquiterpene and lignan constituents of *Magnolia kobus*. *Phytochemistry* **1982**, *21*, 673–675. [CrossRef]
22. Asikin, Y.; Takahashi, M.; Mizu, M.; Takara, K.; Okua, H.; Wada, K. DNA damage protection against free radicals of two antioxidant neolignan glucosides from sugarcane molasses. *J. Sci. Food Agric.* **2016**, *96*, 1209–1215. [CrossRef] [PubMed]
23. Calis, I.; Kirmizibekmez, H.; Beutler, J.A.; Donmez, A.A.; Yalc, F.N.; Kilic, I.E.; Ozlap, M.; Ruedi, P.; Tasdemir, D. Secondary metabolites of *Phlomis viscosa* and their biological activities. *Turk. J. Chem.* **2005**, *29*, 71–81.
24. Sugiyama, M.; Kikuchi, M. Phenylethanoid glycosides from *Osmanthus asiaticus*. *Phytochemistry* **1993**, *32*, 1553–1555. [CrossRef]
25. Seki, K.; Sasaki, T.; Wano, S.; Haga, K.; Kaneko, R. Linderanolides and isolinderanolides, ten butanolides from *Lindera glauca*. *Phytochemistry* **1995**, *40*, 1175–1181. [CrossRef]
26. Anderson, J.E.; Ma, W.; Smith, D.L.; Chang, C.J.; Mclaughlin, J.L. Biologically active γ-lactones and methylketoalkenes from *Lindera benzoin*. *J. Nat. Prod.* **1992**, *55*, 71–83. [CrossRef]
27. Tamura, S.; Doke, S.; Murakami, N. Total synthesis of peumusolide A, NES non-antagonistic inhibitor for nuclear export of MEK. *Tetrahedron* **2010**, *66*, 8476–8480. [CrossRef]
28. Tamura, S.; Tonokawa, M.; Murakami, N. Stereo-controlled synthesis of analogs of peumusolide A, NES non-antagonistic inhibitor for nuclear export of MEK. *Tetrahedron Lett.* **2010**, *51*, 3134–3137. [CrossRef]
29. Tsenga, M.; Su, Y.S.; Cheng, M.J.; Liu, T.W.; Chen, I.S.; Wu, M.D.; Chang, H.S.; Yuan, G.F. Chemical constituents from a soil-derived actinomycete, Actinomadura miaoliensis BCRC 16873, and their inhibitory activities on lipopolysaccharide-induced tumor necrosis factor production. *Chem. Biodivers.* **2013**, *10*, 303–312. [CrossRef]
30. Tanaka, H.; Takaya, Y.; Toyoda, J.; Yasuda, T.; Sato, M.; Murata, J.; Murata, H.; Kaburagi, K.; Iida, O.; Sugiyama, K.; et al. Two new butanolides from the roots of *Litsea acuminate*. *Phytochemistry Lett.* **2015**, *11*, 32–36. [CrossRef]
31. Cheng, H.I.; Lin, W.Y.; Duh, C.Y.; Lee, K.H.; Tsai, I.L.; Chen, I.S. New cytotoxic butanolides from *Litsea acutivena*. *J. Nat. Prod.* **2001**, *64*, 1502–1505. [CrossRef] [PubMed]
32. Juan, C.; Martinez, V.; Yoshida, M.; Gottlieb, O.R. The chemistry of Brazilian Lauraceae. Part LXI. ω-Ethyl, ω-ethenyl and ω-ethynyl-α-alkylidene-γ-lactones from *Clinostemon mahuba*. *Phytochemistry* **1981**, *20*, 459–464. [CrossRef]
33. Takeda, K.I.; Sakurawi, K.; Ishi, H. Components of the Lauracea family. I. New lactonic compounds from *Litsea japonica*. *Tetrahedron* **1972**, *28*, 3757–3766. [CrossRef]
34. Li, X.J.; Dong, J.W.; Cai, L.; Wang, J.P.; Yu, N.X.; Ding, Z.T. Illigerones A and B, two new long-chain secobutanolides from *Illigera henryi* W. W. Sm. *Phytochem. Lett.* **2017**, *19*, 181–186. [CrossRef]
35. Yang, Y.N.; Huang, X.Y.; Feng, Z.M.; Jiang, J.S.; Zhang, P.C. Hepatoprotective Activity of Twelve Novel 7′-Hydroxy Lignan Glucosides from Arctii Fructus. *J. Agric. Food Chem.* **2014**, *62*, 9095–9102. [CrossRef] [PubMed]
36. Greca, M.D.; Molinaro, A.; Monaco, P.; Previtera, L. Neolignans from *Arum italicum*. *Phytochemistry* **1994**, *35*, 777–779. [CrossRef]
37. Arnoldi, A.; Merlini, L. Asymmetric synthesis of 3-methyl-2-phenyl-1,4-benzodioxanes. Absolute configuration of the neolignans eusiderin and eusiderin C and D. *J. Chem. Soc. Perkin Trans. I* **1985**, 2555–2557. [CrossRef]
38. Gan, M.; Zhang, Y.L.; Lin, S.; Liu, M.T.; Song, W.X.; Zi, J.C.; Yang, Y.C.; Fan, X.N.; Shi, J.G.; Hu, J.F.; et al. Glycosides from the root of *Iodes cirrhosa*. *J. Nat. Prod.* **2008**, *71*, 647–654. [CrossRef]
39. Pascitelli, G.; Bruhn, T. Good Computational Practice in the Assignment of Absolute Configurations by TDDFT Calculations of ECD Spectra. *Chirality* **2016**, *28*, 466–474. [CrossRef]
40. Nakagawa-Goto, K.; Oda, A.; Hamel, E.; Ohkoshi, E.; Lee, K.H.; Goto, M. Development of a novel class of tubulin inhibitors from desmosdumotin B with a hydroxylated bicyclic B-ring. *J. Med. Chem.* **2015**, *58*, 2378–2389. [CrossRef]

9

Antiangiogenic Effects of Coumarins against Cancer: From Chemistry to Medicine

Mohammad Bagher Majnooni [1], Sajad Fakhri [2], Antonella Smeriglio [3], Domenico Trombetta [3], Courtney R. Croley [4], Piyali Bhattacharyya [5], Eduardo Sobarzo-Sánchez [6,7], Mohammad Hosein Farzaei [2,*] and Anupam Bishayee [4,*]

1 Student Research Committee, Kermanshah University of Medical Sciences, Kermanshah 6714415153, Iran; mb.majnooni64@yahoo.com

2 Pharmaceutical Sciences Research Center, Health Institute, Kermanshah University of Medical Sciences, Kermanshah 6734667149, Iran; pharmacy.sajad@yahoo.com

3 Department of Chemical, Biological, Pharmaceutical and Environmental Sciences, University of Messina, Viale Palatucci, 98168 Messina, Italy; asmeriglio@unime.it (A.S.); domenico.trombetta@unime.it (D.T.)

4 Lake Erie College of Osteopathic Medicine, Bradenton, FL 34211, USA; CCroley48578@med.lecom.edu

5 Escuela de Ciencias de la Salud, Universidad Ana G. Méndez, Recinto de Gurabo, Gurabo, PR 00778, USA; pbhattacharyya@suagm.edu

6 Laboratory of Pharmaceutical Chemistry, Department of Organic Chemistry, Faculty of Pharmacy, University of Santiago de Compostela, 15782 Santiago de Compostela, Spain; e.sobarzo@usc.es or eduardo.sobarzo@ucentral.cl

7 Instituto de Investigación e Innovación en Salud, Facultad de Ciencias de la Salud, Universidad Central de Chile, Santiago 8330507, Chile

* Correspondence: mh.farzaei@gmail.com (M.H.F.); abishayee@lecom.edu or abishayee@gmail.com (A.B.)

Academic Editor: Kyoko Nakagawa-Goto

Abstract: Angiogenesis, the process of formation and recruitment of new blood vessels from pre-existing vessels, plays an important role in the development of cancer. Therefore, the use of antiangiogenic agents is one of the most critical strategies for the treatment of cancer. In addition, the complexity of cancer pathogenicity raises the need for multi-targeting agents. Coumarins are multi-targeting natural agents belonging to the class of benzopyrones. Coumarins have several biological and pharmacological effects, including antimicrobial, antioxidant, anti-inflammation, anticoagulant, anxiolytic, analgesic, and anticancer properties. Several reports have shown that the anticancer effect of coumarins and their derivatives are mediated through targeting angiogenesis by modulating the functions of vascular endothelial growth factor as well as vascular endothelial growth factor receptor 2, which are involved in cancer pathogenesis. In the present review, we focus on the antiangiogenic effects of coumarins and related structure-activity relationships with particular emphasis on cancer.

Keywords: coumarins; antiangiogenic; cancer; natural agents; chemistry; medicine

1. Introduction

Angiogenesis (also known as neovascularization), the growth of blood vessels from the existing vasculature, has been shown to play a critical role in the development of various diseases, including rheumatoid arthritis, diabetic retinopathy, asthma, endometriosis, psoriasis, obesity, and cancer [1–3]. Inflammation, tissue ischemia, and hypoxia which cause the release of the angiogenesis factors, such as vascular endothelial growth factor (VEGF), cytokines, cell adhesion molecules, and nitric oxide (NO), are among the most important triggers of angiogenesis [4]. In 1971, Folkman reported that tumor metastasis occurs as a consequence of angiogenesis [5]. This was the starting point for the design and use of bevacizumab, thalidomide, sunitinib, and axitinib as antiangiogenic drugs in the treatment of a variety of cancers [6–8]. Considering the crucial role of angiogenesis in the progression of cancer, investigating novel and potential antiangiogenic compounds is of great importance to combat cancer. Several naturally occurring compounds, including vinblastine, vincristine, paclitaxel, were reported as antiangiogenic and anticancer agents. Besides, other natural compounds with antiangiogenic activities, such as resveratrol, artemisinin, boswellic acid, and cannabidiol, have shown enormous potential for cancer prevention and therapy [9–13]. For instance, endocannabinoid 2-arachidonoyl-glycerol showed a promising anticancer effect in several cell lines [14]. Overall, cancer remains a clinical challenge, despite advancements in its treatment. This raises the need to investigate novel multi-target agents to attenuate multiple signaling pathways involved in tumor progression.

Growing evidence has introduced coumarins as potential multi-targeting agents with various pharmacological effects and medicinal uses [15]. Coumarins, with their 2H-1-benzopyran-2-one structure, are natural compounds that exist in various plant families, including Apiaceae, Asteraceae, Fabaceae, Rutaceae, Moraceae, Oleaceae, and Thymelaeaceae [16]. Apiaceae is the greatest family of plants containing coumarin compounds [16]. Also, due to the antioxidant [17], anti-inflammatory [18], anxiolytic [19], analgesic [20], neuroprotective [21], cardioprotective [22], antidiabetic [23], and anticancer [24] activities of coumarins [25], researchers have studied the synthesis of various coumarin derivatives, in addition to their purification from natural sources [26]. Both synthetic and natural coumarins have shown noticeable anticancer effects in vitro and in vivo through various mechanisms [27], including the inhibition of angiogenesis [28,29]. From a mechanistic point of view, some coumarins have shown promising antiangiogenic effects through the interaction with and repression of signaling mediators involved in angiogenesis [30,31].

In this review, we focus on the cellular signaling pathways of angiogenesis and recent pharmacological antiangiogenic agents, emphasizing natural and synthetic coumarins with antiangiogenic effects as well as their pharmacological mechanisms and structure-activity relationship in cancer.

2. Angiogenesis: Biology and Cellular Signaling

Angiogenesis could be controlled by achieving a balance among activating cytokines and growth factors on one hand and inhibiting agents on the other, which stimulate or inhibit endothelial cells (ECs), respectively. Proangiogenic agents include growth factors, namely, VEGF, fibroblast growth factors, epidermal growth factor (EGF), transforming growth factor-β (TGF-β), platelet-derived growth factor (PDGF), placental growth factor (PGF), hepatocyte growth factor/scatter factor (HGF/SF), and cytokines, such as tumor necrosis factor-α (TNF-α), colony-stimulating factor-1 (CSF-1), and interleukin-8 (IL-8) [32–35]. ECs, fibroblasts, platelets, smooth muscle cells, inflammatory cells, and cancer cells are involved in producing angiogenic growth factors and cytokines [4].

VEGF and FGF have been considered as promising antiangiogenic targets [35]. VEGF mainly acts through tyrosine kinase VEGF receptor 2 (VEGFR2) [36]. Furthermore, bioactive lipids, such as prostaglandin E_2 (PGE_2), and sphingosine-1-phosphate (S1P), matrix degenerating enzymes, namely, matrix metalloproteinases (MMP) and heparinases, small mediators (e.g., NO, peroxynitrite, serotonin, and histamine), angiopoietins (Ang), and erythropoietin are among other activators of angiogenesis [35]. In order to attract other angiogenesis-stimulating factors, cancer cells induce a situation of hypoxia by increasing the demand for nutrients and oxygen. In the hypoxic condition, hypoxia-inducible factor-1α (HIF-1α), together with released anti-apoptotic factors, growth factors, and cytokines, provokes angiogenesis [4,37].

On the other hand, angiogenesis could be suppressed by inhibiting proteins, which are classified into either direct or indirect angiogenesis inhibitors. The first class of inhibitors directly suppress ECs in the growing vasculature, while the second class indirectly suppress either tumor cells or other tumor-associated stromal cells [35,38]. This direct inhibitory effect could also be mediated by integrin receptors through several intracellular signaling pathways [39]. Angiostatin, endostatin, arrestin, canstatin, and tumstatin are released by the proteolysis of distinct endothelial cell-matrix molecules and prevent vascular ECs from proliferating and migrating in response to angiogenesis inducers [40]. Interferons, retinoic acid, IL-1, IL-12, tissue inhibitor of metalloproteinases, and multimerin 2 are other angiogenesis inhibitors [41,42].

As previously mentioned, angiogenesis is controlled by a balance between activators and inhibitors of angiogenesis. Hypoxia, as a critical determinant, causes an imbalance between activators and inhibitors by inducing the upregulation of HIF-1α, which elevates the expression of pro-angiogenesis agents as well as suppresses the expression of angiogenesis inhibitors [43]. Therefore, all the mediators in these pathways could be therapeutic targets to inhibit angiogenesis.

3. Recent Advancement in Pharmacological Antiangiogenic Agents

Several angiogenesis inhibitors have been found since Folkman first presented the concept of introducing angiogenesis inhibitors as anticancer drugs [5]. RNA interference (RNAi) therapy, chimeric antigen receptor T cell therapy, gene therapy, and pharmacological agents are auspicious antiangiogenic interventions [44]. According to the United States Food and Drug Administration (FDA), approved antiangiogenic agents are classified into two major groups, namely, monoclonal antibodies (mAbs) and small molecules [45].

VEGF receptors (VEGFRs) and related downstream signaling pathways are crucial targets of mAbs. Small molecules also target receptors, including PDGFR, VEGFR, Fms-like tyrosine kinase 3, and c-Kit receptor, and signaling proteins such as Raf, mitogen-activated protein kinase (MAPK), mammalian target of rapamycin (mTOR), and phosphoinositide 3-kinases (PI3K). Besides, the antiangiogenic/anticancer effects of FDA-approved herbal drugs, including vinca [46], taxan [47], camptothecins [48], podophyllotoxins [49], and homoharringtonine [50], related receptors, and downstream signaling pathways have now been confirmed [13].

VEGF (A–D), PDGF (A–D), HGF [51,52], and FGF [53,54] bind to VEGFR (1 and 2), PDGFR (α and β), MET [55,56], and FGFR (1-4) tyrosine kinase receptors, respectively, and activate downstream signaling pathways, thereby regulating cell growth, differentiation, and angiogenesis [54,57–59]. Their overactivation is attributed to several mutations promoting tumor vascularization in different types of cancers [60,61], while their inhibitors exert antitumor effects [62]. Bevacizumab, aflibercept, and ramucirumab have been developed as antiangiogenic agents to target the VEGF/VEGFR signaling pathway [63].

Angiopoietins (Ang1–4) bind to the Tie2 receptor. While Ang1 helps the vessels stabilize, Ang2 is secreted by ECs in response to proangiogenic factors, including hypoxia, cytokines, and inflammation [64]. Ang/Tie2-targeted therapy is challenging, since it could be either antitumor or protumor, depending on the context [65].

The rearranged during transfection (RET) protein binds receptor tyrosine kinases (RTKs) associated with normal development, maintenance, and maturation of cells and tissues [66]. However, its mutation is related to the growth and progression of tumors [66,67]. Therefore, RET inhibition could be of great importance in combating cancer.

Multi-targeting antiangiogenic drugs are shown in Figure 1. These drugs exert anticancer effects through simultaneously modulating several signaling pathways involved in angiogenesis.

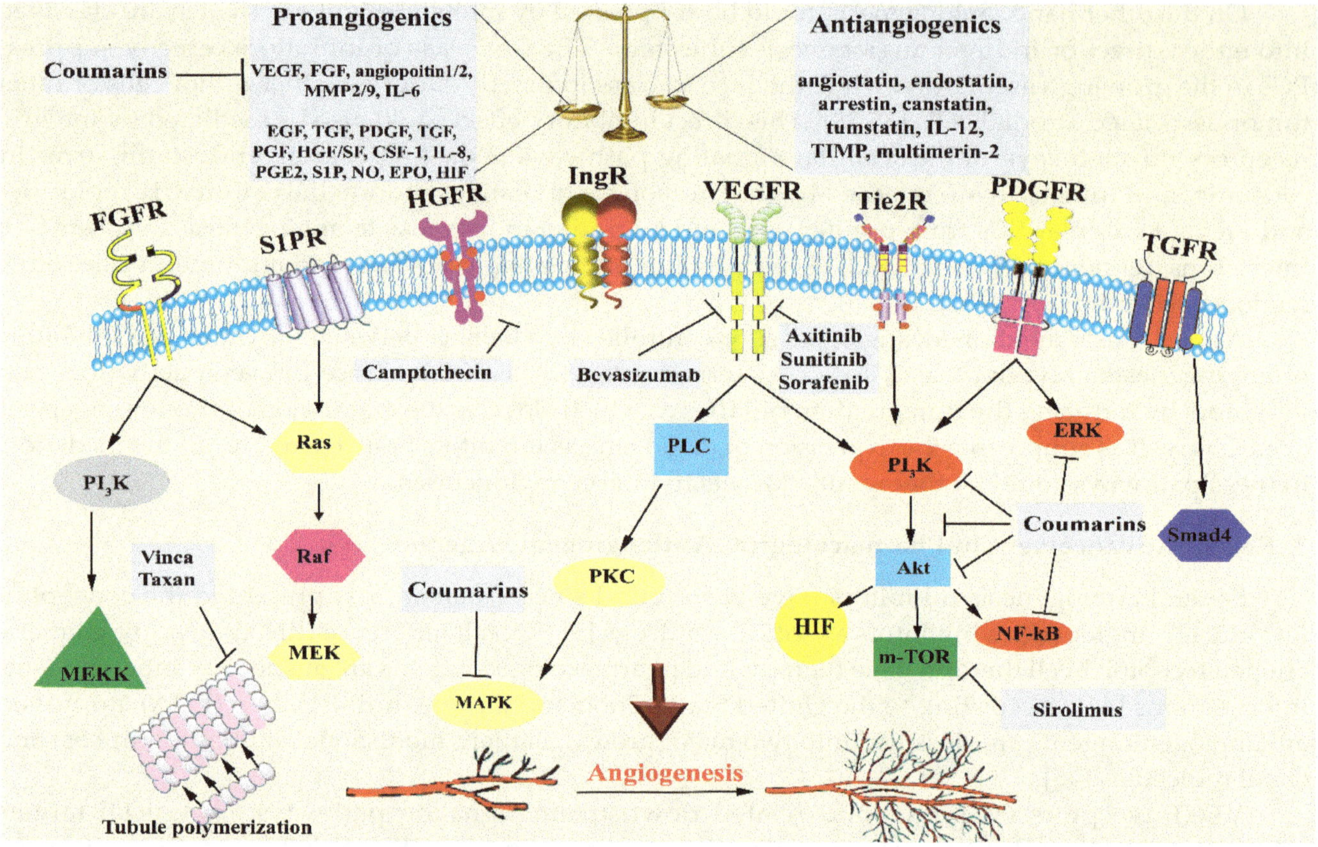

Figure 1. Signaling pathways and therapeutic targets of antiangiogenic and anticancer drugs and agents. VEGF, vascular endothelial growth factor; FGF, fibroblast growth factor; EGF, epidermal growth factor; TGF-β, transforming growth factor-β; PDGF, platelet-derived growth factor; PGF, placental growth factor; HGF/SF, hepatocyte growth factor/scatter factor; TNF-α, tumor necrosis factor-α; CSF-1, colony-stimulating factor-1; IL, interleukin; MMP, matrix metalloproteinase; TIMPs, tissue inhibitors of metalloproteinases; S1PR, sphingosine-1-phosphate receptor; NO, nitric oxide; PI3K:,phosphatidylinositol-3-kinase; PLC, phospholipase C; PKC, protein kinase C; HIF, hypoxia-inducible factor; and m-TOR: mammalian target of rapamycin.

4. Coumarins

4.1. Chemical Structure and Sources

Coumarin ($C_9H_6O_2$, 2H-1-benzopyran-2-one, 146.145 g/mol) and its derivatives (Figure 2) are a large class of natural compounds that are widely distributed in the plant kingdom and are biosynthesized from ortho-hydroxy-cinnamic acid in the shikimic acid pathways [68]. In terms of chemical structure, coumarins are subdivided into four main groups: (a) simple coumarins, such as heparin and scopoletin; (b) furanocoumarins (linear and angular), such as bergapten and imperatorin; (c) pyranocoumarins, such as grandivittin and agasyllin; (d) dicoumarins and pyrone-substituted coumarins, such as phenylcoumarins (Figure 2) [69–71].

Coumarins are isolated and purified from fruits, leaves, stems, roots, and flowers of more than 40 plant families. The Apiaceae represents a family of plants with the highest number of species producing coumarins, including *Anethum graveolens*, *Angelica dahurica*, *Apium graveolens*, *Petroselinum crispum* and *Heracleum mantegazzianum*. Other plant families producing coumarins are Rutaceae (*Citrus aurantium*, *Citrus sinensis*, and *Melicope glabra*), Asteraceae (*Matricaria recutita* and *Achillea millefolium*), Fabaceae (*Melilotus officinalis* and *Glycyrriza glabra*), and Moraceae (*Ficus carica*) [16,72–76].

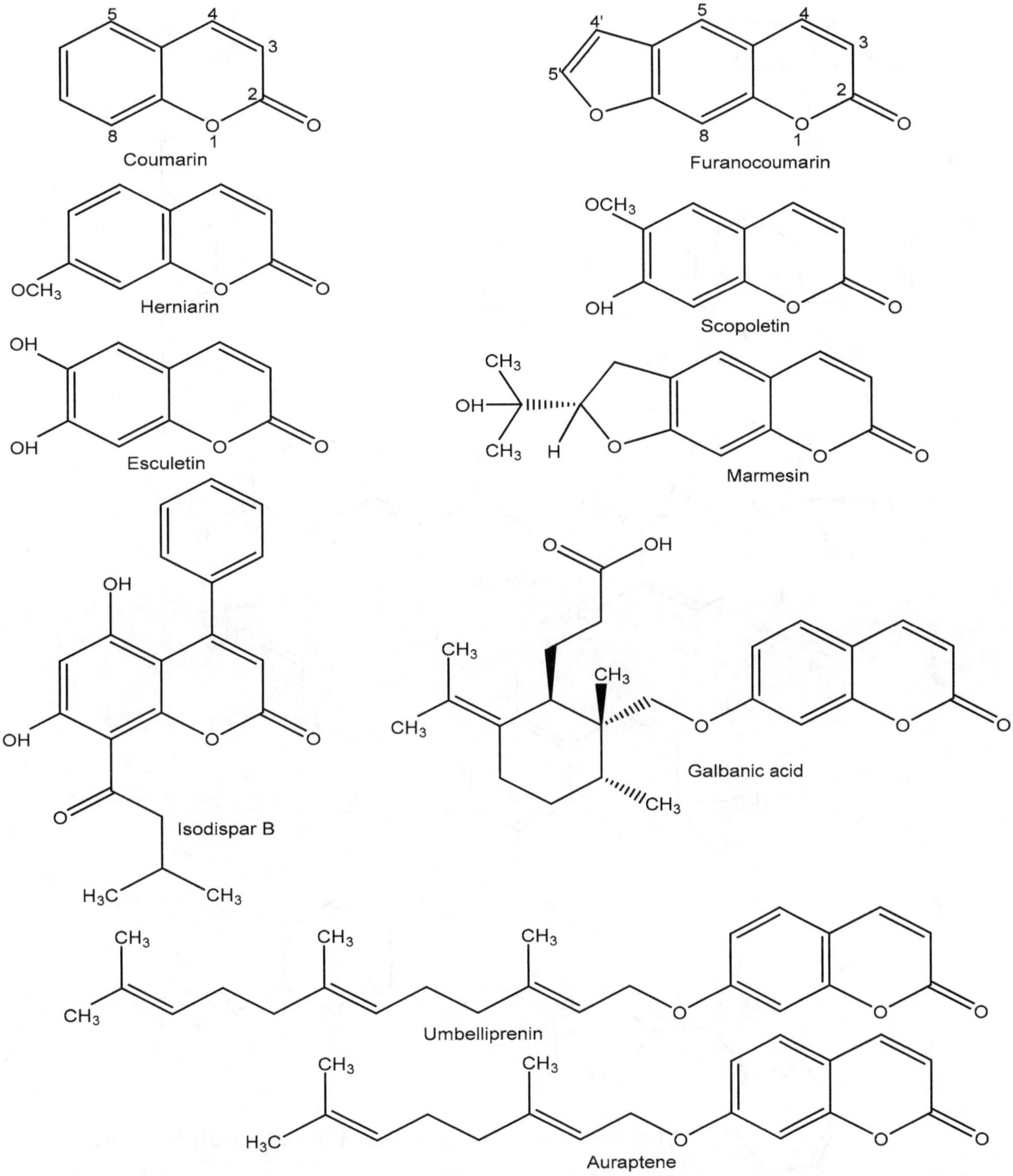

Figure 2. *Cont.*

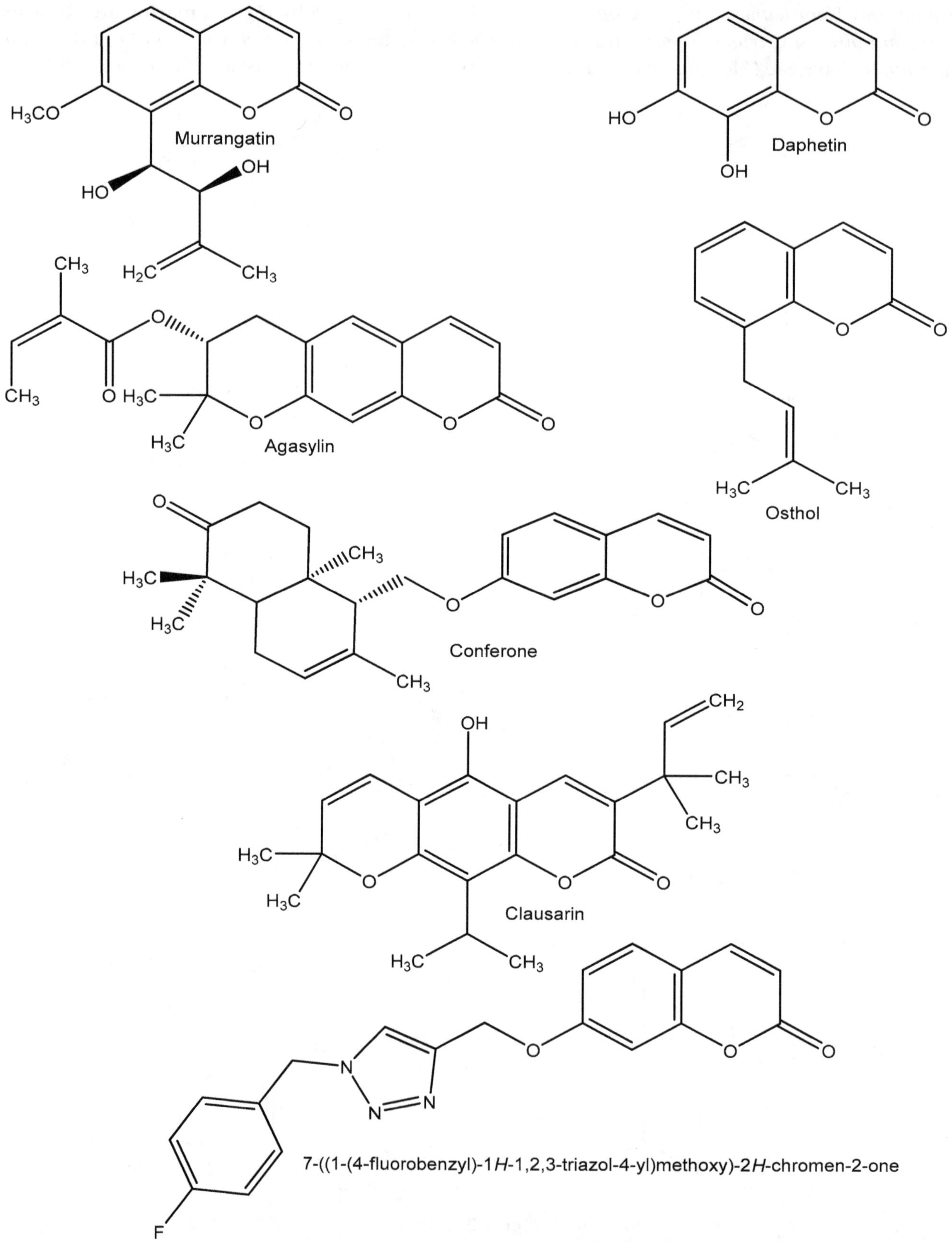

Figure 2. Chemical structures of coumarins with antiangiogenic effects.

4.2. Biological and Pharmacological Effects of Coumarins

Coumarins have several biological and pharmacological effects. For example, coumarins isolated from the bark of *M. glabra* showed antioxidant properties [73]. In this line, antimicrobial effects of coumarins from the fruits of *H. mantegazzianum* Sommier & Levier as well as *Peucedanum luxurians* Tamamsch were reported [76,77]. Antiviral effects of coumarins isolated from *Prangos ferulacea* L. have been shown by Shokoohinia et al. [78]. In addition, anxiolytic effects of coumarin derivatives, purified from the root of *Biebersteinia multifida* DC, have been demonstrated [79]. Other coumarins, such as umbelliferone and pimpinellin, were isolated from the root of *Zosima absinthifolia* and these compounds showed anti-Alzheimer effects [80]. Kontogiorgis and co-workers [81] designed and synthesized coumarin derivatives based on azomethine, with anti-inflammatory activities. Synthesized coumarins based on 3,4-dihydro-2H-benzothiazines showed analgesic effects in formalin- and acetic acid-induced writhing tests [82]. Additionally, various coumarins have shown antiulcerogenic [83], spasmolytic [84], anticoagulant [85], vasorelaxant [86], cytotoxic, and anticancer activities [87].

On the other hand, hepatotoxicity, nausea, and diarrhea were reported as the side effects of coumarin derivatives [88,89].

4.3. Coumarins as Anticancer Agents

As the second leading cause of death worldwide, cancer is one of the most critical diseases that threaten public health and imposes a high cost on countries' health systems each year. Because of the resistance of cancer cells to conventional drugs used in chemotherapy as well as the side effects of these drugs, it is necessary to find new anticancer agents. Undoubtedly, medicinal plants are one of the richest sources of biologically active compounds and potential novel anticancer drugs. Coumarins are natural compounds with low to moderate side effects, which have been introduced by researchers as promising anticancer compounds [29,90–92]. Several coumarins also inhibit cytochrome P450, thereby affecting the blood concentration of various anticancer drugs. In this line, bergamottin inhibits cytochrome P450 and reduces the effects of various carcinogenic agents [93].

The anticancer and cytotoxic activities of synthetic and natural coumarins with different functional groups on their basic structure (Figure 2) have been reported by several investigators. These studies showed the anticancer activity of coumarins against breast cancer [89], colon cancer [94], lung cancer [24], ovarian cancer [95], hepatocellular carcinoma [96], bladder carcinoma [97], leukemia [98], and other types of cancer in vitro and in vivo, via different mechanisms, including free-radical scavenging, antioxidant activity [99], induction of cell cycle arrest [100], interaction with various signaling pathways with important role in cell differentiation and proliferation [101], telomerase and carbonic anhydrase inhibition [102,103], and antiangiogenic activity [104]. For example, Taniguchi and co-workers [105] isolated eight coumarins from the leaves of *Rhizophora mucronata* and reported the anticancer effects of methoxyinophyllum P, calocoumarin B, and calophyllolide against HeLa cells (cervical cancer), with IC_{50} equal to 3.8, 29.9, and 36.4 μM, respectively, and HL-60 cells (promyelocytic leukemia cells) with IC_{50} of 12.9, 2.6, and 2.2 μM, respectively. Also, three hemiterpene ether coumarins, isolated from *Artemisia armeniaca* Lam, showed cytotoxic effects in HL-60 and K562 cells (chronic myelogenous leukemia cells). In their study, armenin showed the highest cytotoxic effect through cycle arrest, with IC_{50} equal to 22.5 and 71.1 μM for K562 and HL-60 cells, respectively [106].

Among coumarins, clausarin, nordentatin, dentatin, and xanthoxyletin, isolated from dichloromethane extraction of root bark of *Clausena harmandiana*, showed high cytotoxic activities [107]. In this study, clausarin (Figure 2) showed the highest cytotoxic activity, which was superior to that of cisplatin used as a positive control, against hepatocellular carcinoma (HepG2, $IC_{50} = 17.6 \pm 2.1$ μM), colorectal carcinoma (HCT116, $IC_{50} = 44.9 \pm 1.4$ μM), and lung adenocarcinoma (SK-LU-1, $IC_{50} = 6.9 \pm 1.6$ μM) cell lines. Clausarin also showed the highest antioxidant activity in the 2,2-diphenyl-1-picryl-hydrazyl-hydrate scavenging assay. From a mechanistic point of view, apoptosis induction was reported as an anticancer mechanism of coumarins [107].

On the other hand, several studies have been carried out on the synthesis of coumarins to produce coumarin derivatives with improved anticancer effects. Among them, synthetic scopoletin derivatives have shown promising antitumor activities. In their study, out of 20 synthesized derivatives of scopoletin, 5 compounds showed the greatest effects ($IC_{50} < 2$ μM) in MCF-7 and MDA-MB 231 cells (human breast adenocarcinoma cell line) as well as in HT29 cells (human colorectal adenocarcinoma cell line). The relationship between the increase in Log P value and the increase in cytotoxic activity was established in this investigation. Cell cycle arrest was also suggested as the anticancer mechanism of these compounds [108].

Besides, Zang et al. [105] synthesized novel anticancer analogs of geiparvarin using a bioisosteric transformation method. In their study, it was also shown that adding electron-withdrawing substituents to the benzene rings, such as 7-((1-(4-fluorobenzyl)-1*H*-1,2,3-triazol-4-yl)methoxy)-4Hchromen-4-one (Figure 2), increased their cytotoxic effects in a human hepatoma cell line (QGY-7701, $IC_{50} = 14.37 \pm 9.93$) and a colon carcinoma cell line (SW480, $IC_{50} = 11.18 \pm 2.16$) compared with geiparvarin ($IC_{50} = 17.68 \pm 0.40$ and 20.34 ± 0.75, respectively) [109]. Additionally, Cui and co-workers [110] showed the anticancer effects of three synthesized coumarins derived from triphenylethylene, occurring through the inhibition of angiogenesis.

Considering the above investigations on the anticancer effects of coumarin derivatives, these compounds could be developed as anticancer drugs.

5. Coumarin and Angiogenesis Inhibition

Inhibition of angiogenesis is one of the most critical anticancer mechanisms of secondary plant metabolites, including coumarins. Natural and synthetic coumarins with different structures can inhibit the factors involved in angiogenesis, migration, proliferation, and differentiation of endothelial cells in vitro and in vivo. Coumarins act by blocking various molecular signaling pathways, involving growth factors (e.g., VEGFs, TNF-α, and FGF-2), cytokines (e.g., IL-1 and IL-6), angiogenic enzymes (e.g., MMP), endothelial-specific receptor tyrosine kinases (e.g., Tie2), and adhesion molecules (e.g., intercellular adhesion molecule-1) [30,111,112].

5.1. Natural Coumarins with Antiangiogenic Effects

The antiangiogenic effects of coumarins from natural sources, especially isolated and purified from plants, are reported in several studies. Scopoletin [113,114], esculetin [104], herniarin [115], decursin, and decursinol [116] with coumarin structure, as well as imperatorin [117] and psoralidine [118] with furanocoumarin structure (Figure 2), are among the natural antiangiogenic coumarins.

Pan and co-workers [119] showed the antiangiogenic effects of scopoletin, isolated from *Erycibe obtusifolia* Benth stem, in vitro and in vivo. In their study, scopoletin markedly reduced the number of blood vessel branch points after a 48-h treatment with the dose of 100 nmol/egg in the chick chorioallantoic membrane (CAM) model. Additionally, the inhibitory effects of scopoletin on migration, proliferation, and tube formation of human umbilical vein endothelial cells (HUVECs) induced by VEGF (10 ng/mL) were observed. These investigators showed that the proliferation of HUVECs was significantly inhibited by 100 μM scopoletin after 72 h, and tube formation and migration of HUVECs were inhibited following treatment with 100 μM scopoletin by 52.4% and 38.1%, respectively [119].

Decursin and decursinol angelate, isolated from *Angelica gigas* root, showed substantial antiangiogenic effects in vitro and in vivo [120]. These natural coumarins significantly decreased the development of blood vessels in transgenic zebrafish embryos at 20 μM concentration as well as in the CAM model at 6 μM/egg. In their study, the inhibition of VEGFR2 (one of the most important receptors of VEGF) and other angiogenesis signaling pathway related to VGEF, such as phosphorylated extracellular signal-regulated kinase (p-ERK) and MAPK as well as phosphorylated-c-Jun N-terminal kinase (JNK) in ECs were observed [116].

The antiangiogenic effect of marmesin (Figure 2), a furanocoumarin isolated from ethanolic extract of the twigs of *Broussonetia kazinoki*, was reported by Kim et al. [121]. They showed that marmesin at 10 μM significantly inhibited the expression and activity of MMP-2 in response to VEGF-A (10 ng/mL) in HUVECs. Besides, marmesin reduced EC proliferation, migration, invasion, tube formation and also induced cell cycle arrest in a concentration-dependent manner. Marmesin at 10 μM also inhibited the development of angiogenesis in the rat aortic ring model. VEGF-A stimulated various critical molecules of angiogenesis signaling pathways, such as focal adhesion kinase (FAK), Src kinase, MEK, ERK, Akt, and p70S6K. These pathways were inhibited by 10 μM marmesin [121]. In another study, osthol, columbianadin and columbianetin acetate, three coumarins isolated from *Angelicae Pubescentis* Radix, showed inhibitory effects on the secretion of monocyte chemoattractant protein-1, a pro-inflammation factor and one of the most important migration-regulating chemokines [122]. On the other hand, conferone, a sesquiterpene coumarin isolated from *Ferula szwitziana*, showed antiangiogenic and cytotoxic effects on a human colorectal adenocarcinoma cell line (HT-29) through reducing proangiogenic factors, including angiopoietin 1 and 2 [123]. Besides, daphnetin (7,8-hydroxy coumarin), another natural coumarin, inhibited the expression of MAPK, VEGFR2, ERK1/2, AKT, FAK, and cSrc, which are involved in angiogenesis [124] (Table 1). Also, inhibiting PI3K/AKT activity, another angiogenesis inducer pathway, is one of the antiangiogenic mechanisms of murrangatin purified from *Micromelum falcatum* [125]. Moreover, reducing and blocking VEGF and MMPs are among the most important antiangiogenic mechanisms of coumarins such as galbanic acid [126], umbelliprenin [127], imperatorin [117], auraptene [128], esculetin [31], osthole [129], and scopolin [130] (Table 1).

Table 1. Natural coumarins with antiangiogenic effects and their mechanisms.

Coumarin	Sources	Mechanism of Action	Concentrations	Reference
Galbanic acid	*Ferula assafoetida*	Decreases molecular angiogenesis pathways including VEGF, MAPK, JNK, and AKT	5, 10, 20, 40 μM for in vitro study and 0.1, 1 mg/Kg for Lewis lung cancer (LLC) mouse model, intraperitoneally (i.p.) injected once daily for 18 days	[126]
Umbelliprenin	*Ferula* species	Reduces and blocks angiogenesis marker activity including Ki-67, CD31, VEGF, MMP2, MMP9, and E-cadherin	3, 6.25, 12.5, 25, 50, 100, and 200 μg/mL	[127]
Murrangatin	*Micromelum falcatum*	Inhibition of phosphoinositol 3-kinase (PI3K)/AKT activity as angiogenic inducer	10, 50, 100 μM	[125]
Imperatorin	*Angelica dahurica* and *Angelica archangelica*	Blocks the expression of nuclear factor (NF-κB) target genes, such as MMP-9, VEGF, IL-6 that are induced by TNF-α	50, 100, 150 μM	[117]
Auraptene	*Citrus sinensis*	Inhibition of angiogenesis via suppression of MMP-2,9	12.5, 25, 50, 100 μM	[128]
Esculetin	*Artemisia scoparia*	Inhibition of angiogenesis via decreasing MMP expression and blocking phosphorylation of VEGFR-2, ERK1/2, Akt, and endothelial nitric oxide synthase (eNOS) induced by VEGF (20 ng/mL)	12.5, 25, 50 μg/ml	[31]
Osthol	*Cnidium monnieri*	Reduction of microvessel density (MVD) with blocked expression of VEGF and NF-κB	61, 122, and 244 mg/kg, i.p, once daily for two weeks in a mouse model of hepatocellular carcinoma (HCC)	[129]
Conferone	*Ferula szwitsiana*	Reduction of the production of the pro-angiogenic factors VEGF, Angiopoietin-1, and Angiopoietin -2	20 μM	[123]
Daphnetin	*Changbai daphne*	Inhibition of the expression of proteins involved in angiogenesis induced by VEGF such as MAPK, VEGFR2, ERK1/2, AKT, focal adhesion kinase (FAK), cSrc, and MMP and inhibition of NF-κB induced by TNF-α	37.5, 75, 150 μM	[124]
Scopolin	*Erycibe obtusifolia* Benth	Decreases VEGF, FGF-2 and IL-6 expressions	25, 50, 100 mg/kg, i.p, once daily for 10 days	[130]

5.2. Synthetic Coumarins with Antiangiogenic Effects

Angiogenesis is a critical process in the development and progression of cancer, as demonstrated by various pre-clinical and clinical evidence. Among natural-based entities, coumarins present little cytotoxicity, while demonstrating more powerful antiangiogenic effects than conventional cytotoxic drugs [131,132]. Semi-synthesized and synthesized products from natural coumarins, used as lead compounds, led to the discovery of interesting antiangiogenic and non-cytotoxic molecules. Coumarins with interesting antiangiogenic and non-cytotoxic properties almost entirely mimic the behavior of the physiological ligands of the main therapeutic targets [132]. Recently, several sulfonyl derivatives of coumarins have been studied as cytotoxic and antiangiogenic agents against HepG2 hepatocellular carcinoma cells in vitro. All synthesized coumarins showed no cytotoxic effect but exhibited a high antimigration activity through the inhibition of MMP-2. CD105 was over-expressed in all cases and, therefore, was not involved in the antimigration activity [132]. In other cases, no statistically significant difference in gene expression of CD44 was found. A synthesized coumarin, 2-oxo-2*H*-chromene-6-sulfonyl derivative, was found to be the most promising antiangiogenic agent, since it was able to inhibit the migratory activity mediated by MMP-2 and down-regulate CD105; however, it did not show any effect on CD44.

On the other hand, the antiangiogenic capacity of several sulfonyl derivatives of coumarins was evaluated using molecular docking studies. In these studies, it was also observed that the compounds showed better docking scores with respect to the I52 ligand, with the nitro derivatives being the best, due to the ability of the nitro group to better coordinate the Zn^{++} ion within the binding site. However, the in vitro antiangiogenic activity of sulfonyl derivatives of coumarins was not statistically significant. Only the 2-oxo-2H-chromene-6-sulfonyl derivative with *N*-acetylpyrazolone substitution at the 6-position showed a promising antiangiogenic activity, exhibiting better binding interactions with the active site and a docking score comparable to that of the inhibitor I52 (−16.22 vs. 18.18 kJmol-1, respectively) [132].

NF-κB is another protein factor, which plays a pivotal role in gene expression and, therefore, is involved in proliferation, angiogenesis, and metastasis, as well as in drug resistance in cancer. In light of this, the development of angiogenesis inhibitors is of significant importance in the treatment of many cancers. Recently, the effects of 26 new synthetic coumarins were tested against hepatocellular carcinoma cells [133]. The investigators identified (7-carbethoxyamino-2-oxo-2*H*-chromen-4-yl)-methylpyrrolidine-1-carbodithioate as the most promising one, because it was cytotoxic in a time- and concentration-dependent manner and it was able to hinder the binding of NF-κB to DNA, therefore inhibiting the expression of several genes, such as *cyclin D1*, *Bcl-2*, *survivin*, *MMP12*, and c-*Myc*. Furthermore, it was able to reduce cell migration and invasion induced by CXCL12, a cytokine that plays a pivotal role in angiogenesis by recruiting endothelial progenitor cells from the bone marrow [133].

Analysis of data present in the existing literature shows that it is possible to identify, through structure-activity analysis, coumarin derivatives more suitable for a given type of tumor. The coumarin derivatives that possess an N-aryl carboxamide, a phenyl substitution at the C-3 position, and 1, 2, 3-triazolyl, trihydroxystilbene, and amino substitutions at the C-4 position were the most effective in targeting lung cancer [24].

Preliminary in vitro results revealed that some coumarin-tethered isoxazolines exhibited significant antiproliferative effect against a human melanoma cancer cell line (UACC 903). Only one derivative with a 3,4-dimethoxy substitution did not show any cytotoxicity against a normal fibroblast cell line (FF2441) in the same concentration range. These results were corroborated in the Ehrlich ascites carcinoma animal model, highlighting significantly lowered cell viability, body weight, ascites volume as well as a down-regulation of angiogenesis and tumor growth [134].

Histone deacetylase 1 (HDAC1), a key element in the control of cell proliferation and differentiation as well as in angiogenesis, represents an attractive therapeutic target for new inhibitors of angiogenesis. In this regard, the benzamidic derivatives of coumarins were found to be the most promising candidates. Four compounds of *N*-(4-((2-aminophenyl)carbamoyl) benzyl)-2-oxo-2*H*-chromene-3-carboxamide derivatives showed the most promising cytotoxic effect, calculated as IC_{50} in the range of 0.53–57.59 μM, on several cancer cells, including HCT116, A2780, MCF7, PC-3, HL60, and A549, without any effects on a human normal cell line (HUVEC, IC_{50} > 100 μM). Moreover, they showed a strong HDAC1-inhibitory activity (IC_{50} 0.47–0.87 μM) with *N*-(4-((2-aminophenyl) carbamoyl) benzyl)-7-((3,4-dichlorobenzyl)oxy)-2-oxo-2*H*-chromene-3-carboxamide, showing an IC_{50} value similar to that of the reference drug entinostat (0.47 ± 0.02 μM vs. 0.41 ± 0.06 μM) [135].

Another interesting coumarin derivative investigated is (*E*)-2-(4-methoxybenzyloxy)-3-prenyl-4-methoxy-N-hydroxycinamide (BMX), a semisynthetic derivative of osthole and a coumarin found in several plant species, such as *Cnidium monnieri* L, *Angelica archangelica* L, and *Angelica pubescens* Maxim. BMX was found to inhibit VEGF-induced proliferation, migration, and endothelial tube formation in HUVECs. These activities were also corroborated by ex vivo and in vivo studies decreasing VEGF-induced microvessel sprouting from aortic rings and HCT116 colorectal cancer cells. Moreover, BMX inhibited HCT116 cell proliferation and the growth of xenografts of HCT116 cells in vivo [136].

Scopoletin is a well-known natural coumarin with antiangiogenic properties. To develop new and robust angiogenesis inhibitors, several scopoletin derivatives were designed and synthesized. According to the study of Tabana et al. [137], scopoletin inhibited VEGF-A, ERK1, and FGF-2, and is thereby considered a strong antiangiogenic agent. In another study, among several scopoletin analogs, three compounds, including 4-bromo-phenyl and 4-chloro-phenyl scopoletin derivatives and 2-hydroxy-3-(piperidin-1-yl)-propoxy)-6-methoxy-2*H*-chromen-2-one, were able to inhibit VEGF-stimulated proliferation, migration, and tube formation of HUVECs. These results showed a significant decrease in the VEGF-triggered phosphorylated forms of ERK1/2 and Akt, which was corroborated by in vivo observations on chick chorioallantoic membrane [138]. Luo and co-workers also showed that 3-aryl-4-anilino/aryloxy-2*H*-chromen-2-one analogues significantly affected breast cancer through the inhibition of estrogen receptor-α and VEGFR-2 [139]. In another study, coumarin-conjugated benzophenone analogs showed promising antitumor activity against Ehrlich ascites carcinoma and Dalton's lymphoma ascites cell lines. In this study, a compound with a bromo group in the benzophenone structure markedly showed antiangiogenic effects through the inhibition of VEGF [28]. In a more recent study by Makowska et al. [140], a series of 2-imino-2*H*-chromen-3-yl-1,3,5-triazine compounds were synthesized. Among them, 4-[7-(diethylamino)-2-imino-2*H*-chromen-3-yl]-6-(4-phenylpiperazin-1-yl)-1,3,5-triazin-2-amine showed the greatest cytotoxic effects against several human cancer cell lines, which underscores the promising role of synthetic coumarins in combating cancer. Figure 1 illustrates how coumarins inhibit various angiogenic signaling pathways.

6. Conclusions

Considering the crucial role of angiogenesis in cancer development, antiangiogenic agents have significant potential to fight cancer. Thus, investigating novel drugs to attenuate or prevent angiogenesis-associated complications in cancer is of great importance. The several clinical limitations and side effects related to the administration of current antiangiogenic agents for cancer treatment raise the need to find alternative treatments. Natural and synthetic coumarins have shown a variety of pharmacological properties. They have demonstrated prominent anticancer effects by targeting multiple signaling pathways involved in several types of cancer.

Recently, studies have focused on the antiangiogenic effects of coumarins according to their structure-activity relationships. The present review reports the currently available literature data on the signaling and regulatory pathways of angiogenesis, as well as on antiangiogenic and anticancer mechanisms of natural and synthetic coumarins, critically analyzing and highlighting their use as possible therapeutic strategies. These studies are essential to identify novel and effective anticancer agents with fewer side effects than conventional drugs. It is also critical to identify potential synergies that may allow reducing the side effects of cytotoxic medicines and increasing the quality of life of patients. Additional studies should focus on additional in vitro and in vivo experiments followed by well-controlled clinical trials to reveal the exact signaling pathways involved in cancer angiogenesis as well as the precise pharmacological mechanisms of coumarins. In addition, there is a need to investigate and adjust novel antiangiogenic coumarin lead compounds to develop more potent and efficient anticancer drugs with lower toxicity. In addition, an appropriate drug delivery system should be introduced to overcome the existing pharmacokinetic challenges of coumarin administration. Such research will unveil the potential of coumarins in the prevention, attenuation, and treatment of angiogenesis in cancer.

Author Contributions: Conceptualization, M.B.M., and M.H.F.; drafting the manuscript, M.B.M., S.F., A.S., D.T., and M.H.F.; review and editing the paper: M.B.M., S.F., E.S.-S., M.H.F., C.R.C., P.B., and A.B.; revising, M.B.M., S.F., M.H.F., and A.B.

Acknowledgments: The authors thank Yalda Shokoohinia for her excellent and helpful suggestions.

References

1. Carmeliet, P.; Jain, R.K. Angiogenesis in cancer and other diseases. *Nature* **2000**, *407*, 249. [CrossRef] [PubMed]
2. Ribatti, D.; Puxeddu, I.; Crivellato, E.; Nico, B.; Vacca, A.; Levi-Schaffer, F. Angiogenesis in asthma. *Clin. Exp. Allergy* **2009**, *39*, 1815–1821. [CrossRef] [PubMed]
3. Rodríguez-Caso, L.; Reyes-Palomares, A.; Sánchez-Jiménez, F.; Quesada, A.R.; Medina, M.Á. What is known on angiogenesis-related rare diseases? A systematic review of literature. *J. Cell. Mol. Med.* **2012**, *16*, 2872–2893. [CrossRef] [PubMed]
4. Ucuzian, A.A.; Gassman, A.A.; East, A.T.; Greisler, H.P. Molecular mediators of angiogenesis. *J. Burn. Care. Res.* **2010**, *31*, 158–175. [CrossRef]
5. Folkman, J. Tumor angiogenesis: Therapeutic implications. *N. Engl. J. Med.* **1971**, *285*, 1182–1186.
6. Al-Abd, A.M.; Alamoudi, A.J.; Abdel-Naim, A.B.; Neamatallah, T.A.; Ashour, O.M. Anti-angiogenic agents for the treatment of solid tumors: Potential pathways, therapy and current strategies–a review. *J. Adv. Res.* **2017**, *8*, 591–605. [CrossRef]
7. EL-Meghawry, E.; Rahman, H.; Abdelkarim, G.; Najda, A. Natural products against cancer angiogenesis. *Tumor. Biol.* **2016**, *37*, 14513–14536.
8. Quesada, A.R.; Muñoz-Chápuli, R.; Medina, M.A. Anti-angiogenic drugs: From bench to clinical trials. *Med. Res. Rev.* **2006**, *26*, 483–530. [CrossRef]
9. Aviello, G.; Romano, B.; Borrelli, F.; Capasso, R.; Gallo, L.; Piscitelli, F.; Di Marzo, V.; Izzo, A.A. Chemopreventive effect of the non-psychotropic phytocannabinoid cannabidiol on experimental colon cancer. *J. Mol. Med.* **2012**, *90*, 925–934. [CrossRef]
10. Wang, Z.; Dabrosin, C.; Yin, X.; Fuster, M.M.; Arreola, A.; Rathmell, W.K.; Generali, D.; Nagaraju, G.P.; El-Rayes, B.; Ribatti, D.; et al. Broad targeting of angiogenesis for cancer prevention and therapy. *Sem. Can. Biol.* **2015**, *35*, S224–S243. [CrossRef]
11. Bishayee, A.; Darvesh, A.S. Angiogenesis in hepatocellular carcinoma: A potential target for chemoprevention and therapy. *Curr. Cancer Drug Targets* **2012**, *12*, 1095–1118.
12. Rajasekar, J.; Perumal, M.K.; Vallikannan, B. A critical review on anti-angiogenic property of phytochemicals. *J. Nutr. Biochem.* **2019**, *71*, 1–15. [CrossRef] [PubMed]
13. Fakhri, s.; Abbaszadeh, F.; Jorjani, M.; Pourgholami, M.H. The effects of anticancer medicinal herbs on vascular endothelial growth factor based on pharmacological aspects: A review study. *Nutr. Cancer* **2019**, *25*, 1–15. [CrossRef] [PubMed]
14. Pagano, E.; Borrelli, F.; Orlando, P.; Romano, B.; Monti, M.; Morbidelli, L.; Aviello, G.; Imperatore, R.; Capasso, R.; Piscitelli, F. Pharmacological inhibition of MAGL attenuates experimental colon carcinogenesis. *Pharmacol. Res.* **2017**, *119*, 227–236. [CrossRef]

15. Kumar, S.; Kumari, R.; Mishra, S. Pharmacological properties and their medicinal uses of Cinnamomum: A review. *J. Pharm. Pharmacol.* **2019**, *71*, 1735–1761. [CrossRef]
16. Ribeiro, C.V.C.; Kaplan, M.A.C. Tendências evolutivas de famílias produtoras de cumarinas em Angiospermae. *Química Nova* **2002**, *25*, 533–538. [CrossRef]
17. Borges Bubols, G.; da Rocha Vianna, D.; Medina-Remon, A.; von Poser, G.; Maria Lamuela-Raventos, R.; Lucia Eifler-Lima, V.; Cristina Garcia, S. The antioxidant activity of coumarins and flavonoids. *Mini. Rev. Med. Chem.* **2013**, *13*, 318–334.
18. Gagliotti Vigil de Mello, S.V.; Frode, T.S. In Vitro and In Vivo Experimental Model-based Approaches for Investigating Anti-inflammatory Properties of Coumarins. *Curr. Med. Chem.* **2018**, *25*, 1446–1476. [CrossRef]
19. Orhan, I.E. Potential of Natural Products of Herbal Origin as Monoamine Oxidase Inhibitors. *Curr. Pharm. Des.* **2016**, *22*, 268–276. [CrossRef]
20. Ghate, M.; Kusanur, R.A.; Kulkarni, M.V. Synthesis and in vivo analgesic and anti-inflammatory activity of some bi heterocyclic coumarin derivatives. *Eur. J. Med. Chem.* **2005**, *40*, 882–887. [CrossRef]
21. Jameel, E.; Umar, T.; Kumar, J.; Hoda, N. Coumarin: A privileged scaffold for the design and development of antineurodegenerative agents. *Chem. Biol. Drug. Des.* **2016**, *87*, 21–38. [CrossRef]
22. Najmanova, I.; Dosedel, M.; Hrdina, R.; Anzenbacher, P.; Filipsky, T.; Riha, M.; Mladenka, P. Cardiovascular effects of coumarins besides their antioxidant activity. *Curr. Top. Med. Chem.* **2015**, *15*, 830–849. [CrossRef] [PubMed]
23. Li, H.; Yao, Y.; Li, L. Coumarins as potential antidiabetic agents. *J. Pharm. Pharmacol.* **2017**, *69*, 1253–1264. [CrossRef] [PubMed]
24. Kumar, M.; Singla, R.; Dandriyal, J.; Jaitak, V. Coumarin derivatives as anticancer agents for lung cancer therapy: A review. *Anti-Cancer Agents Med. Chem.* **2018**, *18*, 964–984. [CrossRef] [PubMed]
25. Ren, Q.-C.; Gao, C.; Xu, Z.; Feng, L.-S.; Liu, M.-L.; Wu, X.; Zhao, F. Bis-coumarin derivatives and their biological activities. *Curr. Top. Med. Chem.* **2018**, *18*, 101–113. [CrossRef] [PubMed]
26. Pereira, T.M.; Franco, D.P.; Vitorio, F.; Kummerle, A.E. Coumarin Compounds in Medicinal Chemistry: Some Important Examples from the Last Years. *Curr. Top. Med. Chem.* **2018**, *18*, 124–148. [CrossRef]
27. Kaur, M.; Kohli, S.; Sandhu, S.; Bansal, Y.; Bansal, G. Coumarin: A promising scaffold for anticancer agents. *Anti-Cancer Agents Med. Chem.* **2015**, *15*, 1032–1048. [CrossRef]
28. Vijay Avin, B.R.; Thirusangu, P.; Lakshmi Ranganatha, V.; Firdouse, A.; Prabhakar, B.T.; Khanum, S.A. Synthesis and tumor inhibitory activity of novel coumarin analogs targeting angiogenesis and apoptosis. *Eur. J. Med. Chem.* **2014**, *75*, 211–221. [CrossRef]
29. Thakur, A.; Singla, R.; Jaitak, V. Coumarins as anticancer agents: A review on synthetic strategies, mechanism of action and SAR studies. *Eur. J. Med. Chem.* **2015**, *101*, 476–495. [CrossRef]
30. Pan, R.; Gao, X.; Lu, D.; Xu, X.; Xia, Y.; Dai, Y. Prevention of FGF-2-induced angiogenesis by scopoletin, a coumarin compound isolated from Erycibe obtusifolia Benth, and its mechanism of action. *Int. Immunopharmacol.* **2011**, *11*, 2007–2016. [CrossRef]
31. Park, S.L.; Won, S.Y.; Song, J.-H.; Lee, S.-Y.; Kim, W.-J.; Moon, S.-K. Esculetin inhibits VEGF-induced angiogenesis both in vitro and in vivo. *Am. J. Chin. Med.* **2016**, *44*, 61–76. [CrossRef] [PubMed]
32. Amini, A.; Masoumi, M.S.; Morris, L.D.; Pourgholami, H.M. The critical role of vascular endothelial growth factor in tumor angiogenesis. *Curr. Cancer Drug Targets.* **2012**, *12*, 23–43. [CrossRef] [PubMed]
33. Simons, M.; Gordon, E.; Claesson-Welsh, L. Mechanisms and regulation of endothelial VEGF receptor signalling. *Nat. Rev. Mol. Cell Biol.* **2016**, *17*, 611. [CrossRef] [PubMed]
34. Bergers, G.; Benjamin, L.E. Angiogenesis: Tumorigenesis and the angiogenic switch. *Nat. Rev. Can.* **2003**, *3*, 401. [CrossRef]
35. El-Kenawi, A.E.; El-Remessy, A.B. Angiogenesis inhibitors in cancer therapy: Mechanistic perspective on classification and treatment rationales. *Brit. J. Pharmacol.* **2013**, *170*, 712–729. [CrossRef]
36. Pourgholami, M.H.; Khachigian, L.M.; Fahmy, R.G.; Badar, S.; Wang, L.; Chu, S.W.L.; Morris, D.L. Albendazole inhibits endothelial cell migration, tube formation, vasopermeability, VEGF receptor-2 expression and suppresses retinal neovascularization in ROP model of angiogenesis. *Bioch. Bioph. Res. Commun.* **2010**, *397*, 729–734. [CrossRef]
37. Folkman, J. Angiogenesis and Apoptosis, Seminars in cancer biology, Semin. *Cancer Biol.* **2003**, *13*, 159–167. [CrossRef]

38. Folkman, J. Opinion: Angiogenesis: An organizing principle for drug discovery? *Nat. Rev. Drug Discov.* **2007**, *6*, 273. [CrossRef]
39. Mundel, T.M.; Kalluri, R. Type IV collagen-derived angiogenesis inhibitors. *Microvasc. Res.* **2007**, *74*, 85–89. [CrossRef]
40. Ribatti, D. Endogenous inhibitors of angiogenesis: A historical review. *Leuk. Res.* **2009**, *33*, 638–644. [CrossRef]
41. Rajabi, M.; Mousa, S. The role of angiogenesis in cancer treatment. *Biomedicines* **2017**, *5*, 34. [CrossRef] [PubMed]
42. Kerbel, R.S. Tumor angiogenesis. *N. Engl. J. Med.* **2008**, *358*, 2039–2049. [CrossRef] [PubMed]
43. Pugh, C.W.; Ratcliffe, P.J. Regulation of angiogenesis by hypoxia: Role of the HIF system. *Nat. Med.* **2003**, *9*, 677. [CrossRef] [PubMed]
44. Ohlfest, J.R.; Demorest, Z.L.; Motooka, Y.; Vengco, I.; Oh, S.; Chen, E.; Scappaticci, F.A.; Saplis, R.J.; Ekker, S.C.; Low, W.C. Combinatorial antiangiogenic gene therapy by nonviral gene transfer using the sleeping beauty transposon causes tumor regression and improves survival in mice bearing intracranial human glioblastoma. *Mol. Ther.* **2005**, *12*, 778–788. [CrossRef]
45. Abdalla, A.M.; Xiao, L.; Ullah, M.W.; Yu, M.; Ouyang, C.; Yang, G. Current challenges of cancer anti-angiogenic therapy and the promise of nanotherapeutics. *Theranostics* **2018**, *8*, 533. [CrossRef]
46. Marimpietri, D.; Brignole, C.; Nico, B.; Pastorino, F.; Pezzolo, A.; Piccardi, F.; Cilli, M.; Di Paolo, D.; Pagnan, G.; Longo, L. Combined therapeutic effects of vinblastine and rapamycin on human neuroblastoma growth, apoptosis, and angiogenesis. *Clin. Can. Res.* **2007**, *13*, 3977–3988. [CrossRef]
47. Li, W.; Tang, Y.-X.; Wan, L.; Cai, J.-H.; Zhang, J. Effects of combining Taxol and cyclooxygenase inhibitors on the angiogenesis and apoptosis in human ovarian cancer xenografts. *Oncol. Lett.* **2013**, *5*, 923–928. [CrossRef]
48. Nakashio, A.; Fujita, N.; Tsuruo, T. Topotecan inhibits VEGF-and bFGF-induced vascular endothelial cell migration via downregulation of the PI3K-Akt signaling pathway. *Int. J. Cancer* **2002**, *98*, 36–41. [CrossRef]
49. Sang, C.-Y.; Xu, X.-H.; Qin, W.-W.; Liu, J.-F.; Hui, L.; Chen, S.-W. DPMA, a deoxypodophyllotoxin derivative, induces apoptosis and anti-angiogenesis in non-small cell lung cancer A549 cells. *Bioorg. Med. Chem. Lett.* **2013**, *23*, 6650–6655. [CrossRef]
50. Xiu-jin, Y.; Mao-fang, L. Homoharringtonine induces apoptosis of endothelium and down-regulates VEGF expression of K562 cells. *J. Zhejiang. Univ. Sci. A* **2004**, *5*, 230–234.
51. Graveel, C.R.; Tolbert, D.; Woude, G.F.V. MET: A critical player in tumorigenesis and therapeutic target. *Cold. Spring. Harb. Perspect. Biol.* **2013**, *5*, a009209. [CrossRef]
52. You, W.-K.; McDonald, D.M. The hepatocyte growth factor/c-Met signaling pathway as a therapeutic target to inhibit angiogenesis. *BMB. Rep.* **2008**, *41*, 833. [CrossRef] [PubMed]
53. Beenken, A.; Mohammadi, M. The FGF family: Biology, pathophysiology and therapy. *Nat. Rev. Drug Discov.* **2009**, *8*, 235. [CrossRef] [PubMed]
54. Turner, N.; Pearson, A.; Sharpe, R.; Lambros, M.; Geyer, F.; Lopez-Garcia, M.A.; Natrajan, R.; Marchio, C.; Iorns, E.; Mackay, A. FGFR1 amplification drives endocrine therapy resistance and is a therapeutic target in breast cancer. *Cancer Res.* **2010**, *70*, 2085–2094. [CrossRef] [PubMed]
55. Lu, K.V.; Chang, J.P.; Parachoniak, C.A.; Pandika, M.M.; Aghi, M.K.; Meyronet, D.; Isachenko, N.; Fouse, S.D.; Phillips, J.J.; Cheresh, D.A. VEGF inhibits tumor cell invasion and mesenchymal transition through a MET/VEGFR2 complex. *Cancer Cell* **2012**, *22*, 21–35. [CrossRef] [PubMed]
56. Jahangiri, A.; De Lay, M.; Miller, L.M.; Carbonell, W.S.; Hu, Y.-L.; Lu, K.; Tom, M.W.; Paquette, J.; Tokuyasu, T.A.; Tsao, S. Gene expression profile identifies tyrosine kinase c-Met as a targetable mediator of antiangiogenic therapy resistance. *Clin. Cancer Res.* **2013**, *19*, 1773–1783. [CrossRef]
57. Cao, Y.; Cao, R.; Hedlund, E.-M. R Regulation of tumor angiogenesis and metastasis by FGF and PDGF signaling pathways. *J. Mol. Med.* **2008**, *86*, 785–789. [CrossRef]
58. Heldin, C.-H. Targeting the PDGF signaling pathway in tumor treatment. *Cell Commun. Signal.* **2013**, *11*, 97. [CrossRef]
59. Wu, E.; Palmer, N.; Tian, Z.; Moseman, A.P.; Galdzicki, M.; Wang, X.; Berger, B.; Zhang, H.; Kohane, I.S. Comprehensive dissection of PDGF-PDGFR signaling pathways in PDGFR genetically defined cells. *PLoS ONE* **2008**, *3*, e3794. [CrossRef]

60. Cao, Y. Multifarious functions of PDGFs and PDGFRs in tumor growth and metastasis. *Trend. Mol. Med.* **2013**, *19*, 460–473. [CrossRef]
61. Levitzki, A. PDGF receptor kinase inhibitors for the treatment of PDGF driven diseases. *Cytokine Growth Factor Rev.* **2004**, *15*, 229–235. [CrossRef] [PubMed]
62. Lu, C.; Shahzad, M.M.; Moreno-Smith, M.; Lin, Y.; Jennings, N.B.; Allen, J.K.; Landen, C.N.; Mangala, L.S.; Armaiz-Pena, G.N.; Schmandt, R. Targeting pericytes with a PDGF-B aptamer in human ovarian carcinoma models. *Cancer Biol. Ther.* **2010**, *9*, 176–182. [CrossRef] [PubMed]
63. Zhao, Y.; Adjei, A.A. Targeting angiogenesis in cancer therapy: Moving beyond vascular endothelial growth factor. *Oncologist* **2015**, *20*, 660–673. [CrossRef] [PubMed]
64. Cascone, T.; Heymach, J.V. Targeting the angiopoietin/Tie2 pathway: Cutting tumor vessels with a double-edged sword? *J. Clin. Oncol.* **2011**, *30*, 441–444. [CrossRef] [PubMed]
65. Gerald, D.; Chintharlapalli, S.; Augustin, H.G.; Benjamin, L.E. Angiopoietin-2: An attractive target for improved antiangiogenic tumor therapy. *Cancer Res.* **2013**, *73*, 1649–1657. [CrossRef] [PubMed]
66. Mulligan, L.M. RET revisited: Expanding the oncogenic portfolio. *Nat. Rev. Cancer* **2014**, *14*, 173. [CrossRef] [PubMed]
67. Ibáñez, C.F. Structure and physiology of the RET receptor tyrosine kinase. *Cold Spring Harb. Perspect. Biol.* **2013**, *5*, a009134. [CrossRef]
68. Santos-Sánchez, N.F.; Salas-Coronado, R.; Hernández-Carlos, B.; Villanueva-Cañongo, C. Shikimic Acid Pathway in Biosynthesis of Phenolic Compounds. In *Plant Physiological Aspects of Phenolic Compounds*; IntechOpen: London, UK, 2019.
69. Jain, P.; Joshi, H. Coumarin: Chemical and pharmacological profile. *JAPS* **2012**, *2*, 236–240.
70. Stefanachi, A.; Leonetti, F.; Pisani, L.; Catto, M.; Carotti, A. Coumarin: A natural, privileged and versatile scaffold for bioactive compounds. *Molecules* **2018**, *23*, 250. [CrossRef]
71. Venugopala, K.N.; Rashmi, V.; Odhav, B. Review on natural coumarin lead compounds for their pharmacological activity. *BioMed. Res. Int.* **2013**, *2013*, 963248. [CrossRef]
72. Hroboňová, K.; Machyňáková, A.; Čižmárik, J. Determination of dicoumarol in Melilotus officinalis L. by using molecularly imprinted polymer solid-phase extraction coupled with high performance liquid chromatography. *J. Chromatogr. A* **2018**, *1539*, 93–102. [CrossRef] [PubMed]
73. Kassim, N.K.; Rahmani, M.; Ismail, A.; Sukari, M.A.; Ee, G.C.L.; Nasir, N.M.; Awang, K. Antioxidant activity-guided separation of coumarins and lignan from Melicope glabra (Rutaceae). *Food Chem.* **2013**, *139*, 87–92. [CrossRef] [PubMed]
74. Pfeifer, I.; Murauer, A.; Ganzera, M. Determination of coumarins in the roots of Angelica dahurica by supercritical fluid chromatography. *J. Pharm. Biomed. Anal.* **2016**, *129*, 246–251. [CrossRef] [PubMed]
75. Teixeira, D.M.; Patão, R.F.; Coelho, A.V.; da Costa, C.T. Comparison between sample disruption methods and solid–liquid extraction (SLE) to extract phenolic compounds from Ficus carica leaves. *J. Chromatogr. A* **2006**, *1103*, 22–28. [CrossRef]
76. Walasek, M.; Grzegorczyk, A.; Malm, A.; Skalicka-Woźniak, K. Bioactivity-guided isolation of antimicrobial coumarins from Heracleum mantegazzianum Sommier & Levier (Apiaceae) fruits by high-performance counter-current chromatography. *Food Chem.* **2015**, *186*, 133–138.
77. Widelski, J.; Luca, S.V.; Skiba, A.; Chinou, I.; Marcourt, L.; Wolfender, J.-L.; Skalicka-Wozniak, K. Isolation and Antimicrobial Activity of Coumarin Derivatives from Fruits of Peucedanum luxurians Tamamsch. *Molecules* **2018**, *23*, 1222. [CrossRef]
78. Shokoohinia, Y.; Sajjadi, S.-E.; Gholamzadeh, S.; Fattahi, A.; Behbahani, M. Antiviral and cytotoxic evaluation of coumarins from Prangos ferulacea. *Pharm. Biol.* **2014**, *52*, 1543–1549. [CrossRef]
79. Monsef-Esfahani, H.R.; Amini, M.; Goodarzi, N.; Saiedmohammadi, F.; Hajiaghaee, R.; Faramarzi, M.A.; Tofighi, Z.; Ghahremani, M.H. Coumarin compounds of Biebersteinia multifida roots show potential anxiolytic effects in mice. *DARU* **2013**, *21*, 51. [CrossRef]
80. Karakaya, S.; Koca, M.; Yılmaz, S.V.; Yıldırım, K.; Pınar, N.M.; Demirci, B.; Brestic, M.; Sytar, O. Molecular docking studies of coumarins isolated from extracts and essential oils of Zosima absinthifolia Link as potential inhibitors for Alzheimer's disease. *Molecules* **2019**, *24*, 722. [CrossRef]

81. Kontogiorgis, C.A.; Savvoglou, K.; Hadjipavlou-Litina, D.J. Antiinflammatory and antioxidant evaluation of novel coumarin derivatives. *J. Enzym. Inhib. Med. Chem.* **2006**, *21*, 21–29. [CrossRef]
82. Alipour, M.; Khoobi, M.; Emami, S.; Fallah-Benakohal, S.; Ghasemi-Niri, S.F.; Abdollahi, M.; Foroumadi, A.; Shafiee, A. Antinociceptive properties of new coumarin derivatives bearing substituted 3, 4-dihydro-2 H-benzothiazines. *DARU* **2014**, *22*, 9. [CrossRef] [PubMed]
83. Bighetti, A.; Antonio, M.; Kohn, L.; Rehder, V.; Foglio, M.; Possenti, A.; Vilela, L.; Carvalho, J. Antiulcerogenic activity of a crude hydroalcoholic extract and coumarin isolated from Mikania laevigata Schultz Bip. *Phytomedicine* **2005**, *12*, 72–77. [CrossRef] [PubMed]
84. Sadraei, H.; Shokoohinia, Y.; Sajjadi, S.; Ghadirian, B. Antispasmodic effect of osthole and Prangos ferulacea extract on rat uterus smooth muscle motility. *Res. Pharm. Sci.* **2012**, *7*, 141. [PubMed]
85. Chen, I.-S.; Chang, C.-T.; Sheen, W.-S.; Teng, C.-M.; Tsai, I.-L.; Duh, C.-Y.; Ko, F.-N. Coumarins and antiplatelet aggregation constituents from Formosan Peucedanum japonicum. *Phytochemistry* **1996**, *41*, 525–530. [CrossRef]
86. Dongmo, A.; Azebaze, A.; Nguelefack, T.; Ouahouo, B.; Sontia, B.; Meyer, M.; Nkengfack, A.; Kamanyi, A.; Vierling, W. Vasodilator effect of the extracts and some coumarins from the stem bark of Mammea africana (Guttiferae). *J. Ethnopharmacol.* **2007**, *111*, 329–334. [CrossRef]
87. Sakunpak, A.; Matsunami, K.; Otsuka, H.; Panichayupakaranant, P. Isolation of new monoterpene coumarins from Micromelum minutum leaves and their cytotoxic activity against Leishmania major and cancer cells. *Food Chem.* **2013**, *139*, 458–463. [CrossRef]
88. Lake, B.G.; Grasso, P. Comparison of the hepatotoxicity of coumarin in the rat, mouse, and Syrian hamster: A dose and time response study. *Fundam. Appl. Toxicol.* **1996**, *34*, 105–117. [CrossRef]
89. Musa, M.A.; Cooperwood, J.S.; Khan, M.O.F. A review of coumarin derivatives in pharmacotherapy of breast cancer. *Curr. Med. Chem.* **2008**, *15*, 2664–2679. [CrossRef]
90. Amaral, R.; dos Santos, S.; Andrade, L.; Severino, P.; Carvalho, A. Natural Products as Treatment against Cancer: A Historical and Current Vision. *Clin. Oncol.* **2019**, *4*, 1562.
91. Devji, T.; Reddy, C.; Woo, C.; Awale, S.; Kadota, S.; Carrico-Moniz, D. Pancreatic anticancer activity of a novel geranylgeranylated coumarin derivative. *Bioorganic Med. Chem. Lett.* **2011**, *21*, 5770–5773. [CrossRef]
92. Siegel, R.L.; Miller, K.D.; Jemal, A. Cancer statistics, 2019. CA. *Cancer J. Clin.* **2019**, *69*, 7–34. [CrossRef] [PubMed]
93. Foroozesh, M.; Sridhar, J.; Goyal, N.; Liu, J. Coumarins and P450s, Studies Reported to-Date. *Molecules* **2019**, *24*, 1620. [CrossRef]
94. Saidu, N.E.B.; Valente, S.; Bana, E.; Kirsch, G.; Bagrel, D.; Montenarh, M. Coumarin polysulfides inhibit cell growth and induce apoptosis in HCT116 colon cancer cells. *Bioorganic Med. Chem.* **2012**, *20*, 1584–1593. [CrossRef] [PubMed]
95. Nordin, N.; Fadaeinasab, M.; Mohan, S.; Hashim, N.M.; Othman, R.; Karimian, H.; Iman, V.; Ramli, N.; Ali, H.M.; Majid, N.A. Pulchrin A, a new natural coumarin derivative of Enicosanthellum pulchrum, induces apoptosis in ovarian cancer cells via intrinsic pathway. *PLoS ONE* **2016**, *11*, e0154023. [CrossRef] [PubMed]
96. Wang, J.; Lu, M.; Dai, H.; Zhang, S.; Wang, H.; Wei, N. Esculetin, a coumarin derivative, exerts in vitro and in vivo antiproliferative activity against hepatocellular carcinoma by initiating a mitochondrial-dependent apoptosis pathway. *Braz. J. Med. Biol. Res.* **2015**, *48*, 245–253. [CrossRef] [PubMed]
97. Haghighitalab, A.; Matin, M.M.; Bahrami, A.R.; Iranshahi, M.; Saeinasab, M.; Haghighi, F. In vitro investigation of anticancer, cell-cycle-inhibitory, and apoptosis-inducing effects of diversin, a natural prenylated coumarin, on bladder carcinoma cells. *Z. Nat. C J. Biosci.* **2014**, *69*, 99–109. [CrossRef] [PubMed]
98. Hejchman, E.; Taciak, P.; Kowalski, S.; Maciejewska, D.; Czajkowska, A.; Borowska, J.; Śladowski, D.; Młynarczuk-Biały, I. Synthesis and anticancer activity of 7-hydroxycoumarinyl gallates. *Pharm. Rep.* **2015**, *67*, 236–244. [CrossRef]
99. Zahri, S.; Razavi, S.M.; Moatamed, Z. Antioxidant activity and cytotoxic effect of aviprin and aviprin-3″-O-d-glucopyranoside on LNCaP and HeLa cell lines. *Nat. Prod. Res.* **2012**, *26*, 540–547. [CrossRef]
100. Chuang, J.-Y.; Huang, Y.-F.; Lu, H.-F.; Ho, H.-C.; Yang, J.-S.; Li, T.-M.; Chang, N.-W.; Chung, J.-G. Coumarin induces cell cycle arrest and apoptosis in human cervical cancer HeLa cells through a mitochondria-and caspase-3 dependent mechanism and NF-κB down-regulation. *In Vivo* **2007**, *21*, 1003–1009.

101. Aas, Z.; Babaei, E.; Feizi, M.A.H.; Dehghan, G. Anti-proliferative and apoptotic effects of dendrosomal farnesiferol C on gastric cancer cells. *Asian. Pac. J. Cancer Prev.* **2015**, *16*, 5325–5329. [CrossRef]
102. Lv, N.; Sun, M.; Liu, C.; Li, J. Design and synthesis of 2-phenylpyrimidine coumarin derivatives as anticancer agents. *Bioorg. Med. Chem. Lett.* **2017**, *27*, 4578–4581. [CrossRef] [PubMed]
103. Maresca, A.; Temperini, C.; Pochet, L.; Masereel, B.; Scozzafava, A.; Supuran, C.T. Deciphering the mechanism of carbonic anhydrase inhibition with coumarins and thiocoumarins. *J. Med. Chem.* **2009**, *53*, 335–344. [CrossRef] [PubMed]
104. Mokdad-Bzeouich, I.; Kovacic, H.; Ghedira, K.; Chebil, L.; Ghoul, M.; Chekir-Ghedira, L.; Luis, J. Esculin and its oligomer fractions inhibit adhesion and migration of U87 glioblastoma cells and in vitro angiogenesis. *Tumor. Biol.* **2016**, *37*, 3657–3664. [CrossRef] [PubMed]
105. Taniguchi, K.; Funasaki, M.; Kishida, A.; Sadhu, S.K.; Ahmed, F.; Ishibashi, M.; Ohsaki, A. Two new coumarins and a new xanthone from the leaves of Rhizophora mucronata. *Bioorg. Med. Chem. Lett.* **2018**, *28*, 1063–1066. [CrossRef] [PubMed]
106. Mojarrab, M.; Emami, S.A.; Delazar, A.; Tayarani-Najaran, Z. Cytotoxic Properties of Three Isolated Coumarin-hemiterpene Ether Derivatives from Artemisia armeniaca Lam. *IJPR* **2017**, *16*, 221. [PubMed]
107. Jantamat, P.; Weerapreeyakul, N.; Puthongking, P. Cytotoxicity and Apoptosis Induction of Coumarins and Carbazole Alkaloids from Clausena Harmandiana. *Molecules* **2019**, *24*, 3385. [CrossRef]
108. Liu, W.; Hua, J.; Zhou, J.; Zhang, H.; Zhu, H.; Cheng, Y.; Gust, R. Synthesis and in vitro antitumor activity of novel scopoletin derivatives. *Bioorg. Med. Chem. Lett.* **2012**, *22*, 5008–5012. [CrossRef]
109. Zhang, Y.; Lv, Z.; Zhong, H.; Geng, D.; Zhang, M.; Zhang, T.; Li, Y.; Li, K. Convenient synthesis of novel geiparvarin analogs with potential anti-cancer activity via click chemistry. *Eur. J. Med. Chem.* **2012**, *53*, 356–363. [CrossRef]
110. Cui, N.; Lin, D.-D.; Shen, Y.; Shi, J.-G.; Wang, B.; Zhao, M.-Z.; Zheng, L.; Chen, H.; Shi, J.-H. Triphenylethylene-Coumarin Hybrid TCH-5c Suppresses Tumorigenic Progression in Breast Cancer Mainly Through the Inhibition of Angiogenesis. *Anti-Cancer Agents. Med. Chem.* **2019**, *19*, 1253–1261. [CrossRef]
111. Nishida, N.; Yano, H.; Nishida, T.; Kamura, T.; Kojiro, M. Angiogenesis in cancer. *Vasc. Health. Risk Manag.* **2006**, *2*, 213. [CrossRef]
112. Sandhiutami, N.M.D.; Moordiani, M.; Laksmitawati, D.R.; Fauziah, N.; Maesaroh, M.; Widowati, W. In vitro assesment of anti-inflammatory activities of coumarin and Indonesian cassia extract in RAW264.7 murine macrophage cell line. *Iran. J. Basic. Med. Sci.* **2017**, *20*, 99. [PubMed]
113. Pan, R.; Dai, Y.; Yang, J.; Li, Y.; Yao, X.; Xia, Y. Anti-angiogenic potential of scopoletin is associated with the inhibition of ERK1/2 activation. *Drug. Dev. Res.* **2009**, *70*, 214–219. [CrossRef]
114. Pan, R.; Gao, X.H.; Li, Y.; Xia, Y.F.; Dai, Y. Anti-arthritic effect of scopoletin, a coumarin compound occurring in Erycibe obtusifolia Benth stems, is associated with decreased angiogenesis in synovium. *Fundam. Clin. Pharm.* **2010**, *24*, 477–490. [CrossRef] [PubMed]
115. Anegundi, N.; Pancharatna, K. 7-Hydroxycoumarin Elicit Anti-Angiogenic Effects Through Cellular Apoptosis in Developing Embryos of Zebrafish (Danio Rerio). *Eur. Sci. J.* **2017**, *13*, 53. [CrossRef]
116. Jung, M.H.; Lee, S.H.; Ahn, E.-M.; Lee, Y.M. Decursin and decursinol angelate inhibit VEGF-induced angiogenesis via suppression of the VEGFR-2-signaling pathway. *Carcinogenesis* **2009**, *30*, 655–661. [CrossRef]
117. Wang, K.S.; Lv, Y.; Wang, Z.; Ma, J.; Mi, C.; Li, X.; Xu, G.H.; Piao, L.X.; Zheng, S.Z.; Jin, X. Imperatorin efficiently blocks TNF-α-mediated activation of ROS/PI3K/Akt/NF-κB pathway. *Oncol. Rep.* **2017**, *37*, 3397–3404. [CrossRef]
118. Bronikowska, J.; Szliszka, E.; Jaworska, D.; Czuba, Z.P.; Krol, W. The coumarin psoralidin enhances anticancer effect of tumor necrosis factor-related apoptosis-inducing ligand (TRAIL). *Molecules* **2012**, *17*, 6449–6464. [CrossRef]
119. Pan, R.; Dai, Y.; Gao, X.-H.; Lu, D.; Xia, Y.-F. Inhibition of vascular endothelial growth factor-induced angiogenesis by scopoletin through interrupting the autophosphorylation of VEGF receptor 2 and its downstream signaling pathways. *Vascul. Pharm.* **2011**, *54*, 18–28. [CrossRef]
120. Zhang, J.; Li, L.; Jiang, C.; Xing, C.; Kim, S.-H.; Lu, J. Anti-cancer and other bioactivities of Korean *Angelica gigas* Nakai (AGN) and its major pyranocoumarin compounds. *Anticancer. Agents. Med. Chem.* **2012**, *12*, 1239–1254. [CrossRef]

121. Kim, J.H.; Kim, J.K.; Ahn, E.K.; Ko, H.J.; Cho, Y.R.; Lee, C.H.; Kim, Y.K.; Bae, G.U.; Oh, J.S.; Seo, D.W. Marmesin is a novel angiogenesis inhibitor: Regulatory effect and molecular mechanism on endothelial cell fate and angiogenesis. *Cancer Lett.* **2015**, *369*, 323–330. [CrossRef]
122. Yang, Y.; Zhu, R.; Li, J.; Yang, X.; He, J.; Wang, H.; Chang, Y. Separation and Enrichment of Three Coumarins from Angelicae Pubescentis Radix by Macroporous Resin with Preparative HPLC and Evaluation of Their Anti-Inflammatory Activity. *Molecules* **2019**, *24*, 2664. [CrossRef] [PubMed]
123. Cheraghi, O.; Dehghan, G.; Mahdavi, M.; Rahbarghazi, R.; Rezabakhsh, A.; Charoudeh, H.N.; Iranshahi, M.; Montazersaheb, S. Potent anti-angiogenic and cytotoxic effect of conferone on human colorectal adenocarcinoma HT-29 cells. *Phytomedicine* **2016**, *23*, 398–405. [CrossRef] [PubMed]
124. Kumar, A.; Sunita, P.; Jha, S.; Pattanayak, S.P. Daphnetin inhibits TNF-α and VEGF-induced angiogenesis through inhibition of the IKK s/IκBα/NF-κB, Src/FAK/ERK 1/2 and Akt signalling pathways. *Clin. Exp. Pharm. Physiol.* **2016**, *43*, 939–950. [CrossRef] [PubMed]
125. Long, W.; Wang, M.; Luo, X.; Huang, G.; Chen, J. Murrangatin suppresses angiogenesis induced by tumor cell-derived media and inhibits AKT activation in zebrafish and endothelial cells. *Drug Des. Devel. Ther.* **2018**, *12*, 3107–3115. [CrossRef]
126. Kim, K.H.; Lee, H.J.; Jeong, S.J.; Lee, H.J.; Lee, E.O.; Kim, H.S.; Zhang, Y.; Ryu, S.Y.; Lee, M.H.; Lü, J.; et al. Galbanic acid isolated from Ferula assafoetida exerts in vivo anti-tumor activity in association with anti-angiogenesis and anti-proliferation. *Pharm. Res.* **2011**, *28*, 597–609. [CrossRef]
127. Alizadeh, M.N.; Rashidi, M.; Muhammadnejad, A.; Zanjani, T.M.; Ziai, S.A. Antitumor effects of umbelliprenin in a mouse model of colorectal cancer. *Iran. J. Pharm. Res.* **2018**, *17*, 976–985.
128. Jamialahmadi, K.; Salari, S.; Alamolhodaei, N.S.; Avan, A.; Gholami, L.; Karimi, G. Auraptene Inhibits Migration and Invasion of Cervical and Ovarian Cancer Cells by Repression of Matrix Metalloproteinasas 2 and 9 Activity. *J. Pharm.* **2018**, *21*, 177.
129. Yao, F.; Zhang, L.; Jiang, G.; Liu, M.; Liang, G.; Yuan, Q. Osthole attenuates angiogenesis in an orthotopic mouse model of hepatocellular carcinoma via the downregulation of nuclear factor-κB and vascular endothelial growth factor. *Oncol. Lett.* **2018**, *16*, 4471–4479. [CrossRef]
130. Pan, R.; Dai, Y.; Gao, X.; Xia, Y. Scopolin isolated from Erycibe obtusifolia Benth stems suppresses adjuvant-induced rat arthritis by inhibiting inflammation and angiogenesis. *Int. Immunopharmacol.* **2009**, *9*, 859–869. [CrossRef]
131. Lee, S.; Sivakumar, K.; Shin, W.-S.; Xie, F.; Wang, Q. Synthesis and anti-angiogenesis activity of coumarin derivatives. *Bioorg. Med. Chem. Lett.* **2006**, *16*, 4596–4599. [CrossRef]
132. El-Sawy, E.R.; Ebaid, M.S.; Rady, H.M.; Shalby, A.B.; Ahmed, K.M.; Abo-Salem, H.M. Synthesis and molecular docking of novel non-cytotoxic anti-angiogenic sulfonyl coumarin derivatives against hepatocellular carcinoma cells in vitro. *J. App. Pharm. Sci.* **2017**, *7*, 049–066.
133. Neelgundmath, M.; Dinesh, K.R.; Mohan, C.D.; Li, F.; Dai, X.; Siveen, K.S.; Paricharak, S.; Mason, D.J.; Fuchs, J.E.; Sethi, G. Novel synthetic coumarins that targets NF-κB in hepatocellular carcinoma. *Bioorganic Med. Chem. Lett.* **2015**, *25*, 893–897. [CrossRef] [PubMed]
134. Lingaraju, G.S.; Balaji, K.S.; Jayarama, S.; Anil, S.M.; Kiran, K.R.; Sadashiva, M.P. Synthesis of new coumarin tethered isoxazolines as potential anticancer agents. *Bioorganic Med. Chem. Lett.* **2018**, *28*, 3606–3612. [CrossRef] [PubMed]
135. Abdizadeh, T.; Kalani, M.R.; Abnous, K.; Tayarani-Najaran, Z.; Khashyarmanesh, B.Z.; Abdizadeh, R.; Ghodsi, R.; Hadizadeh, F. Design, synthesis and biological evaluation of novel coumarin-based benzamides as potent histone deacetylase inhibitors and anticancer agents. *Eur. J. Med. Chem.* **2017**, *132*, 42–62. [CrossRef]
136. Yang, H.Y.; Hsu, Y.F.; Chiu, P.T.; Ho, S.J.; Wang, C.H.; Chi, C.C.; Huang, Y.H.; Lee, C.F.; Li, Y.S.; Ou, G.; et al. Anti-Cancer Activity of an Osthole Derivative, NBM-T-BMX-OS01: Targeting Vascular Endothelial Growth Factor Receptor Signaling and Angiogenesis. *PLoS ONE* **2013**, *8*, e81592. [CrossRef]
137. Tabana, Y.M.; Hassan, L.E.A.; Ahamed, M.B.K.; Dahham, S.S.; Iqbal, M.A.; Saeed, M.A.; Khan, M.S.S.; Sandai, D.; Majid, A.S.A.; Oon, C.E. Scopoletin, an active principle of tree tobacco (Nicotiana glauca) inhibits human tumor vascularization in xenograft models and modulates ERK1, VEGF-A, and FGF-2 in computer model. *Microvasc. Res.* **2016**, *107*, 17–33. [CrossRef]

138. Cai, X.; Yang, J.; Zhou, J.; Lu, W.; Hu, C.; Gu, Z.; Huo, J.; Wang, X.; Cao, P. Synthesis and biological evaluation of scopoletin derivatives. *Bioorganic Med. Chem.* **2013**, *21*, 84–92. [CrossRef]
139. Luo, G.; Li, X.; Zhang, G.; Wu, C.; Tang, Z.; Liu, L.; You, Q.; Xiang, H. Novel SERMs based on 3-aryl-4-aryloxy-2H-chromen-2-one skeleton-A possible way to dual ERα/VEGFR-2 ligands for treatment of breast cancer. *Eur. J. Med. Chem.* **2017**, *140*, 252–273. [CrossRef]
140. Makowska, A.; Sączewski, F.; Bednarski, P.; Sączewski, J.; Balewski, Ł. Hybrid Molecules Composed of 2, 4-Diamino-1, 3, 5-triazines and 2-Imino-Coumarins and Coumarins. Synthesis and Cytotoxic Properties. *Molecules* **2018**, *23*, 1616. [CrossRef]

10

Cytotoxic Effects of Diterpenoid Alkaloids Against Human Cancer Cells

Koji Wada * and Hiroshi Yamashita

Department of Medicinal Chemistry, Faculty of Pharmaceutical Sciences, Hokkaido University of Science, 4-1, Maeda 7-jo 15-choume, Teine-ku, Sapporo 006-8590, Japan; yama@hus.ac.jp
* Correspondence: kowada@hus.ac.jp

Academic Editor: Kyoko Nakagawa-Goto

Abstract: Diterpenoid alkaloids are isolated from plants of the genera *Aconitum*, *Delphinium*, and *Garrya* (Ranunculaceae) and classified according to their chemical structures as C_{18}-, C_{19}- or C_{20}-diterpenoid alkaloids. The extreme toxicity of certain compounds, e.g., aconitine, has prompted a thorough investigation of how structural features affect their bioactivities. Therefore, natural diterpenoid alkaloids and semi-synthetic alkaloid derivatives were evaluated for cytotoxic effects against human tumor cells [A549 (lung carcinoma), DU145 (prostate carcinoma), MDA-MB-231 (triple-negative breast cancer), MCF-7 (estrogen receptor-positive, HER2-negative breast cancer), KB (identical to cervical carcinoma HeLa derived AV-3 cell line), and multidrug-resistant (MDR) subline KB-VIN]. Among the tested alkaloids, C_{19}-diterpenoid (e.g., lipojesaconitine, delcosine and delpheline derivatives) and C_{20}-diterpenoid (e.g., kobusine and pseudokobusine derivatives) alkaloids exhibited significant cytotoxic activity and, thus, provide promising new leads for further development as antitumor agents. Notably, several diterpenoid alkaloids were more potent against MDR subline KB-VIN cells than the parental drug-sensitive KB cells.

Keywords: diterpenoid alkaloids; cytotoxicity; human tumor cells; lipojesaconitine; delcosine; delpheline; kobusine; pseudokobusine

---

1. Introduction

Cancer therapy mainly involves surgery, chemotherapy, radiation therapy, immunotherapy, monoclonal antibody therapy, and hormone therapy. Chemotherapy generally refers to the use of cytotoxic drugs to treat cancer. Plant alkaloids are one major class of chemotherapeutic drugs [1–9]. Chemotherapeutic drugs that affect cell division by preventing the normal functioning of micro-tubules include the vinca alkaloids.

Numerous diterpenoid alkaloids have been isolated from various *Aconitum*, *Delphinium*, and *Garrya* (Family Ranunculaceae) species and are classified according to their chemical structures as C_{18}-, C_{19}- or C_{20}-diterpenoid alkaloids (Figure 1) [10,11]. The C_{19}-diterpenoid alkaloids may be divided into six types: aconitine, lycoctonine, pyro (C_8=C_{15} or C_{15}=O), lactone (δ-valerolactone rather than cyclopentyl C-ring), 7,17-*seco*, and rearranged ones [10,11]. Most of the isolated C_{19}-diterpenoid alkaloids are aconitine- and lycoctonine-types and include aconitine, mesaconitine, hypaconitine and jesaconitine, all of which are extremely toxic. The C_{20}-diterpenoid alkaloids may be divided into ten types: atisine, denudatine, hetidine, hetisine, vakognavine, napelline, kusnezoline, racemulosine, arcutine, and tricalysiamide [10,11]. Most of the isolated C_{20}-diterpenoid alkaloids are atisine-, hetisine-, and napelline-types and include atisine, kobusine, pseudokobusine and lucidusculine, which are far less toxic [12].

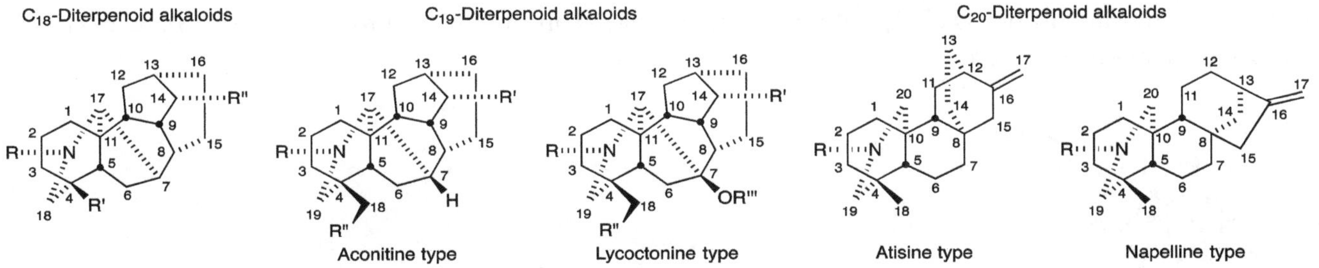

Figure 1. Classifications, general structures and numbering systems for C_{18}-, C_{19}-, and C_{20}-diterpenoid alkaloids.

The pharmacological properties of the C_{19}-diterpenoid alkaloids have been studied extensively and reviewed [12]. Aconitine is a toxin that exhibits activity both centrally and peripherally, acting predominantly on the cardiovascular and respiratory systems by preventing the normal closing of sodium channels [12]. This extreme toxicity resulted in the use of *Aconitum* extracts as poisons in hunting and warfare [13], although extracts were also used as traditional medicines by oral and topical routes. For example, the roots of *Aconitum* plants have been used as "bushi", an herbal drug in some prescriptions of traditional Japanese medicine for the treatment of hypometabolism, dysuria, cardiac weakness, chills, neuralgia, gout, and certain rheumatic diseases [14]. However, proper processing is essential to reduce the content of toxic alkaloids and avoid inadvertent poisoning [15–17]. Such obstacles encourage a good understanding of the relationships between structure and cytotoxic activity of aconitine and related compounds before they can be considered for modification and development as chemotherapeutic agents.

Our previous study demonstrated the effects of various naturally occurring and semi-synthetic C_{19}- and C_{20}-diterpenoid alkaloids on the growth of the A172 human malignant glioma cell line [18]. Antitumor properties and radiation-sensitizing effects of various types of novel derivatives prepared from C_{19}- and C_{20}-diterpenoid alkaloids were also investigated [19]. Two novel hetisine-type C_{20}-diterpenoid derivatives showed significant suppressive effects against the Raji non-Hodgkin's lymphoma cell line [20]. In addition, the effects of various semi-synthetic novel hetisine-type C_{20}-diterpenoid alkaloids on the growth of the A549 human lung cancer cell line were examined and subsequent structure-activity relationships for the antiproliferative effects against A549 cells were considered [21]. Since 2012, several diterpenoid alkaloid components and their derivatives exhibited antiproliferative activity against human tumor cell lines, including A549 (lung carcinoma), DU145 (prostate carcinoma), MDA-MB-231 (estrogen and progesterone receptor-negative & HER2-negative triple-negative breast cancer), MCF-7 (estrogen receptor-positive, HER2-negative breast cancer), KB (identical to cervical carcinoma HeLa derived AV-3 cell line), and multidrug-resistant (MDR) subline KB-VIN [P-glycoprotein (P-gp) overexpressing vincristine-resistant KB subline]. Among such alkaloids, C_{19}-diterpenoid (e.g., lipojesaconitine, delpheline, and delcosine derivative) and C_{20}-diterpenoid (e.g., kobusine and pseudokobusine derivatives) alkaloids have shown significant antiproliferative activity, as well as provided promising new leads for further development as antitumor agents.

2. Antiproliferative Activity of C_{19}-Diterpenoid Alkaloid Derivatives

2.1. *Aconitine-Type C_{19}-Diterpenoid Alkaloids*

The tested aconitine-type C_{19}-diterpenoid alkaloids included 21 natural alkaloids, aconitine (**1**), deoxyaconitine (**2**), jesaconitine (**3**), deoxyjesaconitine (**4**), aljesaconitine A (**5**), secojesaconitine (**6**), mesaconitine (**8**), hypaconitine (**9**), hokbusine A (**10**), 14-anisoyllasianine (**12**), *N*-deethylaljesaconitine A (**13**), aconine (**14**), lipomesaconitine (**15**), lipoaconitine (**16**), lipojesaconitine (**17**), neolinine (**18**), neoline (**19**), 14-benzoylneoline (**20**), isotalatizidine (**21**), karacoline (**22**), and 3-hydroxykaracoline (**23**), isolated from the rhizoma of *Aconitum japonicum* THUNB. subsp. *subcuneatum* (NAKAI) KADOTA [22–28] (Figure 2). Two synthetic aconitine-type C_{19}-diterpenoid alkaloids, 3,15-diacetyljesaconitine (**7**) [26] and 3-acetylmesaconitine (**11**) [29] prepared from secojesaconitine (**6**) and mesaconitine (**8**), respectively (Figure 2), were also tested.

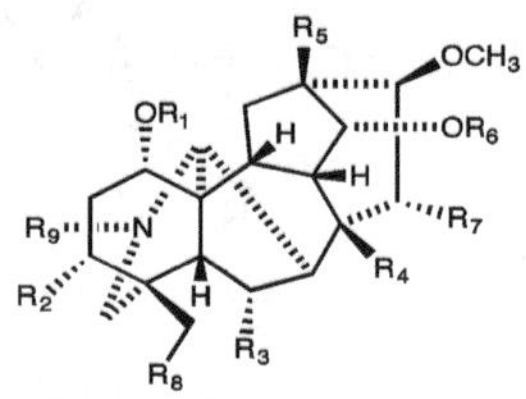

		R_1	R_2	R_3	R_4	R_5	R_6	R_7	R_8	R_9
1 *	aconitine	CH_3	OH	OCH_3	$OCOCH_3$	OH	Bz	OH	OCH_3	CH_2CH_3
2 *	deoxyaconitine	CH_3	H	OCH_3	$OCOCH_3$	OH	Bz	OH	OCH_3	CH_2CH_3
3 *	jesaconitine	CH_3	OH	OCH_3	$OCOCH_3$	OH	As	OH	OCH_3	CH_2CH_3
4 *	deoxyjesaconitine	CH_3	H	OCH_3	$OCOCH_3$	OH	As	OH	OCH_3	CH_2CH_3
5 *	aljesaconitine A	CH_3	OH	OCH_3	OCH_2CH_3	OH	As	OH	OCH_3	CH_2CH_3
6 *	see structure below									
7	3,15-diacetyljesaconitine	CH_3	$OCOCH_3$	OCH_3	$OCOCH_3$	OH	As	$OCOCH_3$	OCH_3	CH_2CH_3
8 *	mesaconitine	CH_3	OH	OCH_3	$OCOCH_3$	OH	Bz	OH	OCH_3	CH_3
9 *	hypaconitine	CH_3	H	OCH_3	$OCOCH_3$	OH	Bz	OH	OCH_3	CH_3
10 *	hokbusine A	CH_3	OH	OCH_3	OCH_3	OH	Bz	OH	OCH_3	CH_3
11	3-acetylmesaconitine	CH_3	$OCOCH_3$	OCH_3	$OCOCH_3$	OH	Bz	OH	OCH_3	CH_3
12 *	14-anisoyllasianine	CH_3	OH	OCH_3	NH_2	OH	As	OH	OCH_3	CH_2CH_3
13 *	*N*-deethylaljesaconitine A	CH_3	OH	OCH_3	OCH_2CH_3	OH	As	OH	OCH_3	H
14 *	aconine	CH_3	OH	OCH_3	OH	OH	H	OH	OCH_3	CH_2CH_3
15 *	lipomesaconitine	CH_3	OH	OCH_3	Olipo	OH	Bz	OH	OCH_3	CH_3
16 *	lipoaconitine	CH_3	OH	OCH_3	Olipo	OH	Bz	OH	OCH_3	CH_2CH_3
17 *	lipojesaconitine	CH_3	OH	OCH_3	Olipo	OH	As	OH	OCH_3	CH_2CH_3
18 *	neolinine	H	H	OCH_3	OH	H	H	H	OH	CH_2CH_3
19 *	neoline	H	H	OCH_3	OH	H	H	H	OCH_3	CH_2CH_3
20 *	14-benzoylneoline	H	H	OCH_3	OH	H	Bz	H	OCH_3	CH_2CH_3
21 *	isotalatizidine	H	H	H	OH	H	H	H	OCH_3	CH_2CH_3
22 *	karacoline	H	H	H	OH	H	H	H	H	CH_2CH_3
23 *	3-hydroxykaracoline	H	OH	H	OH	H	H	H	H	CH_2CH_3

Bz = COC_6H_5
As = $COC_6H_4OCH_3$ (*p*)
lipo = linoleoyl, palmitoyl, oleoyl, stearoyl, linolenoyl

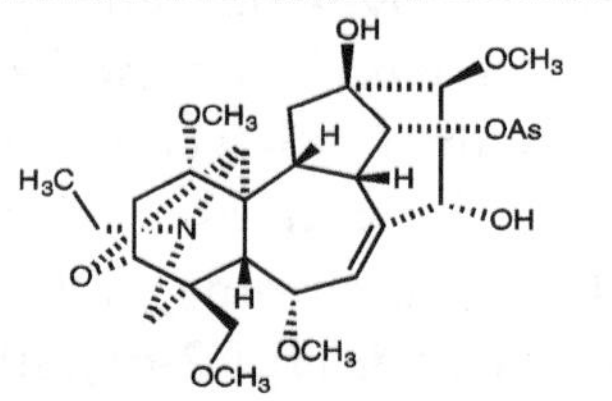

6 *	secojesaconitine

*: Natural alkaloid

Figure 2. Chemical structures of aconitine-type C_{19}-diterpenoid alkaloids **1–23**.

Eighteen of the 23 tested aconitine-type C_{19}-diterpenoid alkaloids, both natural alkaloids (**1~6, 8~10, 12~14, 18~23**) and synthetic analogs (**7** and **11**), were inactive (IC_{50} > 20 or 40 μM) [27,28,30] (Table 1). Three natural diterpenoid alkaloids (**15~17**) exhibited cytotoxic activity against five human tumor cell lines (A549, MDA-MB-231, MCF-7, KB, and MDR KB subline KB-VIN) (Table 1). Lipojesaconitine (**17**) showed significant cytotoxicity against four tested cell lines with IC_{50} values of 6.0 to 7.3 μM, but weak cytotoxicity against KB-VIN (IC_{50} = 18.6 μM) [28]. Lipomesaconitine (**15**) showed moderate cytotoxicity against the KB cell line (IC_{50} = 9.9 μM), but weak cytotoxicity against the other four human tumor cell lines (IC_{50} =17.2 ~ 21.5 μM) [27]. Lipoaconitine (**16**) was weakly cytotoxic (IC_{50} = 13.7 ~ 20.3 μM) against all five human tumor cell lines [28]. Based on the results, the fatty acid ester at C-8 and the anisoyl group at C-14 found in **17** may be important to the cytotoxic activity of aconitine-type C_{19}-diterpenoid alkaloids.

Table 1. Cytotoxic activity data for aconitine-type C_{19}-diterpenoid alkaloids and derivatives **1–23**.

	Cell Line/IC_{50} (μM) [1]					
Alkaloids	**A549**	**DU145**	**MDA-MB-231**	**MCF-7**	**KB**	**KB-VIN**
Aconitine (**1**)	>20	>20	-	-	>20	>20
Deoxyaconitine (**2**)	>20	>20	-	-	>20	>20
Jesaconitine (**3**)	>20	>20	-	-	>20	>20
Deoxyjesaconitine (**4**)	>20	>20	-	-	>20	>20
Aljesaconitine A (**5**)	>20	>20	-	-	>20	>20
Secojesaconitine (**6**)	>20	>20	-	-	>20	>20
7	>20	>20	-	-	>20	>20
Mesaconitine (**8**)	>20	>20	-	-	>20	>20
Hypaconitine (**9**)	>20	>20	-	-	>20	>20
Hokbusine A (**10**)	>20	>20	-	-	>20	>20
11	>20	>20	-	-	>20	>20
14-Anisoyllasianine (**12**)	>40	-	>40	>40	>40	>40
N-Deethylaljesaconitine A (**13**)	>40	-	>40	>40	>40	>40
Aconine (**14**)	>40	-	>40	>40	>40	>40
Lipomesaconitine (**15**)	17.2 ± 2.3	-	20.0 ± 0.2	19.0 ± 1.0	10.0 ± 3.3	21.5 ± 0.9
Lipoaconitine (**16**)	17.4 ± 1.1	-	15.5 ± 0.5	16.0 ± 0.3	13.7 ± 1.3	20.3 ± 1.1
Lipojesaconitine (**17**)	7.3 ± 0.3	-	6.0 ± 0.2	6.7 ± 0.2	6.0 ± 0.2	18.6 ± 0.9
Neolinine (**18**)	>40	-	>40	>40	>40	>40
Neoline (**19**)	>20	>20	-	-	>20	>20
14-benzoylneoline (**20**)	>20	>20	-	-	>20	>20
Isotalatizidine (**21**)	>40	-	>40	>40	>40	>40
Karacoline (**22**)	>20	>20	-	-	>20	>20
3-Hydroxykaracoline (**23**)	>40	-	>40	>40	>40	>40
PXL[2] (nM)	4.8 ± 0.6	5.9 ± 1.9	8.4 ± 0.8	10.2 ± 0.9	5.8 ± 0.2	2405.4 ± 44.8

[1] Values are means ± standard deviation; [2] Paclitaxel (PXL; nM) was used as an experimental control.

2.2. Lycoctonine-Type (7,8-diol) C_{19}-Diterpenoid Alkaloids

The tested lycoctonine-type (7,8-diol) C_{19}-diterpenoid alkaloid group included 12 natural alkaloids, namely nevadensine (**24**), *N*-deethylnevadensine (**25**), and virescenine (**27**), purified from rhizoma of *Aconitum japonicum* subsp. *subcuneatum* [27], and 18-methoxygadesine (**26**), delphinifoline (**28**), delcosine (**34**), 14-acetyldelcosine (**34–43**), and 14-acetylbrowniine (**35**), purified from root of *Aconitum yesoense* var. *macroyesoense* (NAKAI) TAMURA [31–34], and andersonidine (**30**), pacifiline (**31**), pacifinine (**32**), and pacifidine (**33**), purified from seeds of *Delphinium elatum* cv. Pacific Giant [35] (Figure 3). The remaining tested C_{19}-diterpenoid alkaloids from this subtype were synthetic alkaloids, *N*-deethyldelsoline (**29**) [18], 1-acetyldelcosine (**34-1**) [36], 1,14-diacetyldelcosine (**34-2**) [37], 1-(4-trifluoromethylbenzoyl)delcosine (**34-24**) [30], delsoline (**34-42**) [37], 1,14-di-(4-nitrobenzoyl)-delcosine (**34-45**) [30], 14-acetyl-1-(4-nitrobenzoyl)delcosine (**34-46**) [30], and 1-acyl or 1,14-diacyldelcosine derivatives (**34-3~34-23**, **34-25~34-41**, **34-44**, and **34-47**) [38], prepared from delcosine (**34**) or delsoline (**34-42**) (Figure 3). These 42 C_{19}-diterpenoid alkaloids were evaluated for antiproliferative activity against four to five human tumor cell lines (A549, DU145, MDA-MB-231, MCF-7, KB, and KB-VIN) [30,38] (Table 2). Several tested lycoctonine-type (7,8-diol) C_{19}-diterpenoid alkaloids, both natural alkaloids (**24~28**, **30~33**) and a synthetic alkaloid (**29**), were inactive (IC_{50} > 20 or 40 μM). All tested delcosine derivatives that contain an acetyl or methoxy group, both natural alkaloids (**34**, **34-43**, **35**) and synthetic analogs (**34-1**, **34-2**, **34-42**), were inactive (IC_{50} > 20 μM). However, acylation, except with an acetyl group, of the C-1 and/or C-14 hydroxy group of **34** led to various degrees of antiproliferative activity. Among the C-1 esterified alkaloids, the synthetic derivatives **34-6**, **34-8**, **34-10**, and **34-18** exhibited significant potency against all cell lines (average IC_{50} 9.3, 5.3, 5.0, and 6.9 μM, respectively). Also, alkaloids **34-3**, **34-16**, **34-17**, **34-21**, **34-25**, **34-27**, **34-31**, **34-32**, **34-38**, and **34-40** showed moderate potency toward all cell lines (average IC_{50} 12.7–20.7 μM). While alkaloid **34-32** displayed good antiproliferative activity (IC_{50} 8.7 μM) against KB cells, it was much less potent against A549, MDA-MB-231, and KB-VIN cells. Alkaloids **34-5**, **34-13**, **34-15**, **34-29**, **34-35**, **34-37**, and **34-41** exhibited only weak potency against all cell lines (average IC_{50} 22.0–26.5 μM). Finally, alkaloids **34-24**, **34-30**, and **34-34** were inactive against all five human tumor cell lines, while **34-12**, **34-33**, and **34-39** showed limited potency.

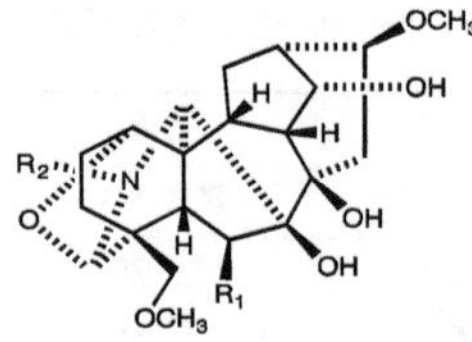

		R1	R2
24 *	nevadensine	H	CH_2CH_3
25 *	*N*-deethylnevadensine	H	H
26 *	18-methoxygadesine	OCH_3	CH_2CH_3

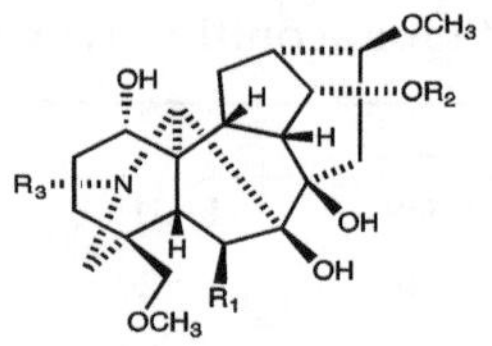

		R1	R2	R3
27 *	virescenine	H	H	CH_2CH_3
28 *	delphinifoline	OH	H	CH_2CH_3
29	*N*-deethyldelsoline	OCH_3	CH_3	H

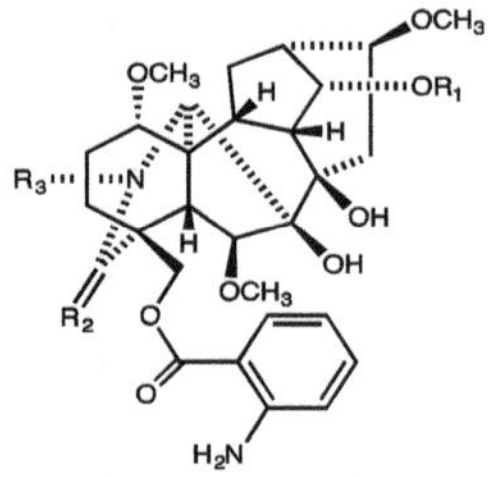

		R1	R2	R3
30 *	andersonidine	$COCH_3$	H_2	CH_2CH_3
31 *	pacifiline	CH_3	O	CH_2CH_3
32 *	pacifinine	CH_3	O	H

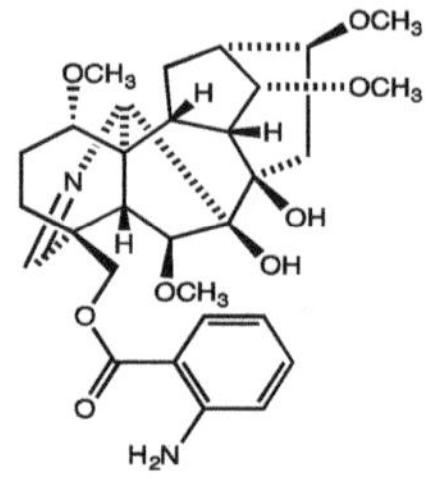

33 *	pacifidine

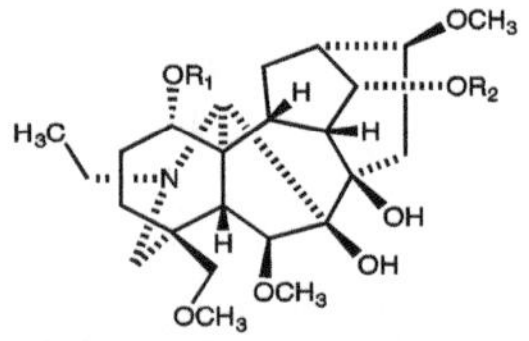

		R1	R2
34 *	delcosine	H	H
34-1	1-acetyldelcosine	$COCH_3$	H
34-2	1,14-diacetyldelcosine	$COCH_3$	$COCH_3$
34-3	1-(4-bromobenzoyl)-delcosine	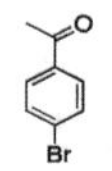	H
34-4	1,14-di-(4-bromobenzoyl)-delcosine	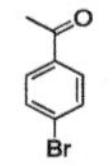	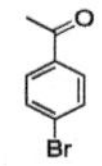
34-5	1-(4-chlorobenzoyl)-delcosine	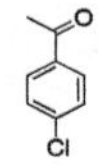	H
34-6	1-(3,5-dichlorobenzoyl)-delcosine	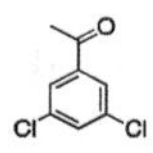	H
34-7	1,14-di-(3,5-dichlorobenzo-yl)delcosine	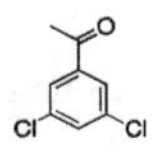	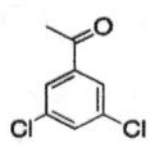
34-8	1-(4-chloro-3-nitro-benzoyl)delcosine	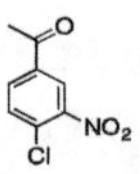	H
34-9	1,14-di-(4-chloro-3-nitro-benzoyl)delcosine	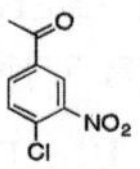	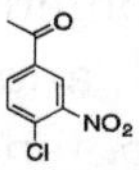
34-10	1-(4-dichloromethyl-benzoyl)delcosine	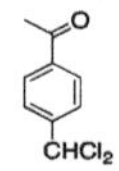	H
34-11	1,14-di-(4-dichloromethyl-benzoyl)delcosine	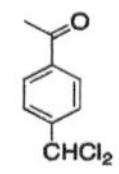	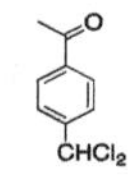
34-12	1-(4-dimethylamino-benzoyl)delcosine	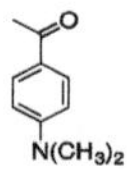	H
34-13	1-(3-chloro-4-fluorobenzoyl)-delcosine	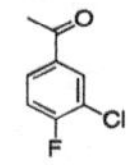	H
34-14	1,14-di-(3-chloro-4-fluoro-benzoyl)delcosine	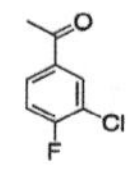	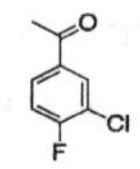
34-15	1-(4-fluoro-3-methyl-benzoyl)delcosine	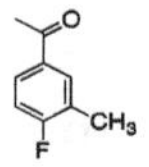	H
34-16	1-(4-fluoro-3-trifluoro-methylbenzoyl)delcosin e	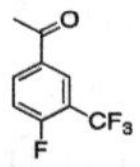	H
34-17	1-(4-methoxy-3-trifluoro-methylbenzoyl)delcosin e	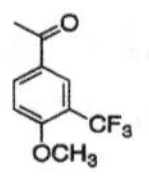	H
34-18	1-(2,3,4,5,6-pentafluoro-benzoyl)delcosine	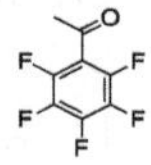	H
34-19	1,14-di-(2,3,4,5,6-penta-fluorobenzoyl)delcosin e	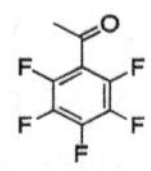	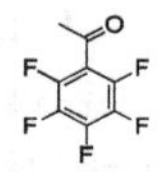
34-20	14-acetyl-1-(2,3,4,5,6-pentafluorobenzoyl) delcosine	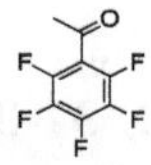	$COCH_3$
34-21	1-(2,4,5-trifluoro-3-methoxybenzoyl)-delcosine	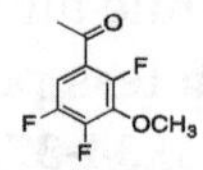	H

Figure 3. *Cont.*

		R_1	R_2			R_1	R_2
34-22	1,14-di-(2,4,5-trifluoro-3-methoxybenzoyl)delcosine	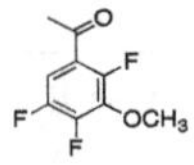	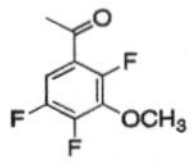	34-36	1,14-di-(2,2-difluoro-1,3-benzodioxole-4-carbonyl)delcosine	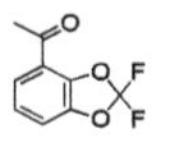	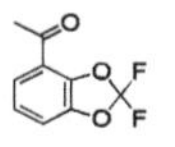
34-23	14-acetyl-1-(2,4,5-tri-fluoro-3-methoxybenzoyl)-delcosine	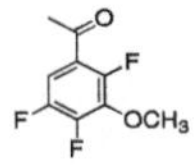	$COCH_3$	34-37	1-(phenylacethyl)-delcosine	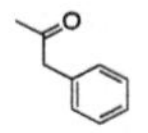	H
34-24	1-(4-trifluoromethyl-benzoyl)delcosine	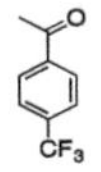	H	34-38	1-(3-trifluoromethyl-cinnamoyl)delcosine	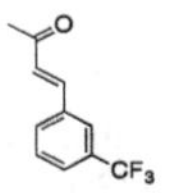	H
34-25	1-(3,5-bis-trifluoromethylbenzoyl)delcosine	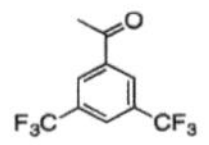	H	34-39	1-(4-nitrocinnamoyl)-delcosine	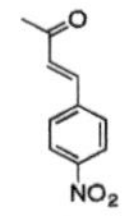	H
34-26	1,14-di-(3,5-bis-trifluoro-methylbenzoyl)delcosine	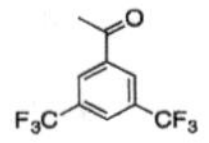	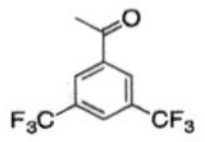	34-40	1-(naphthoyl) delcosine	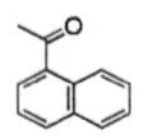	H
34-27	1-(4-trifluoromethyl-thiobenzoyl)delcosine	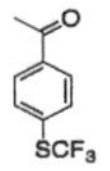	H	34-41	1-(anthraquinone-2-carbonyl)delcosine	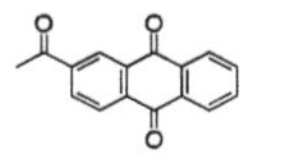	H
34-28	1,14-di-(4-trifluoro-methylthiobenzoyl)-delcosine	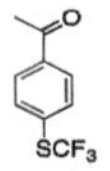	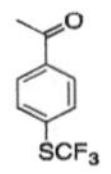	34-42	delsoline	H	CH_3
34-29	1-(3,5-dimethoxy-benzoyl)delcosine	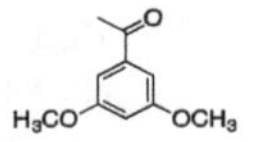	H		14-acetyldelcosine	H	$COCH_3$
34-30	1-(3,4,5-trimethoxy-benzoyl)delcosine	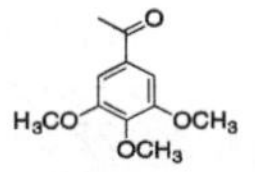	H	34-44	14-benzyldelcosine	H	$CH_2C_6H_5$
34-31	1-(3,5-diethoxybenzoyl)-delcosine	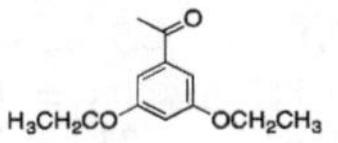	H	34-45	1,14-di-(4-nitro-benzoyl)delcosine	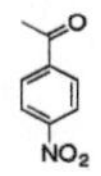	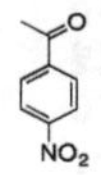
34-32	1-(4-benzyloxybenzoyl)-delcosine	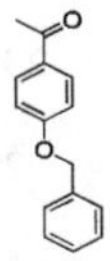	H	34-46	14-acetyl-1-(4-nitro-benzoyl)delcosine	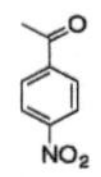	$COCH_3$
34-33	1-(4-cyanobenzoyl)-delcosine	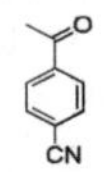	H	34-47	1,14-di-(4-ethoxy-benzoyl)delcosine	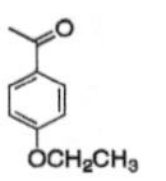	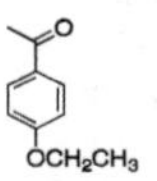
34-34	1-piperonyloyldelcosine	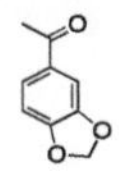	H	35*	14-acetylbrowniine	CH_3	$COCH_3$
34-35	1-(2,2-difluoro-1,3-benzo-dioxole-4-carbonyl)-delcosine	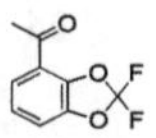	H				

*: Natural alkaloid.

Figure 3. Chemical structures of lycoctonine-type (7,8-diol) C_{19}-diterpenoid alkaloids **24–35.**

Among the derivatives esterified at both C-1 and -14, alkaloids **34-19** and **34-20** exhibited significant potency against all five tested cell lines (average IC_{50} 4.9 and 5.0 μM, respectively). Alkaloid **34-9** (average IC_{50} 11.9 μM) showed significant antiproliferative activity against MDA-MB- 231 and KB cells (IC_{50} 4.7 and 5.8 μM, respectively) comparable with **34-19** and **34-20**, but was less potent against MCF-7 and A549 (IC_{50} 12.2 and 24.8 μM, respectively) and inactive against KB-VIN. Alkaloid **34-23** exhibited only weak potency toward all cell lines (average IC_{50} 23.7 μM). Alkaloids **34-4, 34-7, 34-11, 34-14, 34-26, 34-36, 34-45, 34-46,** and **34-47** were inactive against all five human tumor cell lines, while **34-22** and **34-28** showed limited potency.

Table 2. Cytotoxic activity data for lycoctonine-type (7,8-diol) C_{19}-diterpenoid alkaloids and synthetic analogs of delcosine **24~35**.

	Cell Line/IC_{50} (μM) [1]					
Alkaloids	**A549**	**DU145**	**MDA-MB-231**	**MCF-7**	**KB**	**KB-VIN**
Nevadensine (**24**)	>40	-	>40	>40	>40	>40
N-Deethylnevadensine (**25**)	>40	-	>40	>40	>40	>40
18-Methoxygadesine (**26**)	>20	>20	-	-	>20	>20
Virescenine (**27**)	>40	-	>40	>40	>40	>40
Delphinifoline (**28**)	>20	>20	-	-	>20	>20
N-Deethyldelsoline (**29**)	>20	>20	-	-	>20	>20
Andersonidine (**30**)	>20	>20	-	-	>20	>20
Pacifiline (**31**)	>20	>20	-	-	>20	>20
Pacifinine (**32**)	>20	>20	-	-	>20	>20
Pacifidine (**33**)	>20	>20	-	-	>20	>20
Delcosine (**34**)	>20	>20	-	-	>20	>20
34-1	>20	>20	-	-	>20	>20
34-2	>20	>20	-	-	>20	>20
34-3	20.6 ± 0.3	-	19.4± 1.0	17.9 ± 0.3	14.6 ± 0.6	17.1 ± 0.8
34-4	>40	-	>40	>40	>40	>40
34-5	18.7 ± 0.1	-	29.1 ± 1.6	25.8 ± 1.4	19.6 ± 0.3	21.1 ± 1.5
34-6	7.7 ± 0.9	-	8.6 ± 6.0	15.8 ± 4.2	5.6 ± 1.2	8.6 ± 1.9
34-7	>40	-	>40	>40	>40	>40
34-8	4.5 ± 0.5	-	5.0 ± 0.1	5.9 ± 0.3	5.4 ± 0.3	5.6 ± 0.4
34-9	24.8 ± 0.1	-	4.7 ± 0.1	12.2 ± 0.3	5.8 ± 0.4	>40
34-10	4.8 ± 0.3	-	4.8 ± 0.7	5.7 ± 0.4	4.3 ± 0.5	5.3 ± 0.4
34-11	>40	-	>40	>40	>40	>40
34-12	26.5 ± 0.3	-	>40	40.6 ± 2.5	27.8 ± 1.7	28.1 ± 3.0
34-13	20.8 ± 1.7	-	32.4 ± 1.8	25.9 ± 2.4	23.0 ± 2.4	21.5 ± 1.3
34-14	>40	-	>40	>40	>40	>40
34-15	21.7 ± 1.6	-	30.2 ± 2.7	26.9 ± 1.4	20.7 ± 1.2	21.5 ± 3.6
34-16	14.4 ± 2.1	-	20.1 ± 0.7	16.4 ± 2.1	13.6 ± 1.1	15.7 ± 0.8
34-17	11.4 ± 1.4	-	10.4 ± 1.7	22.5 ± 1.5	10. 8 ± 1.9	11.8 ± 3.2
34-18	4.7 ± 0.1	-	5.3 ± 0.2	9.2 ± 0.4	5.8 ± 0.6	9.5 ± 0.5
34-19	4.9 ± 0.1	-	4.9 ± 0.1	5.3 ± 0.3	4.7 ± 0.1	4.9 ± 0.1
34-20	4.8 ± 0.1	-	4.6 ± 0.3	6.0 ± 0.1	4.8 ± 0.4	4.9 ± 0.4
34-21	20.8 ± 2.1	-	21.5 ± 0.6	21.4± 0.3	18.6 ± 1.7	15.0 ± 0.1
34-22	>40	-	>40	>40	>40	39.1 ± 2.0
34-23	23.8 ± 2.0	-	25.2 ± 1.0	23.3 ± 1.1	23.7 ± 1.1	22. 6 ± 0.3
34-24	>20	>20	-	-	>20	>20
34-25	20.6 ± 1.2	-	21.3 ± 1.3	22.4 ± 1.2	20. 8 ± 2.1	18.0 ± 1.0
34-26	>40	-	>40	>40	>40	>40
34-27	18.6 ± 2.6	-	19.7 ± 2.0	20.6 ± 1.2	22.2± 1.8	19.8 ± 1.9
34-28	33.0 ± 2.1	-	32.4 ± 1.7	31.1 ± 0.8	23.2 ± 1.1	40.0 ± 1.0
34-29	23.8 ± 2.6	-	33.4 ± 1.7	29.8 ± 1.2	22.8 ± 1.7	22.6 ± 2.4
34-30	>40	-	>40	>40	>40	>40
34-31	17. 3 ± 2.2	-	23. 1 ± 0.5	20.0 ± 0.7	16.2 ± 1.8	17.4 ± 1.9
34-32	16.5 ± 1.3	-	22.5 ± 0.8	-	8.71 ± 0.7	15.8 ± 0.8
34-33	40.9 ± 5.3	-	>40	>40	36.3 ± 1.0	29.3 ± 0.6
34-34	>40	-	>40	>40	>40	>40
34-35	21.2 ± 0.1	-	24.8 ± 1.6	24.6 ± 1.0	18.7 ± 1.2	21.7± 0.6
34-36	>40	-	>40	>40	>40	>40
34-37	23.8 ± 0.5	-	32.9 ± 1.0	22.6 ± 1.5	21.2 ± 0.1	19.2 ± 0.1
34-38	11.2 ± 0.7	>20	-	-	21.1 ± 3.9	19.5 ± 8.2
34-39	29.7 ± 0.7	-	43.2 ± 1.8	32.0 ± 0.6	36.0 ± 0.4	45.1 ± 3.4
34-40	18.5 ± 0.5	-	17.9 ± 0.5	15.5± 0.6	13.7± 0.1	14.2 ± 0.5
34-41	22.9± 0.5	-	20.7 ± 2.1	20.5 ± 1.0	21.6 ± 0.1	24.4 ± 0.5
34-42	>20	>20	-	-	>20	>20
14-Acetyldelcosine (**34-43**)	>20	>20	-	-	>20	>20
34-44	>20	>20	-	-	>20	>20
34-45	>20	>20	-	-	>20	>20
34-46	>20	>20	-	-	>20	>20
34-47	>20	>20	-	>20	>20	>20
14-Acetylbrowniine (**35**)	>20	>20	-	-	>20	>20
PXL[2] (nM)	4.8 ± 0.6	5.9 ± 1.9	8.4 ± 0.8	10.2 ± 0.9	5.8 ± 0.2	2405.4 ± 44.8

[1] Values are means ± standard deviation; [2] Paclitaxel (PXL; nM) was used as an experimental control.

Particularly, C-1 monoacylated delcosine derivatives (**34-3**, **34-6**, **34-8**, **34-10**, **34-13**, **34-21**, **34-25**, **34-27**, and **34-35**) were significantly more potent compared with corresponding C-1,14 diacylated delcosine derivatives (**34-4**, **34-7**, **34-9**, **34-11**, **34-14**, **34-22**, **34-23**, **34-26**, **34-28** and **34-36**). Thus, a C-1 acyloxy group and C-14 hydroxy group are crucial for enhanced antiproliferative activity of **1**-derivatives. Regarding alkaloids **34-18** (pentafluorobenzoate at C-1, hydroxy at C-14), **34-19** (pentafluorobenzoate at C-1 and C-14), and **34-20** (pentafluorobenzoate at C-1, acetate at C-14), all three alkaloids were essentially equipotent against three of the five tumor cell lines, while **34-18** was somewhat less potent than the diacylated alkaloids against MCF-7 and KB-VIN cells.

Striking observations from the data in Table 2 were the consistent identities of the most potent alkaloids. Alkaloids **34-8**, **34-10**, **34-19**, and **34-20** exhibited the highest potency against all five tested tumor cell lines with IC_{50} values ranging from 4.3 to 6.0 μM. The same range of potency was found with alkaloid **34-18** against A549 cells, with alkaloids **34-9** and **34-18** against MDA-MB-231 cells, and with **34-6**, **34-9**, and **34-18** against KB cells. The potencies of **34-6** and **34-17** (IC_{50} 5.6−11.8 μM) generally ranked somewhat below those of the most potent alkaloids, except against the MCF-7 cell line, where they were even less active.

The identity of the substituent(s) on the acyl group affected the antiproliferative potency. Notably, among the 1,14-diacyl and 1-acyl-14-acetyl derivatives, only alkaloids **34-19** and **34-20** with one or two pentafluorinated benzoyl esters, respectively, showed significant potency against all five tested cell lines. Alkaloid **34-9** with two 3-nitro-4-chlorobenzoyl groups showed good potency against certain cell lines. Similarly, the 1-monoacylated alkaloids with the highest potency against the five tumor cell lines contained 3-nitro-4-chloro- (**34-8**) and pentafluoro- (**34-18**) as well as 4-dichloro-methyl- (**34-10**) benzoyl esters. The chlorinated alkaloids **34-8** and **34-10** as well as **34-6**, which has 3,5-dichloro substitution on the benzoate ester, were more potent than **34-5** with only a single chloro group or **34-13** with chloro and fluoro groups. Similarly, alkaloid **34-18** showed increased antiproliferative activity against the five tumor cell lines compared with other fluorinated alkaloids **34-13**~**34-17**, **34-21**~**34-27**. Moreover, with some exceptions against certain cell lines, alkaloids with bromo (**34-3** and **34-4**), dimethylamino (**34-12**), dimethoxy (**34-29**), trimethoxy (**34-30**), diethoxy (**34-31**), benzyloxy (**34-32**), cyano (**34-33**), methylenedioxy (**34-34** and **34-35**), nitro (**34-45** and **34-46**), and ethoxy (**34-47**) substituted benzoate esters or phenylacetyl (**34-37**), cinnamoyl (**34-38** and **34-39**), 1-naphthoyl (**34-40**), and anthraquinone-2-carbonyl (**34-41**) esters were less potent or inactive.

Interestingly, the active alkaloids were generally effective against P-gp overexpressing MDR subline KB-VIN, while alkaloids such as vincristine and paclitaxel are ineffective due to excretion from the MDR cells by P-gp. These results suggest that these diterpenoids are not substrates for P-gp.

2.3. *Lycoctonine-Type (7,8-methylenedioxy) C_{19}-Diterpenoid Alkaloids*

The tested lycoctonine-type (7,8-methylenedioxy) C_{19}-diterpenoid alkaloids included 19 natural alkaloids, delcorine (**36**), delpheline (**37**), pacinine (**38**), yunnadelphinine (**39**), melpheline (**40**), bonvalotidine C (**41**), *N*-deethyl-*N*-formylpaciline (**42**), *N*-deethyl-*N*-formylpacinine (**43**), isodel-pheline (**44**), pacidine (**45**), eladine (**46**), *N*-formyl-4,19-secopacinine (**47**), *N*-formyl-4,19-secoyunna-delphinine (**48**), iminoisodelpheline (**49**), iminodelpheline (**50**), laxicyminine (**51**), *N*-deethyl-19-oxo-isodelpheline (**52**), *N*-deethyl-19-oxodelpheline (**53**), and 19-oxoisodelpheline (**54**), purified from seeds of *Delphinium elatum* cv. Pacific Giant [35,39–42] (Figure 4). The remaining 22 tested C_{19}-diterpenoids were synthetic derivatives (**37-1**~**37-22**) [43] prepared from **37** (Figure 4).

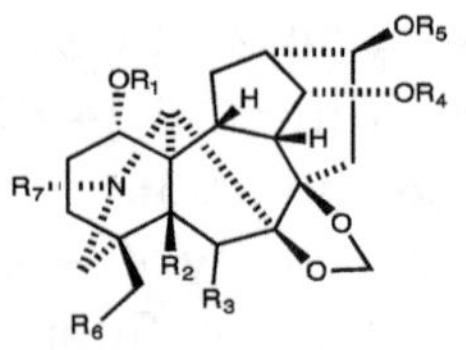

		R1	R2	R3	R4	R5	R6	R7
36 *	delcorine	CH_3	H	β-OH	CH_3	CH_3	OCH_3	CH_2CH_3
37 *	delpheline	CH_3	H	β-OH	CH_3	CH_3	H	CH_2CH_3
38 *	pacinine	CH_3	H	=O	CH_3	CH_3	H	CH_2CH_3
39 *	yunnadelphinine	CH_3	H	=O	H	CH_3	H	CH_2CH_3
40 *	melpheline	CH_3	H	β-OH	CH_3	CH_3	H	CH_3
41 *	bonvalotidine C	CH_3	OH	=O	CH_3	CH_3	H	CH_2CH_3
42 *	*N*-deethyl-*N*-formylpaciline	CH_3	H	β-OCH_3	CH_3	CH_3	H	CHO
43*	*N*-deethyl-*N*-formylpacinine	CH_3	H	=O	CH_3	CH_3	H	CHO
44 *	isodelpheline	CH_3	H	β-OCH_3	H	CH_3	H	CH_2CH_3
45 *	pacidine	H	H	β-OH	CH_3	CH_3	H	CH_2CH_3
46 *	eladine	CH_3	H	β-OH	CH_3	H	H	CH_2CH_3

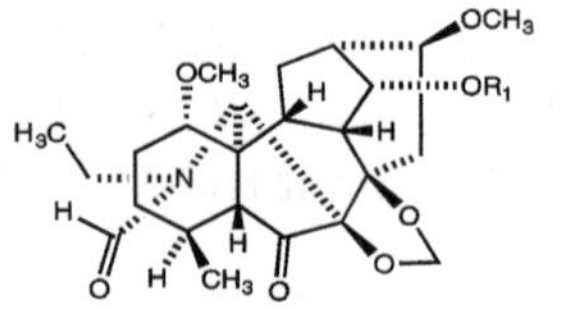

		R1
47 *	*N*-formyl-4,19-secopacinine	CH_3
48 *	*N*-formyl-4,19-secoyunna- delphinine	H

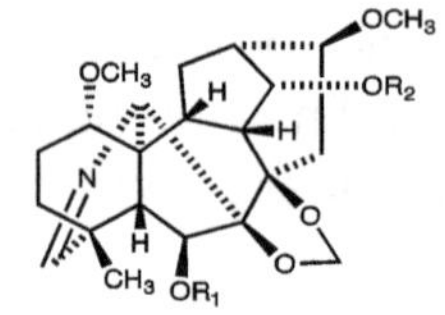

		R1	R2
49 *	iminoisodelpheline	CH_3	H
50 *	iminodelpheline	H	CH_3

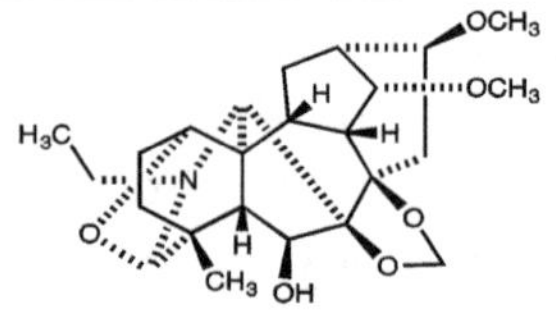

51 *	laxicyminine

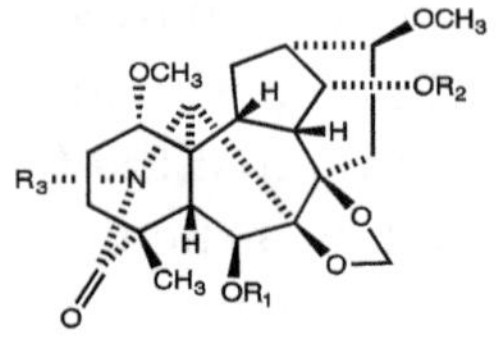

		R1	R2	R3
52*	*N*-deethyl-19-oxoisodelpheline	CH_3	H	H
53*	*N*-deethyl-19-oxodelpheline	H	CH_3	H
54*	19-oxoisodelpheline	CH_3	H	CH_2CH_3
37-22	19-oxodelpheline	H	CH_3	CH_2CH_3

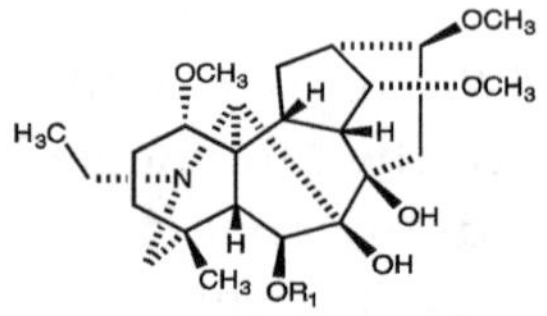

		R1
37-20	7,8-demethylenedelpheline	H
37-21	7,8-demethylene-6-(3-trifluoromethylbenzoyl)delpheline	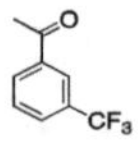

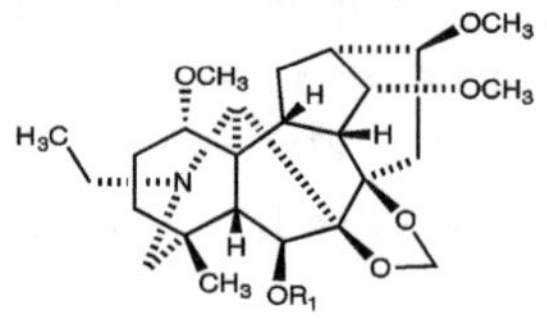

		R1			R1
37-1	6-(4-chlorobenzoyl)delpheline	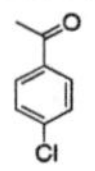	**37-6**	6-(4-trifluoromethoxybenzoyl)-delpheline	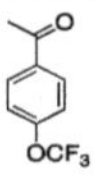
37-2	6-(4-fluorobenzoyl)delpheline	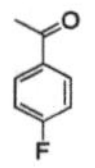	**37-7**	6-(4-trifluoromethylthiobenzoyl)-delpheline	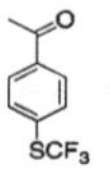
37-3	6-(4-nitrobenzoyl)delpheline	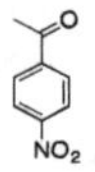	**37-8**	6-(methyl terephthaloyl)delpheline	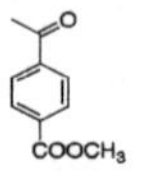
37-4	6-(4-anisoyl)delpheline	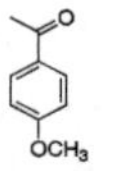	**37-9**	6-(3-trifluoromethylbenzoyl)-delpheline	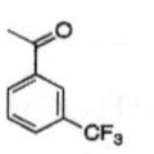
37-5	6-(4-phenylbenzoyl)delpheline	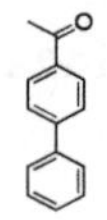	**37-10**	6-(3,5-dinitrobenzoyl)delpheline	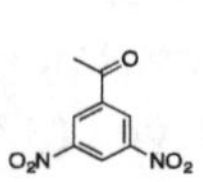

Figure 4. *Cont.*

37-11	6-(3,4,5-trimethoxybenzoyl)-delpheline	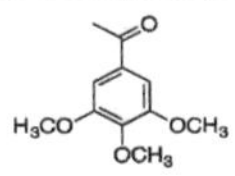	**37-16**	6-(4-ethoxybenzoyl)delpheline	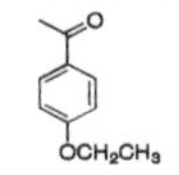
37-12	6-(3,4,5-trifluorobenzoyl)delpheline	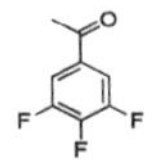	**37-17**	6-(4-benzyloxybenzoyl)delpheline	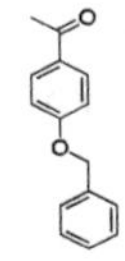
37-13	6-(3-trifluoromethylcinnamoyl)-delpheline	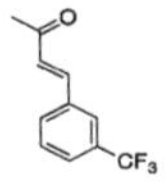	**37-18**	6-(3-fluoro-4-trifluoromethyl-benzoyl)delpheline	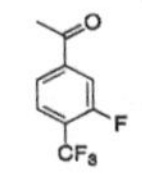
37-14	6-(4-fluorocinnamoyl)delpheline	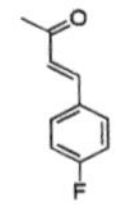	**37-19**	6-(4-fluoro-3-methylbenzoyl)-delpheline	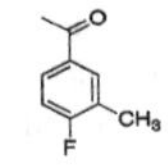
37-15	6-(6-trifluoromethylnicotinoyl)-delpheline	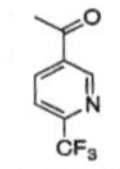			

*: Natural alkaloid

Figure 4. Chemical structures of lycoctonine-type (7,8-methylenedioxy) C_{19}-diterpenoid alkaloids **36-54**.

All tested lycoctonine-type (7,8-methylenedioxy) C_{19}-diterpenoid alkaloids were evaluated for antiproliferative activity against human tumor cell lines [30,40–43] (Table 3). The lycoctonine-type (7,8-methylenedioxy) C_{19}-diterpenoid alkaloids, both the natural alkaloids (**36~54**) and synthetic analogs that did not contain a C-6 ester group (**37-20** and **37-22**), were inactive (IC_{50} > 20 or 40 μM). Among the C-6 esterified alkaloids, **37-1**, **37-17**, and **37-18** exhibited the highest average potency toward four tested cell lines (A549, DU145, KB and KB-VIN; average IC_{50} 9.83, 9.57, and 9.41 μM, respectively). Alkaloids **37-3**, **37-5~37-7**, **37-9**, **37-10**, **37-12**, **37-13**, **37-16**, and **37-19** showed moderate potency against all tested cell lines (average IC_{50} 13.9–20.8 μM). However, alkaloid **37-13** showed significantly increased cytotoxic activity (IC_{50} 10.2 μM) against A549 cells compared with **37-1**, **37-17**, and **37-18**, but was generally less potent against DU145 and KB cells. While alkaloids **37-12**, **37-13**, **37-16**, and **37-19** displayed good antiproliferative activity (IC_{50} 6.8, 9.1, 6.5, and 4.7 μM, respectively) against KB-VIN cells, they were much less potent against A549, DU145, and KB cells. Alkaloids **37-4** and **37-21** were inactive against all tested cancer cell lines, while **37-2**, **37-8**, **37-11**, and **37-14** exhibited only weak potency toward all cell lines (average IC_{50} 23.0–29.2 μM).

The most noticeable observations from the data in Table 3 were the degree and relative ratio of KB/KB-VIN potency. Among the four cancer cell lines tested, the highest potency was found against the KB-VIN cell line by alkaloids **37-17~37-19** (IC_{50} 4.22, 4.40, and 4.71 μM, respectively), followed by alkaloids **37-16**, **37-12**, **37-1**, **37-13**, and **37-9** (IC_{50} 6.50, 6.80, 8.27, 9.10, and 11.9 μM, respectively). Generally, all active alkaloids showed the highest potency against the KB-VIN cell line compared with the other three tested cancer cell lines. Moreover, alkaloids **37-12**, **37-16**, **37-13**, and **37-19** showed over two-fold selectivity between the two cell lines (ratio of IC_{50} KB/IC_{50} KB-VIN: 2.15, 2.28, 2.31, and 2.57, respectively). Alkaloids **37-2**, **37-5**, and **37-17** displayed weak selectivity between the KB and KB-VIN cell lines (ratio of IC_{50} KB/IC_{50} KB-VIN: 1.55, 1.36, and 1.62, respectively). Finally, alkaloids **37-1**, **37-3**, **37-6~37-9**, **37-11**, **37-14**, **37-15**, and **37-18** displayed similar potency against the KB and KB-VIN cell lines (ratio of IC_{50} KB/IC_{50} KB-VIN: 1.07, 1.17, 1.06, 1.21, 1.04, 1.25, 1.07, 1.07, 1.17, and 1.23, respectively).

The identity of the substituent on the C-6 acyl group affected the cytotoxic potency. For instance, the alkaloids with the highest potency against the KB-VIN cell line contained chloro (**37-1**), fluoro (**37-12**, **37-18**, and **37-19**), trifluoromethyl (**37-9**, **37-13**, and **37-18**), ethoxy (**37-16**), or benzyloxy (**37-17**) substituents on the acyl group. Against the KB-VIN cell line, alkaloids **37-18** and **37-19** with both fluoro and trifluoromethyl/methyl groups were more potent than **37-9** with only a single trifluoromethyl group and even more potent than **37-2** with a single fluoro group. Similarly, alkaloid **37-13** showed increased cytotoxic activity against most cell lines compared with the related fluorinated alkaloids **37-14** and **37-15**. Moreover, alkaloids with nitro, methoxy, phenyl, trifluoromethoxy, trifluoromethythio, and methyl carboxylate groups on a C-6 benzoate ester were generally less potent.

Table 3. Cytotoxic activity data for lycoctonine-type (7,8-methylenedioxy) C_{19}-diterpenoid alkaloids and synthetic analogs of delpheline **36~54**.

Alkaloids	Cell Line/IC_{50} (μM) [1]					KB/KB-VIN Ratio
	A549	DU145	MDA-MB-231	KB	KB-VIN	
Delcorine (**36**)	>40	-	>40	>40	>40	-
Delpheline (**37**)	>20	>20	-	>20	>20	-
Pacinine (**38**)	>20	>20	-	>20	>20	-
Yunnadelphinine (**39**)	>20	>20	-	>20	>20	-
Melpheline (**40**)	>40	-	>40	>40	>40	-
Bonvalotidine C (**41**)	>40	-	>40	>40	>40	-
N-Deethyl-*N*-formylpaciline (**42**)	>40	-	>40	>40	>40	-
N-Deethyl-*N*-formylpacinine (**43**)	>40	-	>40	>40	>40	-
Isodelpheline (**44**)	>40	-	>40	>40	>40	-
Pacidine (**45**)	>40	-	>40	>40	>40	-
Eladine (**46**)	>40	-	>40	>40	>40	-
N-Formyl-4,19-secopacinine (**47**)	>40	-	>40	>40	>40	-
N-Formyl-4,19-secoyunnadelphinine (**48**)	>40	-	>40	>40	>40	-
Iminoisodelpheline (**49**)	>40	-	>40	>40	>40	-
Iminodelpheline (**50**)	>40	-	>40	>40	>40	-
Laxicyminine (**51**)	>40	-	>40	>40	>40	-
N-Deethyl-19-oxoisodelpheline (**52**)	>40	-	>40	>40	>40	-
N-Deethyl-19-oxo-delpheline (**53**)	>40	-	>40	>40	>40	-
19-Oxoisodelpheline (**54**)	>40	-	>40	>40	>40	-
37-1	14.8 ± 3.8	7.4 ± 1.2	-	8.9 ± 2.0	8.3 ± 1.6	1.07
37-2	38.1 ± 11.8	15.6 ± 5.4	-	23.3 ± 3.9	15.0 ± 6.5	1.55
37-3	22.7 ± 0.3	17.2 ± 3.3	-	20.7 ± 0.9	17.7 ± 3.5	1.17
37-4	>20	>20	-	>20	>20	-
37-5	24.1 ± 2.7	17.1 ± 11.4	-	23.6 ± 0.4	17.4 ± 7.4	1.36
37-6	18.7 ± 6.6	20.3 ± 7.1	-	20.1 ± 7.6	18.9 ± 5.0	1.06
37-7	21.1 ± 9.2	16.6 ± 12.7	-	21.7 ± 11.6	17.9 ± 4.2	1.21
37-8	28.7 ± 13.6	28.7 ± 7.2	-	24.3 ± 5.7	23.3 ± 3.7	1.04
37-9	21.2 ± 4.7	12.6 ± 3.0	-	14.9 ± 4.9	11.9 ± 3.3	1.25
37-10	20.9 ± 4.3	22.7 ± 6.0	-	19.1 ± 4.8	20.3 ± 2.7	0.94
37-11	30.8 ± 13.3	28.9 ± 4.7	-	29.5 ± 3.5	27.5 ± 3.1	1.07
37-12	19.9 ± 10.1	16.9 ± 6.7	-	14.6 ± 7.1	6.80 ± 5.0	2.15
37-13	10.2 ± 2.6	15.1 ± 6.0	-	21.0 ± 9.4	9.10 ± 1.5	2.31
37-14	22.4 ± 7.1	22.8 ± 8.5	-	25.9 ± 9.3	24.2 ± 4.4	1.07
37-15	29.7 ± 11.6	29.0 ± 5.4	-	21.8 ± 1.4	18.7 ± 5.2	1.17
37-16	20.0 ± 0.9	15.6 ± 2.6	-	14.8 ± 3.3	6.5 ± 2.2	2.28
37-17	14.1 ± 2.9	13.2 ± 5.7	-	6.8 ± 1.7	4.2 ± 1.1	1.62
37-18	16.5 ± 2.2	11.3 ± 7.9	-	5.4 ± 1.8	4.4 ± 0.8	1.23
37-19	25.6 ± 1.2	19.8 ± 4.6	-	12.1 ± 7.8	4.7 ± 1.4	2.57
37-20	>20	>20	-	>20	>20	-
37-21	>20	>20	-	>20	>20	-
37-22	>20	>20	-	>20	>20	-
PXL[2] (nM)	4.8 ± 0.6	5.9 ± 1.9	8.4 ± 0.8	5.8 ± 0.2	2405.4 ± 44.8	-

[1] Values are means ± standard deviation; [2] Paclitaxel (PXL; nM) was used as an experimental control.

3. Antiproliferative Activity of C_{20}-Diterpenoid Alkaloid Derivatives

3.1. *Actaline and Napelline-Type C_{20}-Diterpenoid Alkaloids*

One natural actaline-type C_{20}-diterpenoid alkaloid [44], aconicarchamine A (**55**), isolated from rhizoma of *Aconitum japonicum* subsp. *subcuneatum* [30], (Figure 5) and seven natural napelline-type C_{20}-diterpenoid alkaloids, lucidusculine (**57**), flavadine (**58**), 12-acetyllucidusculine (**59**), 1-acetyl-luciculine (**60**), dehydrolucidusculine (**61**), dehydroluciculine (**62**), and 12-acetyldehydroluciduscu-line (**63**), purified from roots of *Aconitum yesoense* var. *macroyesoense* [31–33], (Figure 5) were tested. Seven synthetic napelline-type C_{20}-diterpenoid alkaloid derivatives (**56-1~56-7**) [18,32,45] were prepared from luciculine (**56**) (Figure 5) and tested also. All tested actaline- and napelline-type C_{20}-diterpenoid alkaloids were evaluated for antiproliferative activity against four to five human tumor cell lines [28,30] (Table 4). Tested actaline- and napelline-type C_{20}-diterpenoid alkaloids, both the natural alkaloids (**55** and **57~63**) and synthetic analogs (**56-1~56-4, 56-6**, and **56-7**), were inactive (IC_{50} > 20 or 40 μM). Among the synthetic alkaloids, alkaloid **56-5** exhibited only weak potency toward the tested cell lines (A549, DU145, KB and KB-VIN; average IC_{50} 27.8 μM). Because the related alkaloids **57, 60, 56-2~56-4, 56-6,** and **56-7** were inactive against all tested cancer cell lines, a C-1 hydroxy group, C-12 acyloxy group, and C-15 acetoxy group found in **56-5** could be needed for antiproliferative activity of luciculine derivatives.

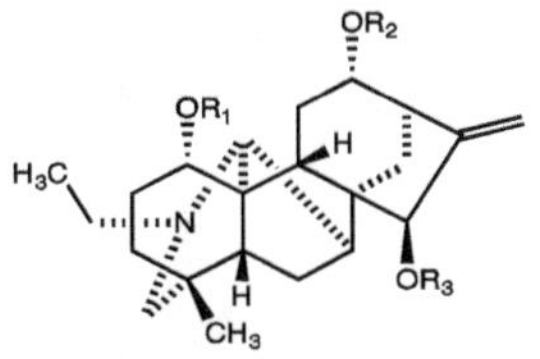

		R1	R2	R3
56 *	luciculine	H	H	H
57 *	lucidusculine	H	H	$COCH_3$
58 *	flavadine: *N*-oxide	H	H	$COCH_3$
59 *	12-acetyllucidusculine	H	$COCH_3$	$COCH_3$
60 *	1-acetylluciculine	$COCH_3$	H	H
56-1	1,12,15-triacetylluciculine	$COCH_3$	$COCH_3$	$COCH_3$
56-2	12-benzoylluciculine	H	Bz	H
56-3	12-anisoylluciculine	H	As	H
56-4	12-veratroylluciculine	H	Vr	H
56-5	12-benzoyllucidsuculine	H	Bz	$COCH_3$
56-6	1,12,15-tribenzoylluciculine	Bz	Bz	Bz
56-7	12,15-dibenzoylluciculine	H	Bz	Bz

Bz = COC_6H_5, As = $COC_6H_4OCH_3$ (*p*)
Vr = $COC_6H_3(OCH_3)_2$ (3,4)

*: Natural alkaloid

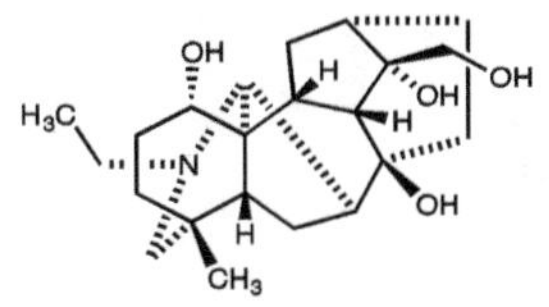

55 *	aconicarchamine A

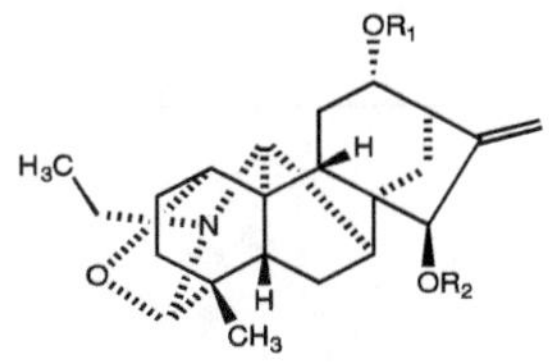

		R1	R2
61 *	dehydrolucidusculine	H	$COCH_3$
62 *	dehydroluciculine	H	H
63 *	12-acetyldehydrolucidusculine	$COCH_3$	$COCH_3$

Figure 5. Chemical structures of actaline and napelline-type C_{20}-diterpenoid alkaloids **55~63**.

Table 4. Cytotoxic activity data for actaline and napelline-type C_{20}-diterpenoid alkaloids **55~63** and synthetic analogs **56-1~56-7** of luciculine.

	Cell Line/IC_{50} (μM) [1]					
Alkaloids	**A549**	**DU145**	**MDA-MB-231**	**MCF-7**	**KB**	**KB-VIN**
Aconicarchamine A (**55**)	>40	-	>40	>40	>40	>40
Lucidusculine (**57**)	>20	>20	-	-	>20	>20
Flavadine (**58**)	>20	>20	-	-	>20	>20
12-Acetyllucidusculine (**59**)	>20	>20	-	-	>20	>20
1-Acetylluciculine (**60**)	>20	>20	-	-	>20	>20
Dehydrolucidusculine (**61**)	>20	>20	-	-	>20	>20
Dehydroluciculine (**62**)	>20	>20	-	-	>20	>20
12-Acetyldehydrolucidusculine (**63**)	>20	>20	-	-	>20	>20
56-1	>20	>20	-	-	>20	>20
56-2	>20	>20	-	-	>20	>20
56-3	>20	>20	-	-	>20	>20
56-4	>20	>20	-	-	>20	>20
56-5	23.3 ± 6.1	28.1 ± 11.1	-	-	31.8 ± 10.5	27.8 ± 1.9
56-6	>20	>20	-	-	>20	>20
56-7	>20	>20	-	-	>20	>20
PXL[2] (nM)	4.8 ± 0.6	5.9 ± 1.9	8.4 ± 0.8	10.2 ± 0.9	5.8 ± 0.2	2405.4 ± 44.8

[1] Values are means ± standard deviation; [2] Paclitaxel (PXL; nM) was used as an experimental control.

3.2. *Hetisine-Type (Analogs of Kobusine) C_{20}-Diterpenoid Alkaloids*

Tested hetisine-type (analogs of kobusine) C_{20}-diterpenoid alkaloids included four natural alkaloids, ryosenamine (**64**), 9-hydroxynominine (**65**), and torokonine (**66**), isolated from rhizoma of *Aconitum japonicum* subsp. *subcuneatum* [27,28] (Figure 6) and kobusine (**67**), purified from roots of *Aconitum yesoense* var. *macroyesoense* [31] (Figure 6). Nineteen synthetic derivatives (**67-1~67-19**) [18,21, 30,46,47] (Figure 6) prepared from **67** were tested also.

All tested hetisine-type (kobusine analogs) C_{20}-diterpenoid alkaloids were evaluated for antiproliferative activity against four human tumor cell lines [27,28,30] (Table 5). Fifteen of the 23 alkaloids, both natural (**64~67**) and synthetic (**67-1~67-4, 67-6, 67-9, 67-11, 67-12, 67-15~67-17**), were inactive (IC_{50} > 20 or 40 μM). Kobusine derivatives **67-5, 67-7, 67-10, 67-18,** and **67-19** exhibited the highest average potency over the four tested cell lines (A549, DU145, KB and KB-VIN; average IC_{50} 7.8, 6.1, 6.2, 6.8, and 4.7 μM, respectively), and alkaloids **67-8, 67-13,** and **67-14** showed moderate potency (average IC_{50} 16.6, 14.3, and 11.6 μM, respectively). However, while alkaloid **67-14** showed good cytotoxic activity (IC_{50} 9.6 μM) against DU145 cells, it was much less potent against A549, KB, and KB-VIN cells.

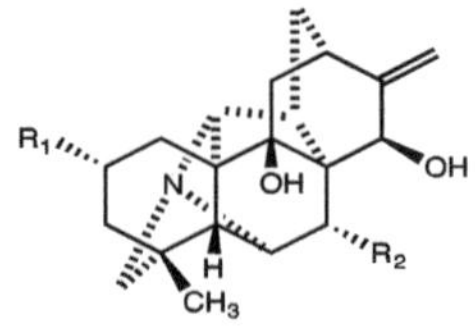

		R1	R2
64 *	ryosenamine	OBz	H
65 *	9-hydroxynominine	H	H
66 *	torokonine	OBz	OH

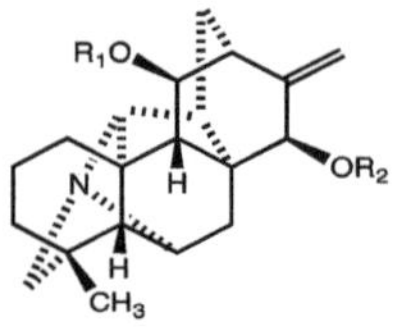

		R1	R2			R1	R2
67 *	kobusine	H	H	**67-10**	11,15-di-(4-nitrobenzoyl)kobusine	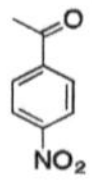	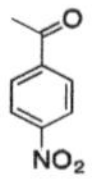
67-1	15-acetylkobusine	H	$COCH_3$	**67-11**	11-(2-trifluorometylbenzoyl)-kobusine	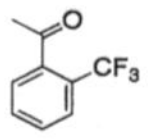	H
67-2	11,15-diacetylkobusine	$COCH_3$	$COCH_3$	**67-12**	11-(3-trifluoromethylbenzoyl)-kobusine	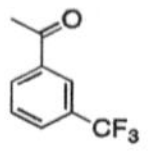	H
67-3	11-benzoylkobusine	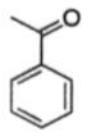	H	**67-13**	11-(4-trifluoromethylbenzoyl)-kobusine	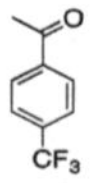	H
67-4	15-benzoylkobusine	H	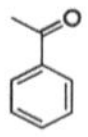	**67-14**	11-(4-trifluoromethoxybenzoyl)-kobusine	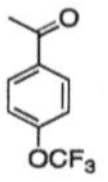	H
67-5	11,15-dibenzoylkobusine	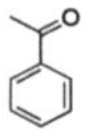	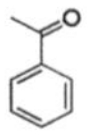	**67-15**	11-nicotinoylkobusine	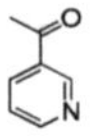	H
67-6	11-anisoylkobusine	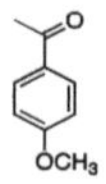	H	**67-16**	11-(4-fluorobenzoyl)kobusine	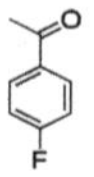	H
67-7	11,15-dianisoylkobusine	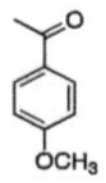	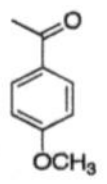	**67-17**	15-(4-fluorobenzoyl)kobusine	H	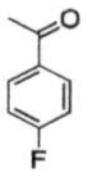
67-8	11-(4-nitrobenzoyl)kobusine	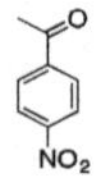	H	**67-18**	11,15-di-(4-fluorobenzoyl)kobusine	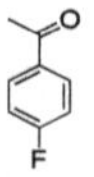	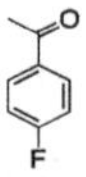
67-9	15-(4-nitrobenzoyl)kobusine	H	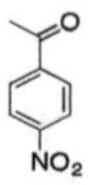	**67-19**	11,15-di-(3-trifluoromethylcinna-moyl)kobusine	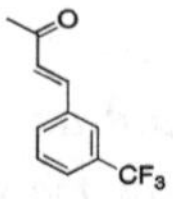	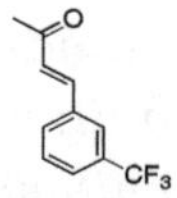

*: Natural alkaloid

Figure 6. Chemical structures of hetisine-type (analogs of kobusine) C_{20}-diterpenoid alkaloids **64~67-19**.

Table 5. Cytotoxic activity data for hetisine-type C_{20}-diterpenoid alkaloids **64~67** and synthetic derivatives **67-1~67-19** of kobusine.

	Cell Line/IC_{50} (μM) [1]						KB/KB-VIN Ratio
Alkaloids	**A549**	**DU145**	**MDA-MB-231**	**MCF-7**	**KB**	**KB-VIN**	
Ryosenamine (**64**)	>40	-	>40	>40	>40	>40	
9-Hydroxynominine (**65**)	>40	-	>40	>40	>40	>40	
Torokonine (**66**)	>40	-	>40	>40	>40	>40	
Kobusine (**67**)	>20	>20	-	-	>20	>20	
67-1	>20	>20	-	-	>20	>20	
67-2	>20	>20	-	-	>20	>20	
67-3	>20	>20	-	-	>20	>20	
67-4	>20	>20	-	-	>20	>20	
67-5	8.4 ± 1.4	9.3 ± 3.0	-	-	6.0 ± 0.8	7.5 ± 3.7	0.80
67-6	>20	>20	-	-	>20	>20	
67-7	6.7 ± 2.4	7.1 ± 2.0	-	-	5.3 ± 0.3	5.2 ± 1.2	1.02
67-8	19.5 ± 3.3	15.3 ± 5.6	-	-	13.9 ± 2.8	17.9 ± 1.8	0.78
67-9	>20	>20	-	-	>20	>20	
67-10	6.9 ± 1.7	7.0 ± 2.2	-	-	5.3 ± 0.6	5.5 ± 0.7	0.96
67-11	>20	>20	-	-	>20	>20	
67-12	>20	>20	-	-	>20	>20	
67-13	17.2 ± 0.9	13.2 ± 2.8	-	-	12.7 ± 1.1	14.1 ± 1.0	0.90
67-14	14.1 ± 0.7	9.6 ± 2.4	-	-	11.7 ± 0.6	10.9 ± 0.7	1.07
67-15	>20	>20	-	-	>20	>20	
67-16	>20	>20	-	-	>20	>20	
67-17	>20	>20	-	-	>20	>20	
67-18	8.1 ± 4.7	6.8 ± 2.0	-	-	5.2 ± 0.6	7.1 ± 2.6	0.73
67-19	5.5 ± 1.9	6.2 ± 3.1	-	-	4.1 ± 0.7	3.1 ± 1.6	1.32
PXL[2] (nM)	4.8 ± 0.6	5.9 ± 1.9	8.4 ± 0.8	10.2 ± 0.9	5.8 ± 0.2	2405.4 ± 44.8	0.0067

[1] Values are means ± standard deviation; [2] Paclitaxel (PXL; nM) was used as an experimental control.

Among these analogs of **67**, esterification of C-15 in addition to C-11 increased potency significantly (compare **67-8** to **67-10**) or even converted an inactive to an active alkaloid (compare **67-3** to **67-5**, **67-6** to **67-7**, **67-16** to **67-18**). Consequently, all of the most potent analogs (**67-5**, **67-7**, **67-10**, **67-18**, and **67-19**) of **67** were esterified at both C-11 and C-15.

Striking observations from the data in Table 5 were the degree and comparative ratio of KB/KB-VIN potency. Five alkaloids (**67-5**, **67-7**, **67-10**, **67-18**, and **67-19**) were quite potent (IC_{50} < 10 μM) against KB-VIN. Indeed, alkaloid **67-19** exhibited a significantly low IC_{50} value of 3.1 μM. The ratios of KB to KB-VIN (IC_{50} KB/IC_{50} KB-VIN) were greater than 0.73 for all active alkaloids, with many alkaloids displaying comparable potency against the two cell lines, in contrast with paclitaxel (ratio of 0.0067). Alkaloid **67-19** showed over 1.3-fold selectivity with the greatest cytotoxic activity against KB-VIN (IC_{50} KB/IC_{50} KB-VIN: 1.32).

3.3. Hetisine-Type (Analogs of Pseudokobusine) C_{20}-Diterpenoid Alkaloids

The two tested natural hetisine-type (analogs of pseudokobusine) C_{20}-diterpenoid alkaloids pseudokobusine (**68**) and 15-veratroylpseudokobusine (**68-11**) were purified from the roots of *Aconitum yesoense* var. *macroyesoense* [31,32] (Figure 7). The 36 tested synthetic derivatives (**68-1~68-10**, **68-12~68-37**) [18,21,30,32,46–49] (Figure 7) were prepared from **68**.

All tested hetisine-type (**68** analogs) C_{20}-diterpenoid alkaloids were evaluated for antiproliferative activity against four human tumor cell lines [30] (Table 6). Many alkaloids, both natural alkaloids (**68** and **68-11**) and synthetic analogs (**68-1~68-3**, **68-6**, **68-8**, **68-9**, **68-14**, **68-16~68-18**, **68-21**, **68-23**, **68-25~68-31**, **68-33~68-37**), were inactive (IC_{50} > 20 μM). The pseudokobusine derivatives **68-5**, **68-15**, **68-19**, **68-20**, **68-24**, and **68-32** exhibited the highest average potency over the tested cell lines (A549, DU145, KB and KB-VIN; average IC_{50} 7.0, 5.2, 5.3, 7.4, 7.1, and 6.1 μM, respectively). Alkaloids **68-7**, **68-10**, **68-12**, **68-13**, and **68-22** showed moderate potency over all tested cell lines (average IC_{50} 13.5-16.8 μM). However, although alkaloid **68-10** showed good cytotoxic activity (IC_{50} 8.0 μM) against A549 cells, it was much less potent against DU145, KB, and KB-VIN cells.

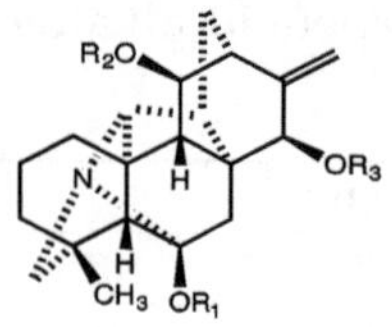

		R1	R2	R3
68*	pseudokobusine	H	H	H
68-1	15-acetylpseudokobusine	H	H	$COCH_3$
68-2	11,15-diacetylpseudokobusine	H	$COCH_3$	$COCH_3$
68-3	6-benzoylpseudokobusine	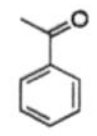	H	H
68-4	6,11-dibenzoylpseudokobusine	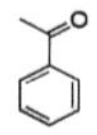	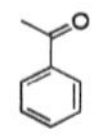	H
68-5	11,15-dibenzoylpseudokobusine	H	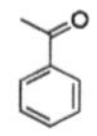	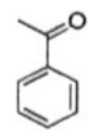
68-6	6-anisoylpseudokobusine	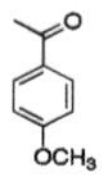	H	H
68-7	11-anisoylpseudokobusine	H	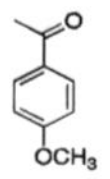	H
68-8	6,11-dianisoylpseudokobusine	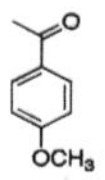	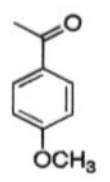	H
68-9	6,15-dianisoylpseudokobusine	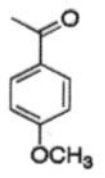	H	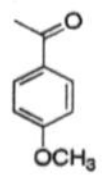
68-10	11-veratroylpseudokobusine	H	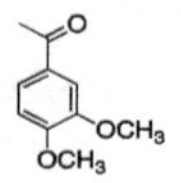	H
68-11*	15-veratroylpseudokobusine	H	H	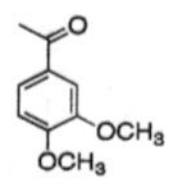
68-12	6,11-diveratroylpseudokobusine	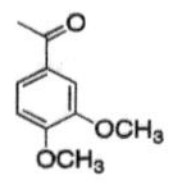	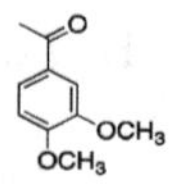	H
68-13	6,15-diveratroylpseudokobusine	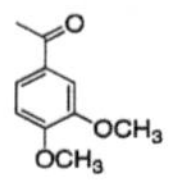	H	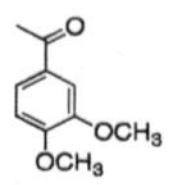
68-14	6-(4-nitrobenzoyl)pseudokobusine	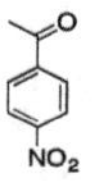	H	H
68-15	11-(4-nitrobenzoyl)pseudokobusine	H	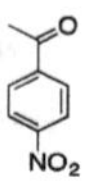	H
68-16	15-(4-nitrobenzoyl)pseudokobusine	H	H	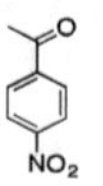
68-17	6,15-di-(4-nitrobenzoyl)pseudokobusine	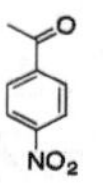	H	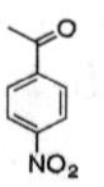
68-18	6,11,15-tri-(4-nitrobenzoyl)pseudokobusine	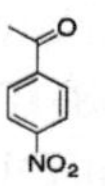	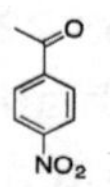	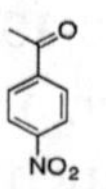

Figure 7. *Cont.*

		R_1	R_2	R_3
68-19	11,15-di-(3-nitrobenzoyl)pseudokobusine	H	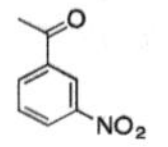	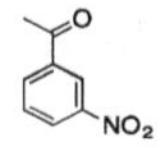
68-20	11-(3-trifluoromethylbenzoyl)pseudokobusine	H	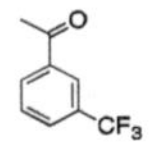	H
68-21	6,11-di-(3-trifluoromethylbenzoyl)pseudokobusine	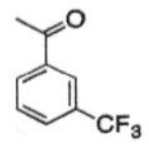	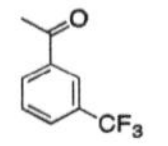	H
68-22	11-(4-trifluoromethylbenzoyl)pseudokobusine	H	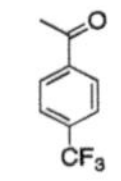	H
68-23	6-cinnamoylpseudokobusine	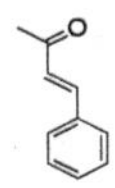	H	H
68-24	11-cinnamoylpseudokobusine	H	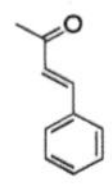	H
68-25	15-cinnamoylpseudokobusine	H	H	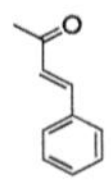
68-26	11-pivaloylpseudokobusine	H	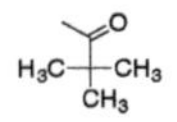	H
68-27	11-nicotinoylpseudokobusine	H	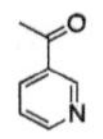	H
68-28	15-nicotinoylpseudokobusine	H	H	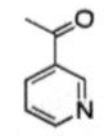
68-29	11,15-dinicotinoylpseudokobusine	H	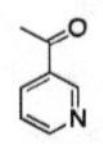	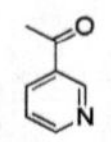
68-30	15-propionylpseudokobusine	H	H	$COCH_2CH_3$
68-31	11,15-dipropionylpseudokobusine	H	$COCH_2CH_3$	$COCH_2CH_3$
68-32	11-tritylpseudokobusine	H	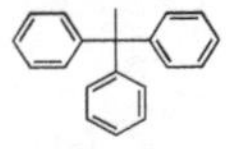	H

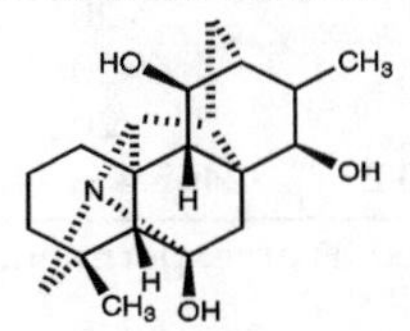

68-33	dihydropseudokobusine

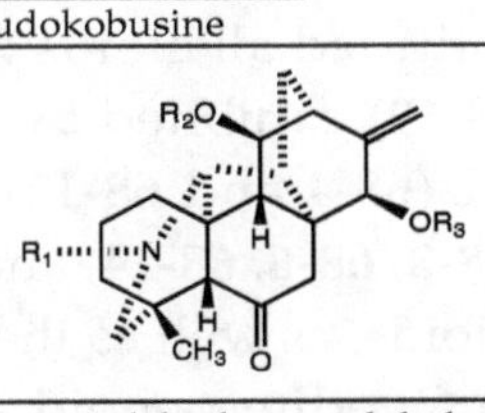

		R_1	R_2	R_3
68-34	*N*-benzyl-*N*,6-seco-6-dehydropseudokobusine	$CH_2C_6H_5$	H	H
68-35	*N*,11,15-triacetyl-*N*,6-seco-6-dehydropseudokobusine	$COCH_3$	$COCH_3$	$COCH_3$
68-36	*N*-acetyl-*N*,6-seco-6-dehydropseudokobusine	$COCH_3$	H	H
68-37	*N*-cinnamoyl-*N*,6-seco-6-dehydropseudokobusine	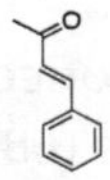	H	H

*: Natural alkaloid

Figure 7. Chemical structures of hetisine-type (analogs of pseudokobusine) C_{20}-diterpenoid alkaloids **68~68-37**.

Table 6. Cytotoxic activity data for hetisine-type C_{20}-diterpenoid alkaloids pseudokobusine (**68**) and its synthetic analogs **68-1~68-37**.

	Cell Line/IC_{50} (μM) [1]				KB/KB-VIN Ratio
Alkaloids	**A549**	**DU145**	**KB**	**KB-VIN**	
Pseudokobusine (**68**)	>20	>20	>20	>20	
68-1	>20	>20	>20	>20	
68-2	>20	>20	>20	>20	
68-3	>20	>20	>20	>20	
68-4	19.3 ± 4.5	15.3 ± 4.3	12.8 ± 1.7	10.2 ± 0.9	1.25
68-5	8.8 ± 4.5	7.6 ± 2.5	5.2 ± 1.3	6.3 ± 0.6	0.83
68-6	>20	>20	>20	>20	
68-7	15.4 ± 3.7	13.2 ± 2.0	11.1 ± 5.5	15.7 ± 1.5	0.70
68-8	>20	>20	>20	>20	
68-9	>20	>20	>20	>20	
68-10	8.0 ± 5.1	15.3 ± 2.9	14.9 ± 3.6	20.1 ± 13.5	0.74
15-Veratroylpseudokobusine (**68-11**)	>20	>20	>20	>20	
68-12	16.0 ± 5.5	16.9 ± 7.8	19.7 ± 3.1	14.7 ± 7.0	1.34
68-13	15.2 ± 6.4	16.6 ± 7.9	18.1 ± 4.3	12.2 ± 5.6	1.48
68-14	>20	>20	>20	>20	
68-15	5.8 ± 0.7	7.2 ± 1.9	6.4 ± 0.8	6.4 ± 1.8	1.00
68-16	>20	>20	>20	>20	
68-17	>20	>20	>20	>20	
68-18	>20	>20	>20	>20	
68-19	5.0 ± 1.1	5.2 ± 1.8	5.6 ± 1.2	5.6 ± 2.9	1.00
68-20	6.8 ± 0.7	7.7 ± 3.8	8.9 ± 3.7	6.2 ± 1.3	1.44
68-21	>20	>20	>20	>20	
68-22	17.9 ± 7.2	14.5 ± 7.2	15.7 ± 4.1	13.9 ± 3.3	1.13
68-23	>20	>20	>20	>20	
68-24	8.4 ± 1.7	6.5 ± 0.5	7.0 ± 1.3	6.4 ± 0.9	1.09
68-25	>20	>20	>20	>20	
68-26	>20	>20	>20	>20	
68-27	>20	>20	>20	>20	
68-28	>20	>20	>20	>20	
68-29	>20	>20	>20	>20	
68-30	>20	>20	>20	>20	
68-31	>20	>20	>20	>20	
68-32	6.4 ± 1.2	6.0 ± 3.3	6.6 ± 3.1	5.2 ± 1.0	1.27
68-33	>20	>20	>20	>20	
68-34	>20	>20	>20	>20	
68-35	>20	>20	>20	>20	
68-36	>20	>20	>20	>20	
68-37	>20	>20	>20	>20	
PXL[2] (nM)	4.8 ± 0.6	5.9 ± 1.9	5.8 ± 0.2	2405.4 ± 44.8	

[1] Values are means ± standard deviation; [2] Paclitaxel (PXL; nM) was used as an experimental control.

Among the analogs of **68**, four C-11 mono-substituted alkaloids (**68-15**, **68-20**, **68-24**, and **68-32**) and two C-11,15 di-esterified alkaloids (**68-5** and **68-19**) exhibited average IC_{50} values of less than 10 μM. Certain C-11 (**68-7**, **68-10**, and **68-22**), C-6,11 (**68-4** and **68-12**) and C-6,15 (**68-13**) esterified alkaloids were generally less potent, while all C-6 (**68-3**, **68-6**, **68-14**, and **68-23**) and C-15 (**68-1**, **68-11**, **68-16**, **68-25**, **68-28**, and **68-30**) mono-substituted alkaloids, as well as the tri-substituted analog (**68-18**), were inactive. Thus, all more active (IC_{50} < 10 μM) C_{20}-diterpenoid alkaloids in this classification had an ester or ether group on the C-11 hydroxy and were 11-monoester/11,15-diester analogs of **68** (OH at C-6).

The data in Table 6 led to noticeable observations about the degree and comparative ratio of KB/KB-VIN potency. Six alkaloids (**68-5**, **68-15**, **68-19**, **68-20**, **68-24**, and **68-32**) were quite potent (IC_{50} < 10 μM) against KB-VIN. Indeed, alkaloid **68-32** exhibited a low IC_{50} value of 5.2 μM. The ratios of KB to KB-VIN (IC_{50} KB/IC_{50} KB-VIN) were greater than 0.70 for all active alkaloids, with many alkaloids displaying comparable potency against the two cell lines, in contrast with paclitaxel (ratio of 0.0067).

Alkaloids **68-12**, **68-13**, and **68-20** showed over 1.3-fold selectivity with their greatest cytotoxic activity against KB-VIN (IC_{50} KB/IC_{50} KB-VIN: 1.34, 1.48, and 1.44, respectively).

In mechanism of action studies on selected diterpenoid alkaloids, the hetisine-type C_{20}-diterpenoid alkaloid derivatives **68-7** and **68-22** showed important suppressive effects against Raji cells. Further study indicated that **68-22** inhibited extracellular signal-regulated kinase phosphorylation but induced enhanced phosphoinositide 3 kinase phosphorylation, leading to accumulation of Raji cells in the G1 or sub G1 phase [20]. More investigation is certainly warranted.

4. Discussion

We have synthesized acylated derivatives of various C_{19}- and C_{20}-diterpenoid alkaloids. Totally, 199 natural alkaloids and their derivatives were evaluated against four to five human tumor cell lines. Among all alkaloids, 128 alkaloids were non-toxic (IC_{50} > 20 or 40 μM) and 51 alkaloids showed moderate antiproliferative effects (average IC_{50} = 10–40 μM). General summaries are described briefly below, and the most active compounds are shown in Figure 8.

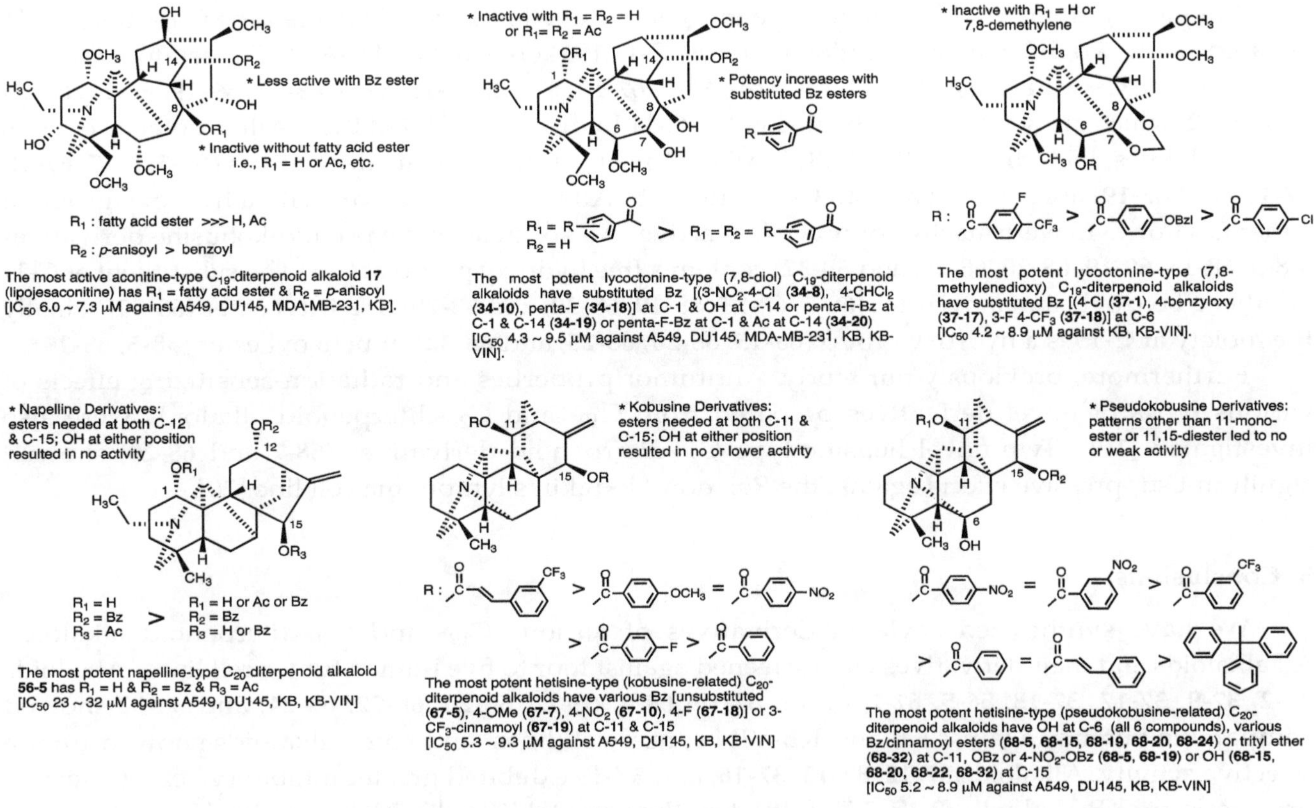

Figure 8. Most potent tested diterpenoid alkaloids & structure-activity correlations.

Among the aconitine-type C_{19}-diterpenoid alkaloids, the fatty acid ester at C-8 and the anisoyl group at C-14 found in **17** may be important to the cytotoxic activity. Compounds without the fatty acid ester at C-8 were inactive, and compounds with an unsubstituted benzoyl group at C-14 were less potent.

Among the C_{19}-diterpenoid alkaloids, the most active alkaloids were lycoctonine-type C_{19}-diterpenoid alkaloids with two different substitution patterns, C-1 (delcosine derivatives) and C-6 (delpheline derivatives). Delcosine derivatives **34-6**, **34-8**, **34-10**, and **34-18**, which are acylated at the C-1 hydroxy, as well as delpheline derivatives **37-1**, **37-17**, and **37-18**, which are acylated at the C-6 hydroxy, exhibited the greatest potency over all tested cell lines, including MDR KB-VIN.

Among the lycoctonine-type (7,8-diol) C_{19}-diterpenoid alkaloids, a C-1 acyloxy group and C-14 hydroxy group were important for improved antiproliferative activity. The C-1,14 diacylated delcosine derivatives were generally less potent than corresponding C-1 monoacylated delcosine derivatives. The 1-monoacylated alkaloids with the highest potency (IC_{50} 4−6 μM) against five tested cell lines contained 3-nitro-4-chloro- (**34-8**) and pentafluoro- (**34-18**) as well as 4-dichloromethyl- (**34-10**) benzoyl esters. Two or one pentafluorinated benzoyl esters were also found in the two most consistently potent alkaloids (**34-19** and **34-20**) among the 1,14-diacyl and 1-acyl-14-acetyl derivatives.

Among the lycoctonine-type (7,8-methylenedioxy) C_{19}-diterpenoid alkaloids, none of the tested compound reached the potency levels of the most active 7,8-diol compounds. However, three 6-acylated delpheline derivatives **37-17~37-19** did show significant potency against the KB-VIN cell line (IC_{50} 4.22, 4.40, and 4.71 μM, respectively). Interestingly, the two latter compounds contained fluorinated benzoyl esters. In addition, among 19 tested delpheline derivatives, four compounds (**37-12**, **37-16**, **37-13**, and **37-19**) showed over two-fold selectivity between the MDR and parental cell lines (ratio of IC_{50} KB/IC_{50} KB-VIN: 2.15, 2.28, 2.31, and 2.57, respectively).

None of the 15 tested actaline- and napelline-type C_{20}-diterpenoid alkaloids showed significant antiproliferative potency. Only 12-benzoyllucidsuculine (**56-5**) with C-1 hydroxy, C-12 acyloxy, and C-15 acetoxy groups showed even weak potency.

Among C_{20}-diterpenoid alkaloids, the most active alkaloids were hetisine-type C_{20}-diterpenoid alkaloids with two different substitution patterns, C-11,15 (kobusine) and C-6,11,15 (pseudo-kobusine). Hetisine-type C_{20}-diterpenoid alkaloids **67-5**, **67-7**, **67-10**, **67-18**, **67-19**, **68-5**, **68-15**, **68-19**, **68-20**, **68-25**, and **68-32**, which are acylated or tritylated at the C-11 hydroxyl, exhibited the greatest potency over all tested cell lines, including MDR KB-VIN. All five most active kobusine derivatives (**67-5**, **67-7**, **67-10**, **67-18**, and **67-19**) are acylated at both C-11 and C-15. All tested derivatives with a hydroxy group at either C-11 or C-15 were inactive or much less active. All six most active pseudo-kobusine derivatives (**68-5**, **68-15**, **68-19**, **68-20**, **68-25**, and **68-32**) contain a free hydroxy group at C-6. The substituent at C-11 is either a benzoyl/cinnamoyl ester (**68-5**, **68-15**, **68-19**, **68-20**, and **68-25**) or a trityl ether (**68-32**). Finally, the moiety at C-15 is a hydroxy group (**68-15**, **68-20**, **68-25**, and **68-32**) or benzoyl ester (**68-5**, **68-19**).

Furthermore, previously our study, Antitumor properties and radiation-sensitizing effects of various types of novel derivatives prepared from C_{19}- and C_{20}-diterpenoid alkaloids were also investigated [19]. Two novel hetisine-type C_{20}-diterpenoid derivatives (**68-7** and **68-20**) showed significant suppressive effects against the Raji non-Hodgkin's lymphoma cell line [20].

5. Conclusions

We have synthesized acylated derivatives of various C_{19}- and C_{20}-diterpenoid alkaloids. All alkaloids and their derivatives were screened against four to five human tumor cell lines. Alkaloids **37-2**, **37-9**, **37-17**, **37-18**, **56-5**, **67-7**, **67-14**, **67-19**, **68-4**, **68-12**, **68-20**, **68-22**, **68-24**, and **68-32** showed comparable potency against KB and KB-VIN cancer cell lines, and some alkaloids showed tumor-selective activity. Alkaloids **37-12**, **37-13**, **37-16**, and **37-19** exhibited greater inhibitory activity against drug-resistant KB-VIN cells (2.15~2.57-fold) than the parental KB cells. These results demonstrate that modified lycoctonine-type C_{19}-diterpenoid alkaloids and hetisine-type C_{20}-diterpenoid alkaloids are not substrates of P-gp and could be effective against P-gp overexpressing MDR tumors. These promising new lead alkaloids merit continued studies to evaluate their potential as antitumor agents, particularly with enhanced resistant tumor selectivity. In addition, our results from modification-based antitumor activity studies can be used for further development of anticancer drugs overcoming an MDR phenotype.

Acknowledgments: The author gratefully acknowledges Lee, K.H., Goto, M., Morris-Natschke, S.L., Ohkoshi, E., Zhao, Yu., Li, K.P., Bastow, K.F., Natural Products Research Laboratories, UNC Eshelman School of Pharmacy, University of North Carolina at Chapel Hill; and Mizukami, M., Kaneda, K., Suzuki, Y., Shimizu, T., Kusanagi, N., Takeda, K., Haraguchi, M., Abe, Y., Kuwahara, N., Suzuki, S., Terui, A., Masaka, T., Munakata, N., Uchida, M., Nunokawa, M., Chiba, R., Kanazawa, R., Matsuoka, K., Suzuki, M., Ikuta, M., Asakawa, E., Tosho, Y., Nakata, A., Hasegawa, Y., Katoh, M., Kokubun, A., Uchimura, A., Mikami, S., Takeuchi, A., Department of Medicinal

Chemistry, Faculty of Pharmaceutical Sciences, Hokkaido University of Science, for their helpful advice and support throughout this work.

References

1. Dzubak, P.; Hajduch, M.; Vydra, D.; Hustova, A.; Kvasnica, M.; Biedermann, D.; Markova, L.; Urban, J.; Sarek, J. Pharmacological activities of natural triterpenoids and their therapeutic implications. *Nat. Prod. Rep.* **2006**, *23*, 394–411. [CrossRef]
2. Cragg, G.M.; Newman, D.J. Nature: A vital source of leads for anticancer drug development. *Phytochem. Rev.* **2009**, *8*, 313–331. [CrossRef]
3. Kingston, D.G. Tubulin-interactive natural products as anticancer agents. *J. Nat. Prod.* **2009**, *72*, 507–515. [CrossRef]
4. Lee, K.H. Discovery and development of natural products-derived chemotherapeutic agents based on a medicinal chemistry approach. *J. Nat. Prod.* **2010**, *73*, 500–516. [CrossRef]
5. Grothaus, P.G.; Cragg, G.M.; Newman, D.J. Plant natural products in anticancer drug discovery. *Curr. Org. Chem.* **2010**, *14*, 1781–1791. [CrossRef]
6. Kinghorn, A.D.; Pan, L.; Fletcher, J.N.; Chai, H. The relevance of higher plants in lead compound discovery programs. *J. Nat. Prod.* **2011**, *74*, 1539–1555. [CrossRef]
7. Dall'Acqua, S. Natural products as antimitotic agents. *Curr. Top. Med. Chem.* **2014**, *14*, 2272–2285. [CrossRef]
8. Hussain, M.; Khera, R.A.; Iqbal, J.; Khalid, M.; Hanif, M.A. Phytochemicals: Key to effective anticancer drugs. *Mini-Rev. Org. Chem.* **2019**, *16*, 141–158. [CrossRef]
9. Agarwal, G.; Carcache, P.J.B.; Addo, E.M.; Kinghorn, A.D. Current status and contemporary approaches to the discovery of antitumor agents from higher plants. *Biotechnol. Adv.* **2019**. [CrossRef]
10. Wang, F.P.; Chen, Q.H. *The diterpenoid alkaloids. The Alkaloids: Chemistry and Biology*; Cordell, G.A., Ed.; Academic Press: San Diego, CA, USA, 2010; Volume 69, pp. 1–577.
11. Wang, F.P.; Chen, Q.H.; Liu, X.Y. Diterpenoid alkaloids. *Nat. Prod. Rep.* **2010**, *27*, 529–570. [CrossRef]
12. Benn, M.H.; Jacyno, J.M. The toxicology and pharmacology of diterpenoid alkaloids. In *Alkaloids: Chemical and Biological Perspectives*; Pelletier, S.W., Ed.; Wiley-Interscience: New York, NY, USA, 1983; Volume 1, pp. 153–210.
13. Bock, J.H.; Norris, D.O. Introduction to forensic plant science. In *Forensic Plant Science*; Elsevier Academic Press: Boston, MA, USA, 2016; pp. 1–22.
14. Amiya, T.; Bando, H. Aconitum alkaloids. In *The Alkaloids*; Brossi, A., Ed.; Academic Press: San Diego, CA, USA, 1988.
15. Chan, T.Y.K. Aconite poisoning. *Clin. Toxicol.* **2009**, *47*, 279–285. [CrossRef]
16. Chan, T.Y.K. Aconite poisoning following the percutaneous absorption of *Aconitum* alkaloids. *Forensic Sci. Int.* **2012**, *223*, 25–27. [CrossRef]
17. Povšnar, M.; Koželj, G.; Kreft, S.; Lumpert, M. Rare tradition of the folk medicinal use of *Aconitum* spp. is kept alive in Solčavsko, Slovenia. *J. Ethnobiol. Ethnomed.* **2017**, *13*, 45. [CrossRef]
18. Wada, K.; Hazawa, M.; Takahashi, K.; Mori, T.; Kawahara, N.; Kashiwakura, I. Inhibitory effects of diterpenoid alkaloids on the growth of A172 human malignant cells. *J. Nat. Prod.* **2007**, *70*, 1854–1858. [CrossRef]
19. Hazawa, M.; Wada, K.; Takahashi, K.; Mori, T.; Kawahara, N.; Kashiwakura, I. Suppressive effects of novel derivatives prepared from *Aconitum* alkaloids on tumor growth. *Invest. New Drugs* **2009**, *27*, 111–119. [CrossRef]
20. Hazawa, M.; Wada, K.; Takahashi, K.; Mori, T.; Kawahara, N.; Kashiwakura, I. Structure-activity relationships between the *Aconitum* C_{20}-diterpenoid alkaloid derivatives and the growth suppressive activities of non-Hodgkin's lymphoma Raji cells and human hematopoietic stem/progenitor cells. *Invest. New Drugs* **2011**, *29*, 1–8. [CrossRef]
21. Wada, K.; Hazawa, M.; Takahashi, K.; Mori, T.; Kawahara, N.; Kashiwakura, I. Structure-activity relationships and the cytotoxic effects of novel diterpenoid alkaloid derivatives against A549 human lung carcinoma cells. *J. Nat. Med.* **2011**, *65*, 43–49. [CrossRef]
22. Bando, H.; Kanaiwa, Y.; Wada, K.; Mori, T.; Amiya, T. Structure of deoxyjesaconitine. A new diterpene alkaloid from *Aconitum subcuneatum* Nakai. *Heterocycles* **1981**, *16*, 1723–1725.

23. Mori, T.; Bando, H.; Kanaiwa, Y.; Wada, K.; Amiya, T. Studies on the constituents of *Aconitum* Species. II. Structure of deoxyjesaconitine. *Chem. Pharm. Bull.* **1983**, *31*, 2884–2886. [CrossRef]
24. Wada, K.; Bando, H.; Mori, T.; Wada, R.; Kanaiwa, Y.; Amiya, T. Studies on the constituents of *Aconitum* Species. III. On the components of *Aconitum subcuneatum* Nakai. *Chem. Pharm. Bull.* **1985**, *33*, 3658–3661. [CrossRef]
25. Bando, H.; Wada, K.; Watanabe, M.; Mori, T.; Amiya, T. Studies on the constituents of *Aconitum* Species. IV. On the components of *Aconitum japonicum* Thunb. *Chem. Pharm. Bull.* **1985**, *33*, 4717–4722. [CrossRef]
26. Bando, H.; Wada, K.; Amiya, T.; Fujimoto, Y.; Kobayashi, K. Structures of secojesaconitine and subdesculine, two new diterpenoid alkaloids from *Aconitum japonicum* Thunb. *Chem. Pharm. Bull.* **1988**, *36*, 1604–1606. [CrossRef]
27. Yamashita, H.; Takeda, K.; Haraguchi, M.; Abe, Y.; Kuwahara, N.; Suzuki, S.; Terui, A.; Masaka, T.; Munakata, N.; Uchida, M.; et al. Four new diterpenoid alkaloids from *Aconitum japonicum* subsp. *subcuneatum*. *J. Nat. Med.* **2018**, *72*, 230–237. [CrossRef]
28. Yamashita, H.; Miyao, M.; Hiramori, K.; Kobayashi, D.; Suzuki, Y.; Mizukami, M.; Goto, M.; Lee, K.H.; Wada, K. Cytotoxic diterpenoid alkaloid from *Aconitum japonicum* subsp. *subcuneatum*. *J. Nat. Med.* **2019**, submitted.
29. Wada, K.; Bando, H.; Kawahara, N.; Mori, T.; Murayama, M. Determination and quantitative analysis of *Aconitum japonicum* by liquid chromatography atomospheric pressure chemical ionization mass spectrometry. *Biol. Mass Spectrom.* **1994**, *23*, 97–102. [CrossRef]
30. Wada, K.; Ohkoshi, E.; Zhao, Y.; Goto, M.; Morris-Natschke, S.L.; Lee, K.H. Evaluation of *Aconitum* diterpenoid alkaloids as antiproliferative agents. *Bioorg. Med. Chem. Lett.* **2015**, *25*, 1525–1531. [CrossRef]
31. Wada, K.; Bando, H.; Amiya, T. Two new C_{20}-diterpenoid alkaloids from *Aconitum yesoense* var. *macroyesoense* (NAKAI) TAMURA. Structures of dehydrolucidusculine and *N*-deethyldehydrolucidusculine. *Heterocycles* **1985**, *23*, 2473–2477.
32. Bando, H.; Wada, K.; Amiya, T.; Fujimoto, Y.; Kobayashi, K.; Sakurai, T. Studies on *Aconitum* Species. V. Constituents of *Aconitum yesoense* var. *macroyesoense* (Nakai) Tamura. *Heterocycles* **1987**, *26*, 2623–2637.
33. Wada, K.; Bando, H.; Kawahara, N. Studies on *Aconitum* species. XI. Two new diterpenoid alkaloids from *Aconitum yesoense* var. *macroyesoense* (Nakai) Tamura V. *Heterocycles* **1989**, *29*, 2141–2148.
34. Wada, K.; Kawahara, N. Diterpenoid and norditerpenoid alkaloids from the roots of *Aconitum yesoense* var. *macroyesoense*. *Helvetica Chimica Acta* **2009**, *92*, 629–637. [CrossRef]
35. Wada, K.; Yamamoto, T.; Bando, H.; Kawahara, N. Four diterpenoid alkaloids from *Delphinium elatum*. *Phytochemistry* **1992**, *31*, 2135–2138. [CrossRef]
36. Wada, K.; Ishizuki, S.; Mori, T.; Bando, H.; Murayama, M.; Kawahara, N. Effects of alkaloids from *Aconitum yesoense* var. *macroyesoense* on cutaneous blood flow in mice. *Biol. Pharm. Bull.* **1997**, *20*, 978–982.
37. Wada, K.; Mori, T.; Kawahara, N. Application of liquid chromatography−atmospheric pressure chemical ionization mass spectrometry to the differentiation of stereoisomeric C_{19}-norditerpenoid alkaloids. *Chem. Pharm. Bull.* **2000**, *48*, 660–668. [CrossRef]
38. Wada, K.; Goto, M.; Shimizu, T.; Kusanagi, N.; Lee, K.-H.; Yamashita, H. Structure-activity relationships and evaluation of esterified diterpenoid alkaloid derivatives as antiproliferative agents. *J. Nat. Med.* **2019**. [CrossRef]
39. Bando, H.; Wada, K.; Tanaka, J.; Kimura, S.; Hasegawa, E.; Amiya, T. Two new alkaloids from *Delphinium pacific giant* and revised ^{13}C-NMR assignment of delpheline. *Heterocycles* **1989**, *29*, 1293–1300. [CrossRef]
40. Wada, K.; Chiba, R.; Kanazawa, R.; Matsuoka, K.; Suzuki, M.; Ikuta, M.; Goto, M.; Yamashita, H.; Lee, K.H. Six new norditerpenoid alkaloids from *Delphinium elatum*. *Phytochem. Lett.* **2015**, *12*, 79–83. [CrossRef]
41. Wada, K.; Asakawa, E.; Tosho, Y.; Nakata, A.; Hasegawa, Y.; Kaneda, K.; Goto, M.; Yamashita, H.; Lee, K.H. Four new norditerpenoid alkaloids from *Delphinium elatum*. *Phytochem. Lett.* **2016**, *17*, 190–193. [CrossRef]
42. Yamashita, H.; Katoh, M.; Kokubun, A.; Uchimura, A.; Mikami, S.; Takeuchi, A.; Kaneda, K.; Suzuki, Y.; Mizukami, M.; Goto, M.; et al. Four new C_{19}-diterpenoid alkaloids from *Delphinium elatum*. *Phytochem. Lett.* **2018**, *24*, 6–9. [CrossRef]
43. Wada, K.; Ohkoshi, E.; Morris-Natschke, S.L.; Bastow, K.F.; Lee, K.H. Cytotoxic esterified diterpenoid alkaloid derivatives with increased selectivity against a drug-resistant cancer cell line. *Bioorg. Med. Chem. Lett.* **2012**, *22*, 249–252. [CrossRef]

44. Wang, F.P.; Liang, X.T. C_{20}-Diterpenoid alkaloids. In *The Alkaloids: Chemistry and Biology*; Cordell, G.A., Ed.; Academic Press: San Diego, CA, USA, 2002; Volume 59, pp. 1–280.
45. Wada, K.; Mori, T.; Kawahara, N. Application of liquid chromatography-atmospheric pressure chemical ionization mass spectrometry to the differentiation of stereoisomeric diterpenoid alkaloids. *Chem. Pharm. Bull.* **2000**, *48*, 1065–1074. [CrossRef]
46. Wada, K.; Ishizuki, S.; Mori, T.; Fujihira, E.; Kawahara, N. Effects of *Aconitum* alkaloid kobusine and pseudokobusine derivatives on cutaneous blood flow in mice. *Biol. Pharm. Bull.* **1998**, *21*, 140–146. [CrossRef] [PubMed]
47. Wada, K.; Ishizuki, S.; Mori, T.; Fujihira, E.; Kawahara, N. Effects of *Aconitum* alkaloid kobusine and pseudokobusine derivatives on cutaneous blood flow in mice; II. *Biol. Pharm. Bull.* **2000**, *23*, 607–615. [CrossRef] [PubMed]
48. Wada, K.; Bando, H.; Kawahara, N. Studies on *Aconitum* Species. XIII. Two new diterpenoid alkaloids from *Aconitum yesoense* var. *macroyesoense* (Nakai) Tamura VI. *Heterocycles* **1990**, *31*, 1081–1088. [CrossRef]
49. Wada, K.; Bando, H.; Wada, R.; Amiya, T. Analgesic activity of main components from *Aconitum yesoense* var. *macroyesoense* (Nakai) Tamura and pseudokobusine derivatives. *Shouyakugaku Zasshi* **1989**, *43*, 50–54.

11

Synthesis and Cytotoxicity Evaluation of DOTA-Conjugates of Ursolic Acid

Michael Kahnt [1], Sophie Hoenke [1], Lucie Fischer [1], Ahmed Al-Harrasi [2] and René Csuk [1,*]

[1] Organic Chemistry, Martin-Luther-University Halle-Wittenberg, Kurt-Mothes-Str. 2, D-06120 Halle (Saale), Germany; michael.kahnt@chemie.uni-halle.de (M.K.); sophie.hoenke@chemie.uni-halle.de (S.H.); lucie.fischer2018@gmx.de (L.F.)

[2] Natural and Medical Sciences Research Center, University of Nizwa, PO Box 33, Birkat Al-Mauz, Nizwa 616, Oman; aharrasi@unizwa.edu.om

* Correspondence: rene.csuk@chemie.uni-halle.de

Academic Editor: Kyoko Nakagawa-Goto

Abstract: In this study, we report the synthesis of several amine-spacered conjugates of ursolic acid (UA) and 1,4,7,10-tetraazacyclododecane-1,4,7,10-tetraacetic acid (DOTA). Thus, a total of 11 UA-DOTA conjugates were prepared holding various oligo-methylene diamine spacers as well as different substituents at the acetate units of DOTA including *tert*-butyl, benzyl, and allyl esters. Furthermore, three synthetic approaches were compared for the ethylenediamine-spacered conjugate **29** regarding reaction steps, yields, and precursor availability. The prepared conjugates were investigated regarding cytotoxicity using SRB assays and a set of human tumor cell lines. The highest cytotoxicity was observed for piperazinyl spacered compound **22**. Thereby, EC_{50} values of 1.5 μM (for A375 melanoma) and 1.7 μM (for A2780 ovarian carcinoma) were determined. Conjugates **22** and **24** were selected for further cytotoxicity investigations including fluorescence microscopy, annexin V assays and cell cycle analysis.

Keywords: ursolic acid; DOTA; triterpenoids; cytotoxicity

1. Introduction

Despite all medical advances in tumor therapy, cancer is still one of the most prevalent diseases worldwide, with 9.6 million cancer-related deaths counted in 2018 [1]. The research of novel therapeutic approaches and potent chemotherapeutic agents are important contributions in the battle against cancer. However, diagnosis is a prerequisite for successful treatment since an early detection of cancer cells can often significantly reduce the pathogenicity of a tumor and increase the healing rate. One molecule, which made significant impact on the field of diagnostic imaging in the past decades, is the EDTA-related macrocyclic chelator 1,4,7,10-tetraazacyclododecane-1,4,7,10-tetraacetic acid (DOTA, Figure 1) [2,3].

DOTA-derivatives and complexes thereof are widely used for molecular imaging, especially for the medical diagnosis of cancer [2,3]. By variation of the coordinated metal ion or substituents, they are applicable for a number of imaging techniques, such as magnetic resonance imaging (MRI) [2–4], positron emission tomography (PET) [2,3,5,6] and single photon emission computed tomography (SPECT) [2,3,7]. Because of this versatility, a crossover application of DOTA-derivatives as multimodal contrast agents for combined imaging modalities such as PET/MRI or PET/CT is possible and has already been described in the literature [2,3].

Although DOTA and derivatives thereof have a wide range of uses in diagnostic imaging, there are virtually no references for applications in the therapy of cancer. Therefore, we decided to prepare possible cytotoxic DOTA-derivatives by linkage with an ursolic acid backbone. Ursolic acid (UA, Figure 1) is a natural occurring triterpenoic acid with promising pharmacological properties, being widely distributed in various plants and fruits, such as rosemary [8], sage [8], oleander [9], and apples [10,11]. A wide range of biological activities, including antidiabetic, anti-inflammatory, antibacterial, and anticancer effects have been credited to UA and structurally-related derivatives [12–14]. Many structural modifications have been described in the literature starting from ursolic acid with various impacts on cytotoxic properties [12,15–18]. Structure activity investigations concerning modifications at C-3 of UA revealed the presence of an acetyloxy group to be beneficial for obtaining high anti-tumor activity [18]. Furthermore, it has been shown that the modification of C-28 with a piperazine moiety had a positive influence on the cytotoxic properties of ursolic acid [19,20]. Previously, we also have shown oligo-methylene diamine derived carboxamides of ursolic acid to be of high cytotoxicity [21]. Keeping these structure activity relationships in mind, we considered 3-acetyloxy protected and C-28 modified UA derivatives a convenient starting point for the preparation of cytotoxic oligo-methylene diamine spacered DOTA conjugates.

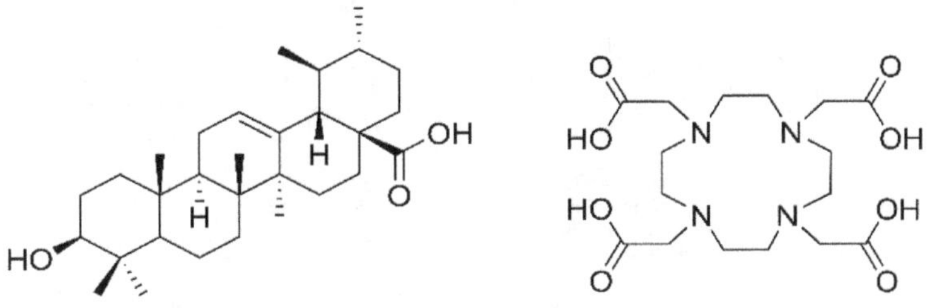

Figure 1. Structures of ursolic acid (UA) and 1,4,7,10-tetraazacyclododecane-1,4,7,10-tetraacetic acid (DOTA).

2. Results and Discussion

The synthesis of UA-DOTA conjugates started with the structural modification of cyclen (**2**) as illustrated in Scheme 1. Treatment of **2** with 3 equiv. of sodium bicarbonate and 3 equiv. of the respective bromoacetic ester (**3–5**) in dry acetonitrile yielded triple substituted cyclen derivatives **6–8**, being ready to be coupled with ursolic acid. We decided to use *tert*-butyl, benzyl and allyl esters as protecting groups. Benzyl, as well as *tert*-butyl bromoacetate, were bought from commercial suppliers. Allyl bromoacetate was prepared from allylic alcohol and bromoacetyl bromide.

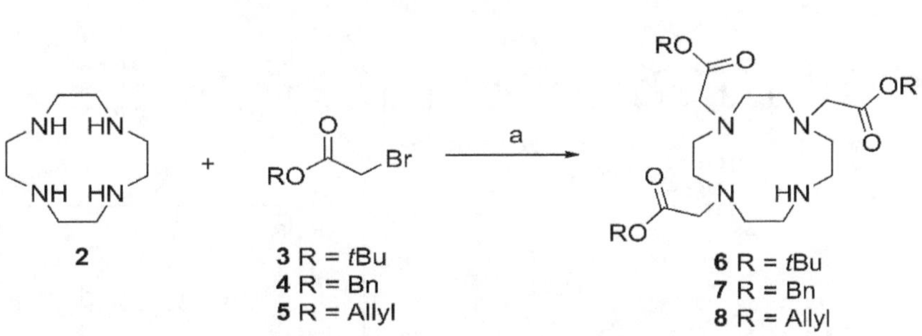

Scheme 1. Synthesis of DOTA precursors **6–8**: (a) $NaHCO_3$, MeCN, 25 °C, 48 h, yield: 50% (**6**), 68% (**7**), 63% (**8**).

Ursolic acid has also been modified before coupling with the DOTA precursors (Scheme 2). Derivatization started with the attachment of a spacer moiety using oxalyl chloride and 1-(2-aminoethyl)piperazine in dry dichloromethane affording compound **10**. The terminal amino moiety was further substituted with chloroacetyl chloride in dry dichloromethane to furnish the ursolic acid precursor **11** in excellent yield. Linkage of both precursors was performed in dry acetonitrile in the presence of potassium carbonate and potassium iodide yielding UA-DOTA conjugates **12–14**. Allylic esters of the acetate groups were removed by treating compound **14** with [$(PPh_3)_4Pd$], triphenylphosphane and pyrrolidine in acetonitrile at 25 °C for 3 days; this procedure gave **15** in almost quantitative yield. Purification of **15** was performed by reversed phase chromatography using MeOH/MeCN/TFA as eluent since the compound was difficult to eluate from normal silica phases. Furthermore, a synthetic approach for **15** starting from either **12** or **13** failed. Hydrogenation of **13** employing palladium catalysis retained the benzyl esters, and the deprotection of tert-butyl esters (as in compound **12**) using TFA/DCM resulted in a partial degradation of the triterpenoic backbone.

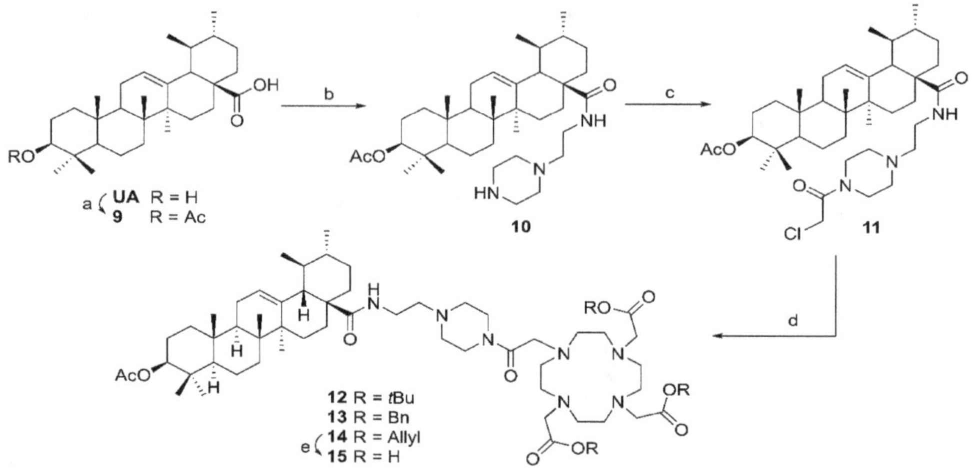

Scheme 2. Synthesis of ursolic acid chelator conjugates **12–15**: (**a**) Ac_2O, CH_2Cl_2, NEt_3, 25 °C, 2 days, 82%; (**b**) oxalyl chloride, CH_2Cl_2, DMF, 0–25 °C, 1 h, then 1-(2-Aminoethyl)piperazine, CH_2Cl_2, 25 °C, 2 h, yield: 82%; (**c**) chloroacetyl chloride, CH_2Cl_2, NEt_3, 25 °C, 30 min, yield: 91%; (**d**) K_2CO_3, KI, **6** (for **12**) or **7** (for **13**) or **8** (for **14**), MeCN, 25 °C, 48 h, yield: 54% (**12**), 82% (**13**), and 80% (**14**); (**e**) $[(PPh_3)_4Pd]$, PPh_3, pyrrolidine, MeCN, 25 °C, 3 days, yield: 96%.

The synthetic approach summarized in Scheme 2 can also be applied to various other spacer units. Thus, we decided to alter the amino component. Therefore, ursolic acid was treated with piperazine, ethylene diamine and 2,2'-oxybis(ethylamine), to furnish ursolic carboxamides **16–18** (Scheme 3), respectively. Chloroacetyl derivatives **19–21** and UA-DOTA conjugates **22–27** were prepared analogous to Scheme 2.

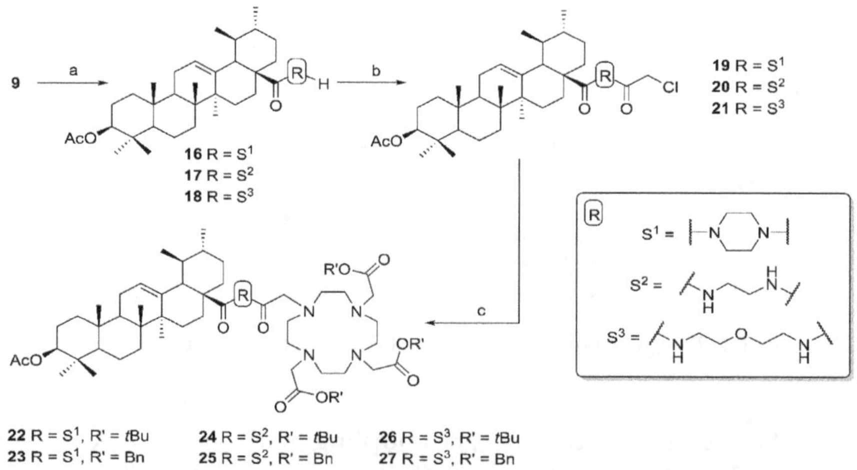

Scheme 3. Synthesis of ursolic acid DOTA conjugates **22–27**: (**a**) oxalyl chloride, CH_2Cl_2, DMF, 0–25 °C, 1 h, then amine, CH_2Cl_2, 25 °C, 2 h, yield: 80% (**16** and **17**), and 78% (**18**); (**b**) chloroacetyl chloride, CH_2Cl_2, NEt_3, 25 °C, 0.5–4 h, yield: 94% (**19**), and 91% (**20** and **21**); (**c**) K_2CO_3, KI, **6** (for **22, 24** and **26**) or **7** (for **23, 25** and **27**), MeCN, 25 °C, 5 days, yield: 88% (**22**), 72% (**23**), 73% (**24**), 75% (**25**), 74% (**26**), and 62% (**27**).

Additionally, an alternative synthetic approach was established for the preparation of the ethylene diamine-spacered UA-DOTA conjugate **29** (Scheme 4). Therefore carboxamide **28** was prepared either by deacetylation of **17** or directly from UA by amidation with ethylene diamine using EDC and HOBt in dry DMF. In the next step, DOTA-tris(*tert*-butyl ester) (DOTA-3T) was activated by preparing its HOBt ester. Adding **28** to this freshly prepared ester furnished UA-DOTA conjugate **29**. For comparison, compound **29** was also synthesized from **24** by removing the C-3 acetyloxy moiety. Due to the presence of an unprotected hydroxyl moiety at this position, compound **29** offers the possibility for a set of modifications and is therefore considered to be a good starting material for further modifications.

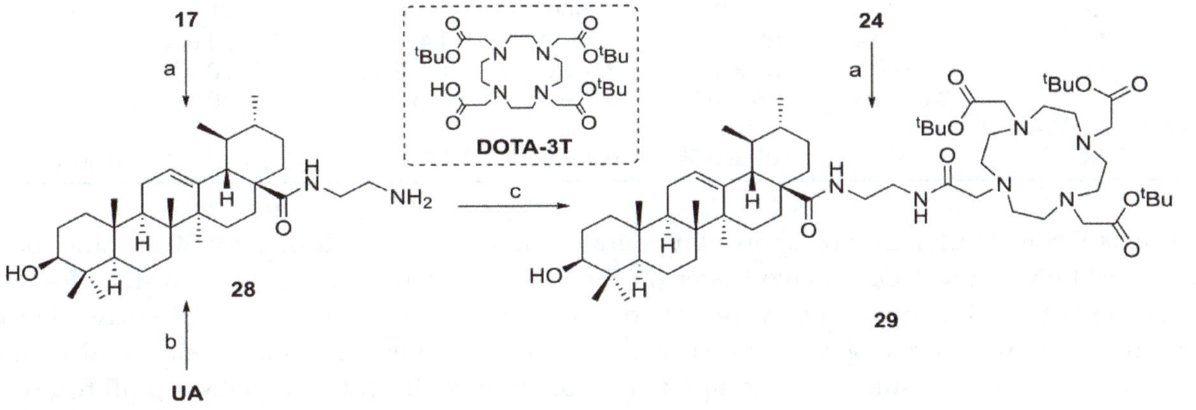

Scheme 4. Synthesis of ursolic acid derivative **29**: (**a**) KOH, MeOH, 25 °C, 48 h (for **28**) or 24 h (for **29**), yield: 85% (**28**) or 86% (**29**); (**b**) ethylene diamine, HOBt·H_2O, EDC·HCl, DMF, 25 °C, 24 h, yield: 46% (**c**) DOTA-3T, HOBt·H_2O, EDC·HCl, DMF, 25 °C, 5 days, yield: 49%.

Both synthetic approaches for the preparation of **29** (Figure 2) hold advantages but also some disadvantages. Although route A (5 steps) is significantly longer than B, but the former route gave the highest overall yield (44%). Approach B is a rather short and quick way to synthesize **29** (2 steps only), but the overall yield (23%) is barely half as high as in route A. Combining routes A and B, as shown in approach C led to compound **29** in 4 steps with an overall yield of 32%. A major difference between the approaches A and B is the availability and preparation of the DOTA precursors. Both, DOTA-tris(tert-butyl ester) and DO3A-tert-butyl ester (**6**) are available from commercial suppliers, with DOTA-3T being almost twice as expensive as **6**. Most advantageous is the one-step synthesis of **6** starting from cylcen (**2**), since **2** is commercially available for a price, being almost tenfold lower than that of **6**.

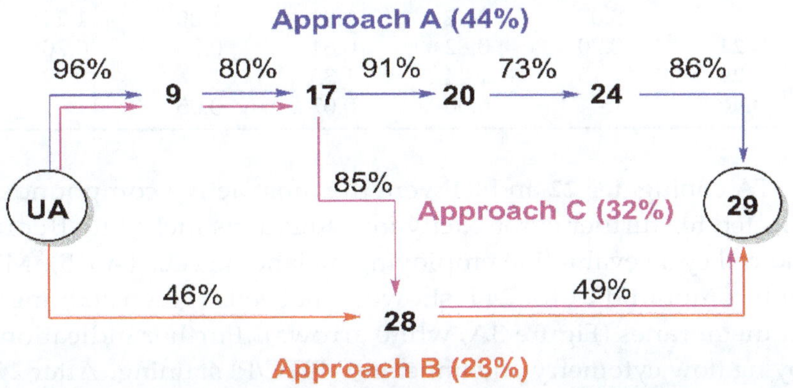

Figure 2. Comparison of synthetic routes **A**, **B**, and **C** for the preparation of UA-DOTA conjugate **29**.

Due to cytotoxicity evaluation, the prepared UA-DOTA conjugates were screened in rhodamine B assays employing a series of human tumor cell lines and non-malignant mouse fibroblasts (NIH 3T3). Results of this investigation are summarized in Table 1.

Table 1. Cytotoxicity of UA-DOTA conjugates (**12–15, 22–27, 29**), DOTA precursors (**6,7**), ursolic acid (UA), and doxorubicin hydrochloride (DRC): EC_{50} values from SRB assays after 72 h of treatment are given in μM (n.d. not detected; n.s. not soluble); the values are averaged from three independent experiments each performed in triplicate; confidence interval CI = 95%.

	A375	A2780	HT29	MCF-7	FaDu	NIH 3T3
UA	n.d.	11.7 ± 0.6	10.6 ± 0.7	12.7 ± 0.1	n.d.	13.1 ± 1.1
6	12.4 ± 2.7	10.5 ± 3.0	8.7 ± 2.7	11.3 ± 2.3	9.5 ± 0.9	17.3 ± 0.1
7	4.7 ± 0.3	3.8 ± 0.3	2.0 ± 0.2	4.1 ± 0.5	3.9 ± 0.7	4.5 ± 0.3
13	n.d.	2.1 ± 0.4	4.0 ± 0.4	3.3 ± 0.2	6.0 ± 0.1	3.6 ± 0.5
15	>60	>60	>60	>60	>60	>60
22	1.5 ± 0.4	1.9 ± 0.3	5.7 ± 0.5	4.4 ± 0.7	3.7 ± 0.6	4.6 ± 1.0
24	2.0 ± 0.1	1.7 ± 0.1	2.3 ± 0.3	1.8 ± 0.1	2.0 ± 0.2	1.4 ± 0.1
29	2.0 ± 0.3	1.6 ± 0.5	1.7 ± 0.4	n.d.	2.9 ± 0.4	2.3 ± 0.7
12, 14, 23, 25–27	n.s.	n.s	n.s	n.s.	n.s.	n.s.
DRC	n.d.	0.01 ± 0.01	0.9 ± 0.2	1.1 ± 0.3	n.d.	0.06 ± 0.03

The DO3A-tert-butyl ester (**6**) showed moderate cytotoxicity as indicated by EC_{50} values between 10 μM and 14 μM, while DO3A-benzyl ester (**7**) showed EC_{50} values lower than 5 μM. Unfortunately, most of the UA-DOTA conjugates were not soluble in solvents suitable for SRB assays. However, combining **7** with ursolic acid gave cytotoxic conjugate **13**, showing EC_{50} values below 6 μM. Removal of ester units (as in **15**) resulted in a complete loss of cytotoxicity (EC_{50} >60 μM for all tumor cells). Compounds **22** and **24**, both holding tert-butyl esters but different spacer units were also highly cytotoxic. Piperazine-spacered conjugate **22** showed the highest cytotoxicity observed in this screening for A375 tumor cells (EC_{50} = 1.5 ± 0.4 μM), while being quite selective, too (SI (NIH 3T3/A375) = 3.07, Table 2). EC_{50} values of ethylenediamine-spacered conjugate **24** were below 2.5 μM for all tumor cell lines. The highest cytotoxicity was observed for ovarian carcinoma (A2780, EC_{50} = 1.7 ± 0.1 μM). Removal of the acetyloxy moiety of **24** (as in **29**) had almost no significant impact on cytotoxicity.

Table 2. Selectivity of selected UA-DOTA conjugates (**13, 22, 24,** and **29**), DOTA precursors (**6, 7**), ursolic acid (UA) and doxorubicin hydrochloride (DRC): Selectivity index (SI) is defined as: SI = EC_{50} (NIH 3T3)/EC_{50} (tumor cell line).

	A375	A2780	HT29	MCF-7	FaDu
UA	-	1.12	1.24	1.03	-
6	1.40	1.65	1.99	1.53	1.82
7	0.96	1.18	2.25	1.10	1.15
13	-	1.71	0.90	1.09	0.60
22	3.07	2.42	0.81	1.05	1.24
24	0.70	0.82	0.61	0.78	0.70
29	1.15	1.44	1.35	-	0.79
DRC	-	6.00	0.07	0.05	-

Because UA-DOTA conjugates **22** and **24** were the most active compounds of this study, these compounds were selected for further cytotoxicity investigations including fluorescence microscopy, annexin V assays, and cell cycle evaluation employing melanoma cells (A375). Microscopic images of A375 cells treated with compound **24** for 24 h showed vital cells (green staining) with some of them having ruptured cell membranes (Figure 3A, white arrows). Further indications of apoptosis have been detected employing flow cytometry and annexin V-FITC/PI staining. After 24 h 63% of the tumor cells treated with **24** were annexin V-FITC-positive, and 51.9% of all cells having died by apoptosis. Additionally, the number of vital cells decreased in comparison to the control from 86.1% to 36.7 % (Figure 3B). An extra investigation of the cell cycle showed a decreased number of cells in G1/G0, G2/M, as well as in S phase. Additionally, a large population of cells has been shifted into the subG1 region (Figure 3C).

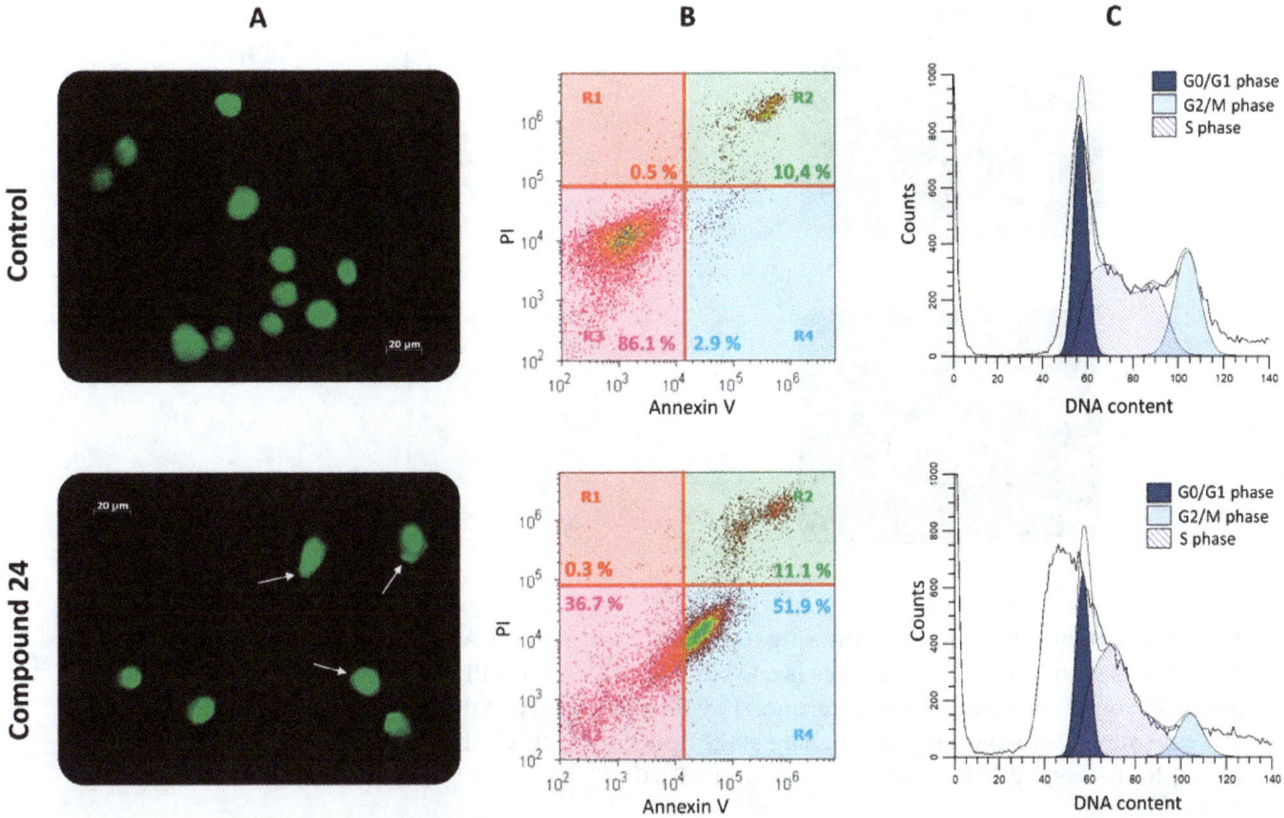

Figure 3. Extended cytotoxicity investigation after treatment of A375 cells with **24** (4.0 µM) for 24 h: (**A**) Fluorescence microscopic images (scale bar 20 µm), AO and PI were used; (**B**) Annexin V-FITC/PI assay. Examples of density plots determined by flow cytometry (Attune® Cytometric Software v 1.2.5), R1: necrotic, R2: secondary necrotic/late stage apoptotic, R3: vital, R4: apoptotic; (**C**) Representative examples for cell cycle evaluation via ModFit LT 5.0.

Fluorescence microscopic images and density plots of A375 cells treated with **22** for 24 h showed no significant differences in comparison to the control (Supplementary material, Figure S1). Therefore, further investigations were performed with a prolonged incubation time of 48 h. After treating A375 cells with compound **22** for 48 h, subsequent fluorescence microscopic investigations using AO/PI staining showed ruptures of the plasma membrane (Figure 4A, white arrows). Additionally, some necrotic/late stage apoptotic cells were observed, indicated by slightly orange stained nuclei (Figure 4 A, orange arrow). The density plot of A375 cells treated with **22** for 48 h showed a decreased number of vital cells (66.3%) compared to the control (86.0%), while 32.9% of the cells were considered annexin V-FITC-positive. Nearly half of them (17.4% of all cells) have died by apoptosis, and the remaining cells (15.5% of all cells) were secondary necrotic/late stage apoptotic (Figure 4 B). During extra investigations of the cell cycle, some differences compared to the control have been observed. Cells treated with **22** for 48 h showed a quite broad and flat DNA distribution. G1/G0, G2/M, and S phase were drastically reduced, while an increased population of cells with reduced DNA content has been observed in the subG1 region (Figure 4C).

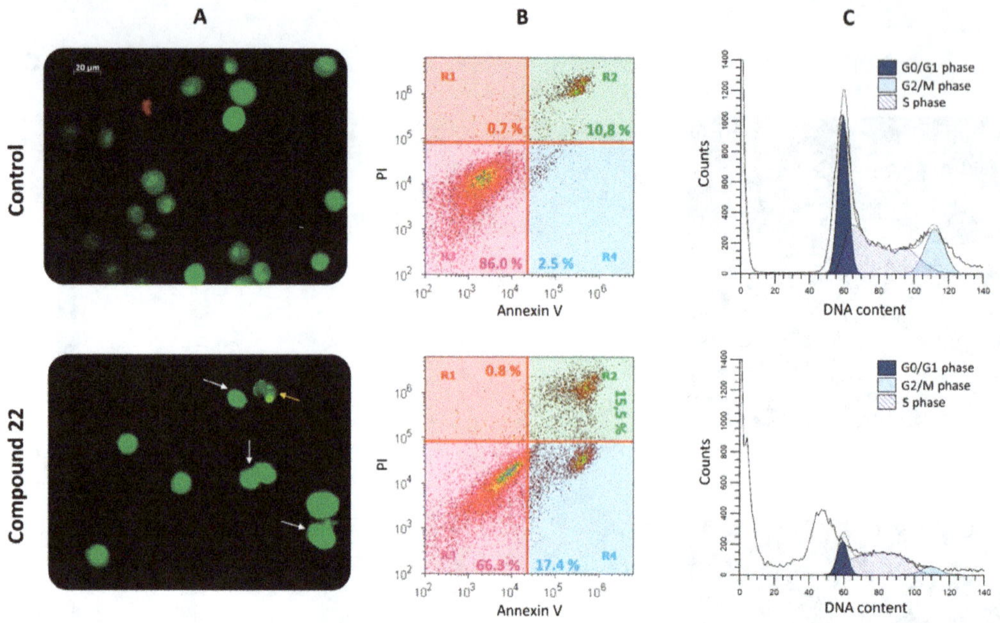

Figure 4. Extended cytotoxicity investigation after treatment of A375 cells with **22** (3.0 µM) for 48 h: (**A**) Fluorescence microscopic images (scale bar 20 µm), AO and PI were used; (**B**) Annexin V-FITC/PI assay. Examples of density plots determined by flow cytometry (Attune® Cytometric Software vl 1.2.5), R1: necrotic, R2: secondary necrotic/late stage apoptotic, R3: vital, R4: apoptotic; (**C**) Representative examples for cell cycle evaluation via ModFit LT 5.0.

3. Conclusions

In this study, a series of overall 11 amine-spacered UA-DOTA conjugates have been prepared starting from the natural occurring triterpenoid ursolic acid (UA). We hereby report a synthetic approach to UA-DOTA conjugates, which is applicable for several amine spacers and other triterpenoic backbones, too. Additionally, we compared three synthetic approaches for the preparation of compound **29** in terms of yield, number of steps and precursor availability. This conjugate offers the possibility for further modifications at the C-3 hydroxylic group, which is known to influence cytotoxicity. All of the prepared DOTA conjugates were screened in SRB assays showing some compounds to be of good cytotoxicity. EC_{50} values were determined to range from 17.3 µM to 1.4 µM. The most active compound of this series was a piperazinyl spacered conjugate **22** showing low EC_{50} values such as 1.5 ± 0.4 µM for A375 tumor cells and 1.9 ± 0.3 µM for A2780 tumor cells, respectively, while showing good selectivity (SI (NIH 3T3(A375) = 3.07), too. Unfortunately, the selectivity of the other screened conjugates was quite low. Additional cytotoxicity investigations such as fluorescence microscopy, annexin V assays, and cell cycle analyses were performed employing the UA-DOTA conjugates **22** and **24** to gain information about their mode of action. The results of these extended biological testing indicate **24** to induce death of A375 cancer cells by apoptosis. These results hold some starting points for further studies. Conjugate **15** and structural related compounds (holding free carboxylic acids at the DOTA unit) are currently subjects of ongoing investigations regarding their ability to form complexes with metal ions or radioactive isotopes like ^{68}Ga to examine possible future uses as tracer or contrast agents in molecular imaging techniques, such as positron emission tomography (PET) [22].

4. Materials and Methods

4.1. General

NMR spectra were recorded using the Varian spectrometers Gemini 2000 or Unity 500 (Varian GmbH, Darmstadt, Germany) δ given in ppm, *J* in Hz; typical experiments: APT, H-H-COSY,

HMBC, HSQC, NOESY), MS spectra were taken on a Finnigan MAT LCQ 7000 (ThermoFisher Scientific, Braunschweig, Germany) electrospray, voltage 4.1 kV, sheath gas nitrogen) instrument. The optical rotations were measured on a Perkin-Elmer polarimeter (Perkin Elmer LAS, Rodgau, Germany) or on a Jasco P-2000 polarimeter (Jasco Germany, Pfungstadt, Germany) at 20 °C; TLC was performed on NP or RP18 silica gel (Macherey-Nagel, detection with cerium molybdate or Dragendorff's reagent). Melting points are uncorrected (*Leica* hot stage microscope, or BUCHI melting point M-565), and elemental analyses were performed on a Foss-Heraeus Vario EL (CHNS, Elementar Analysensysteme GmbH, Langenselbold, Germany) unit. IR spectra were recorded on a Perkin Elmer FT-IR spectrometer Spectrum 1000 or on a Perkin-Elmer Spectrum Two (UATR Two Unit; both instruments from Perkin Elmer LAS, Rodgau, Germany). UV-VIS spectra were taken on a Perkin-Elmer Lambda 14 spectrometer or on a Perkin-Elmer Lambda 750 S (UV/VIS/NIR) spectrometer (both instruments from Perkin Elmer LAS, Rodgau, Germany). The solvents were dried according to usual procedures. The purity of the compounds was determined by HPLC and found to be >96%.

4.2. Cytotoxicity

4.2.1. Cell Lines and Culture Conditions

The cell lines used are human cancer cell lines: A2780 (ovarian carcinoma), HT29 (colon adenocarcinoma), MCF-7 (breast adenocarcinoma), A375 (melanoma), FaDu (pharynx squamous cell carcinoma) and non-malignant mouse fibroblasts NIH 3T3; all cell lines were obtained from the Department of Oncology (Martin-Luther-University Halle-Wittenberg). Cultures were maintained as monolayers in RPMI 1640 medium with L-glutamine (Capricorn Scientific GmbH, Ebsdorfergrund, Germany) supplemented with 10% heat inactivated fetal bovine serum (Sigma-Aldrich Chemie GmbH, Steinheim, Germany) and penicillin/streptomycin (Capricorn Scientific GmbH, Ebsdorfergrund, Germany) at 37 °C in a humidified atmosphere with 5% CO_2.

4.2.2. Cytotoxic Assay (SRB)

The cytotoxicity of the compounds was evaluated using the sulforhodamine-B (Kiton-Red S, ABCR) micro culture colorimetric assay. Cells were seeded into 96-well plates on day 0 at appropriate cell densities to prevent confluence of the cells during the period of experiment. After 24 h, the cells were treated with six different concentrations (1, 3, 7, 12, 20, and 30 μM) minimum. The final concentration of DMSO/DMF never exceeded 0.5%, which was non-toxic to the cells. After a 72-h treatment, the supernatant medium from the 96-well plates was discarded, the cells were fixed with 10% trichloroacetic acid (TCA) and allowed to rest at 4 °C. After 24 h fixation, the cells were washed in a strip washer and dyed with SRB solution (100 μL, 0.4%, in 1% acetic acid) for about 20 min. After dying, the plates were washed four times with 1% acetic acid to remove the excess of the dye and allowed to air-dry overnight. Tris base solution (200 μL, 10 mM) was added to each well and absorbance was measured at λ = 570 nm using a 96 well plate reader (Tecan Spectra, Crailsheim, Germany). The EC_{50} values were averaged from three independent experiments performed each in triplicate calculated from semi logarithmic dose response curves applying a non-linear 4P Hills-slope equation (GraphPad Prism5; variables top and bottom were set to 100 and 0, respectively).

4.2.3. AO/PI Dye Exclusion Test

Morphological characteristics of cell death were analyzed employing an AO/PI assay using human cancer cell line A375. Approx. 2×10^5 cells were seeded in cell culture flasks (25 cm^2), and the cells were allowed to grow up for 24 h. After removing of the used medium, the substance loaded fresh medium was reloaded (or a blank new medium as a control). After 24 h and 48 h, the content of the flask was collected and centrifuged (1200 rpm, 4 °C), the pellet was gently suspended in phosphate-buffered saline (PBS (w/Ca^{2+} and Mg^{2+}), 1 mL) and centrifuged again. The PBS was removed, and the pellet gently suspended in PBS (150 μL) again. The analysis of the cells was performed using a fluorescence microscope after having mixed the cell suspension (10 μL) with a solution of AO/PI (5 μg/mL, 10 μL).

4.2.4. Annexin V-FITC/PI Assay

Approximately 2×10^5 cells (A375) were seeded in cell culture flasks (25 cm^2), and the cells were allowed to grow up for 24 h. After removing of the used medium, the substance loaded fresh medium was reloaded (or a blank fresh medium as a control). After 24 h and 48 h, the cells were harvested, centrifuged (1200 rpm, 4 °C), and washed twice with PBS (w/Ca^{2+} and Mg^{2+}, 1 mL). The cells were counted and approximately $1{\cdot}10^6$ cells were washed with Annexin V binding buffer (BioLegend®, San Diego, USA) and treated with propidium iodide solution (3 μL, 1 mg/mL) and Annexin V-FITC (5 μL, BioLegend®, San Diego, CA, USA) for 15 min in the dark at room temperature. After adding Annexin V binding buffer (400 μL) the suspension was analyzed using Attune® FACS machine. After gating for living cells, the data from detectors BL-1A and BL-3A were collected (20,000 events) in technical triplicates. The assay was performed in duplicates; cell distribution was calculated using Attune® Software (ThermoFisher Scientific, Braunschweig, Germany).

4.2.5. Cell Cycle Investigations

Approximately 2×10^5 cells (A375) were seeded in cell culture flasks (25 cm^2), and the cells were allowed to grow up for 24 h. After removing of the used medium, the substance loaded fresh medium was reloaded (or a blank fresh medium as a control). After 24 h or 48 h, respectively, only the adherent cells were harvested, centrifuged (1200 rpm, 4 °C), and washed twice with PBS ((*w*/*w*), 1 mL). The cells were counted and approximately 1×10^6 cells were fixed with ethanol (70%, 4 °C, 24 h). After centrifugation (4500 rpm, 4 °C) the cells were washed with PBS ((*w*/*w*), 1 mL) and centrifuged. The pellet was resuspended in 1 mL RNAse A containing PI buffer (100μL RNAse (100 mg/mL), 15 μL PI solution (1 mg/mL)) and after incubating for 30 min at room temperature in the dark, cells were analyzed using the Attune® FACS machine; collecting data from the BL-2A channel. Doublet cells were excluded from the measurements by plotting BL-2A against BL-2H. For each cell cycle distribution 20,000 events were collected in technical triplicates, each sample was measured in duplicates. Cell cycle distribution was calculated using ModFitLT™ (Verity Software House, Topsham, ME, USA).

4.3. *Syntheses*

4.3.1. General

Ursolic acid (**1**) was obtained from betulinines (Stříbrná Skalice, Czech Republic). 1,4,7,10-Tetraazacyclododecane (cyclen, **2**) was bought from abcr GmbH (Karlsruhe, Germany) in 95% purity. Benzyl bromoacetate (96%) and tert-Butyl bromoacetate (98%) were both purchased from Sigma-Aldrich Chemie GmbH (Steinheim, Germany). DOTA-tris(*tert*-butyl ester) was obtained from TCI Deutschland GmbH (Eschborn, Germany) in 97% purity. Ursolic acid derivatives **10**, **16–18** and **28** have been synthesized as previously reported [20,21]. Experimental procedures and full analytical data of these compounds can be found in the supplementary material [23,24].

4.3.2. General Procedure A for the Synthesis of DOTA Precursors (**6–8**)

To a suspension of cyclen (5.81 mmol) and sodium bicarbonate (17.43 mmol) in dry acetonitrile (100 mL), a solution of the respective bromoacetate (**3–5**, 17.43 mmol) in dry acetonitrile (10 mL) was added dropwise under argon atmosphere. The mixture was stirred for 48 h at 25 °C. After usual aqueous work-up, the solvent was removed under reduced pressure, and the crude products were subjected to column chromatography (silica gel, chloroform/methanol mixtures) affording DOTA precursors **6–8** (50–68%).

4.3.3. General Procedure B for the Synthesis of Carboxamides (**10**, **16–18**)

Compound **9** (0.5 mmol) was dissolved in dry DCM (10 mL), cooled to 0 °C and oxalyl chloride (3.2 mmol) and dry DMF (2 drops) were added. After warming to 25 °C, the mixture was stirred for 1 h. The solvent was removed under reduced pressure, re-evaporated with dry THF (4 × 15 mL), and the residue was immediately resolved in dry DCM (10 mL). This mixture was then added dropwise to a solution of the amine (3.0 mmol) in dry DCM (2 mL) and stirred at 25 °C for 2 h. After usual aqueous work-up, the solvent was removed under reduced pressure, and the crude products were subjected to column chromatography (silica gel, chloroform/methanol mixtures). Compounds **10** and **16–18** were each obtained as colorless solids (78–82%).

4.3.4. General Procedure C for the Alkylation with Chloroacetyl Chloride (**11**, **19–21**)

Chloroacetyl chloride (2.20 mmol) was added dropwise to a solution of the respective carboxamide (**10**, **16–18**; 1.43 mmol) and triethylamine (0.71 mmol) in dry dichloromethane (75 mL). The mixture was stirred at 25 °C for 0.5–4 h. After usual aqueous work-up, the solvent was removed under reduced pressure, and the crude products were subjected to column chromatography (silica gel, chloroform/acetone mixtures). Compounds **11** and **19–21** were each obtained as colorless solids (91%–94%).

4.3.5. General Procedure D for the Synthesis of Ursolic Acid Chelator Conjugates (**12–14**, **22–27**)

To a solution of the respective chloroacetyl derivative (**11**, **19–21**; 0.44 mmol) and freshly grounded potassium carbonate (0.83 mmol) in dry acetonitrile (15 mL) was added potassium iodide (0.35 mmol) and the respective DOTA precursor (**6–8**, 0.41 mmol in 5 mL dry acetonitrile). The mixture was stirred for 2–5 days at 25 °C. After completion of the reaction (as indicated by TLC) the mixture was filtered, and the solvent was removed under reduced pressure. The crude products were subjected to column chromatography (silica gel, chloroform/methanol mixtures) to afford compounds **12–14** and **22–27** (yield: 54–88%), respectively.

Allyl bromoacetate (**5**), To a solution of allyl alcohol (0.62 mol), bromo acetylbromide (0.1 mol) was added dropwise over a period of 30 min at 0 °C under argon atmosphere. The mixture was stirred for 1 h at 0 °C, warmed to 25 °C and stirred for another 3 h. The solvent was removed under reduced pressure and the residue was dissolved in dichloromethane. After usual aqueous work-up, the solvent was removed under reduced pressure, and the crude product was purified by vacuum distillation affording allyl bromoacetate as colorless oil (68%). ^{1}H NMR (400 MHz, $CDCl_3$): δ = 5.88 (*ddt*, *J* = 16.5, 11.0, 5.8 Hz, 1H, $CH{=}CH_2$), 5.38–5.17 (*m*, 2H, $CH{=}CH_2$), 4.61 (*dt*, *J* = 5.8, 1.4 Hz, 2H, $CH_2CH{=}CH_2$), 3.82 (*s*, 2H, $BrCH_2$) ppm; ^{13}C NMR (101 MHz, $CDCl_3$): δ = 166.8 (C=O), 131.2 ($CH{=}CH_2$), 119.0 ($CH{=}CH_2$), 66.6 ($CH_2CH{=}CH_2$), 25.8 ($BrCH_2$) ppm.

Tri-tert-butyl 2,2′,2″-(1,4,7,10-tetraazacyclododecane-1,4,7-triyl)triacetate (**6**), Compound **6** was prepared from **2** according to general procedure A using *tert*-butyl bromoacetate (**3**). Column chromatography (SiO_2, $CHCl_3$/MeOH 9:1) gave **6** (yield: 50%); m.p. 180–182 °C (lit.: 181–183 °C [25]); R_f = 0.27 ($CHCl_3$/MeOH 95:5); IR (ATR): ν = 2974*w*, 2943*w*, 2912*w*, 2853*w*, 2736*w*, 1718*s*, 1576*w*, 1466*w*, 1453*w*, 1412*w*, 1392*w*, 1368*m*, 1330*w*, 1255*m*, 1218*w*, 1147*s*, 1117*m*, 1099*m*, 1050*w*, 935*m*, 873*m*, 848*m* cm^{-1}; ^{1}H NMR (400 MHz, $CDCl_3$): δ = 3.36 (*s*, 4H, 2 × CH_2 (acetate)), 3.28 (*s*, 2H, CH_2 (acetate)), 3.12–3.06 (*m*, 4H, 2 × CH_2 (cyclen)), 2.95–2.84 (*m*, 12H, 6 × CH_2 (cyclen)), 1.45 (*s*, 18H, 6 × CH_3 (*t*-butyl)), 1.45 (*s*, 9H, 3 × CH_3 (*t*-butyl)) ppm; ^{13}C NMR (101 MHz, $CDCl_3$): δ = 170.6 (2 × CO, acetate), 169.8 (CO, acetate), 81.9 (C_q, *t*-butyl), 81.8 (2 × C_q, *t*-butyl), 58.4 (2 × CH_2, acetate), 51.5 (2 × CH_2, cyclen), 51.4 (2 × CH_2, cyclen), 49.4 (2 × CH_2, cyclen), 49.0 (CH_2, acetate), 47.7 (2 × CH_2, cyclen), 28.4 (3 × CH_3, *t*-butyl), 28.3 (6 × CH_3, *t*-butyl) ppm; MS (ESI, MeOH): *m*/*z* = 515.3 (100%, $[M + H]^+$), 537.3 (10%, $[M + Na]^+$); analysis calcd for $C_{26}H_{50}N_4O_6$ (514.71): C 60.67, H 9.79, N 10.89; found: C 60.51, H 9.98, N 10.67.

Tribenzyl 2,2′,2″-(1,4,7,10-tetraazacyclododecane-1,4,7-triyl)triacetate (**7**). Compound **7** was prepared from **2** according to general procedure A using benzyl bromoacetate (**4**). Column chromatography (SiO_2, $CHCl_3$/MeOH 9:1) gave **7** (yield: 68%); R_f = 0.32 ($CHCl_3$/MeOH 95:5); IR (KBr): ν = 2948*w*, 2857*w*, 2738*w*, 1732*s*, 1586*w*, 1498*w*, 1455*m*, 1418*w*, 1381*w*, 1314*w*, 1169*s*, 1096*m*, 1049*m*, 994*m*, 739*s*, 697*s* cm^{-1}; UV-Vis ($CHCl_3$): λ_{max} (logε) = 251 nm (2.87), 258 nm (2.86), 263 nm (2.76); ^1H NMR (400 MHz, $CDCl_3$): δ = 7.40–7.29 (*m*, 15H, 15 × CH (Bn)), 5.13 (*s*, 4H, 2 × CH_2 (Bn)), 5.13 (*s*, 2H, CH_2 (Bn)), 3.48 (*s*, 4H, 2 × CH_2 (acetate)), 3.41 (*s*, 2H, CH_2 (acetate)), 3.12–3.05 (*m*, 4H, 2 × CH_2 (cyclen)), 2.93–2.79 (*m*, 12H, 6 × CH_2 (cyclen)) ppm; ^{13}C NMR (101 MHz, $CDCl_3$): δ = 171.1 (2 × CO, acetate), 170.3 (CO, acetate), 135.5 (C_i, Bn), 128.8 (CH, Bn), 128.8 (CH, Bn), 128.7 (CH, Bn), 128.7 (CH, Bn), 128.6 (CH, Bn), 66.8 (CH_2, Bn), 57.4 (2 × CH_2, acetate), 51.9 (2 × CH_2, cyclen), 51.7 (2 × CH_2, cyclen), 49.6 (2 × CH_2, cyclen), 48.8 (CH_2, acetate), 47.5 (2 × CH_2, cyclen) ppm; MS (ESI, MeOH): *m/z* = 309.0 (10%, $[M + 2H]^{2+}$), 617.4 (100%, $[M + H]^+$), 639.3 (10%, $[M + Na]^+$); analysis calcd for $C_{35}H_{44}N_4O_6$ (616.76): C 68.16, H 7.19, N 9.08; found: C 67.84, H 7.39, N 8.81.

Triallyl 2,2′,2″-(1,4,7,10-tetraazacyclododecane-1,4,7-triyl)triacetate (**8**), Compound **8** was prepared from **2** according to general procedure A using allyl bromoacetate (**5**). Column chromatography (SiO_2, $CHCl_3$/MeOH 95:5) gave **8** (yield: 63%); R_f = 0.27 ($CHCl_3$/MeOH 95:5); IR (KBr): ν = 2945*w*, 2858*w*, 2743*w*, 1731*s*, 1673*w*, 1648*w*, 1455*w*, 1420*w*, 1364*w*, 1314*w*, 1179*s*, 1095*m*, 985*s*, 928*s* cm^{-1}; ^1H NMR (400 MHz, $CDCl_3$): δ = 5.93–5.81 (*m*, 3H, 3 × CH (allyl)), 5.32–5.20 (*m*, 6H, 3 × CH_2 (allyl)), 4.60–4.53 (*m*, 6H, 3 × CH_2 (allyl)), 3.49 (*s*, 4H, 2 × CH_2 (acetate)), 3.41 (*s*, 2H, CH_2 (acetate)), 3.12–3.06 (*m*, 4H, 2 × CH_2 (cyclen)), 2.96–2.81 (*m*, 12H, 6 × CH_2 (cyclen)) ppm; ^{13}C NMR (101 MHz, $CDCl_3$): δ = 170.8 (2 × CO, acetate), 170.0 (CO, acetate), 131.7 (2 × CH, allyl), 131.7 (CH, allyl), 119.2 (CH_2, allyl), 119.0 (2 × CH_2, allyl), 65.5 (2 × CH_2, allyl), 65.4 (CH_2, allyl), 57.3 (2 × CH_2, acetate), 51.7 (2 × CH_2, cyclen), 51.6 (2 × CH_2, cyclen), 49.4 (2 × CH_2, cyclen), 48.5 (CH_2, acetate), 47.4 (CH_2, cyclen) ppm; MS (ESI, MeOH): *m/z* = 234.1 (18%, $[M + 2H]^{2+}$), 467.3 (100%, $[M + H]^+$), 489.3 (10%, $[M + Na]^+$); analysis calcd for $C_{23}H_{38}N_4O_6$ (466.6): C 59.21, H 8.21, N 12.01; found: C 59.03, H 8.44, N 11.78.

(3β) 3-Acetyloxy-urs-12-en-28-oic acid (**9**), Compound **1** was prepared from ursolic acid according to the procedure given in the literature [26]. Yield: 96%; m.p. 287–290 °C (lit.: 289–290 °C [27]).

(3β) N-(2-(4-(2-Chloroacetyl)piperazin-1-yl)ethyl)-3-acetyloxy-urs-12-en-28-amide (**11**). Compound **11** was synthesized from **10** according to general procedure C. Column chromatography (SiO_2, $CHCl_3$/acetone 4:1) furnished compound **11** (91%); m.p. 124–129 °C; $[\alpha]_D$ = +32.3° (*c* 0.320, $CHCl_3$); R_f = 0.38 ($CHCl_3$/acetone 4:1); IR (KBr): ν = 3423*s*, 2947*s*, 1734*m*, 1654*s*, 1522*m*, 1458*m*, 1370*m*, 1247*s*, 1150*w*, 1027*m* cm^{-1}; ^1H NMR (400 MHz, $CDCl_3$): δ = 6.32 (*t*, *J* = 5.0 Hz, 1H, N*H*), 5.28 (*t*, *J* = 3.6 Hz, 1H, 12-H), 4.49 (*dd*, *J* = 10.4, 5.4 Hz, 1H, 3-H), 4.06 (*s*, 2H, 36-H), 3.72–3.47 (*m*, 4H, 34-H, 34′-H), 3.47–3.36 (*m*, 1H, 31-H_a), 3.25–3.15 (*m*, 1H, 31-H_b), 2.58–2.39 (*m*, 6H, 33-H, 32-H, 33′-H), 2.04 (*s*, 3H, Ac), 2.02–1.80 (*m*, 5H, 11-H_a, 11-H_b, 16-H_a, 22-H_a, 18-H), 1.79–1.70 (*m*, 1H, 16-H_b), 1.69–1.21 (*m*, 13H, 15-H_a, 1-H_a, 2-H_a, 2-H_b, 9-H, 6-H_a, 21-H_a, 7-H_a, 22-H_b, 19-H, 6-H_b, 21-H_b, 7-H_b), 1.09 (*s*, 3H, 27-H), 1.08–1.01 (*m*, 2H, 1-H_b, 15-H_b), 0.96–0.94 (*m*, 4H, 20-H, 30-H), 0.93 (*s*, 3H, 25-H), 0.89–0.86 (*m*, 3H, 29-H), 0.86 (*s*, 3H, 23-H), 0.85 (*s*, 3H, 24-H), 0.84–0.79 (*m*, 1H, 5-H), 0.78 (*s*, 3H, 26-H) ppm; ^{13}C NMR (101 MHz, $CDCl_3$): δ = 178.1 (C-28), 171.1 (Ac), 165.2 (C-35), 140.0 (C-13), 125.3 (C-12), 80.9 (C-3), 56.7 (C-32), 55.4 (C-5), 54.2 (C-18), 53.0 (C-33), 52.5 (C-33′), 48.0 (C-17), 47.6 (C-9), 46.5 (C-34), 42.6 (C-14), 42.4 (C-34′), 40.9 (C-36), 39.9 (C-19), 39.7 (C-8), 39.3 (C-20) 38.4 (C-1), 37.8 (C-4), 37.5 (C-22), 37.0 (C-10), 35.9 (C-31), 32.8 (C-7), 31.0 (C-21), 28.2 (C-23), 28.0 (C-15), 25.0 (C-16), 23.6 (C-2), 23.6 (C-11), 23.4 (C-27), 21.4 (Ac), 21.3 (C-30), 18.3 (C-6), 17.5 (C-29), 17.1 (C-26), 16.9 (C-24), 15.8 (C-25) ppm; MS (ESI, MeOH): m/z = 686.5 (100%, $[M + H]^+$); analysis calcd for $C_{40}H_{64}ClN_3O_4$ (686.42): C 69.99, H 9.40, N 6.12; found: C 69.70, H 9.63, N 6.02.

Tris-t-butyl 2′,2″-[10-[2-[4-[2-(3β-acetyloxy-urs-12-en-28-oylamino)ethyl]piperazin-1-yl]-2-oxoethyl]-1,4,7,10-tetraazacyclododecane-1,4,7-triyl]triacetate (**12**), Compound **12** was synthesized from **6** and **11** according to general procedure D. Column chromatography (SiO_2, $CHCl_3$/MeOH 9:1) furnished compound

12 (54%). m.p. 247–250 °C (decomp.); $[\alpha]_D$ = +18.9° (c 0.345, $CHCl_3$); R_f = 0.30 ($CHCl_3$/MeOH 9:1); IR (KBr): ν = 2931*m*, 1727*s*, 1644*s*, 1529*w*, 1455*m*, 1425*w*, 1368*s*, 1306*m*, 1228*s*, 1159*s*, 1105*s*, 1005*m*, 755*m* cm^{-1}; ^1H NMR (400 MHz, $CDCl_3$): δ = 6.38 (*s*, 1H, NH), 5.26 (*t*, *J* = 3.4 Hz, 1H, 12-H), 4.46 (*dd*, *J* = 10.5, 5.2 Hz, 1H, 3-H), 3.92–2.04 (*m*, 36H, 34-H, 34′-H, 36-H, 3 × CH_2 (acetate), 31-H_a, 31-H_b, 8 × CH_2 (cyclen), 32-H, 33-H, 33′-H), 2.01 (*s*, 3H, Ac), 2.00–1.68 (*m*, 4H, 16-H_a, 11-H_a, 11-H_b, 18-H), 1.69–1.14 (*m*, 14H, 16-H_b, 22-H_b, 15-H_a, 1-H_a, 2-H_a, 2-H_b, 9-H, 6-H_a, 21-H_a, 7-H_a, 19-H, 6-H_b, 21-H_b, 7-H_b), 1.42 (*s*, 27H, 9 × CH_3 (t-Butyl)), 1.05 (*s*, 3H, 27-H), 1.11–0.95 (*m*, 3H, 1-H_b, 15-H_b, 20-H), 0.91 (*d*, *J* = 6.1 Hz, 3H, 30-H), 0.90 (*s*, 3H, 25-H), 0.85 (*d*, *J* = 6.5 Hz, 3H, 29-H), 0.83 (*s*, 3H, 23-H), 0.82 (*s*, 3H, 24-H), 0.80–0.75 (*m*, 1H, 5-H), 0.74 (*s*, 3H, 26-H) ppm; ^{13}C NMR (100 MHz, $CDCl_3$): δ = 178.0 (C-28), 172.8 (CO, acetate), 171.0 (Ac), 169.8 (C-35), 139.8 (C-13), 125.3 (C-12), 81.9 (C_q, *t*-Butyl), 81.7 (2 × C_q, *t*-Butyl), 80.9 (C-3), 56.8 (C-32), 55.8 (3 × CH_2, acetate), 55.3 (C-5), 55.2 (C-36), 53.9 (C-18), 53.4 (8 × CH_2, cyclen), 52.2 (C-33, C-33′), 47.8 (C-17), 47.5 (C-9), 44.3 (C-34, C-34′), 42.5 (C-14), 39.8 (C-19), 39.7 (C-8), 39.1 (C-20), 38.4 (C-1), 37.8 (C-4), 37.4 (C-22), 36.9 (C-10), 35.7 (C-31), 32.8 (C-7), 31.0 (C-21), 28.2 (C-23), 28.0 (9 × CH_3, t-Butyl), 27.9 (C-15), 24.8 (C-16), 23.6 (C-2), 23.5 (C-11), 23.4 (C-27), 21.4 (Ac), 21.3 (C-30), 18.3 (C-6), 17.4 (C-29), 17.1 (C-26), 16.8 (C-24), 15.7 (C-25) ppm; MS (ESI, MeOH): *m/z* = 593.9 (100%, $[M + Na + H]^+$), 1186.7 (95%, $[M + Na]^+$); analysis calcd for $C_{66}H_{113}N_7O_{10}$ (1164.67): C 68.06, H 9.78, N 8.42; found: C 67.75, H 9.97, N 8.51.

Tribenzyl 2,2′,2″-[10-[2-[4-[2-(3β-acetyloxy-urs-12-en-28-oylamino)ethyl]piperazin-1-yl]-2-oxoethyl]-1,4,7,10-tetraazacyclododecane-1,4,7-triyl]triacetate (**13**). Compound **13** was synthesized from **7** and **11** according to general procedure D. Column chromatography (SiO_2, $CHCl_3$/MeOH 95:5) furnished compound **13** (82%). m.p. 142–146 °C; $[\alpha]_D$ = +14.5° (c 0.300, $CHCl_3$); R_f = 0.50 ($CHCl_3$/MeOH 9:1); IR (KBr): ν = 3440*s*, 2947*m*, 1734*s*, 1641*s*, 1456*m*, 1371*m*, 1310*w*, 1247*m*, 1197*s*, 1105*m*, 1006*w*, 750*m* cm^{-1}; UV-Vis ($CHCl_3$): λ_{max} (logε) = 257 nm (3.99); ^1H NMR (400 MHz, $CDCl_3$): δ = 7.36–7.24 (*m*, 15H, CH_{Ar}), 6.36–6.28 (*m*, 1H, NH), 5.27 (*t*, *J* = 3.7 Hz, 1H, 12-H), 5.21–5.13 (*m*, 4H, 2 × CH_2Bn), 5.12–5.05 (*m*, 2H, CH_2Bn), 4.47 (*dd*, *J* = 10.7, 5.1 Hz, 1H, 3-H), 3.72–2.81 (*m*, 12H, 34-H, 34′-H, 36-H, 3 × CH_2 (acetate)), 3.40–3.30 (*m*, 1H, 31-H_a), 3.22–3.14 (*m*, 1H, 31-H_b), 2.46–2.33 (*m*, 6H, 32-H, 33-H, 33′-H), 2.81–2.06 (*m*, 16H,8 × CH_2 (cyclen)), 2.03 (*s*, 3H, Ac), 2.00–1.68 (*m*, 6H, 16-H_a, 11-H_a, 11-H_b, 18-H, 22-H_a, 16-H_b), 1.68–1.20 (*m*, 13H, 15-H_a, 1-H_a, 2-H_a, 2-H_b, 9-H, 6-H_a, 21-H_a, 7-H_a, 22-H_b, 19-H, 6-H_b, 21-H_b, 7-H_b), 1.06 (*s*, 3H, 27-H), 1.05–0.94 (*m*, 3H, 1-H_b, 15-H_b, 20-H), 0.93 (*brs*, 3H, 30-H), 0.91 (*s*, 3H, 25-H), 0.85 (*d*, *J* = 5.7 Hz, 3H, 29-H), 0.85 (*s*, 3H, 23-H), 0.83 (*s*, 3H, 24-H), 0.82–0.77 (*m*, 1H, 5-H), 0.76 (*s*, 3H, 26-H) ppm; ^{13}C NMR (101 MHz, $CDCl_3$): δ = 177.9 (C-28), 173.5 (CO, acetate), 170.9 (Ac), 170.0 (C-35), 139.7 (C-13), 135.4 (C_{Ar}), 135.3 (C_{Ar}), 135.2 (C_{Ar}), 128.7 (CH_{Ar}), 128.6 (CH_{Ar}), 128.5 (CH_{Ar}), 128.3 (CH_{Ar}), 128.3 (CH_{Ar}), 128.2 (CH_{Ar}), 125.3 (CH_{Ar}), 80.8 (C-3), 67.0 (CH_2, Bn), 66.8 (CH_2, Bn), 56.7 (C-32), 55.4 (C-36), 55.3 (CH_2, acetate), 55.2 (C-5), 53.9 (C-18), 53.4 (CH_2, cyclen), 52.7 (C-33, C-33′), 47.7 (C-17), 47.4 (C-9), 42.4 (C-14), 39.7 (C-19), 39.5 (C-8), 39.0 (C-20), 38.3 (C-1), 37.6 (C-4), 37.3 (C-22), 36.8 (C-10), 35.8 (C-31), 32.7 (C-7), 30.9 (C-21), 28.0 (C-23), 27.8 (C-15), 24.8 (C-16), 23.5 (C-2), 23.4 (C-11), 23.2 (C-27), 21.3 (Ac), 21.2 (C-30), 18.1 (C-6), 17.3 (C-29), 17.0 (C-26), 16.7 (C-24), 15.6 (C-25) ppm; MS (ESI, MeOH): *m/z* = 634 (20%, $[M + 2H]^{2+}$), 645 (100%, $[M + H + Na]^{2+}$), 1289 (62%, $[M + Na]^+$); analysis calcd for $C_{75}H_{107}N_7O_{10}$ (1266.72): C 71.11, H 8.51, N 7.74; found: C 70.73, H 8.70, N 7.49.

Triallyl 2,2′,2″-[10-[2-[4-[2-(3β-acetyloxy-urs-12-en-28-oylamino)ethyl]piperazin-1-yl]-2-oxoethyl]-1,4,7,10-tetraazacyclododecane-1,4,7-triyl]triacetate (**14**). Compound **14** was synthesized from **8** and **11** according to general procedure D. Column chromatography (SiO_2, $CHCl_3$/MeOH 95:5) furnished compound **14** (80%); m.p. 159–163 °C (decomp.); $[\alpha]_D$ = +14.8° (c 0.310, $CHCl_3$); R_f = 0.35 (SiO_2, CHC13/MeOH 9:1); IR (KBr): ν = 3342*s*, 2946*m*, 2852*w*, 1734*s*, 1642*s*, 1522*w*, 1456*m*, 1386*w*, 1310*w*, 1246*m*, 1202*m*, 1106*m*, 1026*w* cm^{-1}; ^1H NMR (400 MHz, $CDCl_3$): δ = 6.35 (*s*, 1H, NH), 5.97 – 5.83 (*m*, 3H, 3 × CH (allyl)), 5.34–5.19 (*m*, 7H, 12-H, 3 × CH_2 (allyl)), 4.67–4.55 (*m*, 6H, 3 × CH_2 (allyl)), 4.47 (*dd*, *J* = 10.6, 5.3 Hz, 1H, 3-H), 3.72–2.97 (*m*, 14H, 34-H, 34′-H, 36-H, 3 × CH_2 (acetate), 31-H_a, 31-H_b), 2.97–2.14 (*m*, 22H, 8 × CH_2 (cyclen), 32-H, 33-H, 33′-H), 2.03 (*s*, 3H, Ac), 2.01–1.68 (*m*, 6H, 16-H_a, 11-H_a, 11-H_b, 18-H, 22-H_a, 16-H_b), 1.68–1.19 (*m*, 13H, 15-H_a, 1-H_a, 2-H_a, 2-H_b, 9-H, 6-H_a, 21-H_a, 7-H_a, 22-H_b, 19-H, 6-H_b,

21-H_b, 7-H_b), 1.07 (*s*, 3H, 27-H), 1.06–0.94 (*m*, 3H, 1-H_b, 15-H_b, 20-H), 0.94 (*d*, *J* = 6.5 Hz, 3H, 30-H), 0.92 (*s*, 3H, 25-H), 0.87 (*d*, *J* = 6.5 Hz, 3H, 29-H), 0.85 (*s*, 3H, 23-H), 0.83 (*s*, 3H, 24-H), 0.82–0.78 (*m*, 1H, 5-H), 0.76 (*s*, 3H, 26-H) ppm; ^{13}C NMR (101 MHz, $CDCl_3$): δ = 178.0 (C-28), 173.4 (2 × CO, acetate), 173.3 (CO, acetate), 171.1 (Ac), 170.0 (C-35), 139.8 (C-13), 131.9 (2 × CH, allyl), 131.7 (CH, allyl), 125.4 (C-12), 119.0 (CH_2, allyl), 118.8 (2 × CH_2, allyl), 80.9 (C-3), 66.0 (CH_2, allyl), 65.9 (2 × CH_2, allyl), 56.8 (C-32), 55.4 (C-36), 55.3 (C-5), 55.2 (3 × CH_2, acetate), 53.9 (C-18), 53.6 (8 x CH_2, cyclen), 52.7 (C-33, C-33′), 47.9 (C-17), 47.5 (C-9), 45.0 (C-34, C-34′), 42.6 (C-24), 39.8 (C-19), 39.7 (C-8), 39.1 (C-20), 38.4 (C-1), 37.8 (C-4), 37.4 (C-22), 37.0 (C-10), 35.9 (C-31), 32.8 (C-7), 31.0 (C-21), 28.2 (C-23), 27.9 (C-15), 24.9 (C-16), 23.6 (C-2), 23.6 (C-11), 23.3 (C-27), 21.4 (Ac), 21.3 (C-30), 18.3 (C-6), 17.4 (C-29), 17.1 (C-26), 16.8 (C-24), 15.7 (C-25) ppm; MS (ESI, MeOH): *m/z* = 569.8 (100%, $[M + Na + H]^+$), 1138.8 (52%, $[M + Na]^+$); analysis calcd for $C_{63}H_{101}N_7O_{10}$ (1116.54): C 67.77, H 9.12, N 8.78; found: C 67.50, H 9.37, N 8.43.

2,2′,2″-[10-[2-[4-[2-(3β-Acetyloxy-urs-12-en-28-oylamino)ethyl]piperazin-1-yl]-2-oxoethyl]-1,4,7,10-tetraazacyclododecane-1,4,7-triyl]triacetic acid (**15**). Triphenylphosphane (0.038 mmol), $[(PPh_3)_4Pd]$ (0.013 mmol) and pyrrolidine (0.290 mmol) were added to a solution of compound **14** (0.128 mmol) in acetonitrile (4 mL), and the mixture was stirred for 6 days at 25 °C. After filtration, the solvent was removed under reduced pressure, and the crude product was subjected to column chromatography (RP18, MeCN/MeOH/TFA 60:40:0.1) affording compound **15** as colorless solid (96%); m.p. 206–210 °C (decomp.); $[\alpha]_D$ = +17.1° (c 0.315, MeOH); R_f = 0.35 (RP18, ACN/TFA 100:1); IR (ATR): ν = 2925*w*, 1634*s*, 1371*m*, 1245*s*, 1199*s*, 1127*s*, 1026*m*, 829*m*, 800*m*, 719*m* cm^{-1}; ^{1}H NMR (400 MHz, CD_3OD): δ = 5.35 (*t*, *J* = 3.6 Hz, 1H, 12-H), 4.47 (*dd*, *J* = 11.0, 5.3 Hz, 1H, 3-H), 3.72–2.93 (*m*, 14H, 34-H, 34′-H, 36-H, 31-H_a, 31-H_b, 3 × CH_2 (acetate)), 2.91–2.20 (*m*, 22H, 32-H, 33-H, 33′-H, 8 × CH_2 (cyclen)), 2.09–2.06 (*m*, 1H, 18-H), 2.03 (*s*, 3H, Ac), 2.02–1.93 (*m*, 3H, 11-H_a, 11-H_b, 16-H_a), 1.84–1.23 (*m*, 15H, 15-H_a, 22-H_a, 1-H_a, 16-H_b, 2-H_a, 2-H_b, 9-H, 7-H_a, 6-H_a, 21-H_a, 22-H_b, 19-H, 6-H_b, 21-H_b, 7-H_b), 1.15 (*s*, 3H, 27-H), 1.12–0.96 (*m*, 3H, 15-H_b, 1-H_b, 20-H), 0.99 (*s*, 3H, 25-H), 0.97 (*brs*, 3H, 30-H), 0.92 (*d*, *J* = 6.4 Hz, 3H, 29-H), 0.89 (*s*, 3H, 24-H), 0.88 (*s*, 3H, 23-H), 0.87–0.84 (*m*, 1H, 5-H), 0.83 (*s*, 3H,26-H) ppm; ^{13}C NMR (101 MHz, CD_3OD): δ = 180.1 (C-28), 172.8 (Ac), 172.5 (CO, acetate), 172.1 (2 × CO, acetate), 171.2 (C-35), 140.2 (C-13), 127.0 (C-12), 82.4 (C-3), 59.8 (CH_2, acetate), 59.7 (CH_2, acetate), 59.1 (CH_2, acetate), 57.7 (C-32), 56.7 (C-5), 55.3 (C-36), 54.4 (C-18), 54.2 (8 × CH_2, cyclen), 53.8 (C-33, C-33′), 49.0 (C-17), 48.8 (C-9), 46.2 (C-34. C-34′), 43.4 (C-14), 40.9 (C-8), 40.9 (C-19), 40.3 (C-20), 39.4 (C-1), 38.7 (C-4), 38.7 (C-22), 38.1 (C-10), 37.3 (C-31), 34.0 (C-7), 31.9 (C-21), 29.0 (C-15), 28.6 (C-23), 25.4 (C-16), 24.6 (C-2), 24.5 (C-11), 24.0 (C-27), 21.6 (C-30), 21.1 (Ac), 19.3 (C-6), 18.0 (C-26), 17.8 (C-29), 17.2 (C-24), 16.1 (C-25) ppm; MS (ESI, MeOH, positive ion mode): *m/z* = 1018.6 (27%, $[M + Na]^+$), 1034.7 (100%, $[M + K]^+$); MS (ESI, MeOH, negative ion mode): *m/z* = 1017.7 (13%, $[M - 2H + Na]^-$), 1032.6 (100%, $[M - 2H + K]^-$); analysis calcd for $C_{54}H_{89}N_7O_{10}$ (996.35): C 65.10, H 9.00, N 9.84; found: C 64.82, H 9.21, N 9.61.

1-(3β-Acetyloxy-urs-12-en-28-oyl)-4-(2-chloroacetyl) piperazine (**19**). Compound **19** has been synthesized from **16** according to general procedure C. Column chromatography (SiO_2, $CHCl_3$/acetone/hexanes 95:5:20) furnished compound **19** (94%); m.p. 155–158 °C; $[\alpha]_D$ = +34.3° (*c* 0.370, $CHCl_3$); R_f = 0.66 ($CHCl_3$/acetone 9:1); IR (ATR): ν = 2924*m*, 2871*w*, 1731*m*, 1658*s*, 1455*m*, 1392*m*, 1370*m*, 1243*s*, 1200*m*, 1145*m*, 1025*m*, 985*m*, 752*m* cm^{-1}; ^{1}H NMR (400 MHz, $CDCl_3$): δ = 5.21 (*t*, *J* = 3.6 Hz, 1H, 12-H), 4.52–4.45 (*m*, 1H, 3-H), 4.06 (*s*, 2H, 34-H), 3.73–3.46 (*m*, 8H, 31-H, 31′-H, 32-H, 32′-H), 2.41 (*d*, *J* = 11.6 Hz, 1H, 18-H), 2.24–2.11 (*m*, 1H, 16-H_a), 2.03 (*s*, 3H, Ac), 1.91 (*dd*, *J* = 8.9, 3.6 Hz, 2H, 11-H_a, 11-H_b), 1.80–1.24 (*m*, 15H, 15-H_a, 16-H_b, 22-H_a, 1-H_a, 2-H_a, 2-H_b, 22-H_b, 9-H, 6-H_a, 21-H_a, 7-H_a, 19-H, 6-H_b, 21-H_b, 7-H_b), 1.07 (*s*, 3H, 27-H), 1.12–0.98 (*m*, 3H, 1-H_b, 15-H_b, 20-H), 0.95 (*d*, *J* = 6.2 Hz, 3H, 30-H), 0.93 (*s*, 3H, 25-H), 0.88 (*d*, *J* = 6.4 Hz, 3H, 29-H), 0.85 (*s*, 3H, 23-H), 0.84 (*s*, 3H, 24-H), 0.84–0.77 (*m*, 1H, 5-H), 0.73 (*s*, 3H, 26-H) ppm; ^{13}C NMR (101 MHz, $CDCl_3$): δ = 175.8 (C-28), 171.1 (Ac), 165.5 (C-33), 138.6 (C-13), 125.5 (C-12), 81.0 (C-3), 55.5 (C-5), 55.1 (C-18), 48.8 (C-17), 47.7 (C-9), 46.3 (C-31), 45.5 (C-31′), 45.1 (C-32), 42.3 (C-32′, C-14), 40.9 (C-34), 39.6 (C-19), 39.6 (C-8), 38.9 (C-20), 38.4 (C-1), 37.8 (C-4), 37.1 (C-10), 34.6 (C-22), 33.1 (C-7), 30.6 (C-21), 28.3 (C-15), 28.2 (C-23), 23.9 (C-27), 23.7 (C-2, C-16), 23.4 (C-11), 21.4 (Ac), 21.4 (C-30), 18.3 (C-6), 17.6 (C-29), 17.0 (C-26), 16.9 (C-24), 15.6 (C-25) ppm; MS

(ESI, MeOH): m/z = 643.5 (100%, $[M + H]^+$), 665.4 (56%, $[M + Na]^+$), 1307.3 78%, $[2M + Na]^+$); analysis calcd for $C_{38}H_{59}ClN_2O_4$ (643.4): C 70.94, H 9.24, N 4.35; found: C 70.72, H 9.51, N 4.09.

(3β) N-(2-(2-Chloroacetyl)aminoethyl)-3-acetyloxy-urs-12-en-28-amide (**20**). Compound **20** was synthesized from **17** according to general procedure C. Column chromatography (SiO_2, $CHCl_3$/acetone/hexanes 95:5:20) furnished compound **20** (91%); m.p. 103–107 °C; $[\alpha]_D$ = +25.2° (*c* 0.300, $CHCl_3$); R_f = 0.40 ($CHCl_3$/acetone 9:1); IR (KBr): ν = 3422*br s*, 2948*s*, 2872*m*, 1734*s*, 1640*s*, 1532*s*, 1456*m*, 1370*m*, 1246*s*, 1148*w*, 1092*w*, 1028*m*, 756*m* cm^{-1}; ^1H NMR (400 MHz, $CDCl_3$): δ = 7.43 (*t*, *J* = 5.1 Hz, 1H, NH), 6.28 (*t*, *J* = 5.7 Hz, 1H, NH), 5.32 (*t*, *J* = 3.6 Hz, 1H, 12-H), 4.48 (*dd*, *J* = 9.7, 6.1 Hz, 1H, 3-H), 4.00 (*s*, 2H, 34-H), 3.56–3.46 (*m*, 1H, 31-H_a), 3.41–3.35 (*m*, 2H, 32-H), 3.26–3.18 (*m*, 1H, 31-H_b), 2.04 (*s*, 3H, Ac), 2.03–1.80 (*m*, 5H, 16-H_a, 11-H_a, 11-H_b, 18-H, 22-H_a), 1.80–1.22 (*m*, 14H, 16-H_b, 2-H_a, 2-H_b, 1-H_a, 15-H_a, 9-H, 6-H_a, 21-H_a, 7-H_a, 22-H_b, 19-H, 6-H_b, 21-H_b, 7-H_b), 1.08 (*s*, 3H, 27-H), 1.08–0.95 (*m*, 3H, 1-H_b, 15-H_b, 20-H), 0.94 (*s*, 3H, 30-H), 0.93 (*s*, 3H, 25-H), 0.87 (*d*, *J* = 6.5 Hz, 3H, 29-H), 0.86 (*s*, 3H, 23-H), 0.84 (*s*, 3H, 24-H), 0.84–0.79 (*m*, 1H, 5-H), 0.75 (*s*, 3H, 26-H) ppm; ^{13}C NMR (101 MHz, $CDCl_3$): δ = 180.0 (C-28), 171.1 (Ac), 167.0 (C-33), 139.7 (C-13), 125.9 (C-12), 81.0 (C-3), 55.4 (C-5), 53.8 (C-18), 48.0 (C-17), 47.6 (C-9), 42.6 (C-14), 42.6 (C-34), 41.3 (C-32), 39.9 (C-19), 39.7 (C-8), 39.2 (C-31), 39.2 (C-20), 38.4 (C-1), 37.8 (C-4), 37.4 (C-22), 37.0 (C-10), 32.8 (C-7), 31.0 (C-21), 28.2 (C-23), 27.9 (C-15), 24.9 (C-16), 23.7 (C-2), 23.5 (C-11), 23.4 (C-27), 21.4 (Ac), 21.3 (C-30), 18.3 (C-6), 17.4 (C-29), 17.0 (C-26), 16.8 (C-24), 15.7 (C-25) ppm; MS (ESI, MeOH): m/z = 617.3 (48%, $[M + H]^+$), 639.5 (52%, $[M + Na]^+$), 1255.4 (100%, $[2M + Na]^+$); analysis calcd for $C_{36}H_{57}ClN_2O_4$ (617.31): C 70.04, H 9.31, N 4.54; found: C 69.83, H 9.52, N 4.11.

(3β) N-(2-(2-(2-Chloroacetyl)aminoethoxy)ethyl)-3-acetyloxy-urs-12-en-28-amide (**21**). Compound **21** has been synthesized from **18** according to general procedure C. Column chromatography (SiO_2, $CHCl_3$/acetone/hexanes 95:5:20) furnished compound **21** (91%); m.p. 94–97 °C; $[\alpha]_D$ = +33.7° (*c* 0.335, $CHCl_3$); R_f = 0.35 ($CHCl_3$/acetone 9:1); IR (KBr): ν = 3426*br s*, 2928*m*, 2872*m*, 1734*m*, 1638*s*, 1528*m*, 1458*w*, 1386*w*, 1248*s*, 1124*w*, 1028*m* cm^{-1}; ^1H NMR (400 MHz, $CDCl_3$): δ = 7.00–6.90 (*m*, 1H, NH), 6.22 (*t*, *J* = 5.0 Hz, 1H, NH), 5.30 (*t*, *J* = 3.6 Hz, 1H, 12-H), 4.49 (*dd*, *J* = 10.0, 5.7 Hz, 1H, 3-H), 4.06 (*s*, 2H, 36-H), 3.57–3.47 (*m*, 7H, 32-H, 31-H_a, 33-H, 34-H), 3.31–3.21 (*m*, 1H, 31-H_b), 2.04 (*s*, 3H, Ac), 2.02–1.76 (*m*, 5H, 16-H_a, 11-H_a, 11-H_b, 18-H, 22-H_a), 1.77–1.21 (*m*, 14H, 16-H_b, 15-H_a, 1-H_a, 2-H_a, 2-H_b, 9-H, 6-H_a, 21-H_a, 7-H_a, 22-H_b, 19-H, 6-H_b, 21-H_b, 7-H_b), 1.09 (*s*, 3H, 27-H), 1.08–0.95 (*m*, 3H, 1-H_b, 15-H_b, 20-H), 0.94 (*d*, *J* = 6.2 Hz, 3H, 30-H), 0.93 (*s*, 3H, 25-H), 0.88 (*d*, *J* = 6.2 Hz, 3H, 29-H), 0.86 (*s*, 3H, 23-H), 0.85 (*s*, 3H, 24-H), 0.84–0.80 (*m*, 1H, 5-H), 0.78 (*s*, 3H, 26-H) ppm; ^{13}C NMR (101 MHz, $CDCl_3$): δ = 178.4 (C-28), 171.1 (Ac), 166.1 (C-35), 139.9 (C-13), 125.6 (C-12), 80.9 (C-3), 70.0 (C-33), 69.4 (C-32), 55.4 (C-5), 54.0 (C-18), 48.0 (C-17), 47.6 (C-9), 42.8 (C-36), 42.6 (C-14), 39.9 (C-29), 39.8 (C-34), 39.7 (C-8), 39.2 (C-31), 39.2 (C-20), 38.5 (C-1), 37.8 (C-4), 37.4 (C-22), 37.0 (C-10), 32.8 (C-7), 31.0 (C-21), 28.2 (C-23), 28.0 (C-15), 25.0 (C-16), 23.7 (C-2), 23.6 (C-11), 23.4 (C-27), 21.4 (Ac), 21.4 (C-30), 18.3 (C-6), 17.4 (C-29), 17.1 (C-26), 16.9 (C-24), 15.7 (C-25) ppm; MS (ESI, MeOH): m/z = 661.4 (60%, $[M + H]^+$), 685.5 (86%, $[M + Na]^+$), 1343.3 (100%, $[2M + Na]^+$); analysis calcd for $C_{38}H_{61}ClN_2O_5$ (661.37): C 69.01, H 9.30, N 4.24, Cl 5.36; found: C 68.80, H 9.61, N 4.01.

Tri-tert-butyl 2,2′,2″-[10-[2-[4-(3β-acetyloxy-urs-12-en-28-oyl)piperazin-1-yl]-2-oxoethyl]-1,4,7,10-tetraazacyclododecane-1,4,7-triyl]triacetate (**22**). Compound **22** was synthesized from **6** and **19** according to general procedure D. Column chromatography (SiO_2, $CHCl_3$/MeOH 95:5) furnished compound **22** (88%); m.p. 237–240 °C (decomp.); $[\alpha]_D$ = +15.0° (c 0.3, $CHCl_3$); R_f = 0.42 ($CHCl_3$/MeOH 9:1); IR (ATR): ν = 2927*w*, 2928*w*, 2871*w*, 2829*w*, 1726*s*, 1646*m*, 1453*m*, 1424*w*, 1368*s*, 1305*m*, 1227*s*, 1160*s*, 1105*s*, 1004*m*, 975*m*, 754*m* cm^{-1}; ^1H NMR (400 MHz, $CDCl_3$): δ = 5.19 (*t*, *J* = 3.5 Hz, 1H, 12-H), 4.47 (*dd*, *J* = 9.8, 6.0 Hz, 1H, 3-H), 3.93 – 2.05 (*m*, 32H, 31-H, 31′-H, 32-H, 32′-H, 8 × CH_2 (cyclen), 3 × CH_2 (acetate), 34-H), 2.40 (*d*, *J* = 11.0 Hz, 1H, 18-H), 2.19–2.09 (*m*, 1H, 16-H_a), 2.02 (*s*, 3H, Ac), 1.93–1.85 (*m*, 2H, 11-H_a, 11-H_b), 1.82–1.67 (*m*, 3H, 15-H_a, 16-H_b, 22-H_a), 1.65–1.21 (*m*, 12H, 2-H_a, 2-H_b, 22-H_b, 1-H_a, 9-H, 21-H_a, 6-H_a, 7-H_a, 19-H, 21-H_b, 6-H_b, 7-H_b), 1.43 (*s*, 9H, CH_3 (*t*Butyl)), 1.42 (*s*, 9H; CH_3 (*t*Butyl)), 1.42 (*s*, 9H, CH_3 (*t*Butyl)), 1.10–0.96 (*m*, 3H, 1-H_b, 15-H_b, 20-H), 1.05 (*s*, 3H, 27-H), 0.92 (*d*, *J* = 6.3 Hz, 3H, 30-H), 0.91 (*s*, 3H, 25-H), 0.86 (*d*, *J* = 6.3 Hz, 3H, 29-H), 0.84 (*s*, 3H, 23-H), 0.82

(*s*, 3H, 24-H), 0.82–0.76 (*m*, 1H, 5-H), 0.71 (*s*, 3H, 26-H) ppm; ^{13}C NMR (101 MHz, $CDCl_3$): δ = 175.9 (C-28), 172.8 (CO, acetate), 172.7 (CO, acetate), 171.0 (Ac), 170.7 (C-33), 138.7 (C-13), 125.1 (C-12), 81.9 (C_q, *t*Butyl), 81.7 (C_q, *t*Butyl), 81.7 (C_q, *t*Butyl), 81.0 (C-3), 55.8 (CH_2, acetate), 55.8 (CH_2, acetate), 55.7 (CH_2, cyclen), 55.4 (C-5), 55.1 (C-18), 48.8 (C-17), 47.6 (C-9), 44.6 (C-31, C-31′, C-32, C-32′), 42.3 (C-14), 41.7 (C-34), 39.5 (C-8), 39.4 (C-19), 38.8 (C-20), 38.3 (C-1), 37.8 (C-4), 37.0 (C-10), 34.4 (C-22), 33.1 (C-7), 30.5 (C-21), 28.3 (C-15), 28.2 (C-23), 28.1 (CH_3, *t*Butyl), 28.0 (CH_3, *t*Butyl), 23.8 (C-27), 23.6 (C-2, C-16), 23.4 (C-11), 21.4 (Ac), 21.3 (C-30), 18.2 (C-6), 17.5 (C-29), 17.0 (C-26), 16.8 (C-24), 15.6 (C-25) ppm; MS (ESI, MeOH): *m*/*z* = 1143.7 (100%, $[M + Na]^+$); analysis calcd for $C_{64}H_{108}N_6O_{10}$ (1121.60): C 68.54, H 9.71, N 7.49; found: C 68.31, H 10.03, N 7.27.

Tribenzyl 2,2′,2″-[10-[2-[4-(3β-acetyloxy-urs-12-en-28-oyl)piperazin-1-yl]-2-oxoethyl]-1,4,7,10-tetraazacyclododecane-1,4,7-triyl]triacetate (**23**). Compound **23** was synthesized from **19** and **7** according to general procedure D. Column chromatography (SiO_2, $CHCl_3$/MeOH 95:5) furnished compound **23** (72%); m.p. 157–161 °C; $[\alpha]_D$ = +4.2° (c 0.300, $CHCl_3$); R_f = 0.37 ($CHCl_3$/MeOH 9:1); IR (ATR): ν = 2945*w*, 2836*w*, 1730*s*, 1638*m*, 1454*m*, 1424*w*, 1392*m*, 1370*m*, 1302*m*, 1243*s*, 1194*s*, 1105*s*, 1005*m*, 966*m*, 743*m*, 697*s* cm^{-1}; UV-Vis ($CHCl_3$): λ_{max} (logε) = 246 nm (3.96), 294 nm (3.47), 364 nm (3.23); ^{1}H NMR (400 MHz, $CDCl_3$): δ = 7.39–7.26 (*m*, 15H, 15 × CH (Bn)), 5.33–4.97 (*m*, 7H, 12-H, 3 × CH_2 (Bn)), 4.45 (*dd*, *J* = 10.1, 5.9 Hz, 1H, 3-H), 4.02–2.05 (*m*, 34H, 31-H, 31′-H, 32-H, 32′-H, 8 × CH_2 (cyclen), 3 × CH_2 (acetate), 34-H, 16-H_a, 18-H), 2.02 (*s*, 3H, Ac), 1.95–1.65 (*m*, 5H, 11-H_a, 11-H_b, 15-H_a, 16-H_b, 22-H_a), 1.65–1.09 (*m*, 12H, 2-H_a, 2-H_b, 22-H_b, 1-H_a, 9-H, 21-H_a, 6-H_a, 7-H_a, 19-H, 21-H_b, 6-H_b, 7-H_b), 1.03 (*s*, 3H, 27-H), 1.08–0.95 (*m*, 3H, 1-H_b, 15-H_b, 20-H), 0.93 (*d*, *J* = 6.0 Hz, 3H, 30-H), 0.85 (*d*, *J* = 6.3 Hz, 3H, 29-H), 0.85 (*s*, 3H, 25-H), 0.82 (*s*, 3H, 23-H), 0.79 (*s*, 3H, 24-H), 0.79–0.71 (*m*, 1H, 5-H), 0.66 (*s*, 3H, 26-H) ppm; ^{13}C NMR (101 MHz, $CDCl_3$): δ = 175.9 (C-28), 173.6 (CO, acetate), 171.0 (Ac), 170.8 (C-33), 138.6 (C-13), 135.5 (C_i, Bn), 135.3 (C_i, Bn), 128.7 (CH, Bn), 128.7 (CH, Bn), 128.6 (CH, Bn), 128.6 (CH, Bn), 128.4 (CH, Bn), 128.4 (CH, Bn), 125.1 (C-12), 81.0 (C-3), 67.1 (CH_2, Bn), 66.9 (CH_2, Bn), 55.7 (CH_2, acetate), 55.4 (CH_2, cyclen), 55.2 (C-5), 55.1 (C-18), 48.7 (C-17), 47.6 (C-9), 44.8 (C-31, C-31′, C-32, C-32′), 42.2 (C-14), 42.0 (C-34), 39.5 (C-19), 39.5 (C-8), 38.8 (C-20), 38.3 (C-1), 37.7 (C-4), 36.9 (C-10), 34.5 (C-22), 33.1 (C-7), 30.6 (C-21), 28.2 (C-15), 28.1 (C-23), 23.6 (C-2, C-16), 23.5 (C-27), 23.4 (C-11), 21.4 (Ac), 21.3 (C-30), 18.2 (C-6), 17.5 (C-29), 17.0 (C-26), 16.8 (C-24), 15.5 (C-25) ppm; MS (ESI, MeOH): *m*/*z* = 1245.8 (100%, $[M + Na]^+$); analysis calcd for $C_{73}H_{102}N_6O_{10}$ (1223.65): C 71.65, H 8.40, N 6.87; found: C 71.42, H 8.69, N 6.56.

Tri-tert-butyl 2,2′,2″-[10-[2-[2-(3β-acetyloxy-urs-12-en-28-oylamino)ethyl]amino-2-oxoethyl]-1,4,7,10-tetraazacyclododecane-1,4,7-triyl]triacetate (**24**). Compound **24** was synthesized from **20** and **6** according to general procedure D. Column chromatography (SiO_2, $CHCl_3$/MeOH 95:5) furnished compound **24** (73%); m.p. 254–257 °C (decomp.); $[\alpha]_D$ = +33.8° (c 0.300, $CHCl_3$); R_f = 0.40 ($CHCl_3$/MeOH 9:1); IR (KBr): ν = 2971*m*, 2929*m*, 2829*w*, 1727*s*, 1668*m*, 1520*m*, 1454*m*, 1426*w*, 1368*s*, 1307*m*, 1228*s*, 1159*s*, 1106*s*, 1027*m*, 1006*m*, 975*m*, 755*m* cm^{-1}; ^{1}H NMR (400 MHz, $CDCl_3$): δ = 8.03 (*s*, 1H, NH), 7.08 (*s*, 1H, NH), 5.46 (*t*, *J* = 3.4 Hz, 1H, 12-H), 4.47 (*dd*, *J* = 9.8, 6.1 Hz, 1H, 3-H), 3.80–2.05 (*m*, 28H, 31-H, 32-H, 34-H, 3 × CH_2 (acetate), 8 × CH_2 (cyclen)), 2.44–2.38 (*m*, 1H, 18-H), 2.02 (*s*, 3H, Ac), 2.00–1.67 (*m*, 6H, 15-H_a, 11-H_a, 11-H_b, 16-H_a, 16-H_b, 22-H_a), 1.66–1.19 (*m*, 12H, 1-H_a, 2-H_a, 2-H_b, 22-H_b, 9-H, 6-H_a, 7-H_a, 21-H_a, 19-H, 6-H_b, 21-H_b, 7-H_b), 1.44 (*s*, 9H, CH_3 (*t*Butyl)), 1.43 (*s*, 9H, CH_3 (*t*Butyl)), 1.43 (*s*, 9H, CH_3 (*t*Butyl)), 1.15–0.98 (*m*, 3H, 20-H, 1-H_b, 15-H_b), 1.04 (*s*, 3H, 27-H), 0.91 (*s*, 3H, 25-H), 0.90 (*d*, *J* = 6.1 Hz, 3H, 30-H), 0.88 (*d*, *J* = 6.1 Hz, 3H, 29-H), 0.84 (*s*, 3H, 23-H), 0.83 (*s*, 3H, 24-H), 0.82–0.77 (*m*, 1H, 5-H), 0.74 (*s*, 3H, 26-H) ppm; ^{13}C NMR (101 MHz, $CDCl_3$): δ = 178.7 (C-28), 172.4 (CO, acetate), 171.7 (C-33), 171.1 (Ac), 139.0 (C-13), 125.5 (C-12), 82.1 (C_q, *t*Butyl), 82.1 (C_q, *t*Butyl), 82.1 (C_q, *t*Butyl), 81.1 (C-3), 56.4 (3 × CH_2, acetate), 55.8 (C-34), 55.8 (CH_2, cyclen), 55.4 (C-5), 52.3 (C-18), 47.7 (C-9), 47.6 (C-17), 42.2 (C-14), 40.0 (C-32), 39.7 (C-19), 39.7 (C-8), 38.5 (C-20), 38.4 (C-31, C-1), 37.8 (C-4), 37.4 (C-22), 37.0 (C-10), 32.9 (C-7), 31.2 (C-21), 28.2 (C-23), 28.2 (CH_3, *t*Butyl), 28.1 (CH_3, *t*Butyl), 28.1 (CH_3, *t*Butyl), 27.9 (C-15), 24.4 (C-16), 23.7 (C-2), 23.5 (C-27), 23.4 (C-11), 21.5 (C-30), 21.4 (Ac), 18.4 (C-6), 17.2 (C-29), 17.0

(C-26), 16.9 (C-24), 15.7 (C-25) ppm; MS (ESI, MeOH): m/z = 1117.7 (100%, $[M + Na]^+$); analysis calcd for $C_{62}H_{106}N_6O_{10}$ (1095.56): C 67.97, H 9.75, N 7.67; found: C 67.68, H 10.02, N 7.41.

Tribenzyl 2,2′,2″-[10-[2-[2-(3β-acetyloxy-urs-12-en-28-oylamino)ethyl]amino-2-oxoethyl]-1,4,7,10-tetraazacyclododecane-1,4,7-triyl]triacetate (**25**). Compound **25** was synthesized from **7** and **20** according to general procedure D. Column chromatography (SiO_2, $CHCl_3$/MeOH 95:5) furnished compound **25** (75%); m.p. 142–146 °C; $[\alpha]_D$ = +20.5° (c 0.390, $CHCl_3$); R_f = 0.36 ($CHCl_3$/MeOH 9:1); IR (ATR): ν = 2945*w*, 2832*w*, 1732*s*, 1663*m*, 1519*w*, 1454*m*, 1370*m*, 1305*m*, 1245*s*, 1194*s*, 1176*s*, 1105*s*, 1007*m*, 965*m*, 747*m*, 697*s* cm^{-1}; UV-Vis ($CHCl_3$): λ_{max} (logε) = 241 nm (3.89), 295 nm (3.29), 364 nm (3.08); ^1H NMR (400 MHz, $CDCl_3$): δ = 8.20 (*t*, *J* = 4.5 Hz, 1H, NH), 7.39–7.27 (*m*, 15H, CH (Bn)), 7.01 (*t*, *J* = 4.9 Hz, 1H, NH), 5.48 (*s*, 1H, 12-H), 5.26–5.05 (*m*, 6H, CH_2 (Bn)), 4.47 (*dd*, *J* = 10.0, 5.7 Hz, 1H, 3-H), 3.77–2.07 (*m*, 28H, 31-H_a, 31-H_b, 32-H, 34-H, 3 × CH_2 (acetate),8 × CH_2 (cyclen)), 2.41 (*d*, *J* = 10.7 Hz, 1H, 18-H), 2.02 (*s*, 3H, Ac), 2.00–1.64 (*m*, 6H, 16-H_a, 16-H_b, 11-H_a, 11-H_b, 22-H_a, 15-H_a), 1.64–1.19 (*m*, 12H, 1-H_a, 2-H_a, 2-H_b, 22-H_b, 9-H, 6-H_a, 7-H_a, 21-H_a, 6-H_b, 19-H, 21-H_b, 7-H_b), 1.17–0.97 (*m*, 3H, 20-H, 1-H_b, 15-H_b), 1.04 (*s*, 3H, 27-H), 0.89 (*d*, *J* = 6.3 Hz, 6H, 29-H, 30-H), 0.87 (*s*, 3H, 25-H), 0.83 (*s*, 3H, 23-H), 0.81 (*s*, 3H, 24-H), 0.80–0.76 (*m*, 1H, 5-H), 0.72 (*s*, 3H, 26-H) ppm; ^{13}C NMR (101 MHz, $CDCl_3$): δ = 178.8 (C-28), 173.2 (CO, acetate), 172.0 (C-33), 171.0 (Ac), 139.0 (C-13), 135.4 (C_i, Bn), 135.4 (C_i, Bn), 135.3 (C_i, Bn), 128.8 (CH, Bn), 128.8 (CH, Bn), 128.7 (CH, Bn), 128.6 (CH, Bn), 125.6 (12-H), 81.0 (3-H), 67.3 (CH_2, Bn), 67.3 (CH_2, Bn), 67.2 (CH_2, Bn), 56.8 (CH_2, acetate), 55.4 (C-34), 55.3 (C-5), 55.3 (CH_2, cyclen), 52.3 (C-18), 47.7 (C-17), 47.6 (C-9), 42.2 (C-14), 40.1 (C-32), 39.8 (C-19), 39.7 (C-8), 38.5 (C-20), 38.5 (C-31, C-1), 37.8 (C-4), 37.4 (C-22), 37.0 (C-10), 32.9 (C-7), 31.2 (C-21), 28.2 (C-23), 28.0 (C-15), 24.5 (C-16), 23.7 (C-2), 23.5 (C-27), 23.4 (C-11), 21.4 (Ac), 21.4 (C-30), 18.4 (C-6), 17.2 (C-29), 17.1 (C-26), 16.8 (C-24), 15.6 (C-25) ppm; MS (ESI, MeOH): m/z = 1219.8 (100%, $[M + Na]^+$); analysis calcd for $C_{71}H_{100}N_6O_{10}$ (1197.61): C 71.21, H 8.42, N 7.02; found: 70.93, H 8.56, N 6.82.

Tri-tert-butyl 2,2′,2″-[10-[2-[2-[2-(3β-acetyloxy-urs-12-en-28-oylamino)ethoxy]ethyl]amino-2-oxoethyl]-1,4,7,10-tetraazacyclododecane-1,4,7-triyl]triacetate (**26**). Compound **26** was synthesized from **6** and **21** according to general procedure D. Column chromatography (SiO_2, $CHCl_3$/MeOH 95:5) furnished compound **26** (74%); m.p. 263–266 °C (decomp.); $[\alpha]_D$ = +21.9° (c 0.315, $CHCl_3$); R_f = 0.38 ($CHCl_3$/MeOH 9:1); IR (ATR): ν = 2972*m*, 2930*m*, 1726*s*, 1166*m*, 1523*w*, 1453*m*, 1368*s*, 1307*m*, 1228*s*, 1160*s*, 1106*s*, 1026*m*, 1006*m*, 975*m*, 755*m* cm^{-1}; ^1H NMR (400 MHz, $CDCl_3$): δ = 7.82 (*t*, *J* = 5.6 Hz, 1H, NH), 6.46 (*t*, *J* = 5.1 Hz, 1H, NH), 5.33 (*t*, *J* = 3.7 Hz, 1H, 12-H), 4.47 (*dd*, *J* = 10.2, 5.9 Hz, 1H, 3-H), 3.56–3.30 (*m*, 9H, 32-H, 31-H_a, 33-H, 36-H, 34-H), 3.28–3.16 (*m*, 1H, 31-H_b), 3.15–2.05 (*m*, 22H, 3 × CH_2 (acetate), 8 × CH_2 (cyclen)), 2.02 (*s*, 3H, Ac), 2.02–1.21 (*m*, 19H, 18-H, 16-H_a, 11-H_a, 11-H_b, 22-H_b, 16-H_b, 15-H_a, 1-H_a, 2-H_a, 2-H_b, 9-H, 6-H_a, 21-H_a, 7-H_a, 22-H_b, 19-H, 6-H_b, 21-H_b, 7-H_b), 1.44 (*s*, 9H, CH_3 (*t*Butyl)), 1.43 (*s*, 18H, CH_3 (*t*Butyl)), 1.06 (*s*, 3H, 27-H), 1.05–0.94 (*m*, 3H, 1-H_b, 15-H_b, 20-H), 0.92 (*s*, 3H, 25-H), 0.92 (*d*, *J* = 6.2 Hz, 3H, 30-H), 0.86 (*d*, *J* = 6.5 Hz, 3H, 29-H), 0.84 (*s*, 3H, 23-H), 0.83 (*s*, 3H, 24-H), 0.82–0.77 (*m*, 1H, 5-H), 0.76 (*s*, 3H, 26-H) ppm; ^{13}C NMR (101 MHz, $CDCl_3$): δ = 178.3 (C-28), 173.0 (CO, acetate), 172.5 (CO, acetate), 172.1 (C-35), 171.1 (Ac), 139.3 (C-13), 125.7 (C-12), 82.1 (C_q, *t*Butyl), 82.0 (C_q, *t*Butyl), 81.9 (C_q, *t*Butyl), 81.0 (C-3), 69.5 (C-33), 69.0 (C-32), 56.5 (C-36), 55.9 (CH_2, acetate), 55.8 (CH_2, acetate), 55.7 (CH_2, cyclen), 55.4 (C-5), 53.4 (C-18), 47.8 (C-17), 47.6 (C-9), 42.4 (C-14), 39.8 (C-19), 39.7 (C-8), 39.2 (C-31), 39.0 (C-34), 39.0 (C-20), 38.4 (C-1), 37.8 (C-4), 37.3 (C-22), 37.0 (C-10), 32.9 (C-7), 31.1 (C-21), 28.2 (CH_3, *t*Butyl), 28.0 (CH_3, *t*Butyl), 28.0 (C-23), 28.0 (C-15), 24.9 (C-16), 23.7 (C-2), 23.5 (C-11), 23.4 (C-27), 21.4 (Ac), 21.4 (C-30), 18.3 (C-6), 17.3 (C-29), 17.0 (C-26), 16.8 (C-24), 15.7 (C-25) ppm; MS (ESI, MeOH): m/z = 1161.7 (100%, $[M + Na]^+$); analysis calcd for $C_{64}H_{110}N_6O_{11}$ (1139.6): C 67.45, H 9.73, N 7.37; found: C 67.31, H 9.87, N 7.09.

Tribenzyl 2,2′,2″-[10-[2-[2-[2-(3β-acetyloxy-urs-12-en-28-oylamino)ethoxy]ethyl]amino-2-oxoethyl]-1,4,7,10-tetraazacyclododecane-1,4,7-triyl]triacetate (**27**). Compound **27** has been synthesized from **7** and **21** according to general procedure D. Column chromatography (SiO_2, $CHCl_3$/MeOH 95:5) furnished compound **27** (62%); m.p. 137–141 °C; $[\alpha]_D$ = +15.4° (c 0.350, $CHCl_3$); R_f = 0.35 ($CHCl_3$/MeOH 9:1); IR (ATR): ν = 2945*w*, 2830*w*, 1731*s*, 1662*m*, 1523*w*, 1454*m*, 1390*m*, 1370*m*, 1305*m*, 1245*s*, 1193*s*, 1105*s*,

1026*m*, 1008*m*, 967*m*, 747*m*, 697*m* cm^{-1}; UV-Vis ($CHCl_3$): λ_{max} (logε) = 244 nm (3.73), 294 nm (3.36), 363 nm (3.12); ^{1}H NMR (400 MHz, $CDCl_3$): δ = 8.02 (*t*, *J* = 5.4 Hz, 1H, NH), 7.37–7.27 (*m*, 15H, CH (Bn)), 6.48 (*t*, *J* = 5.1 Hz, 1H, NH), 5.32 (*t*, *J* = 3.5 Hz, 1H, 12-H), 5.24–5.14 (*m*, 4H, CH_2 (Bn)), 5.14–5.05 (*m*, 2H, CH_2 (Bn)), 4.46 (*dd*, *J* = 10.2, 5.7 Hz, 1H, 3-H), 3.59–3.33 (*m*, 9H, 32-H, 33-H, 31-H_a, 34-H, 36-H), 3.33–2.01 (*m*, 23H, 31-H_b, 8 × CH_2 (cyclen), 3 × CH_2 (acetate)), 2.02 (*s*, 3H, Ac), 2.00–1.17 (*m*, 19H, 18-H, 16-H_a, 11-H_a, 11-H_b, 22-H_a, 16-H_b, 15-H_a, 1-H_a, 2-H_a, 2-H_b, 9-H, 6-H_a, 22-H_b, 7-H_a, 21-H_a, 19-H, 6-H_b, 7-H_b, 21-H_b), 1.05 (*s*, 3H, 27-H), 1.04 – 0.94 (*m*, 3H, 1-H_b, 15-H_b, 20-H), 0.90 (*s*, 3H, 25-H), 0.90 (*d*, *J* = 5.8 Hz, 3H, 30-H), 0.85 (*d*, *J* = 6.6 Hz, 3H, 29-H), 0.84 (*s*, 3H, 23-H), 0.82 (*s*, 3H, 24-H), 0.81–0.76 (*m*, 1H, 5-H), 0.75 (*s*, 3H, 26-H) ppm; ^{13}C NMR (101 MHz, $CDCl_3$): δ = 178.3 (C-28), 173.3 (CO, acetate), 173.1 (CO, acetate), 172.3 (C-35), 171.1 (Ac), 139.3 (C-13), 135.4 (C_i, Bn), 135.3 (C_i, Bn), 128.7 (CH, Bn), 128.7 (CH, Bn), 128.7 (CH, Bn), 128.6 (CH, Bn), 128.5 (CH, Bn), 125.7 (C-12), 81.0 (C-3), 69.6 (C-33), 68.9 (C-32), 67.2 (CH_2, Bn), 67.2 (CH_2, Bn), 56.9 (C-36), 55.4 (3 × CH_2, acetate), 55.4 (C-5), 55.3 (8 × CH_2, cyclen), 53.3 (C-18), 47.8 (C-17), 47.6 (C-9), 42.4 (C-14), 39.8 (C-19), 39.7 (C-8), 39.2 (C-31, C-34), 38.9 (C-20), 38.4 (C-1), 37.8 (C-4), 37.3 (C-22), 36.9 (C-10), 32.9 (C-7), 31.1 (C-21), 28.2 (C-23), 28.0 (C-15), 24.8 (C-16), 23.6 (C-2), 23.5 (C-11), 23.4 (C-27), 21.4 (Ac), 21.4 (C-30), 18.3 (C-6), 17.3 (C-29), 17.1 (C-26), 16.8 (C-24), 15.7 (C-25) ppm; MS (ESI, MeOH): *m/z* = 1263.9 (100%, $[M + Na]^+$); analysis calcd for $C_{73}H_{104}N_6O_{11}$ (1241.67): C 70.62, H 8.44, N 6.77; found: C 70.41, H 8.69, N 6.41.

(3β) N-(2-Aminoethyl)-3-hydroxy-urs-12-en-28-amide (**28**). Method A: The synthesis was performed according to the procedure given in the Supplementary material in 82%. *Method B*: Ursolic acid (100 mg, 0.20 mmol), HOBt·H_2O (37 mg, 0.24 mmol) and EDC·HCl (46 mg, 0.24 mmol) were dissolved in dry DMF (5 mL), and the mixture was stirred for 30 min at 25 °C. Ethylene diamine (55 μL, 0.82 mmol) was added to the mixture, and stirring was continued for 24 h at 25 °C. Usual aqueous work-up followed by column chromatography (silica gel, $CHCl_3$/MeOH/NH_4OH 90:10:0.1) gave **28** (46%). Analytical data of this compound can be found in the supplementary material.

Tri-tert-butyl 2,2′,2″-[10-[2-[2-(3β-hydroxy-urs-12-en-28-oylamino)ethyl]amino-2-oxoethyl]-1,4,7,10-tetraazacyclododecane-1,4,7-triyl]triacetate (**29**). Method A: To a solution of DOTA-tris(tert-butyl ester) (58 mg, 0.10 mmol) in dry DMF (8 mL) were added HOBt·H_2O (29 mg, 0.19 mmol) and EDC·HCl (29 mg, 0.15 mmol). After stirring for 30 min at 25 °C, a solution of **28** (71 mg, 0.14 mmol) in dry DMF (2 mL) was added and stirring was continued for 5 days. After usual aqueous work-up, the solvent was removed under reduced pressure and the crude product was subjected to column chromatography (silica gel, $CHCl_3$/MeOH 9:1) yielding compound **29** as colorless solid. Yield: 49%. Method B: Compound **24** (50 mg, 0.10 mmol) was dissolved in methanol (7 mL) and a solution of potassium hydroxide (12 mg, 0.21 mmol) in methanol (1 mL) was added. The mixture was stirred at 25 °C for 24 h. After completion of the reaction (as indicated by TLC) and usual work-up, the solvent was removed under reduced pressure, and the residue was subjected to column chromatography (silica gel, $CHCl_3$/MeOH 9:1) affording **29** (yield: 86%); m.p. 136–139 °C; $[\alpha]_D$ = −44.4° (c 0.330, MeOH); R_f = 0.29 ($CHCl_3$/MeOH 9:1); IR (KBr): ν = 3300*br w*, 2973*w*, 2928*m*, 2869*w*, 1728*s*, 1668*m*, 1525*m*, 1455*m*, 1425*w*, 1368*s*, 1307*m*, 1227*s*, 1159*s*, 1121*m*, 1106*s*, 1047*w*, 1006*w* cm^{-1}; ^{1}H NMR (400 MHz, $CDCl_3$): δ = 8.84 (*s*, 1H, NH), 7.55 (*s*, 1H, NH), 5.36 (*t*, *J* = 3.5 Hz, 1H, 12-H), 3.59–2.05 (*m*, 28H, 31-H, 32-H, 33-H, 3 × CH_2 (acetate), 8 × CH_2 (cyclen)), 3.20 (*dd*, *J* = 11.1, 4.8 Hz, 1H, 3-H), 2.34 (*d*, *J* = 11.0 Hz, 2H, 18-H), 2.03–1.96 (*m*, 1H, 16-H_a), 1.95–1.83 (*m*, 3H, 11-H_a, 11-H_b, 16-H_b), 1.83–1.72 (*m*, 1H, 22-H_a), 1.64–1.21 (*m*, 13H, 1-H_a, 15-H_a, 2-H_a, 2-H_b, 22-H_b, 6-H_a, 9-H, 7-H_a, 21-H_a, 19-H, 6-H_b, 7-H_b, 21-H_b), 1.45 (*s*, 9H, CH_3 (*t*Butyl)), 1.43 (*s*, 18H, CH_3 (*t*Butyl)), 1.05 (*s*, 3H, 27-H), 1.04–0.97 (*m*, 3H, 1-H_b, 15-H_b, 20-H), 0.97 (*s*, 3H, 23-H), 0.89 (*d*, *J* = 6.3 Hz, 3H, 30-H), 0.89 (*s*, 3H, 25-H), 0.85 (*d*, *J* = 6.4 Hz, 3H, 29-H), 0.76 (*s*, 3H, 24-H), 0.75 (*s*, 3H, 26-H), 0.72–0.68 (*m*, 1H, 5-H) ppm; ^{13}C NMR (101 MHz, $CDCl_3$): δ = 178.4 (C-28), 172.4 (CO, acetate), 171.8 (C-33), 138.9 (C-13), 125.3 (C-12), 82.2 (C_q, *t*Butyl), 82.1 (C_q, *t*Butyl), 82.1 (C_q, *t*Butyl), 79.2 (C-3), 56.0 (CH_2, acetate), 55.9 (C-34), 55.8 (CH_2, cyclen), 55.3 (C-5), 52.5 (C-18), 47.8 (C-9), 47.5 (C-17), 42.2 (C-14), 40.0 (C-32), 39.7 (C-8), 39.6 (C-19), 38.9 (C-4), 38.7 (C-20), 38.7 (C-31, C-1), 37.4 (C-22), 37.1 (C-10), 33.2 (C-7), 31.3 (C-21), 28.3 (C-23), 28.2 (CH_3, *t*Butyl), 28.2 (CH_3, *t*Butyl), 28.1 (CH_3, *t*Butyl), 28.0 (C-15), 27.4 (C-2), 24.2 (C-16), 23.6 (C-27), 23.5 (C-11), 21.5 (C-30), 18.6 (C-6), 17.2 (C-29), 17.1 (C-26), 15.8 (C-24), 15.7 (C-25) ppm; MS (ESI, MeOH): m/z = 1075.7 (100%, $[M + Na]^+$); analysis calcd for $C_{60}H_{104}N_6O_9$ (1053.53): C 68.40, H 9.95, N 7.98; found: C 60.09, H 10.11, N 7.83.

Author Contributions: M.K.; and R.C. conceived and designed the experiments; M.K. performed the experiments; S.H. and L.F. performed the biological assays and experiments; M.K.; A.A-H.; and R.C. analyzed the data and wrote the paper.

Acknowledgments: We would like to thank R. Kluge for measuring the ESI-MS spectra and D. Ströhl and his team for the NMR spectra. Thanks are also due to V. Simon for measuring the IR an UV-VIS spectra and optical rotations. The cell lines were kindly provided by Th. Müller (Dept. of Haematology/Oncology, Martin-Luther Universität Halle-Wittenberg).

References

1. Bray, F.; Ferlay, J.; Soerjomataram, I.; Siegel, R.L.; Torre, L.A.; Jemal, A. Global cancer statistics 2018: GLOBOCAN estimates of incidence and mortality worldwide for 36 cancers in 185 countries. *Ca-Cancer J. Clin.* **2018**, *68*, 394–424. [CrossRef] [PubMed]
2. Stasiuk, G.J.; Long, N.J. The ubiquitous DOTA and its derivatives: The impact of 1, 4, 7, 10-tetraazacyclododecane-1, 4, 7, 10-tetraacetic acid on biomedical imaging. *Chem. Commun.* **2013**, *49*, 2732–2746. [CrossRef] [PubMed]
3. Chilla, S.N.M.; Henoumont, C.; Elst, L.V.; Muller, R.N.; Laurent, S. Importance of DOTA derivatives in bimodal imaging. *Isr. J. Chem.* **2017**, *57*, 800–808. [CrossRef]
4. Magerstädt, M.; Gansow, O.A.; Brechbiel, M.W.; Colcher, D.; Baltzer, L.; Knop, R.H.; Girton, M.E.; Naegele, M. Gd (DOTA): An alternative to Gd (DTPA) as a T1, 2 relaxation agent for NMR imaging or spectroscopy. *Magn. Reson. Med.* **1986**, *3*, 808–812. [CrossRef] [PubMed]
5. Jones-Wilson, T.M.; Deal, K.A.; Anderson, C.J.; McCarthy, D.W.; Kovacs, Z.; Motekaitis, R.J.; Sherry, A.D.; Martell, A.E.; Welch, M.J. The in vivo behavior of copper-64-labeled azamacrocyclic complexes. *Nucl. Med. Biol.* **1998**, *25*, 523–530. [CrossRef]
6. Wu, A.M.; Yazaki, P.J.; Tsai, S.-w.; Nguyen, K.; Anderson, A.-L.; McCarthy, D.W.; Welch, M.J.; Shively, J.E.; Williams, L.E.; Raubitschek, A.A. High-resolution microPET imaging of carcinoembryonic antigen-positive xenografts by using a copper-64-labeled engineered antibody fragment. *Proc. Natl. Acad. Sci. USA* **2000**, *97*, 8495–8500. [CrossRef] [PubMed]
7. Deshpande, S.V.; DeNardo, S.J.; Kukis, D.L.; Moi, M.K.; McCall, M.J.; DeNardo, G.L.; Meares, C.F. Yttrium-90-labeled monoclonal antibody for therapy: Labeling by a new macrocyclic bifunctional chelating agent. *J. Nucl. Med.* **1990**, *31*, 473–479.
8. Razboršek, M.I.; Vončina, D.B.; Doleček, V.; Vončina, E. Determination of Oleanolic, Betulinic and Ursolic Acid in Lamiaceae and Mass Spectral Fragmentation of Their Trimethylsilylated Derivatives. *Chromatographia* **2008**, *67*, 433–440. [CrossRef]
9. Fu, L.; Zhang, S.; Li, N.; Wang, J.; Zhao, M.; Sakai, J.; Hasegawa, T.; Mitsui, T.; Kataoka, T.; Oka, S.; et al. Three New Triterpenes from Nerium oleander and Biological Activity of the Isolated Compounds. *J. Nat. Prod.* **2005**, *68*, 198–206. [CrossRef]
10. Cargnin, S.T.; Gnoatto, S.B. Ursolic acid from apple pomace and traditional plants: A valuable triterpenoid with functional properties. *Food Chem.* **2017**, *220*, 477–489. [CrossRef]
11. Yamaguchi, H.; Noshita, T.; Kidachi, Y.; Umetsu, H.; Hayashi, M.; Komiyama, K.; Funayama, S.; Ryoyama, K. Isolation of Ursolic Acid from Apple Peels and Its Specific Efficacy as a Potent Antitumor Agent. *J. Health Sci.* **2008**, *54*, 654–660. [CrossRef]
12. Chen, H.; Gao, Y.; Wang, A.; Zhou, X.; Zheng, Y.; Zhou, J. Evolution in medicinal chemistry of ursolic acid derivatives as anticancer agents. *Eur. J. Med. Chem.* **2015**, *92*, 648–655. [CrossRef] [PubMed]
13. Hussain, H.; Green, I.R.; Ali, I.; Khan, I.A.; Ali, Z.; Al-Sadi, A.M.; Ahmed, I. Ursolic acid derivatives for pharmaceutical use: A patent review (2012-2016). *Expert Opin. Pat.* **2017**, *27*, 1061–1072. [CrossRef] [PubMed]
14. Seo, D.Y.; Lee, S.R.; Heo, J.-W.; No, M.-H.; Rhee, B.D.; Ko, K.S.; Kwak, H.-B.; Han, J. Ursolic acid in health and disease. *Korean J. Physiol. Pharm.* **2018**, *22*, 235–248. [CrossRef] [PubMed]

15. Zou, J.; Lin, J.; Li, C.; Zhao, R.; Fan, L.; Yu, J.; Shao, J. Ursolic Acid in Cancer Treatment and Metastatic Chemoprevention: From Synthesized Derivatives to Nanoformulations in Preclinical Studies. *Curr. Cancer Drug Targets* **2019**, *19*, 245–256. [CrossRef] [PubMed]
16. Ma, C.-M.; Cai, S.-Q.; Cui, J.-R.; Wang, R.-Q.; Tu, P.-F.; Hattori, M.; Daneshtalab, M. The cytotoxic activity of ursolic acid derivatives. *Eur. J. Med. Chem.* **2005**, *40*, 582–589. [CrossRef] [PubMed]
17. Liu, D.; Meng, Y.-q.; Zhao, J.; Chen, L.-g. Synthesis and Anti-tumor Activity of Novel Amide Derivatives of Ursolic Acid. *Chem. Res. Chin. Univ.* **2008**, *24*, 42–46. [CrossRef]
18. Meng, Y.-Q.; Liu, D.; Cai, L.-L.; Chen, H.; Cao, B.; Wang, Y.-Z. The synthesis of ursolic acid derivatives with cytotoxic activity and the investigation of their preliminary mechanism of action. *Bioorg. Med. Chem.* **2009**, *17*, 848–854. [CrossRef]
19. Liu, M.-C.; Yang, S.-J.; Jin, L.-H.; Hu, D.-Y.; Xue, W.; Song, B.-A.; Yang, S. Synthesis and cytotoxicity of novel ursolic acid derivatives containing an acyl piperazine moiety. *Eur. J. Med. Chem.* **2012**, *58*, 128–135. [CrossRef]
20. Sommerwerk, S.; Heller, L.; Kerzig, C.; Kramell, A.E.; Csuk, R. Rhodamine B conjugates of triterpenoic acids are cytotoxic mitocans even at nanomolar concentrations. *Eur. J. Med. Chem.* **2017**, *127*, 1–9. [CrossRef]
21. Kahnt, M.; Fischer, L.; Al-Harrasi, A.; Csuk, R. Ethylenediamine Derived Carboxamides of Betulinic and Ursolic Acid as Potential Cytotoxic Agents. *Molecules* **2018**, *23*, 2558. [CrossRef] [PubMed]
22. Kim, S.-M.; Jeong, I.H.; Yim, M.S.; Chae, M.K.; Kim, H.N.; Kim, D.K.; Kang, C.M.; Choe, Y.S.; Lee, C.; Ryu, E.K. Characterization of oleanolic acid derivative for colon cancer targeting with positron emission tomography. *J. Drug Target.* **2014**, *22*, 191–199. [CrossRef] [PubMed]
23. Yang, X.; Li, Y.; Jiang, W.; Ou, M.; Chen, Y.; Xu, Y.; Wu, Q.; Zheng, Q.; Wu, F.; Wang, L. Synthesis and biological evaluation of novel ursolic acid derivatives as potential anticancer prodrugs. *Chem. Biol. Drug Des.* **2015**, *86*, 1397–1404. [CrossRef]
24. Bai, K.-K.; Yu, Z.; Chen, F.-L.; Li, F.; Li, W.-Y.; Guo, Y.-H. Synthesis and evaluation of ursolic acid derivatives as potent cytotoxic agents. *Bioorg. Med. Chem. Lett.* **2012**, *22*, 2488–2493. [CrossRef] [PubMed]
25. Rami, M.; Cecchi, A.; Montero, J.-L.; Innocenti, A.; Vullo, D.; Scozzafava, A.; Winum, J.-Y.; Supuran, C.T. Carbonic Anhydrase Inhibitors: Design of Membrane-Impermeant Copper(II) Complexes of DTPA-, DOTA-, and TETA-Tailed Sulfonamides Targeting the Tumor-Associated Transmembrane Isoform IX. *ChemMedChem* **2008**, *3*, 1780–1788. [CrossRef]
26. Loesche, A.; Kahnt, M.; Serbian, I.; Brandt, W.; Csuk, R. Triterpene-Based Carboxamides Act as Good Inhibitors of Butyrylcholinesterase. *Molecules* **2019**, *24*, 948. [CrossRef] [PubMed]
27. Deng, S.-L.; Baglin, I.; Nour, M.; Cavé, C. Synthesis of phosphonodipeptide conjugates of ursolic acid and their homologs. *Heteroat. Chem.* **2008**, *19*, 55–65. [CrossRef]

12

Romanian Wormwood (*Artemisia absinthium* L.): Physicochemical and Nutraceutical Screening

Elena-Alina Moacă [1,†], Ioana Zinuca Pavel [2,†], Corina Danciu [2,*], Zorin Crăiniceanu [3,*], Daliana Minda [2], Florina Ardelean [4], Diana Simona Antal [4], Roxana Ghiulai [5], Andreea Cioca [6], Mihnea Derban [6], Sebastian Simu [7], Raul Chioibaş [8], Camelia Szuhanek [9] and Cristina-Adriana Dehelean [1]

1 Department of Toxicology and Drug Industry, Faculty of Pharmacy, "Victor Babes" University of Medicine and Pharmacy, 2 Eftimie Murgu Square, 300041 Timisoara, Romania
2 Department of Pharmacognosy, Faculty of Pharmacy, "Victor Babes" University of Medicine and Pharmacy, 2 Eftimie Murgu Square, 300041 Timisoara, Romania
3 Department of Plastic and Reconstructive Surgery, Faculty of Medicine, "Victor Babes" University of Medicine and Pharmacy, 2 Eftimie Murgu Square, 300041 Timisoara, Romania
4 Department of Botany, Faculty of Pharmacy, "Victor Babes" University of Medicine and Pharmacy, 2 Eftimie Murgu Square, 300041 Timisoara, Romania
5 Department of Pharmaceutical Chemistry, Faculty of Pharmacy, "Victor Babes" University of Medicine and Pharmacy, 2 Eftimie Murgu Square, 300041 Timisoara, Romania
6 Department of Pathology, CFR Clinical Hospital, 13-15, Tudor Vladimirescu, 300173 Timisoara, Romania
7 Department of Physical Chemistry, Faculty of Pharmacy, "Victor Babes" University of Medicine and Pharmacy, 2 Eftimie Murgu Square, 300041 Timisoara, Romania
8 CBS Medcom Hospital, 12 Popa Sapca Street, 300047 Timisoara, Romania
9 Department of Orthodontics, Faculty of Dentistry, "Victor Babes" University of Medicine and Pharmacy, 2 Eftimie Murgu Square, 300041, Timisoara, Romania
* Correspondence: corina.danciu@umft.ro (C.D.); zcrainiceanu@gmail.com (Z.C.)
† These authors contributed equally to this work.

Abstract: *Artemisia* species are used worldwide for their antioxidant, antimicrobial and anti-inflammatory properties. This research was designed to investigate the phytochemical profile of two ethanolic extracts obtained from leaves and stems of *A. absinthium* L. as well as the biological potential (antioxidant activity, cytotoxic, anti-migratory and anti-inflammatory properties). Both plant materials showed quite similar thermogravimetric, FT-IR phenolic profile (high chlorogenic acid) with mild antioxidant capacity [ascorbic acid (0.02–0.1) > leaves (0.1–2.0) > stem (0.1–2.0)]. Alcoholic extracts from these plant materials showed a cytotoxic effect against A375 (melanoma) and MCF7 (breast adenocarcinoma) and affected less the non-malignant HaCaT cells (human keratinocytes) at 72 h post-stimulation and this same trend was observed in the anti-migratory (A375, MCF7 > HaCat) assay. Lastly, extracts ameliorated the pro-inflammatory effect of TPA (12-*O*-tetradecanoylphorbol-13-acetate) in mice ears, characterized by a diffuse neutrophil distribution with no exocytosis or micro-abscesses.

Keywords: *Artemisia absinthium* L.; antioxidants; total phenolic content; cytotoxicity; melanoma and breast cancer cell line; HaCaT cells; inflammation

---

1. Introduction

Common wormwood (*Artemisia absinthium* L., Asteraceae) is a woody-based perennial herb which grows widely in dry, sunny regions of Eurasia, Northern Africa, North and South America [1]. It may be recognized by its silver-grey leaves, which have a soft silk texture. The upper parts of the plant have a distinctive aromatic scent when bruised. From a biochemical point of view, wormwood stands out due to the synthesis of bitter-tasting metabolites and essential oils [2]. Bitterness is conferred by sesquiterpenes (0.15–0.4%), including absinthin, artabsin, anabsinthin, and matricin [3]. Essential oils are secreted by numerous glandular hairs and secretory ducts [4], providing a content of 2–6 mL/kg volatiles in the dried herb [5]. Several chemotypes of volatile oils are known from different parts of the world according to the main constituent: α-and β-thujone, *cis*-epoxyocimene, *trans*-sabinyl acetate and chrysanthenyl acetate [6]. Other secondary metabolites in wormwood include flavonoids (myricetin, quercetin, rutin, hesperidin), hydroxybenzoic acids (salicylic acid, gallic acid), hydroxycinnamic acids (caffeic acids, coumaric acids, ferulic acid), resveratrol, and other [7].

Wormwood leaves and stems have traditionally been employed as a bitter tonic in appetite loss. Preparations are also prescribed as a choleretic in dyspeptic disorders, and in liver diseases due to its hepatoprotective effect. The herb is as well known for its anthelmintic, antipyretic, antibacterial and insecticide properties [5]. The importance of the herb is acknowledged by its inclusion in the European Pharmacopoeia and other official compendia, as well as by the monograph of the Committee on Herbal Medicinal Products of the European Medicine Agency (EMA/HMPC/751484/ 2016).

In recent years, wormwood has attracted considerable attention due to its anti-inflammatory effect. Clinical studies could point out favorable effects in Crohn's disease. Patients receiving an herbal blend containing wormwood as an add-up to standard steroids could afford the lowering of steroid doses; the remission of the disease could be pointed out in 65% of the patients after eight weeks of treatment [8]. The favorable evolution was explained by the suppression of tumor necrosis factor alpha (TNF-α) by some metabolites from *A. absinthium* extracts, and the potential of wormwood to treat diseases with an augmented production of pro-inflammatory cytokines was pointed out [9]. Wormwood extracts proved as well efficient in the supportive treatment of early-stage IgA nephropathy [10].

The current research aims to investigate in depth both the chemical composition as well as the biological activity of ethanolic extracts obtained from leaves and stems of wormwood collected from the Southern part of Romania in order to enhance the knowledge about the phytochemistry and bioactivity of this ancient medicinal plant with important medicinal potential. To this end, ethanol extracts of leaves and stems were investigated by liquid chromatography–mass spectrometry (LC-MS), thermal analysis (TG-DSC) and Fourier-transform infrared spectroscopy (FT-IR). The Total Phenolic Content (TPC) was evaluated spectrophotometrically, and radical scavenging effects as well as the cytotoxic and anti-migratory potential on two tumor cell lines–melanoma and breast adenocarcinoma cells and on a non-tumor cell line–HaCaT–keratinocytes was assessed. The anti-inflammatory effects of the extracts were tested in a mouse ear edema model.

2. Results

2.1. Physicochemical Analysis

After lyophilization, both ethanolic extracts, obtained from leaves and stems of wormwood were characterized by thermal analysis (TG-DSC) and Fourier-transform infrared spectroscopy (FT-IR).

2.1.1. Thermal Analysis

TG-DSC curves of dried and lyophilized extracts of *A. absinthium* L. leaves and stems are depicted in Figure 1A,B. Thermal analysis performed for dried and lyophilized wormwood leaves extract revealed a total mass loss of 94.17% in four stages. In the first stage, the wormwood leaves extract loses 66.30% of the total mass and an endothermic process which can be noticed with a maximum at 122.5 °C. The second stage is located between 450 °C and 600 °C; within this interval the sample loses 4.46% of the total mass and shows an exothermic effect with a maximum at 464.5 °C. In the third stage of extract degradation, four exothermic processes occur between 600 °C and 700 °C, and a total mass loss of 20.06% was measured. In the final stage of extract degradation only a slight mass loss (3.35%) without any thermal effect could be determined.

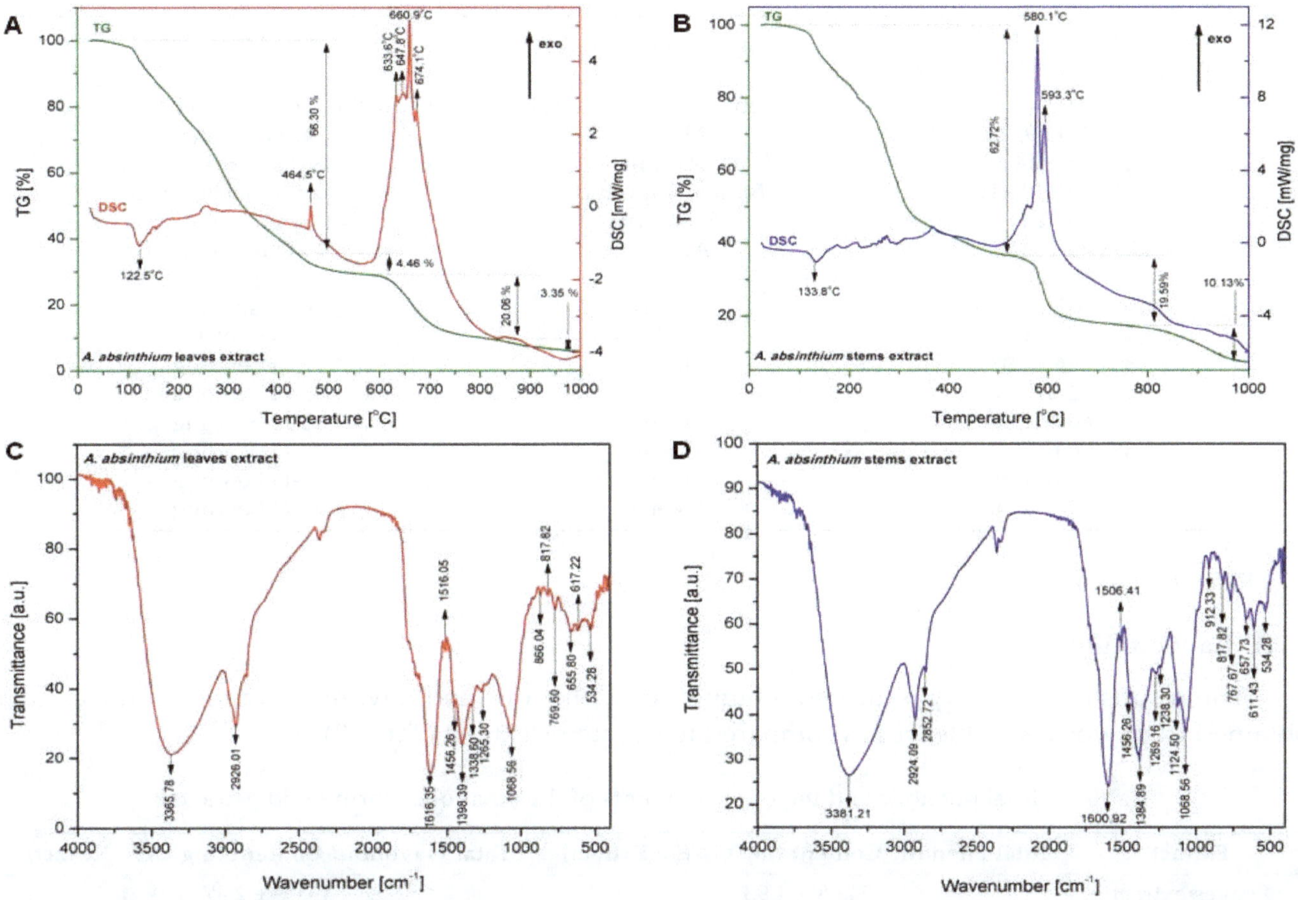

Figure 1. **A**—TG-DSC curves of *A. absinthium* leaves extract, **B**—TG-DSC curves of *A. absinthium* stems extract, **C**—FT-IR spectra of *A. absinthium* leaves extract, **D**—FT-IR spectra of *A. absinthium* stems extract.

Thermal analysis performed for dried and lyophilized wormwood stems extract revealed a total mass loss of 92.44% in three stages. The largest mass loss (about 62.72%) occurs during the first stage; it is accompanied by an endothermic process with a maximum at 133.8 °C. In the second stage (temperature range 500 °C–650 °C) a mass loss of 19.59% was registered, related to two exothermic processes peaking at 580.1 °C and 593.3 °C, respectively. In the final stage of the extract degradation only a mass loss of 10.13% occurred.

2.1.2. FT-IR Investigations

In order to identify the functional groups of the active components which are present in the leaves and stems extracts of *A. absinthium*, the FT-IR analysis was done. The FT-IR analysis is based on the presence of the peak values in the region of IR radiation appeared on different wavenumber. The results of analysis of dried lyophilized leaves and stems extracts based on *A. absinthium* are given in Table 1 and Figure 1C,D. The two lyophilized extracts based on *A. absinthium* exhibited a similar IR profile most probably due to the polar nature of molecules present in both extracts.

Table 1. Peak values and functional groups of *A. absinthium* leaves and stems extracts in the spectrum.

Characteristic Absorptions [cm^{-1}] Leaves Extract/Stems Extract	Functional Group	Bond
3365.78/3381.21	Amines, amide, alcohol	N-H stretching O-H stretch (H-bonded)
2926.01/2924.09; 2852.72	Alkanes	C-H strech
1616.35/1600.92	Amide	N-H bending
1516.05/1506.41	Nitro compounds	N-O asymmetric strech
1456.26	Aromatics	C=C stretch (in ring)
1398.39/1384.89	Alkanes	-C-H bending
1338.60/-	Amines	C-N strech
1265.30/1269.16; 1238.30	Acids	C-O strech
1068.56/1068.56; 1124.50	Alcohols	C-O stretch
866.04/912.33	Alkenes	=C-H bending
817.82/817.82	Alkenes	=C-H bending
769.60/767.67	Alkenes	=C-H bending
655.80/657.73	Alkenes	=C-H bending
617.22/611.43	Alkenes	=C-H bending
534.28/534.28	Alkenes	=C-H bending

2.2. *Phenolic Composition*

2.2.1. Raw Profiling

The results of our study indicated a higher total phenolic and flavonoid content in the extract obtained from wormwood leaves as compared to the stems extract (Table 2).

Table 2. Total phenolic and flavonoid contents of the ethanolic wormwood extracts.

Extract	Total Phenolic Content (mg GAE/g Extract)	Total Flavonoid Content (mg CE/g Extract)
Leaves extract	54.68 ± 1.93	43.08 ± 2.47
Stems extract	44.15 ± 1.12	34.14 ± 2.16

2.2.2. LC-MS Fingerprint

In Table 3 are presented the polyphenolic content of the *A. absinthium* L. leaves and stems, obtained by LC-MS analysis.

Table 3. Polyphenolic content of extracts analysed by LC-MS.

	Compound Name	Rt (min)	$[M - H^+]^+$ (m/z)	*A. absinthium* Leaves (µg/mg d.w.)	*A. absinthium* Stems (µg/mg d.w.)
1.	Gentisic acid	2.67	153	ND	NQ
2.	Chlorogenic acid	6.45	353	1.94	2.03
3.	Caffeic acid	6.97	179	NQ	NQ
4.	*p*-Coumaric acid	10.56	163	NQ	ND
5.	Isoquercitrin	22.50	463	0.04	0.07
6.	Rutin	23.01	609	0.08	0.55
7.	Quercitrin	26.18	447	0.11	0.05
8.	Luteolin	32.78	285	NQ	ND
9.	Apigenin	36.91	269	NQ	ND

Notes: ND—not detected, below the limit of detection; NQ—not quantified, below the limit of quantification.

2.2.3. Antioxidant Activity

In order to evaluate the antioxidant activity (AOA), both wormwood lyophilized extracts were dissolved in ultra-pure distilled water. The values corresponding to the inhibition percentages of the two extracts of *A. absinthium* (leaves and stems) were evaluated in time, and compared to those of ascorbic acid solution (control) are presented in Figure 2A. As it can be noticed from the graph, both extracts of *A. absinthium* show antioxidant effects during the time frame of the evaluation. Moreover, the AOA values of *A. absinthium* stem extract are slightly higher than the AOA values of *A. absinthium* leaves extract.

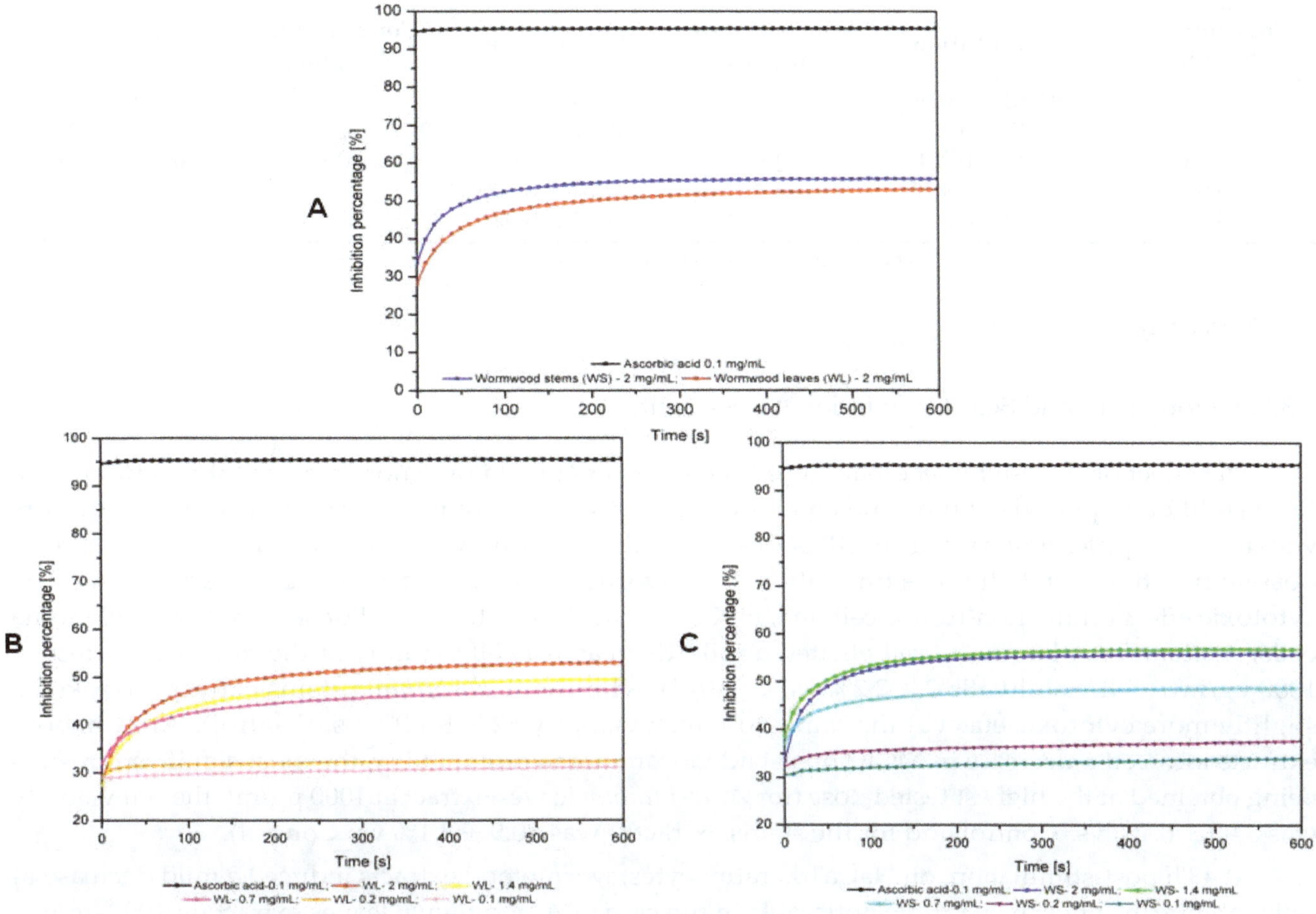

Figure 2. The time dependent inhibition percentage of *A. absinthium* extracts: **A**—*A. absinthium* stock solutions based on leaves and stems vs. ascorbic acid; **B**—extracts of *A. absinthium* leaves vs. ascorbic acid; **C**—extracts of *A. absinthium* stems vs. ascorbic acid.

The reduction rate of DPPH free radical is different for the two extracts. The wormwood stems extract quenches the free radicals after 250 s; subsequently the reaction reaches equilibrium. Wormwood leaves extract quenches the entirety of free radicals after 500 s.

From Figure 2B it can be noted that the antioxidant activity of *A. absinthium* leaves extract is concentration-dependent. In the case of *A. absinthium* stems extracts the values corresponding to inhibition percentages are not directly proportional with their concentration; the maximal inhibition was measured for the sample containing 1.4 mg extract/mL.

Table 4 presents the percent inhibition of leaves and stems extracts. The values were calculated with equation (1) and subsequently used for the determination of IC_{50} values. IC_{50}, characterizing the antioxidant activity as evaluated by the DPPH test, were as follows: for ascorbic acid $IC_{50} = 0.03191 \pm 0.0019$ mg/mL; for wormwood leaves extract $IC_{50} = 0.4993 \pm 0.0201$ mg/mL and for wormwood stems extract $IC_{50} = 0.4865 \pm 0.0182$ mg/mL. The IC_{50} parameter for each sample was determined using GraphPad Prism 8 software. Correlation coefficients were $R^2 = 0.9856$ for wormwood leaves extract and $R^2 = 0.9855$ for wormwood stems extract.

Table 4. The inhibition percentage of *A. absinthium* extracts obtained from leaves and stems, as compared to the inhibition percentage of ascorbic acid [1].

Ascorbic Acid		*A. absinthium* Leaves Extract		*A. absinthium* Stems Extract	
Concentration [mg/mL]	% Inhibition	Concentration [mg/mL]	% Inhibition	Concentration [mg/mL]	% Inhibition
0.1	94.88 ± 0.029	2	53.11 ± 0.014	2	55.77 ± 0.054
0.08	95.47 ± 0.001	1.4	49.47 ± 0.015	1.4	56.84 ± 0.026
0.06	95.06 ± 0.001	0.7	47.32 ± 0.026	0.7	48.79 ± 0.015
0.04	94.85 ± 0.0015	0.2	32.61 ± 0.020	0.2	37.71 ± 0.019
0.02	83.19 ± 0.005	0.1	31.15 ± 0.021	0.1	34.02 ± 0.056

[1] The results are expressed as average ± SD (n = 3).

2.3. Bioactivity

2.3.1. Cytotoxicity and Selectivity Index Assessment

The effect of *A. absinthium* ethanolic extracts was evaluated on a non-tumor and two tumor cell lines at different periods of time and compared to the Control group (cells stimulated with ultrapure water). In Supplementary Figure S1 is described the in vitro cytotoxic effect at 24 h and at 48 h post-stimulation. At 24 h post-stimulation, both wormwood leaves and stems extracts showed no cytotoxic effect on the non-tumor cell line, HaCat, regardless of the tested dose. On A375 melanoma cells, *A. absinthium* leaves extract elicited a mild decrease of cell viability at the higher dose tested, 1000 μg/mL (cell viability 86.2 ± 2.2% vs. Control), whereas *A. absinthium* stems extract provoked a slightly more cytotoxic effect at the same dose (cell viability 82.2 ± 4.9% vs. Control). At 24 h, both extracts induced a decrease in MCF7 breast adenocarcinoma cell viability, the most significant results being obtained at the highest tested dose (for *A. absinthium* leaves extract at 1000 μg/mL the cell viability was 84.3 ± 6.1% vs. Control and for the stems extract it was 80.9 ± 3.1% vs. Control).

At 48 h post-stimulation, on HaCaT keratinocytes, wormwood extracts induced a mild decrease in cell viability, the effect being more noticeable in the case of *A. absinthium* leaves extract (at 1000 μg/mL, cells viability was 92.8 ± 4.6% vs. Control). On the tumor cell lines, both wormwood extracts provoked a dose dependent decrease of cells viability, with the best results obtained after stimulation with the stems extract. For A375 cells, at the highest dose, the stems extract decreased the viability to 68.8 ± 4.3% vs. Control, while the same extract induced a viability of 56.9 ± 4.4% in MCF7 cells vs. Control cells. The obtained data shows that the wormwood extracts affect more the cancer cells than the non-tumor cells, especially at higher doses.

Figure 3 presents the effect of wormwood extracts at 72 h post-stimulation. On HaCaT cells, the extracts induced a decrease in cell viability especially at 1000 μg/mL: cell viability was 71.6 ± 7.3% vs. Control in case of *A. absinthium* leaves extract, and 77.6 ± 9.2% vs. Control in case of *A. absinthium* stems extract. These data show that the leaves extract induced a more pronounced decrease in HaCaT cell viability than wormwood stems extract. Regarding the tumor cell lines, *A. absinthium* extracts elicited a significant cytotoxic effect at all the tested doses. Moreover, *A. absinthium* extracts affect rather the tumor cells than the non-tumor cell line, HaCaT. At 1000 μg/mL, on A375 melanoma cells, *A. absinthium* leaves extract decreased cells viability to 38.2 ± 3.8% vs. Control and *A. absinthium* stems extract to 21.06 ± 1.1% vs. Control. On the breast adenocarcinoma cells, at the same dose, *A. absinthium* leaves extract decreased cells viability to 37.6 ± 4.3% vs. Control and the stems extract to 10.8 ± 2.3% vs. Control. For both tumor cell lines, the most potent cytotoxic effect was obtained in the case of the stems extracts and the highest reduction of tumor cells viability was noticed for MCF7 breast cancer cells.

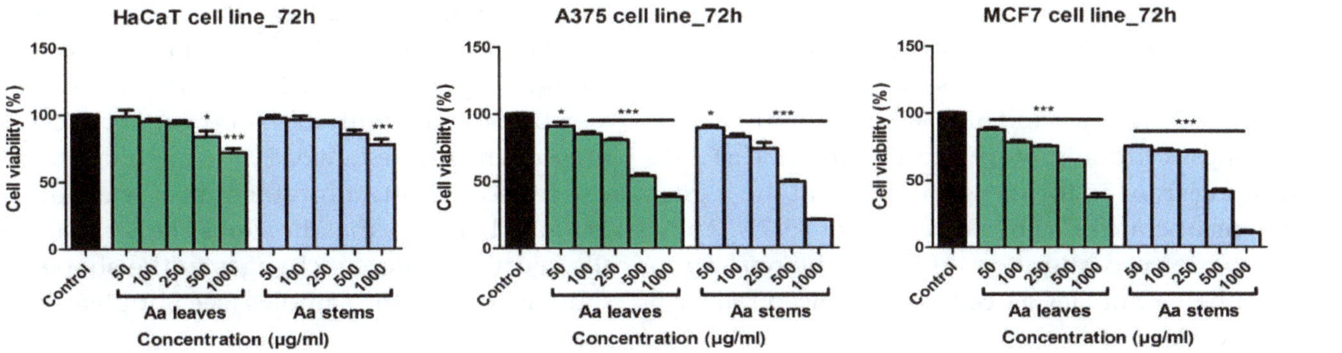

Figure 3. In vitro cytotoxicity assessment of *A. absinthium* leaves and stems ethanolic extracts (50, 100, 250, 500 and 1000 µg/mL) on a non-tumor cell line–HaCaT–human keratinocytes and on two human tumor cell lines A375—melanoma cells and MCF7–breast adenocarcinoma cells at 72 h post-stimulation by the means of Alamar blue assay. The results are expressed as cell viability percentage (%) related to Control (cells stimulated with ultrapure water). The data represent the mean values ± SD of three independent experiments. Comparison among the groups was performed using the One-way ANOVA test followed by Dunnett's post-test. (* $p < 0.05$; *** $p < 0.001$).

The IC_{50} values for the tumor and non-tumor cells following 72 h stimulation with *A. absinthium* extracts are shown in Table 5. The highest IC_{50} value was recorded in the case of HaCaT cells stimulated with *A. absinthium* leaves extract, whereas the lowest values were obtained for the breast cancer cells, MCF7. These data indicate that the tumor cell lines are more affected than the non-cancer cells following stimulation with wormwood extracts.

Table 5. IC_{50} values and selectivity of *A. absinthium* leaves and stems extracts (cancer cells vs. non-malignant HaCaT cells—human keratinocytes) at 72 h post-stimulation.

Extract	HaCaT IC_{50} (µg/mL)	A375 IC_{50} (µg/mL)	MCF7 IC_{50} (µg/mL)	SI *
A. absinthium leaves	397.7 ± 7.2	295.4 ± 7.1	-	1.35
		-	250.6 ± 6.3	1.59
A. absinthium stems	361.8 ± 9.3	312 ± 3.4	-	1.16
		-	246.8 ± 7.2	1.47

* Selectivity index (SI) is calculated as the ratio between the IC_{50} values; IC_{50} [non-malignant HaCaT]/IC_{50} [tumor cell line]. The data represent the mean values ± SD of three independent experiments.

Within this study the Selectivity index (SI) of *A. absinthium* leaves and stems extracts was also determined. The non-malignant HaCaT cells, human keratinocytes, were used as a control in order to evaluate the degree of selectivity of wormwood extracts for the tumor cell lines. The values obtained for the SI range between 1.16 (for A375 cells stimulated 72 h with *A. absinthium* stems extract) and 1.59 (for MCF7 cells stimulated 72 h with *A. absinthium* leaves extract), showing a slightly more active effect of wormwood on the breast adenocarcinoma cells. Following the calculation of SI we can indicate that the extracts did not display a significant selective effect towards the cancer cells.

2.3.2. Scratch Assay Assessment

In order to determine the anti-migratory potential of *A. absinthium* extracts a scratch assay technique was performed. The non-tumor and tumor cell lines were stimulated with different concentrations of wormwood extracts and compared to Control (cells stimulated with ultrapure water).

In Figure 4, the effect of *A. absinthium* leaves and stems extracts on HaCaT, A375 and MCF7 cells is shown. Regarding the effect of *A. absinthium* leaves on HaCaT cells, at low concentrations (50 and 100 µg/mL) stimulation with the extract induced a pro-migratory effect upon the non-tumor cells, the results being similar to those obtained in the Control group. For these concentrations the scratch closure rate after 24 h was 100%. At the concentration of 250 μg/mL, the leaves extract elicited a mild anti-migratory effect, showing a scratch closure rate of 95.4%. On HaCaT cells, at the higher doses tested, *A. absinthium* leaves extract slowed down the migratory effect, showing a scratch closure of 70.8% (500 μg/mL) and 62.7% (1000 μg/mL), respectively. Stimulation with the stems extract elicited a significant pro-migratory effect on the HaCaT cells with scratch closure rate of 100% for concentration ranging from 50 to 500 μg/mL. Only at the highest dose tested, an anti-migratory effect was noticed, having a scratch closure percentage of 85.5%. The data obtained indicate that the stems extract exhibited a superior pro-migratory effect on the non-tumor cells. Furthermore, no changes in the shape and morphology of HaCaT cells were noticed following stimulation with the samples (see Supplementary Figure S2).

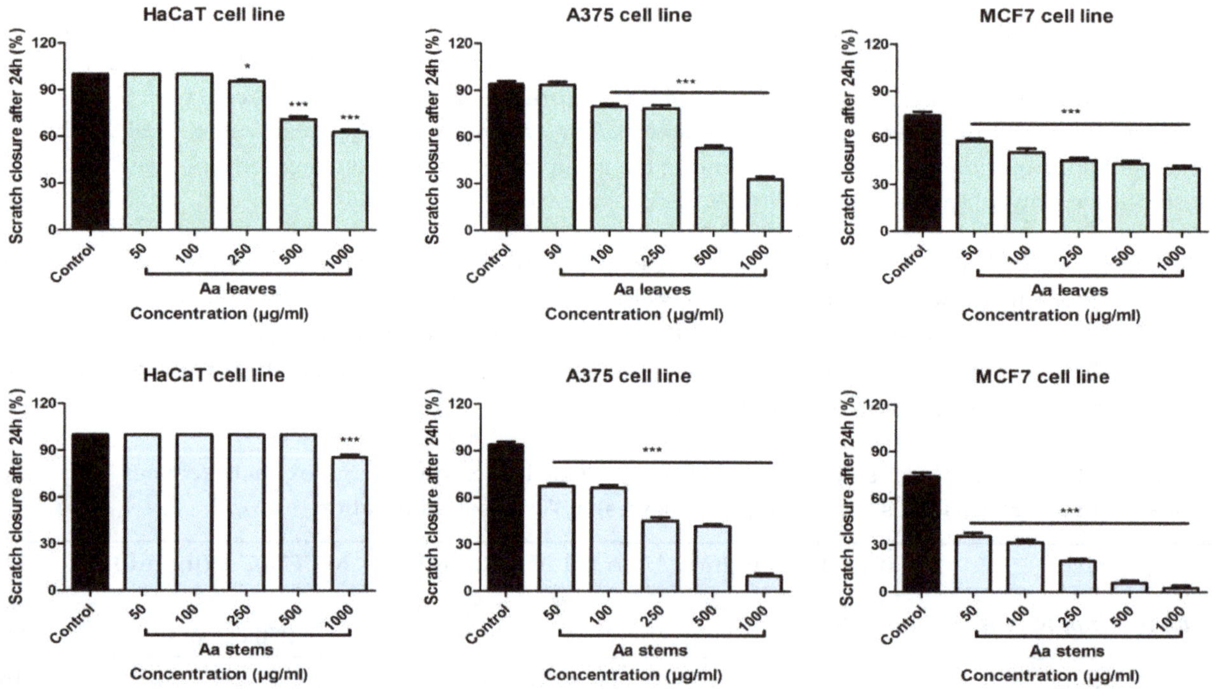

Figure 4. The migratory potential of HaCat, A375 and MCF7 cells following treatment with *A. absinthium* leaves and stems ethanolic extract (50, 100, 250, 500 and 1000 μg/mL). Images were taken by light microscopy at 10× magnification (the scale bars represent 100 μm). The bar graphs are expressed as percentage of scratch closure after 24 h compared to the initial surface. Comparison among the groups was performed using the One-way ANOVA test followed by Dunnett's post-test. (* $p < 0.05$; *** $p < 0.001$ vs. Control-cells stimulated with ultrapure water).

Stimulation of human A375 melanoma cells with *A. absinthium* leaves extract proved to have a dose dependent anti-migratory effect (Figure 4). At the lowest tested dose, 50 μg/mL, the leaves extract provoked a closure of the scratch of 93.3%, similar to the Control group, while at the highest tested dose, 1000 μg/mL, the closure was 32.9%. Moreover, at 24 h post-stimulation, it can be seen in the pictures that at the highest concentration there is a slightly change in the cells shape, some of them displayed round shape, indicating that the leaves extract affects melanoma cells (see Supplementary Figure S2).

A. absinthium stems extract manifested a significant anti-migratory effect on A375 cells at all the tested concentrations. The results show that the stems extract had a stronger inhibitory effect on the migration of melanoma cells. At the highest tested dose, the scratch closure rate was around 9.9%. Furthermore, at this concentration, cells with round shape and detached ones were present, showing the cytotoxic effect of this extract. The results obtained are consistent with the ones from the cell viability assay, proving an anti-migratory and cytotoxic effect of these extracts.

Regarding the anti-migratory effect of *A. absinthium* leaves extract on MCF7 human breast adenocarcinoma cells, at 24 h post-stimulation, all the evaluated concentrations manifested a significant inhibitory effect on cancer cells migration.

The anti-migratory properties on MCF7 cells were more potent after stimulation with *A. absinthium* stems extract compared to the effects obtained in the case of the leaves extract. Application of the stems extract provoked at the concentration of 500 μg/mL a closure percentage of 5.8% and for 1000 μg/mL it was 2.6%. Furthermore, it can be seen in the images from Supplementary Figure S2, that at 500 and 1000 μg/mL, the cells had a modified morphology with round shape and also many cells are detached from the plate (Supplementary Figure S2). These elements suggest that the stems extract had a cytotoxic effect on the breast adenocarcinoma cells.

2.3.3. Anti-Inflammatory Assessment

Skin specimens from the control group had normal histological structures, while the group treated with acetone showed marked edema and congestion of the blood vessels but without inflammation or changes of the epidermal thickness (Figure 5A,B).

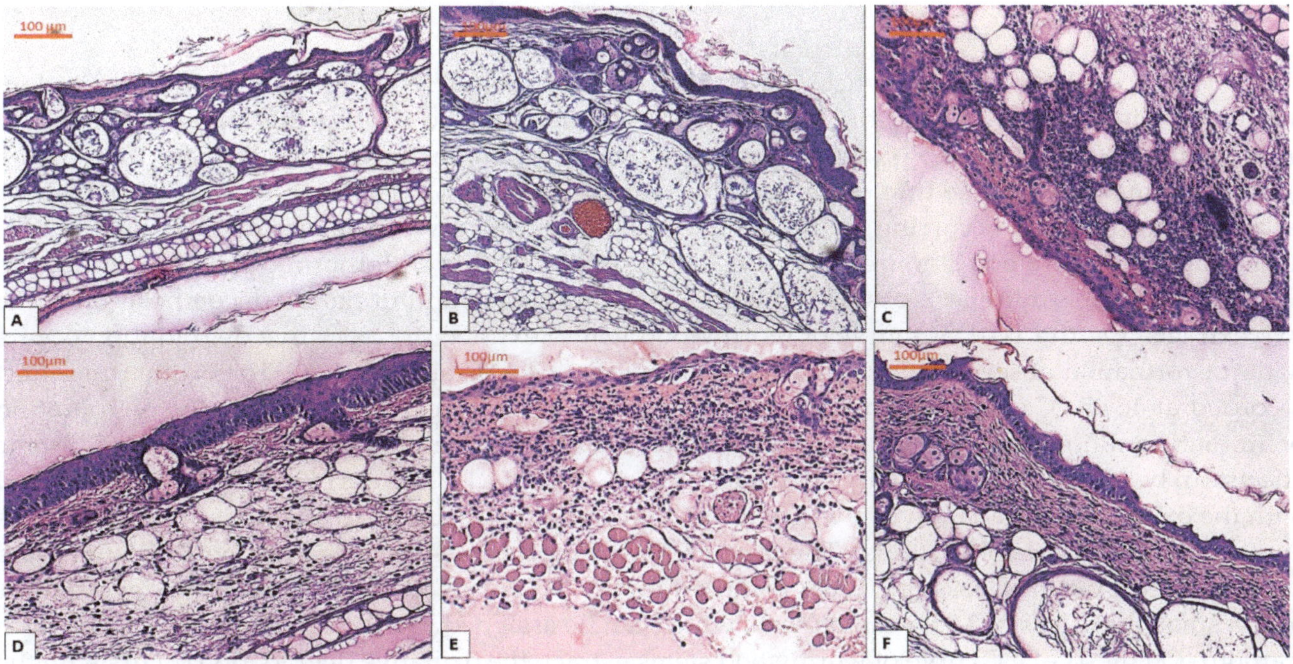

Figure 5. Histological aspects of the skin, H&E stain, **A**: Control group—with no intervention, magnification ×10; **B**: Acetone group showing edema, magnification ×10; **C**: TPA group showing abundant inflammation in the entire dermis with abscess formation, magnification ×20; **D**: TPA + indomethacin group depicting mild inflammation, magnification ×20; **E**: topical application of *A. absinthium* leaves extract indicating moderate inflammation and moderate interstitial edema, magnification ×20; **F**: treatment with *A. absinthium* stems extract having a reduced number of neutrophils and thick collagen fibers in dermis, magnification ×20.

As illustrated in Figure 5C, TPA treatment produced a marked pro-inflammatory action on mice ears. The epidermal thickness was increased and it was accompanied by reactive changes of the cells. We noticed an abundant inflammatory infiltrate composed of neutrophils, disposed in the papillary and reticular dermis and around the dermal appendages. The inflammation showed a diffuse pattern, but it also formed micro-abscesses. In some areas, neutrophils migrated in the epidermal thickness leading to exocytosis. In addition, the blood vessels were congested and some of them displayed leukocytes margination. Intraepidermal and dermal edema was noted in this group.

Topical administration of indomethacin (Figure 5D) provoked a reduction of the inflammatory processes compared to the TPA group. The inflammatory infiltrate was composed of a reduced number of neutrophils that were diffusely disposed in the dermis. Exocytosis and the abcesses were absent in this group and dermal edema was mild.

In the group treated with *A. absinthium* leaves extract (Figure 5E) the epidermis was focally enlarged compared to the untreated group. The inflammation was moderate with a diffuse distribution of the neutrophils in the dermis. No exocytosis or micro-abscesses were observed in this group. Congestion of the blood vessels and interstitial edema were mild and some blood vessels showed leucocytes margination.

In contrast, topical application of the *A. absinthium* stems extract (Figure 5F) showed a clearer anti-inflammatory effect. In this group, the inflammatory infiltrate was mild and diffusely distributed in the dermis and moderate in only few areas. The interstitial edema was mild and focal, while congestion and leucocytes margination of the blood vessels were absent. Moreover, the dermis showed thick collagen fibers organized in compact bundles.

3. Discussion

3.1. Physicochemical Analysis

Thermal analysis is an analytical method used also to characterize the compounds from plant medicine. Figure 1A,B present the TG and DSC signals obtained during thermal decomposition of, lyophilized extracts based on wormwood leaves and stems, in air. In both extracts, there was a substantial mass loss in the first stage of degradation (above 60%). This step was accompanied by an endothermic effect, occurring at: 122.5 °C in the case of wormwood leaves extract and 133.8 °C in the case of wormwood stems extract. We can assume that this endothermic process is in fact an overlap of endothermic effects associated with water elimination and/or partial decomposition of the two extracts. On the TG-DSC curve of wormwood leaves extract, the oxidative degradation occurs with the formation of several exothermic peaks between 464.5 °C and 674.1 °C. The exothermic effect recorded at 464.5 °C, associated with a lower mass loss (4.46%), can be related to the degradation of aromatic amino-acids and/or carbohydrates present in the leaves extract. Continuous exothermic effects can be observed on DSC curve between 633.6 °C and 674.1 °C; these effects could be associated with the oxidative degradation of a wide variety of metabolites, principally phenolics, simple amines and several aromatic compounds. The four exothermic processes recorded on the DSC curve, are accompanied by a mass loss of 20.06% recorded on the TG curve. In the final stage of degradation, only a small mass loss of 3.35% can be seen, which can be assigned to the burning of organic residues (carbon). On the TG-DSC curve of wormwood stems extract, the oxidative degradation occurs with the formation of two exothermic peaks at 580.1 °C and at 593.3 °C, associated with a mass loss of 19.59%. These exothermic effects could be related with the degradation of aromatic compounds, carbohydrates and aromatic amino-acids present in the stems extract.

FT-IR spectroscopy analysis is one of the most widely technique that can be utilized for the qualitative analysis of pharmacologically active compounds from various plant species. The FT-IR spectrum presents unique bands which express the presence of functional groups contained by the molecules in the extracts; it constitutes a chemical fingerprint [11].

Figure 1C,D show that the FT-IR spectra of *A. absinthium* leaves and stems extracts had relevant absorption peaks at 3365.78 cm^{-1} (for leaves) and 3381.21 cm^{-1} (for stems); 2926.01 cm^{-1} (for leaves) and 2924.09 cm^{-1} and 2852.72 cm^{-1} respectively (for stems); 1616.35 cm^{-1} (for leaves) and 1600.92 cm^{-1} (for stems) and at 1068.56 cm^{-1} for both wormwood extracts. The broad bands at 3365.78 (for leaves extract) and 3381.21 cm^{-1} for stems extract correspond both to O-H stretching of hydroxyl groups from alcohols, phenols and carboxylic acids [12] as well as N-H stretching of amines or amides [13]. The peak situated at 2926.01 cm^{-1} for leaves as well as 2924.09 cm^{-1} and 2852.72 cm^{-1} respectively, for stems extract, corresponds to the saturated aliphatic C-H bonds. In the case of stems extract, the two values correspond to C-H stretching which indicate the occurrence of aromatic ring and alkyl group attachment. This may be corresponding to C-C stretching vibration of aromatic amines [14]. Moreover, the band situated at 2926.01 cm^{-1} in case of leaves extract, may correspond to the CH_3 vibrations which exist in the functional groups of chlorophyll present in wormwood extract [15]. The peak at 1616.35 cm^{-1} in the case of leaves extract and the peak at 1600.92 cm^{-1} showed in the case of stems extract, confirm the presence of amide functional groups, like N-H bending vibration [16]. The analysis of C-H out-of plane bending can often distinguish substitution patterns which may correspond to N-O asymmetric stretch of nitro functional groups, with bands situated at 1516.05 cm^{-1} in the case of leaves extract and 1506.41 cm^{-1} in the case of stems extract. These two bands confirm the presence of aromatic ring [13]. The bands situated at 1398.39 cm^{-1} (for leaves extract) and 1384.89 cm^{-1} (for stems extract) are attributed to the C-H bending vibration of alkanes, which refer to the binding of the aromatic ring –C-H for the in-plane bending absorption. The band situated at 1265.30 cm^{-1} (for the leaves extract) and the band from 1269.16 cm^{-1} as well as 1238.30 cm^{-1} respectively, in the case of stems extract, corresponds to the aromatic acid ester C-O stretching vibration [17]. The bands located in the range 1068.56 cm^{-1} and 1124.50 cm^{-1} can be attributed to C-O stretch vibration that may come from alcohol functional groups (primary, secondary and tertiary) [17]. The bands in the range 534.28 cm^{-1} and 912.33 cm^{-1} represent the out of plane bending vibration from aromatics alkenes =C-H [18]. The FT-IR spectra reveal only the structural information of some functional groups presents in the plant extract and can be used for authentification of some constituents, but completing information with other techniques for determining the quantitative analysis and confirm the presence of pharmacologically active compounds are required.

3.2. Phenolic Composition

Phenolic compounds are widely distributed in plants and they are associated with the prevention of several diseases where oxidative stress plays an important role [19]. The total phenolic content of the two wormwood extracts was evaluated due to the importance of this class of compounds for the antioxidant activity. The results showed that the leaves extract have a higher phenolic content (54.68 ± 1.93 mg GAE/g extract) compared to the extract from stems (44.15 ± 1.12 mg GAE/g extract).

The total phenolic content of various wormwood extracts was evaluated in several studies. A higher value was observed for the hydroalcoholic extract obtained from the above ground parts of the plant (9.29 ± 0.51 mg GAE/g dry weight) as compared to the hexane and methanol one [20]. Another study estimated a total phenolic content of 123 ± 0.82 mg GAE/g extract for the methanolic extract obtained from aerial parts of the plant [21].

A variation in the total phenolic content depending on the collecting area was observed. Values of the total phenolic content ranging between 49.39 ± 2.20 mg GAE/g dry weight and 99.89 ± 3.30 mg GAE/g dry weight were determined for methanolic extracts obtained from *A. absinthium* aerial parts [22]. In the plant material collected in Romania, a previous study estimated a total phenolic content of 18.14 mg GAE/g dry weight for aerial parts of the plant [23]. The above ground parts of wormwood collected in Turkey presented a total phenolic content of 9.79 μg GAE/mg [24].

Among polyphenols, flavonoids are known for their antioxidant, anti-inflammatory, antibacterial, antiviral and anticancer properties [25]. The total flavonoid content of wormwood extracts was in agreement with the results obtained for total phenolic content, with a lower value for wormwood stems extract (34.14 ± 2.16 mg CE/g extract) compared to leaves extract (43.08 ± 2.47 mg CE/g extract).

Other studies mentioned higher flavonoid content for the ethanolic extract from wormwood aerial parts as compared to chloroform and aqueous extracts [26]. Variations between 3.02 ± 0.05 and 19.28 ± 0.12 mg quercetin equivalents per gram dry weight were observed for different extracts obtained from the above ground plant material [20]. The highest total flavonoid content estimated for plant material collected in different Tunisian areas was 126.4 ± 2.32 mg catechin equivalent per gram dry weight [22].

Both alcoholic extracts were subjected to LC-MS analysis under identical solution and instrumental conditions which enabled the identification and in some cases quantification, consistent with their

Rt and *m/z* values, of 9 polyphenolic acids: gentisic acid, chlorogenic acid, caffeic acid, *p*-coumaric acid, isoquercitrin, rutin, quercitrin, luteolin and apigenin expressed in μg/mg d.w. (Table 3). Obtained results indicated that chlorogenic acid was the most abundant polyphenolic quantified compound. Isoquercitrin, rutin and quercitrin were also detected but in smaller concentrations, accompanied by traces of gentisic acid, caffeic acid, *p*-coumaric acid, luteolin and apigenin which were below the limit of quantification. In terms of their concentration in the two types of extract, it seems that *A. absinthium* stems extract are somehow similar to *A. absinthium* leaves extract, *A. absinthium* stems extracts being slyghtly richer, with one exception (Table 3). Thus, chlorogenic acid, isoquercitrin and rutin have concentrations a bit higher in *A. absinthium* stems while quercitrin is more abundant in *A. absinthium* leaves extract (Table 3).

In a similar approach, Ivanescu and co-workers have conducted a HPLC-DAD-MS study in order to determine the polyphenols from the aerial part of three *Artemisia* species, namely *A. absinthium*, *A. annua*, and *A. vulgaris* before as well as after acid hydrolysis. Results for *A. absinthium* have shown that in case of the un-hydrolyzed extract ferulic acid (0.608 mg/100 g dry herb) and kaempferol (2.456 mg/100 g dry herb) could be identified. On the other hand in case of the hydrolyzed extract *p*-Coumaric acid (12.6 mg/100 g dry herb), ferulic acid (2.432 mg/100 g dry herb), fisetin (0.792 mg/100 g dry herb) and patuletin (0.616 mg/100 g dry herb) could be detected [27]. Also Craciunescu and co-workers, used maceration as a method of extraction but ethanol 70% as solvent. Among the phenolic and flavonoid screened compounds they have detected gallic acid (0.092 ± 0.005 mg/g dry extract), chlorogenic acid (0.077 ± 0.004 mg/g dry extract), caffeic acid (0.181 ± 0.009 mg/g dry extract), coumaric acid (0.112 ± 0.006 mg/g dry extract), ferulic acid (0.100 ± 0.005 mg/g dry extract), rutin (0.089 ± 0.005 mg/g dry extract), luteolin (0.677 ± 0.036 mg/g dry extract), quercetin (2.707 ± 0.135 mg/g dry extract), myricetin (0.201 ± 0.011 mg/g dry extract), apigenin (0.359 ± 0.019 mg/g dry extract) [28]. In a comprehensive study conducted by Aberham and co-workers, sesquiterpene lactones, flavonoids and lignans were detected from an extract of *A. absinthium* obtained by maceration with dichloromethane by HPLC-MS [29]. Sahin and co-workers have tried to increase the amount of bioactive compounds from *A. absinthium* by optimization of ultrasonic-assisted extraction. HPLC-DAD analysis has shown the presence the following polyphenols: protocatechuic acid (0.10 ± 0.01 mg/g dried plant), chlorogenic acid (5.72 ± 0.11 mg/g dried plant), caffeic acid (2.07 ± 0.01 mg/g dried plant), ferulic acid (19.57 ± 0.44 mg/g dried plant), rosmarinic acid (7.82 ± 0.01 mg/g dried plant) [30].

For the prevention of various types of cell damage, antioxidants are widely employed compounds. Antioxidants are natural products with the ability to eliminate reactive oxygen species (ROS) in enzymatic and nonenzymatic processes. Plants contain potent antioxidants which act as radical scavengers and mitigate the damaging effects of ROS to the human body [31].

Regarding the antioxidant activity presented in this study, it was demonstrated that the wormwood extract obtained from stems showed a slightly increased antioxidant effect compared to the leaves extract. Looking at the wormwood extracts obtained from leaves it was showed that with increasing concentration, antioxidant activity increases. Our results are in agreement with those obtained by Kim and co-workers [32]. Lee and co-workers reported an antiradical activity of *A. absinthium* roots (IC_{50} = 271.34 μg/mL). They also found for *A. annua* high IC_{50} values of antiradical activities (IC_{50} = 190.54 μg/mL for leaves extract and IC_{50} = 22.90 μg/mL for stems extracts). Comparable to our results are the values obtained by the same group of authors for *A. capillaries* leaves extract (IC_{50} = 448.15 μg/mL) and *A. selengensis* stems extract (IC_{50} = 411.85 μg/mL) [33].

Slightly higher values regarding the radical-scavenging activities of wormwood extract were reported by Mahmoudi et al. [34]. These authors found IC_{50} values of 612 μg/mL for the DPPH radical-scavenging activity, in case of an *A. absinthium* extract obtained from aerial parts collected during flowering stage.

3.3. Bioactivity

The in vitro studies performed in this paper demonstrate that *A. absinthium* leaves and stems extracts exhibited a dose dependent anti-migratory and cytotoxic effect on the two tumor cell lines, melanoma and breast adenocarcinoma cells. An important aspect is represented by the data obtained for non-tumor cells (human keratinocytes), where *A. absinthium* extracts had no significant cytotoxic effect at 24 and 48 h post-stimulation; at 72 h after stimulation the cytotoxic effect was lower compared to the effect obtained on cancer cells. The differences between the cytotoxic activity on tumor and non-tumor cells suggest that *A. absinthium* extracts affect more the cancer cells.

Our results regarding the fact that wormwood has a more potent effect on cancer cells, are in accordance with the data found in the literature, where Koyuncu [35] evaluated the anticancer activity of *A. absinthium* methanolic extract on DLD-1 colon cancer cells, ECC-1 endometrium cancer cells and HEK-293 embryonic kidney cells and indicated that it had a cytotoxic effect on the cancer cells while showing low cytotoxicity on the kidney cells. Gordanian et al. [36] tested the effect of five *Artemisia* species (*A. absinthium*, *A. vulgaris*, *A. incana*, *A. fragrans* and *A. spicigera*) harvested from Iran against MCF7 breast adenocarcinoma and HEK-293 embryonic kidney cells. *A. absinthium* L. methanolic extract displayed a stronger cytotoxic effect against MCF7 cells than on HEK-293 cells [36]. The same authors evaluated the anti-cancer effect of various *A. absinthium* L. extracts obtained from different parts of the species—flower, leaf, stem or root and demonstrated that the most potent decrease in MCF7 cells viability was obtained after stimulation with the methanolic extract obtained from flowers, followed by the leaf, stem and finally the root methanolic extract [36]. The present study demonstrated strong cytotoxic and anti-migratory activities against both A375 and MCF7 cancer cells after stimulation with *A. absinthium* stems ethanolic extract.

Another aim of the present study was to determine the degree of selectivity of *A. absinthium* leaves and stems extracts. Even though the results obtained in the cytotoxicity assay evidenced that *A. absinthium* extracts affect more the melanoma and breast adenocarcinoma cells rather than the human keratinocytes, the tested samples did not show a selective effect on the cancer cells after the determination of SI; the values obtained were lower than 2. It is considered that the higher the SI is, the more potent and differential a sample is [37]. According to Peña-Morán et al. [38] for a compound to be considered selective the SI value must be higher than 10. The same authors stated that compounds that have the SI between 1 and 10 are considered non-selective [38].

Shafi and co-workers [39] proved that *A. absinthium* methanolic extract obtained from the aerial parts inhibits cell proliferation and triggers apoptosis in two breast cancer cells, namely MDA-MB-231 and MCF7 cells. In a recent study it was shown that *A. absinthium* ethanolic extract inhibited BEL-7404 human hepatoma and H22 mouse hepatoma cells growth and induced apoptosis without affecting the normal hepatic cells [40].

The TPA model of ear inflammation is a very useful tool for assessing anti-inflammatory compounds. When applied to mice ear skin, TPA provokes an influx of mast cells that release mediators responsible for an increased vascular permeability and for neutrophils infiltration [41]. This is consistent with our results, where topical application of TPA led to a massive pro-inflammatory response in mouse ear such as interstitial edema, diffuse inflammation, exocytosis and micro-abscesses.

The group treated with *A. absinthium* leaves extract showed a mild anti-inflammatory effect. By contrast, topical application of *A. absinthium* stems extract elicited a noticeable anti-inflammatory effect in TPA-induced ear inflammation in mice. Histological evaluation showed that *A. absinthium* stems extract inhibited infiltration of neutrophils into the site of inflammation as there was a mild infiltrate with neutrophils at the dermis level, without micro-abscesses, exocytosis or leucocytes margination.

4. Materials and Methods

4.1. Chemicals and Reagents

Ethanol 80% (*v*/*v*) and distilled water, purchased from Chemical Company SA (Iasi, Romania) were used to obtain the wormwood extracts (leaves and stems). In order to investigate the antioxidant effect, 2,2-diphenyl-1-picrylhydrazyl (DPPH, Batch No: # STBF5255V, purchased from Sigma Aldrich, Steinheim, Germany) was used The ascorbic acid used as etalon for determination of antioxidant effect, was acquired from Lach-Ner Company (Prague, Czech Republic). For the determination of total phenolic content, were used gallic acid 98% and Na_2CO_3 99%, acquired from Roth (Dautphetal, Germany) and Folin-Ciocalteu reagent, purchased from Merck (Darmstadt, Germany). For the determination of total flavonoid content, were used $NaNO_2$ purchased from Merck; $AlCl_3$ 98% acquired from Roth and NaOH pellets, acquired from ChimReactiv SRL (Bucharest, Romania). (+)-Cathechin hydrate 98% used as standard for the determination of flavonoid content was acquired from Sigma-Aldrich.

The chemicals used for LC-MS analysis were as follows: methanol (99.9% purity) and acetic acid (99.9% purity), purchased from Merck. Standard polyphenolic compounds were: gentisic acid, chlorogenic acid, caffeic acid, *p*-coumaric acid, isoquercitrin, rutin, quercitrin, luteolin, and apigenin were purchased from Sigma-Aldrich. Ultrapure deionized water was provided by a MiliQ system Milli-Q® Integral Water Purification System (Merck Millipore, Darmstadt, Germany).

The chemicals used for cell culture were purchased from Sigma-Aldrich (Taufkirchen, Germany) and Thermo Fisher Scientific (Boston, MA, USA). TPA (12-*O*-tetradecanoylphorbol-13-acetate) was acquired from Sigma-Aldrich. For the experimental protocol the substance was dissolved in acetone at a concentration of 8×10^{-4} M. Acetone (analytical purity of 99.92%) was purchased from ChimReactiv SRL.

4.2. Cell Lines

A375-human melanoma cell line (ATCC® CRL-1619 ™) and MCF7—human breast adenocarcinoma cell line (ATCC® HTB-22™) were purchased from the American Type Culture Collection (ATCC, Manassas, VA, USA); HaCaT—human keratinocytes were kindly provided by the University of Debrecen (Debrecen, Hungary). A375 and HaCaT cells were cultured in high glucose Dulbecco's Modified Eagle's Medium (DMEM; Sigma-Aldrich); MCF7 cells were cultured in Eagle's Minimum Essential Medium (EMEM; ATCC). Each cell line was supplemented with 10% fetal bovine serum (FBS; Gibco, Thermo Fisher Scientific) and 1% antibiotic mixture (Penicillin/Streptomycin—Pen/Strep, 10,000 IU/mL; Sigma-Aldrich). The cells were kept under standard conditions (37 °C and humidified atmosphere containing 5% CO_2).

4.3. Plant Material

A. absinthium leaves and stems were collected in June 2018 from Vâlcea county (Romania; coordinates: 44°59′17.46″ N, 23°52′5.59″ E) and identified by Professor DS Antal from the Department of Pharmaceutical Botany. A voucher specimen (no. MA_AA1) was deposited at the Herbarium of the Faculty of Pharmacy, Timisoara. After collection, the samples were dried in a plant dryer at room temperature and conserved in a desiccator at 20 °C in darkness until further uses.

4.4. Preparation of A. absinthium L. Ethanolic Extracts

Ethanolic extracts from *A. absinthium* leaves and stems were obtained according to the method of Mau et al., slightly modified [42]. Procedures were as follows: 1 g of dried and ground sample (leaves/stem) was mixed with 60 mL ethanol 80% and sonicated for 1 h at room temperature (amplitude A = 50% and cycle C = 0.5) with an UP200S Ultrasonic Homogenizer from Hielscher (Wanaque, NJ, USA).

After sonication, both samples were filtered through a Whatman no. 4 filter paper and concentrated under reduced pressure at 35 °C using a rotary evaporator. Each dried crude extract was subsequently lyophilized and stored at −4 °C. Lyophilized extracts were further employed for the preparation of aqueous stock solutions (concentration 10 mg/mL). Dispersion in ultrapure water was enhanced by sonication (50% amplitude) for 10 min; finally the obtained stock solutions were filtered. The schematic protocol is depicted in Figure 6.

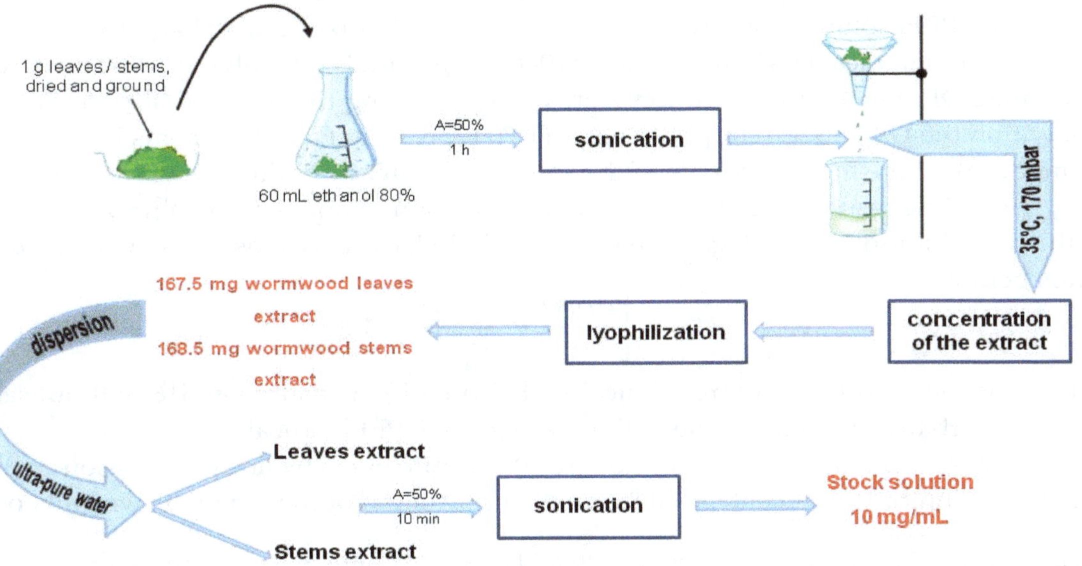

Figure 6. Schematic protocol of *A. absinthium* L. ethanolic extracts preparation.

4.5. Physico-Chemical Characterization

Thermal behavior of the two dried lyophilized extracts was studied using a STA 449C instrument (Netzsch, Selb, Germany) in air atmosphere at a flow rate of 20 mL·min^{-1}. The TG/DSC curves were recorded in the range 25–1000 °C with a heating rate of 10 K·min^{-1}, using alumina crucibles.

The FT-IR spectra of the dried lyophilized of *A. absinthium* leaves and stems extracts were obtained using a Prestige-21 spectrometer (Shimadzu, Duisburg, Germany) at room temperature conditions. The spectral region ranged from 4000–400 cm^{-1} using KBr pellets and a resolution of 4 cm^{-1}.

LC-MS experiments were conducted on an 6120 LC-MS analytical system from Agilent (Santa Clara, CA, USA) consisting of 1260 Infinity HPLC equipped with G1322A degasser, G1311B cuaternary pump, G1316A column thermostat, G1365C MWD detector and G7129A autosampler coupled with a Quadrupolar (Q) mass spectrometer and electrospray ionization source (ESI). LC-MS is connected to a PC computer running the OpenLAB CDS ChemStation Workstation software.

The samples preparation for LC-MS analysis were homogenized with a WisdVM-10vortex mixer (Witeg Labortechnik, Wertheim, Baden-Württemberg, Germany) and centrifuged for 2 min at 10,000 rpm in a ThermoMicro CL17microcentrifuge (Thermo Fisher Scientific). The supernatant was collected and submitted to LC-MS analysis. Polyphenolic compounds were separated on a reverse phase Zorbax Eclipse Plus C18 column (3.0 mm × 100 mm × 3.5 μm). Gradient elution with a mixture of 0.1% acetic acid and methanol as mobile phase consists was performed: the first 5 min 5% methanol, until 38 min in gradient elution up to 42% methanol, proportion kept until 41 min and ending with 5% methanol for 1 more minute as described before [43]. The injection volume was 10 μL, the flow rate was 1 mL/min and the column temperature 40 °C. UV detection was conducted at 330 and 370 nm. MS detection was achieved by electrospray ionization (ESI) in the single ion monitoring mode (SIM) simultaneous for all screened compounds. All mass spectra were recorded in the negative ion mode. Capillary voltage was set at 3500 V, the dry gas flow was 12 L/min at 350 °C, the nebulizer pressure was kept at 55 psi and the fragmentor was set at 70. For the quantification of polyphenolic compounds calibration curves were conducted by the external standard method in the 0.05–2 μg/mL range for a six-point plot for each compound. The *m/z* scale of the mass spectrum was calibrated by use of an external calibration standard ESI Tuning Mix from Agilent.

4.6. Antioxidant Activity Assay

The antioxidant activity of *A. absinthium* extracts was determined by DPPH (2,2-diphenyl-1-picrylhydrazyl) free-radical scavenging assay. The electron donation ability of wormwood leaves and stems extracts was measured spectrophotometrically, leading to the yellow coloration of the initially purple-colored DPPH solution, according to the method of Manzoco et al. [44]. To 0.5 mL ethanolic extract of *A. absinthium* leaves/stems extracts (10–0.5 mg/mL), 2 mL solvent (ultrapure water) and 0.5 mL of 1 mM DPPH ethanolic solution were added. During the incubation period, the extracts were kept within the UV/VIS Spectrophotometer (T 70 type, from PG Instruments Ltd., Leicestershire, United Kingdom) where the absorbance of the samples was read continuously (for 10 min) against a blank at 516 nm. The results were expressed in comparison to an ethanol solution of ascorbic acid 0.1 mg/mL. The inhibition percentage of free radical DPPH, expressed as (IP%), was calculated with the formula below:

$$IP\,\% = \left[\frac{A_{DPPH} - A_{sample}}{A_{DPPH}}\right] * 100 \tag{1}$$

where: A_{DPPH} is the absorbance of free radical DPPH (blank), measured at 516 without sample and A_{sample} is the absorbance of each sample in the presence of DPPH radical.

The half maximal inhibitory concentration (IC_{50}) was calculated by linear regression analysis curve plotting between inhibition percentage (IP%) and concentration of the ethanolic wormwood extracts.

4.7. Determination of Total Phenolic Content and Total Flavonoid Content of A. Absinthium

The total phenolic content of the ethanolic extracts from wormwood leaves and stems was evaluated using the Folin-Ciocalteu method, slightly modified [45]. The method was briefly the following: 0.5 mL of extract solutions (1 mg/mL) were mixed with 2.5 mL Folin-Ciocalteu reagent diluted 1:10. Then 2 mL of 7.5% sodium carbonate solution were added. Samples were kept in the dark for 90 min, then the absorbance was read versus blank at 750 nm using a UviLine 9400 Spectrophotometer from SI Analytics (Deutschland, Germany). The total phenolic content was determined using a gallic acid calibration curve (R^2 = 0.996). To this end, a gallic acid calibration curve was obtained, using gallic acid solutions of different concentrations (0.0025–0.1 mg/mL). The total phenolic content of the two extracts was calculated as milligrams of gallic acid equivalents (GAE) per gram extract.

The total flavonoid content of the two ethanolic extracts was evaluated using the following method [22]: an aliquot of 1 mg/mL extract solution (250 μL) was mixed with 5% $NaNO_2$ (75 μL). After 6 min, 10% $AlCl_3$ (150 μL) and 1M NaOH (500 μL) were added. The volume was adjusted to 2.5 mL with distilled water. The absorbance was read at 510 nm versus blank using a UviLine 9400 Spectrophotometer from SI Analytics. The total flavonoid content was calculated using a (+)-Catechin hydrate calibration curve (R^2 = 0.999) in the range 0.005–0.4 mg/mL. The results were expressed as milligrams catechin equivalents per gram extract (mg CE/g extract).

4.8. Alamar Blue Assay–Cell Viability Assessment

The viability was determined using the Alamar blue assay, a technique meant to evaluate the cytotoxic effect caused by different agents. The cells (1×10^4/well) were cultured in 96-well plates, allowed to adhere overnight and then stimulated with different concentrations of the extractive solutions (50, 100, 250, 500 and 1000 μg/mL) for 24, 48 and 72 h. After the stimulation periods, 20 μL of Alamar blue (10% of the volume of cell culture medium—200 μL/well) was added. The cells were incubated for 3h at 37 °C and then the absorbance was measured at two different wavelengths (570 and 600 nm) with an xMark™ Microplate spectrophotometer (BioRad, xMarkTMMicroplate, Serial No. 10578, Tokyo, Japan). The principle of this technique consists of the natural ability of metabolically active cells (viable cells) to reduce resazurin (dark blue compound) to the fluorescent form, resorufin (pink compound with intense fluorescence).

4.9. Selectivity-Index

In order to determine the selectivity of *A. absinthium* leaves and stems extracts, the selectivity index was calculated according to the following formula [38,46]:

$$Selectivity\,index\,(SI) = \frac{IC_{50\,[non-malignant\,HaCaT]}}{IC_{50\,[tumor\,cell\,line]}} \quad (2)$$

4.10. Scratch Assay–Assessment of the Anti-Migratory Potential

This method is an in vitro technique used to determine a possible inhibitory effect of *A absinthium* extractive solutions on the migration and invasion capacity of the tumor cell lines (A375 and MCF7 cells) and of the non-tumor cells (HaCaT). The protocol was applied as previously described in the literature [47]. Briefly, 2×10^5 cells/well were cultured in 12-well plates until 90% confluence was reached. Using a sterile pipette tip scratches were drawn on well-defined zones of the cells monolayer. The detached cells resulted from the procedure were removed by washing with phosphate-buffered saline (PBS) prior to stimulation. The cells were stimulated with different concentrations of the extractive solutions (50, 100, 250, 500 and 1000 μg/mL). Images of the cells in culture were taken at 0 h and 24 h and compared with the control cells (no stimulation). Pictures were taken with Olympus IX73 inverted microscope provided with DP74 camera (Olympus, Tokyo, Japan) and the analysis of the cell growth was performed with cell Sense Dimension software. The migration percentage was calculated according to the formula previously described by Felice et al. [48]:

$$Scratch\,closure\,rate = \left[\frac{A_{t_0} - A_t}{A_{t_0}}\right] * 100 \quad (3)$$

where: A_{t_0} is the scratch area at time 0; A_t is the scratch area at 24 h.

4.11. In Vivo TPA-Induced Ear Inflammation Protocol

In order to evaluate the effect of *A. absinthium* leaves and stems extracts on ear inflammation were performed *in vivo* experiment using SKH1 female mice (n = 3), 6 months old (weigh = 29.70–32.80 g); purchased from Charles River Laboratory (Budapest, Hungary). The mice were kept in standard conditions: a 20–24 °C temperature, humidity between 45–65%, a 12-h light/dark cycle, food *ad libitum* with free access to water, as recommended by the European Directive 2010/63/EU and the national law 43/2014. The protocol used for the euthanasia of the animals followed the Guidelines described by the American Veterinary Medical Association (AVMA) for the Euthanasia of Animals (2013 Edition). The Bioethical Committee of "Victor Babes" University of Medicine and Pharmacy Timisoara, Romania, approved the performed experiment.

The experimental model of TPA-induced ear inflammation was performed according to the following protocol: female mice were anesthetized with Isoflurane and the TPA solution was topically applied (20 μL/mouse ear) and they were assigned to the subsequent groups (Table 6).

Table 6. In vivo experimental design for the local acute inflammation model.

Group No.	Group Name	Description
1	Control	With no intervention
2	Control + Acetone	Acetone (solvent for TPA)—20 μL/mouse ear
3	TPA	TPA solution (20 μL/mouse ear)
4	TPA + Indomethacin	Indomethacine cream (4%) was topically applied after the TPA solution
5	TPA + *A. absinthium* L. leaves extract	*A. absinthium* leaves extract (~2%) was topically applied after the TPA solution
6	TPA + *A. absinthium* L. stems extract	*A. absinthium* stems extract (~2%) was topically applied after the TPA solution

An electronic caliper was used to measure the diameter and length of mice ears (the results were presented in millimeters) before the TPA application and at the end of the experiment. After 24 h the mice were weighted and after that were anesthetized and sacrificed, the ears were measured and collected for histopathological evaluation.

4.12. Histopathological Assessment of Mice Ears

For histopathological analysis, the mice ears were fixed in 10% buffered formalin for 48 h and then they were embedded in paraffin followed the routine automated flow of this procedure. Four µm-thick sections were cut using a Leica Rotary Microtome (Leica Biosystems Nussloch GmbH, Nussloch, Germany) and mounted on glass slides, deparaffinized in xylene and rehydrated. Finally, the samples were stained with the conventional Hematoxylin & Eosin. The slides were examined by two pathologists in a blinded way. Image acquisition and analysis were performed using a Nikon Eclipse E 600 microscope (Nikon Microscopes/Instruments Division, Vienna, Austria) and Lucia G software (Laboratory Imaging, Prague, Czech Republic) for microscopic image analysis.

4.13. Statistical Analysis

The statistical program used in the present study was GraphPad Prism 5 (GraphPad Software, San Diego, CA, USA). The data obtained were expressed as mean ± SD. Regarding the in vitro results, comparison among the groups was performed using the one-way ANOVA followed by Dunnett's multiple comparison test (* $p < 0.05$; ** $p < 0.01$; *** $p < 0.001$).

5. Conclusions

Results of this study showed that the ethanolic extracts from *A. absinthium* leaves and stems collected from Southern Romania contain chlorogenic acid, quercitrin, isoquercitrin and rutin. The IR profiles of extracts from leaves and stems of *A. absinthium* revealed the presence of active components with various functional groups (acid, alcohol, alkane, amine, amide, aromatic radicals). Leaves displayed a higher content of total phenolics and flavonoids than stems. Regarding the activity against cancer cells, at the check point of 72 h a significant cytotoxic activity against both MCF7 and A375 cell lines was detected. Wormwood stems extract were slightly more active than leaves extract. In the experimental conditions of our study, both leaves and stems extracts showed dose-dependent anti-migratory potential, MCF7 being the most sensitive cell line. Moreover, stems extract elicited a stronger anti-migratory activity. In an *in vivo* model of inflammation, the topical application of stems extract led to a noticeable anti-inflammatory effect, while the activity of the leaves extract was milder. Overall, A. *absinthium* from Southern Romania was proved to possess biological activities that can be exploited in further studies.

Author Contributions: Conceptualization, E.-A.M., F.A. and I.Z.P.; methodology, E.-A.M., F.A., D.M., S.S., R.G. and A.C.; software, I.Z.P., F.A. and R.G.; validation, D.S.A., C.D. and C.-A.D.; formal analysis, D.A., C.D. and E.-A.M; investigation, A.C., M.D., S.S., R.G., I.Z.P., D.M., F.A. and E.-A.M.; resources, C.-A.D., Z.C., C.S. and R.C.; data curation, D.S.A., C.D. and C.-A.D.; writing—original draft preparation, E.-A.M., F.A. and I.Z.P.; writing—review and editing, D.S.A., C.-A.D., C.D., Z.C., R.C. and M.D.; visualization, E.-A.M., F.A. and D.S.A.; supervision, D.S.A., C.-A.D., C.S. and C.D.; project administration, C.-A.D.; funding acquisition, Z.C., R.C. and C.-A.D.

Abbreviations

LC-MS	Liquid chromatography–mass spectrometry
TG-DSC	Thermogravimetry-differential scanning calorimeter analysis
FT-IR	Fourier-transform infrared spectroscopy
Rt	Retention time
DPPH	2,2-Diphenyl-1-picrylhydrazyl
AOA	Antioxidant activity
IC_{50}	Maximal inhibitory concentration

IP	Inhibition percentage
HaCaT	Human keratinocytes
MCF7	Human breast adenocarcinoma cell line
PBS	Phosphate-buffered saline
A375	Human melanoma cell line
ATCC	American Type Culture Collection
DMEM	Dulbecco's Modified Eagle's Medium
EMEM	Eagle's Minimum Essential Medium
FBS	Fetal bovine serum
SD	Standard deviation
TPA	12-*O*-Tetradecanoylphorbol-13-acetate
ROS	Reactive oxygen species
MS	Mass spectroscopy
ESI	Electrospray ionization
SIM	Single ion monitoring mode
SI	Selectivity index
mg GAE	Milligrams of gallic equivalents
mg CE	Milligrams cathechin equivalents

References

1. Deans, S.G.; Kennedy, A.I. *Artemisia absinthium*. In *Artemisia*, 1st ed.; Wright, C.W., Ed.; CRC Press: London, UK, 2001; pp. 79–90.
2. Bora, K.S.; Sharma, A. The Genus Artemisia: A Comprehensive Review. *Pharm. Biol.* **2011**, *49*, 101–109. [CrossRef] [PubMed]
3. European Medicines Agency. Assessment Report on *Artemisia absinthium L.*, herba. Available online: https://docplayer.net/90203895-Assessment-report-on-artemisia-absinthium-l-herba.html (accessed on 24 August 2019).
4. Ivanescu, B.; Miron, A.; Lungu, C. Histo-anatomy of vegetative organs of some Artemisia species. *Med. Surg. J.* **2015**, *119*, 917–924.
5. Bruneton, J. *Pharmacognosie. Phytochimie. Plantes Médicinales*, 5th ed.; Lavoisier: Paris, France, 2016; pp. 767–769.
6. Hänsel, R.; Sticher, O. *Pharmakognosie–Phytopharmazie*, 8th ed.; Springer: Heidelberg, Germany, 2007; pp. 443–445.
7. Lee, Y.J.; Thiruvengadam, M.; Chung, I.M.; Nagella, P. Polyphenol composition and antioxidant activity from the vegetable plant *Artemisia absinthium* L. *AJCS* **2013**, *7*, 1921–1926.
8. Omer, B.; Krebs, S.; Omer, H.; Noor, T.O. Steroid-sparing effect of wormwood (*Artemisia absinthium*) in Crohn's disease: A double-blind placebo-controlled study. *Phytomedicine* **2007**, *14*, 87–95. [CrossRef] [PubMed]
9. Krebs, S.; Omer, T.N.; Omer, B. Wormwood (*Artemisia absinthium*) suppresses tumour necrosis factor alpha and accelerates healing in patients with Crohn's disease—A controlled clinical trial. *Phytomedicine* **2010**, *17*, 305–309. [CrossRef] [PubMed]
10. Krebs, S.; Omer, B.; Omer, T.N.; Fliser, D. Wormwood (*Artemisia absinthium*) for poorly responsive early-stage IgA nephropathy: A pilot uncontrolled trial. *Am. J. Kidney Dis.* **2010**, *56*, 1095–1099. [CrossRef] [PubMed]
11. Easmin, S.; Sarker, M.Z.I.; Ghafoor, K.; Ferdosh, S.; Jaffri, J.; Ali, M.E.; Mirhosseini, H.; Al-Juhaimi, F.Y.; Perumal, V.; Khatib, A. Rapid investigation of α-glucosidase inhibitory activity of Phaleria macrocarpa extracts using FTIR-ATR based fingerprinting. *J. Food Drug Anal.* **2017**, *25*, 306–315. [CrossRef] [PubMed]
12. Szymczycha-Madeja, A.; Welna, M.; Zyrnicki, W. Multi-element analysis, bioavailability and fractionation of herbal tea products. *J. Braz. Chem. Soc.* **2013**, *24*, 777–787. [CrossRef]
13. Mohani, N.; Ahmad, M.; Mehjabeen; Jahan, N. Evaluation of phytoconstituents of three plants Acorus calamus linn. *Artemisia absinthium* Linn and Bergenia himalaica boriss by FTIR spectroscopic analysis. *Pak. J. Pharm. Sci.* **2014**, *27*, 2251–2255. [PubMed]
14. Malaikozhundan, B.; Vaseeharan, B.; Vijayakumar, S.; Sudhakaran, R.; Gobi, N.; Shanthini, G. Antibacterial and antibiofilm assessment of Momordica charantia fruit extract coated silver nanoparticles. *Biocatal. Agric. Biotechnol.* **2016**, *8*, 189–196. [CrossRef]

15. Chang, H.; Kao, M.J.; Chen, T.L.; Chen, C.H.; Cho, K.C.; Lai1, X.R. Characterization of Natural Dye Extracted from Wormwood and Purple Cabbage for Dye-Sensitized Solar Cells. *Int. J. Photoenergy* **2013**, 1–8. [CrossRef]
16. Kumar, P.; SenthamilSelvi, S.; LakshmiPraba, A.; PremKumar, K.; Ganeshkumar, R.S.; Govindaraju, M. Synthesis of silver nanoparticles from Sargassum tenerrimum and screening phytochemcials for its anti-bacterial activity. *Nano Biomed. Eng.* **2012**, *4*, 12–16. [CrossRef]
17. Li, Y.Q.; Kong, D.X.; Wu, H. Analysis and evaluation of essential oil components of cinnamon barks using GC–MS and FTIR spectroscopy. *Ind. Crops Prod.* **2013**, *41*, 269–278. [CrossRef]
18. Heredia-Guerrero, J.A.; Benítez, J.J.; Domínguez, E.; Bayer, I.S.; Cingolani, R.; Athanassiou, A.; Heredia, A. Infrared and Raman spectroscopic features of plant cuticles: A review. *Front. Plant Sci.* **2014**, *5*, 305. [CrossRef] [PubMed]
19. Dai, J.; Mumper, R.J. Plant phenolics: Extraction, analysis and their antioxidant and anticancer properties. *Molecules* **2010**, *15*, 7313–7352. [CrossRef] [PubMed]
20. Bhat, M.Y.; Gul, M.Z.; Lohamror, L.R.; Qureshi, I.A.; Ghazi, I.A. An in vitro Study of the Antioxidant and Antiproliferative Properties of *Artemisia absinthium*—A Potent Medicinal Plant. *Free Radic. Antioxid.* **2018**, *8*, 18–25.
21. Bora, K.S.; Sharma, A. Evaluation of antioxidant and free-radical scavenging potential of *Artemisia absinthium*. *Pharm. Biol.* **2011**, *49*, 1216–1223. [CrossRef] [PubMed]
22. Msaada, K.; Salem, N.; Bachrouch, O.; Bousselmi, S.; Tammar, S.; Alfaify, A.; Al Sane, K.; Ben Ammar, W.; Azeiz, S.; Haj Brahim, A.; et al. Chemical composition and antioxidant and antimicrobial activities of wormwood (*Artemisia absinthium L.*) essential oils and phenolics. *J. Chem.* **2015**, *804658*, 1–12. [CrossRef]
23. Ivanescu, B.; Vlase, L.; Lungu, C.; Corciova, A. HPLC analysis of phenolic compounds from *Artemisia species*. *Eur. Chem. Bull.* **2016**, *5*, 119–123.
24. Sengul, M.; Ercisli, S.; Yildiz, H.; Gungor, N.; Kavaz, A.; Çetin, B. Antioxidant, antimicrobial activity and total phenolic content within the aerial parts of *Artemisia absinthum*, *Artemisia santonicum* and *Saponaria officinalis*. *Iran. J. Pharm. Res.* **2011**, *10*, 49–56.
25. Kumar, S.; Pandey, A.K. Chemistry and biological activities of flavonoids: An overview. *Sci. World J.* **2013**, 1–16. [CrossRef]
26. Singh, R.; Verma, P.K.; Singh, G. Total phenolic, flavonoids and tannin contents in different extracts of *Artemisia absinthium*. *J. Intercult. Ethnopharmacol.* **2012**, *1*, 101–104. [CrossRef]
27. Ivanescu, B.; Vlase, L.; Corciova, A.; Lazar, M.I. HPLC-DAD-MS study of polyphenols from *Artemisia absinthium*, *A. annua*, and *A. vulgaris*. *Chem. Nat. Compd.* **2010**, *46*, 468–470. [CrossRef]
28. Craciunescu, O.; Constantin, D.; Gaspar, A.; Toma, L.; Utoiu, E.; Moldovan, L. Evaluation of antioxidant and cytoprotective activities of Arnica montana L. and *Artemisia absinthium* L. ethanolic extracts. *Chem. Cent. J.* **2012**, *6*, 97. [CrossRef] [PubMed]
29. Aberham, A.; Cicek, S.S.; Schneider, P.; Stuppner, H. Analysis of Sesquiterpene Lactones, Lignans, and Flavonoids in Wormwood (*Artemisia absinthium* L.) Using High-Performance Liquid Chromatography (HPLC)−Mass Spectrometry, Reversed Phase HPLC, and HPLC−Solid Phase Extraction−Nuclear Magnetic Resonance. *J. Agric. Food Chem.* **2010**, *58*, 10817–10823. [CrossRef]
30. Sahin, S.; Aybastıer, O.; Işık, E. Optimisation of ultrasonic-assisted extraction of antioxidant compounds from *Artemisia absinthium* using response surface methodology. *Food Chem.* **2013**, *141*, 1361–1368. [CrossRef]
31. Huang, D. Dietary Antioxidants and Health Promotion. *Antioxidants* **2018**, *7*, 9. [CrossRef]
32. Kim, W.S.; Choi, W.J.; Lee, S.; Kim, W.J.; Lee, D.C.; Sohn, U.D.; Shin, H.S.; Kim, W. Anti-inflammatory, Antioxidant and Antimicrobial Effects of Artemisinin Extracts from *Artemisia annua* L. *Korean J. Physiol. Pharm.* **2015**, *19*, 21–27. [CrossRef]
33. Lee, J.H.; Lee, J.M.; Lee, S.H.; Kim, Y.G.; Lee, S.; Kim, S.M.; Cha, S.W. Comparison of Artemisinin Content and Antioxidant Activity from Various Organs of Artemisia Species. *Hortic. Environ. Biotechnol.* **2015**, *56*, 697–703. [CrossRef]
34. Mahmoudi, M.; Ebrahimzadeh, M.A.; Ansaroudi, F.; Nabavi, S.F.; Nabavi, S.M. Antidepressant and antioxidant activities of Artemisia absinthium L. at flowering stage. *Afr. J. Biotechnol.* **2009**, *8*, 7170–7175.
35. Koyuncu, I. Evaluation of anticancer, antioxidant activity and phenolic compounds of *Artemisia absinthium* L. Extract. *Cell Mol. Biol.* **2018**, *64*, 25–34. [CrossRef]

36. Gordanian, B.; Behbahani, M.; Carapetian, J.; Fazilati, M. In vitro evaluation of cytotoxic activity of flower, leaf, stem and root extracts of five Artemisia species. *Res. Pharm. Sci.* **2014**, *9*, 91–96.
37. Badisa, R.B.; Darling-Reed, S.F.; Joseph, P.; Cooperwood, J.S.; Latinwo, L.M.; Goodman, C.B. Selective cytotoxic activities of two novel synthetic drugs on human breast carcinoma MCF-7 cells. *Anticancer Res.* **2009**, *29*, 2993–2996.
38. Peña-Morán, O.A.; Villarreal, M.L.; Álvarez-Berber, L.; Meneses-Acosta, A.; Rodríguez-López, V. Cytotoxicity, Post-Treatment Recovery, and Selectivity Analysis of Naturally Occurring Podophyllotoxins from Bursera fagaroides var. fagaroides on Breast Cancer Cell Lines. *Molecules* **2016**, *21*, 1013.
39. Shafi, G.; Hasan, T.N.; Syed, N.A.; Al-Hazzani, A.A.; Alshatwi, A.A.; Jyothi, A.; Munshi, A. *Artemisia absinthium* (AA): A novel potential complementary and alternative medicine for breast cancer. *Mol. Biol. Rep.* **2012**, *39*, 7373–7379. [CrossRef]
40. Wei, X.; Xia, L.; Ziyayiding, D.; Chen, Q.; Liu, R.; Xu, X.; Li, J. The Extracts of *Artemisia absinthium* L. Suppress the Growth of Hepatocellular Carcinoma Cells through Induction of Apoptosis via Endoplasmic Reticulum Stress and Mitochondrial-Dependent Pathway. *Molecules* **2019**, *24*, 913. [CrossRef]
41. Bralley, E.E.; Greenspan, P.; Hargrove, J.L.; Wicker, L.; Hartle, D.K. Topical anti-inflammatory activity of Polygonum cuspidatum extract in the TPA model of mouse ear inflammation. *J. Inflamm. (Lond.)* **2008**, *5*, 1. [CrossRef]
42. Mau, J.L.; Chang, C.N.; Huang, S.J.; Chen, C.C. Antioxidant properties of methanolic extracts from Grifola frondosa, Morchella esculenta and Termitomyces albuminosus mycelia. *Food Chem.* **2004**, *87*, 111–118. [CrossRef]
43. Toiu, A.; Mocan, A.; Vlase, L.; Pârvu, A.E.; Vodnar, D.C.; Gheldiu, A.M.; Moldovan, C.; Oniga, I. Comparative Phytochemical Profile, Antioxidant, Antimicrobial and In Vivo Anti-Inflammatory Activity of Different Extracts of Traditionally Used Romanian Ajuga genevensis L. and A. reptans L. (Lamiaceae). *Molecules* **2019**, *24*, 1597. [CrossRef]
44. Manzocco, L.; Anese, M.; Nicoli, M.C. Antioxidant Properties of Tea Extracts as Affected by Processing. *LWT—Food Sci. Technol.* **1998**, *31*, 694–698. [CrossRef]
45. Riahi, L.; Chograni, H.; Elferchichi, M.; Zaouali, Y.; Zoghlami, N.; Mliki, A. Variations in Tunisian wormwood essential oil profiles and phenolic contents between leaves and flowers and their effects on antioxidant activities. *Ind. Crops Prod.* **2013**, *46*, 290–296. [CrossRef]
46. Siewert, B.; Pianowski, E.; Obernauer, A.; Csuk, R. Towards cytotoxic and selective derivatives of maslinic acid. Bioorg. *Med. Chem.* **2014**, *22*, 594–615. [CrossRef]
47. Ghiţu, A.; Schwiebs, A.; Radeke, H.H.; Avram, S.; Zupko, I.; Bor, A.; Pavel, I.Z.; Dehelean, C.A.; Oprean, C.; Bojin, F.; et al. A Comprehensive Assessment of Apigenin as an Antiproliferative, Proapoptotic, Antiangiogenic and Immunomodulatory Phytocompound. *Nutrients* **2019**, *11*, 858. [CrossRef]
48. Felice, F.; Zambito, Y.; Belardinelli, E.; Fabiano, A.; Santoni, T.; Di Stefano, R. Effect of different chitosan derivatives on in vitro scratch wound assay: A comparative study. *Int. J. Biol. Macromol.* **2015**, *76*, 236–241. [CrossRef]

13

Essential Oil of *Mentha aquatica var. Kenting Water Mint* Suppresses Two-Stage Skin Carcinogenesis Accelerated by BRAF Inhibitor Vemurafenib

Chih-Ting Chang [1,2], Wen-Ni Soo [1], Yu-Hsin Chen [3] and Lie-Fen Shyur [1,2,4,*]

1 Agricultural Biotechnology Research Center, Academia Sinica, Taipei 115, Taiwan
2 Department of Biological Science and Technology, National Taiwan University, Taipei 106, Taiwan
3 Taichung District Agricultural Research and Extension Station, Council of Agriculture, Executive Yuan, Taichung 515, Taiwan
4 Graduate Institute of Pharmacognosy, Taipei Medical University, Taipei 110, Taiwan
* Correspondence: lfshyur@ccvax.sinica.edu.tw

Academic Editor: Kyoko Nakagawa-Goto

Abstract: The v-raf murine sarcoma viral homolog B1 (BRAF) inhibitor drug vemurafenib (PLX4032) is used to treat melanoma; however, epidemiological evidence reveals that it could cause cutaneous keratoacanthomas and squamous cell carcinoma in cancer patients with the most prevalent *HRAS*^{Q61L} mutation. In a two-stage skin carcinogenesis mouse model, the skin papillomas induced by 7,12-dimethylbenz[a]anthracene (DMBA)/12-*O*-tetradecanoylphorbol-13-acetate (TPA) (DT) resemble the lesions in BRAF inhibitor-treated patients. In this study, we investigated the bioactivity of *Mentha aquatica var. Kenting Water Mint* essential oil (KWM-EO) against PDV cells, mouse keratinocytes bearing *HRAS*^{Q61L} mutation, and its effect on inhibiting papilloma formation in a two-stage skin carcinogenesis mouse model with or without PLX4032 co-treatment. Our results revealed that KWM-EO effectively attenuated cell viability, colony formation, and the invasive and migratory abilities of PDV cells. Induction of G_2/M cell-cycle arrest and apoptosis in PDV cells was also observed. KWM-EO treatment significantly decreased the formation of cutaneous papilloma further induced by PLX4032 in DT mice (DTP). Immunohistochemistry analyses showed overexpression of keratin14 and COX-2 in DT and DTP skin were profoundly suppressed by KWM-EO treatment. This study demonstrates that KWM-EO has chemopreventive effects against PLX4032-induced cutaneous side-effects in a DMBA/TPA-induced two-stage carcinogenesis model and will be worth further exploration for possible application in melanoma patients.

Keywords: BRAF inhibitor; *Mentha aquatica var. Kenting Water Mint*; essential oil; chemoprevention; two-stage skin carcinogenesis

---

1. Introduction

Cutaneous squamous cell carcinoma (cuSCC) and keratoacanthoma (KA) develop in approximately 20% to 30% of patients who are treated with BRAF (v-raf murine sarcoma viral homolog B1) inhibitors, such as vemurafenib (PLX4032) [1]. Functional studies have demonstrated that these serious side-effects caused during the treatment of PLX4032 are through paradoxical activation of the MAPK signaling pathway of wild-type BRAF cell lines bearing either oncogenic *RAS* mutations or upstream receptor tyrosine kinase activity [2–4]. In a recent study, cuSCC and KAs emerging from patients administrated with BRAF inhibitor were analyzed for oncogenic mutations and activating mutations on *RAS*, especially the *HRAS* isoform was noticed in about 60% of subjects [5]. Among the *RAS* mutants, *HRAS*^{Q61L} was the most prevalent, and thus, the genetic *HRAS*^{Q61L} mutation of cells (e.g., keratinocytes PDV) was selected to investigate the pre-clinical pathological mechanisms [6]. Meanwhile, the mouse skin model of multiple-stage chemical carcinogenesis is a representable in vivo model for understanding the development of cuSCC [7,8]. Topical exposure of carcinogens, 7,12-dimethyl[a]anthracene (DMBA), as a tumor initiator results in $HRAS^{Q61L}$ mutation in mouse skin. Subsequently, topical treatment of tumor promoter, 12-*O*-tetradecanoyl-phorbol-13-acetate (TPA) then leads to the formation of lesions, KAs, and the development of SCC. FVB (Friend Virus B NIH Jackson) mice administrated with DMBA/TPA along with BRAF inhibitor, PLX4720, showed a remarkable acceleration in the appearance of lesions, an increase of incidence, and enhanced progression to KAs and SCC which resemble the papillomas induced by BRAF inhibitors in the clinical setting [5].

Tumor development is correlated with proliferation and expansion of not only cancer cells but also stroma, vessels, and infiltrating inflammatory cells and elements [9]. Neoplastic growth is related to a prolonged inflammatory condition induced by extrinsic or intrinsic pathways. The extrinsic pathways are related to a continued inflammatory condition, while the intrinsic pathways are stimulated by genetic transformations, which result in the activation of oncogenes or inactivation of tumor suppressor genes [10]. Cells with an altered phenotype propagate the secretion of inflammatory mediators, thus triggering the formation of a tumor microenvironment (TME) and development of tumors [11]. Recently, immunoinflammatory cells, such as macrophages, have been identified as critical contributors to malignancies in various tumor types, such as melanoma, lung carcinoma, glioma, gastric cancer, and wound-induced skin cancer [12,13].

Numerous studies have demonstrated that essential oils (EOs) of *Mentha* species have antiviral, antimicrobial, antioxidant, anti-inflammatory, and anti-tumor activities [14–18]. The objective of this study was to investigate the bioefficacy of EO from *Mentha aquatica var. citrata Kenting Water Mint* (KWM-EO) against two-stage skin carcinogenesis, with or without PLX4032 irritation, and the underlying molecular mechanisms. The chemical components of KWM-EO were analyzed using GC×GC-TOF MS, and its effect on *HRAS* mutant PDV keratinocyte activity was further investigated. Our in vitro bioassay results demonstrated that KWM-EO treatment suppressed PDV cell viability, colony formation ability, and induced G_2/M cell-cycle arrest and cell apoptosis in the presence and absence of PLX4032. KWM-EO also inhibited proinflammatory cell infiltration and papilloma formation in DMBA/TPA-induced two-stage skin carcinogenesis facilitated by PLX4032 in mice.

2. Results

2.1. Chemical Compositions of Mentha aquatica var. Kenting Water Mint Essential Oil

KWM-EO was obtained by hydrodistillation of the aerial parts. The chemical profile of KWM-EO was analyzed by GC×GC-TOF MS. Twenty compounds representing 81.86% of the total content were identified in KWM-EO (Table 1). Monoterpene hydrocarbons accounted for 56.01% of KWM-EO with 22.18% β-ocimene as the most abundant component, and β-pinene and α-pinene accounting for 15.41% and 10.49%, respectively. KWM-EO was identified to contain 15.86% oxygenated monoterpenes, of which eucalyptol (12.87%) was the most abundant.

Table 1. Chemical constituents of KWM-EO determined by GC×GC-TOF MS.

	Chemical Compound	CAS no.[a]	RT1[b]	RT2[c]	KI_{exp}[d]	KI_{Lit}[e]	Relative Percentage (%)
1	α-Pinene	7785-70-8	6.27	0.0245	936	929	10.49
2	β-Pinene	127-91-3	7.00	0.0250	981	973	15.41
3	β-Myrcene	123-35-3	7.20	0.0243	992	993	4.86
4	β-Cymene	535-77-3	7.73	0.0253	1027	1031	3.07
5	Eucalyptol	470-82-6	7.93	0.0258	1040	1041	12.87
6	β-Ocimene	3338-55-4	8.07	0.0245	1049	1036	22.18
7	Linalool	78-70-6	8.87	0.0262	1097	1101	0.25
8	Menthone	89-80-5	9.80	0.0325	1160	1154	0.04

Table 1. *Cont.*

	Chemical Compound	CAS no.[a]	RT1[b]	RT2[c]	KI_{exp}[d]	KI_{Lit}[e]	Relative Percentage (%)
9	Menthofuran	494-90-6	9.93	0.0267	1169	1169	0.04
10	Levomenthol	2216-51-5	10.07	0.0277	1178	1172	0.05
11	*p*-Menth-8-en-2-one	5948-4-9	10.60	0.0330	1213	1218	0.07
12	Carveol	1197-07-5	10.73	0.0272	1222	1223	0.13
13	Carvone	6485-40-1	11.13	0.0327	1251	1249	1.59
14	Linalyl acetate	115-95-7	11.20	0.0270	1256	1257	0.08
15	Dihydroedulan I	63335-66-0	11.87	0.0258	1302	1292	0.28
16	β-Bourbonene	5208-59-3	13.13	0.0250	1396	1386	0.78
17	Caryophyllene	87-44-5	13.60	0.0258	1434	1431	2.80
18	Humulene	6753-98-6	14.00	0.0318	1466	1465	0.29
19	Ethyl 4-ethoxybenzoate	23676-09-7	14.73	0.0302	1524	1521	2.37
20	Viridiflorol	552-02-3	15.73	0.0272	1608	1603	3.47
Monoterpene hydrocarbons identified							56.01
Oxygenated monoterpene identified							15.86
Sesquiterpene hydrocarbon identified							3.87
Oxygenated sesquiterpene identified							3.47
Other							2.56
Identified components							81.86

[a] Chemical abstracts service registry number; [b] Retention time of the first column; [c] Retention time of the second column; [d] KI_{exp} = Kovats indices, retention indices relative to C_7–C_{30} n-alkanes based on the retention time of components separated by the 1st dimension Rtx-5MS column; [e] KI_{Lit}: Retention indices reported in the literature.

2.2. *KWM-EO Effect on PDV Cell Proliferation, Invasion, and Migration*

The PDV cell line is a mouse keratinocyte bearing *HRAS*^{Q61L} mutation, which is the most relevant mutation in BRAF inhibitor-induced cutaneous squamous cell carcinoma. The PDV cell viability after treatment with 0 to 100 μg/mL KWM-EO was determined by MTT assay. The cell viability was decreased when KWM-EO concentration increased. When the PDV cells were treated with up to 100 μg/mL of KWM-EO for 24 h, the cell viability was inhibited to 53.31% (Figure 1A). The long-term colony formation ability of PDV cells was determined by treating with KWM-EO alone or in the presence of PLX4032 (PLX). The MEK (mitogen-activated protein kinase kinase) inhibitor, selumetinib (AZD6244), was used as a reference control. As shown in Figure 1B, 0.5 μM PLX4032 treatment promoted the colony formation of PDV cells compared to the vehicle-treated cells. In the presence or absence of PLX4032, KWM-EO treatment showed a dose-dependent effect, and KWM-EO treatment at the high dose of 40 μg/mL revealed a better effect than 0.5 μM AZD6244 treatment. PDV cell invasive ability was investigated by Matrigel coated-transwell assay. The result showed that PLX4032 treatment facilitated cell invasion relative to vehicle treatment, and KWM-EO suppressed the invasive ability on concentration-dependence (Figure 1C). In wound healing assay representing cell migratory ability, 2 μM PLX4032 treatment significantly and time-dependently increased cell migration. The migratory ability of PDV cells was restricted by 50 μg/mL KWM-EO treatment with or without PLX4032 stimulation (Figure 1D).

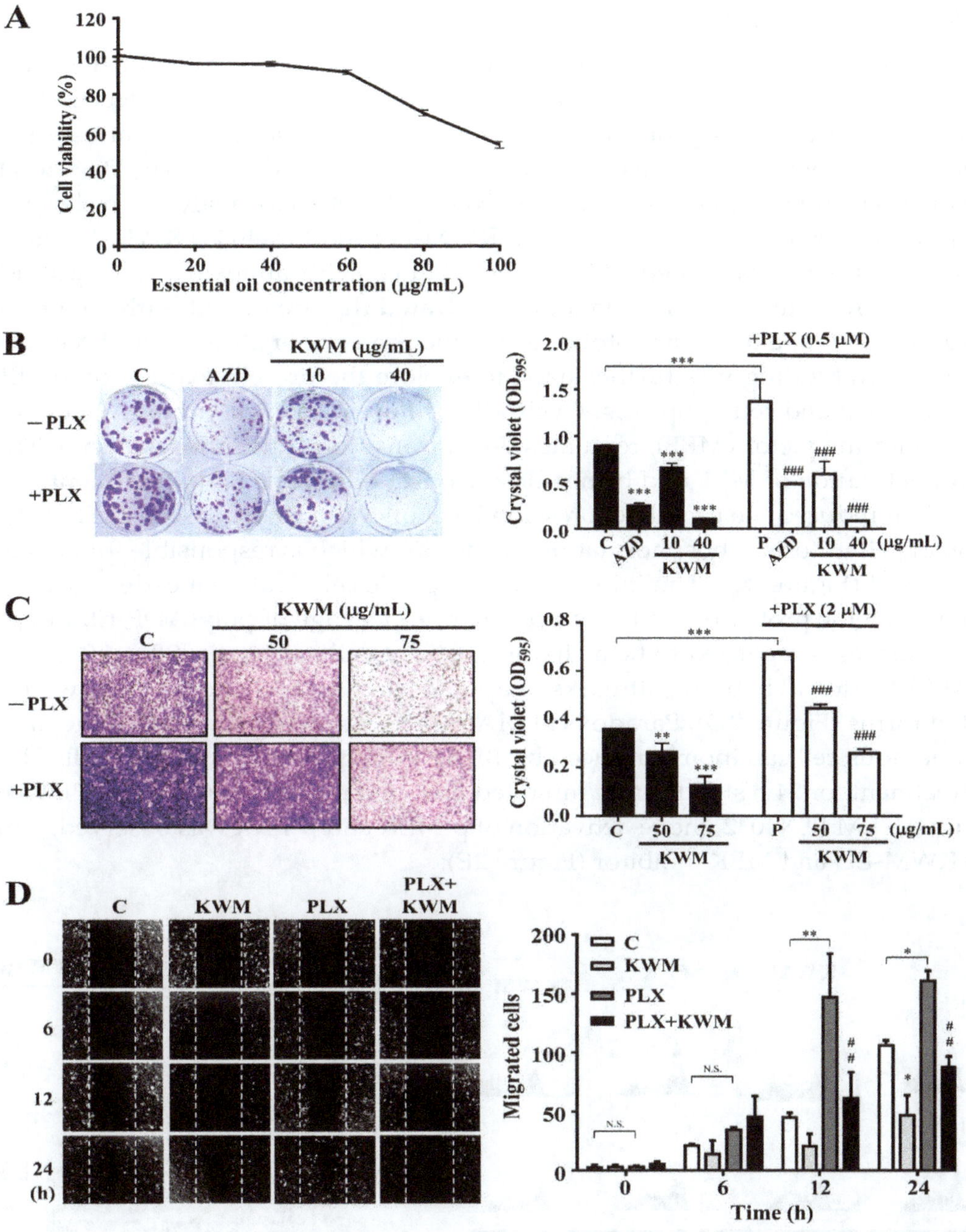

Figure 1. Effect of *Mentha aquatica var. Kenting Water Mint* essential oil (KWM-EO) on PDV cells. (**A**) PDV cells were treated with vehicle or the indicated concentrations of KWM-EO for 24 h. Cell viability (%) was determined by MTT assay. (**B**) PDV cells were incubated with KWM-EO in the presence or absence of 0.5 μM PLX4032 for 6 days, and colony formation was detected by staining cells with crystal violet. (**C**) PDV cells were seeded in Matrigel coated–transwell inserts and incubated with vehicle or KWM-EO in the presence or absence of 2 μM PLX4032 for 24 h. The invasive cells were stained with crystal violet. (**D**) PDV cell migratory ability was examined by wound healing assay. Cells were treated with vehicle or 50 μg/mL KWM-EO in the presence or absence of 2 μM PLX4032, and observed after 0, 6, 12, 24 h. Vehicle controls (C) were obtained from cells treated with 0.5% DMSO. The absorbance at 595 nm was obtained by dissolving crystal violet with 20% acetic acid. The data are representative of three independent experiments and are expressed as mean ± SD. Representative images are shown. $P^{*} < 0.05$, $P^{**} < 0.01$, $P^{***} < 0.001$ compared to vehicle control; $P^{\#\#} < 0.01$, $P^{\#\#\#} < 0.001$ compared to the PLX4032-treated group (ANOVA). AZD: AZD6244 (MEK inhibitor)

2.3. KWM-EO Induces Cell-Cycle Arrest and Apoptosis in PDV Cells

The KWM-EO effect on the PDV cell-cycle machinery was determined using flow cytometry. The analysis demonstrated that PLX4032 treatment alone had no significant effect on the cell-cycle of PDV cells; however, the cell-cycle profile treated with KWM-EO exhibited G_2/M arrest. After KWM-EO treatment for 24 h, the percentage of cells in the G_2/M phase was raised from 33.0–33.6% to 44.3–45.0%, in the presence or absence of PLX4032 (Figure 2A). According to cell-cycle analysis, an elevated percentage of the sub-G_1 population was also observed with KWM-EO and PLX4032+KWM-EO treatment. Thus cell apoptosis was further examined. Cells were stained with annexin V and propidium iodide and analyzed by flow cytometry. The data demonstrated that treatment with 75 μg/mL KWM-EO strongly induced 86.9% and 80.7% apoptotic cells in the presence or absence of PLX4032, respectively (Figure 2B). Western blotting was further used to explore the protein expression profile related to G_2/M cell-cycle arrest and cell apoptosis. Cyclin B1-cell division cycle protein 2 (cdc2), also known as M-phase promoting factor (MPF), regulates G_2/M transition. Phosphorylation of Thr161 in cdc2 is required for activation of MPF and brings on the onset of mitosis [19]. Treatment with 75 μg/mL KWM-EO for 24 h reduced the protein expression level of cyclin B1 and p-cdc 2 (Thr161), suggesting the inhibition of cell mitosis. Phosphorylation of cdc25C, which is responsible for activation of MPF, was also decreased (Figure 2C). The initiation of apoptotic cell death is needed to activate a group of intracellular cysteine proteases, named caspases. The cleavage of poly(ADP-ribose) polymerase-1 (PARP-1) by caspases is regarded to be a characteristic of cell apoptosis [20]. After treatment with 75 μg/mL KWM-EO for 12 h, both hallmarks of apoptosis, caspase 3 and PARP-1, were cleaved into their activated forms (Figure 2D). Paradoxical MAPK activation is known to be the main reason for cutaneous squamous cell carcinoma induced by BRAF inhibitor in *RAS* mutant cells [21]. KWM-EO (75 μg/mL) treatment for 24 h significantly inhibited ERK and p-ERK expression in PDV cells; while in treatment with 0.5 μM PLX4032, the re-activation of p-MEK and p-ERK was observed, which could be reversed by KWM-EO and MEK inhibitor (Figure 2E).

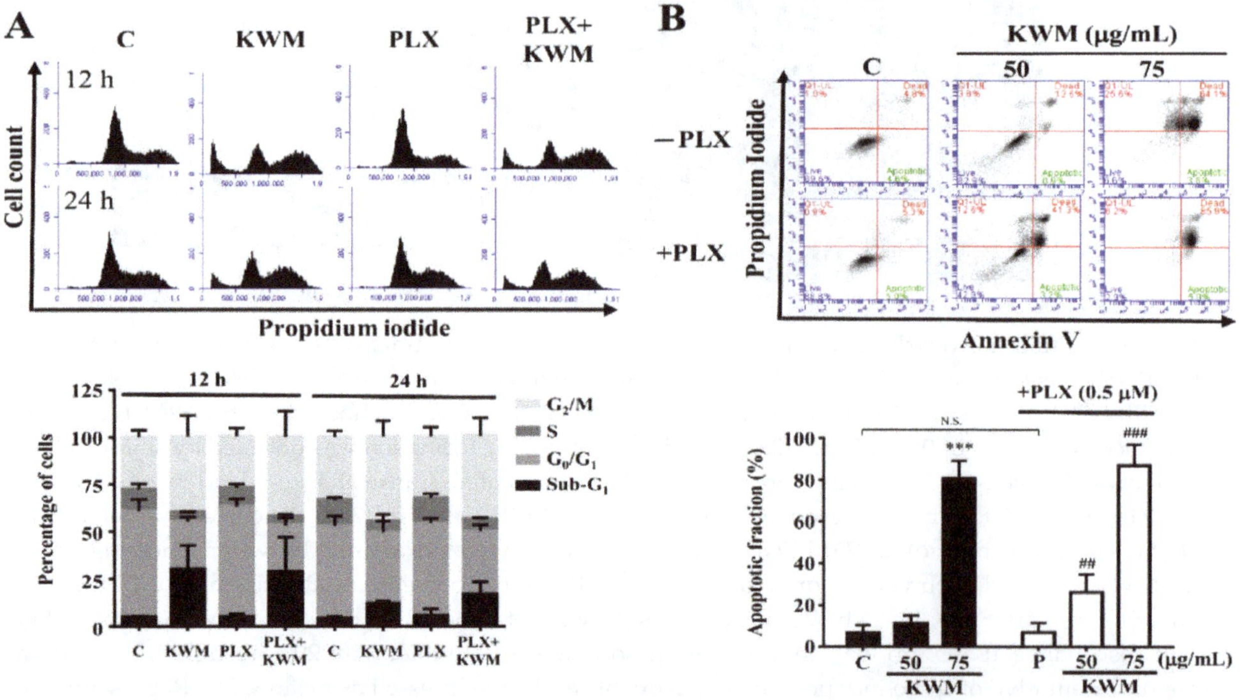

Figure 2. *Cont.*

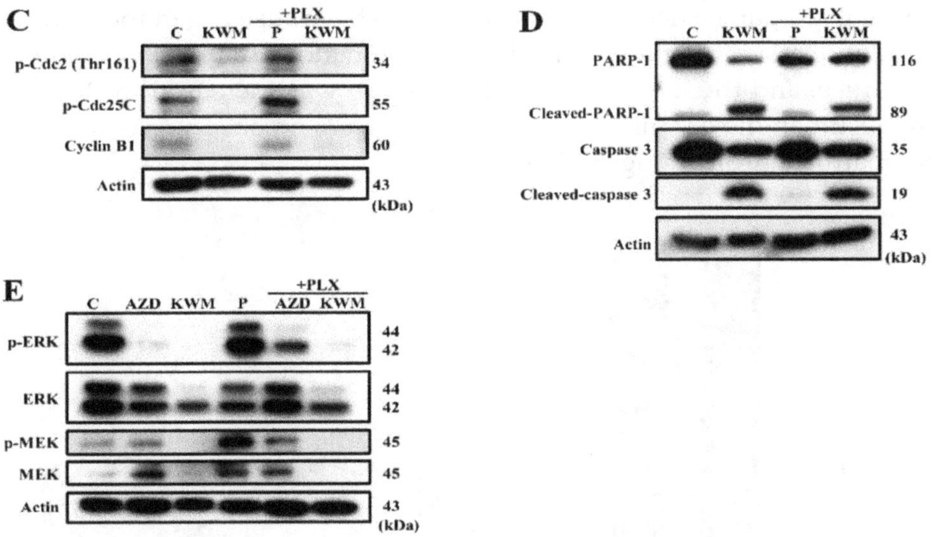

Figure 2. Effect of KWM-EO on cell-cycle and apoptosis in PDV cells. (**A**) PDV cells were exposed to vehicle or 75 μg/mL KWM-EO in the presence or absence of 0.5 μM PLX4032 for 12 or 24 h, then the cell-cycle was analyzed by flow cytometry. (**B**) PDV cells were treated with vehicle or 75 μg/mL KWM-EO in the presence or absence of 0.5 μM PLX4032 for 24 h. Cells were then stained with annexin V and propidium iodide, and the cell apoptosis was detected by flow cytometry. (**C**) PDV cells were treated with 75 μg/mL KWM-EO in the presence or absence of 0.5 μM PLX4032 for 24 h before lysis. The cell lysates were subjected to Western blotting against cell-cycle-related proteins, including p-cdc2 (Thr161), p-cdc25C, and cyclin B1. (**D**) The expression level of apoptosis-related proteins in PDV cells treated with 75 μg/mL KWM-EO in the presence or absence of 0.5 μM PLX4032 for 6 h was examined by Western blotting against PARP-1 and caspase 3. (**E**) Western blotting analysis of MAPK signaling-related proteins (p-ERK, ERK, p-MEK, MEK) in PDV cells treated with 75 μg/mL KWM-EO in the presence or absence of 0.5 μM PLX4032 for 24 h. Actin was used as an internal control in the experiment. Vehicle controls (**C**) were obtained from cells treated with 0.5% DMSO. The data are representative of three independent experiments and are expressed as mean ± SD. N.S. means non significance; $P^{***} < 0.05$ compared to vehicle control; $P^{\#\#} < 0.01$, $P^{\#\#\#\#} < 0.001$ compared to PLX4032-treated group (ANOVA).

2.4. *KWM-EO Inhibits Two-Stage Skin Carcinogenesis in FVB Mice*

To investigate the chemopreventive effect of KWM-EO in BRAF inhibitor-induced cutaneous squamous cell carcinoma, a DMBA-initiated and TPA-promoted two-stage skin carcinogenesis model was established, and the study diagram is shown in Supplementary Figure 1. After topical application of 25 μg DMBA and 4 μg TPA (DT) on mouse dorsal skin for 12 weeks, papillomas were successfully induced. If mice were co-treated with 20 mg/kg/BW PLX4032 (DTP), starting at 6 weeks, bigger and more papillomas occurred (Figure 3A). The DT and DTP groups developed papillomas on the skin as early as 5 weeks after TPA treatment. Within 6 to 7 weeks, the tumor incidence in DTP mice was much higher than in DT mice; at 8 weeks, the tumor incidence in the DT and DTP group reached 100%, while KWM-EO treatment delayed and decreased the tumor incidence (Figure 3B). On average, the DT group developed 15.4 papillomas/mouse at 12 weeks, the topical application of 5 mg KWM-EO reduced the average number of papillomas to 7.9/mouse. Under stimulation of PLX4032 in DTP mice, the average number of papillomas was raised to 22.4/mouse which was ameliorated by KWM-EO to 9.1 papillomas/mouse at 12 weeks ($P < 0.05$) (Figure 3C). The dot histogram shows the distribution of papilloma number per mouse and the median in a group (Figure 3D). The papilloma number was significantly decreased by KWM-EO treatment in DTP mice. Mouse body weights were recorded every week during the experimental period, and the results show that the body weights in all treated mice were similar to the sham control mice (Supplementary Figure 2). To examine the toxicology of these applied compounds and essential oil, mouse organ index was calculated, and H&E staining was executed to observe the organ structure and pathology. The mouse organ index was unchanged for the heart, lung, and kidney within the groups; however, the index of the liver organ was lower in the KWM-EO-treated mice, and the index of the spleen organ was increased in PLX4032-treated mice. The H&E staining result on the organs showed that there were no observable differences between the sham and all the treatment groups (Figure 3F).

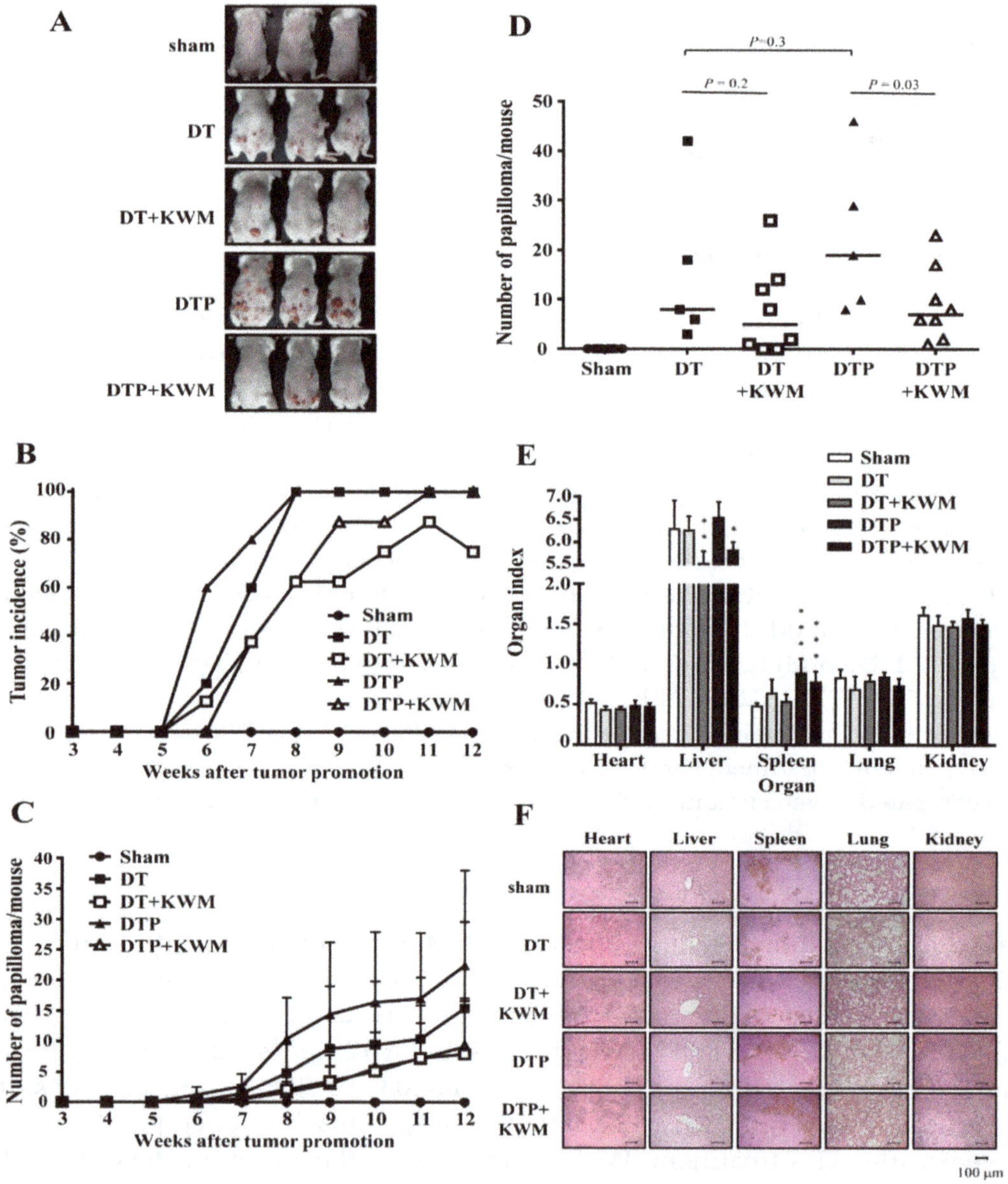

Figure 3. Effect of KWM-EO on two-stage skin carcinogenesis in mice. (**A**) Representative images of mice from each group at week 12 are shown. Tumor incidence (**B**) and mean number of papillomas (**C**) per group during the experimental period are calculated. (**D**) Papilloma numbers per mouse at week 12 are shown in the dot histogram. (**E**) Organ weights were recorded after mice were sacrificed at week 12. Organ index was calculated by the following formula: $organ\ index = (organ\ weight \div body\ weight) \times 100$ empty. $P^* < 0.05$, $P^{**} < 0.01$, $P^{***} < 0.001$ compared to sham group (ANOVA). (**F**) Organ tissues were detected by H&E staining. The DT and DTP groups consisted of 5 mice each. Sham, the DT+KWM, and DTP+KWM groups consisted of 8 mice each. The data are presented as mean ± SD. D: DMBA, T: TPA, P: PLX4032. Scale bar: 100 μm.

2.5. *Skin Histology and Epidermal Cell Proliferation in KWM-EO-Treated Mice*

Effect of topically applied KWM-EO on chemically induced skin tumorigenesis was further observed by skin histologic changes. The skin structure was first examined by H&E staining. With DMBA and TPA treatment in the presence or absence of PLX4032, the thickness of the epidermis was elevated compared to the sham group (Figure 4A), while the epidermal hyperplasia was attenuated by repeated treatment with KWM-EO for 12 weeks. The main cell type responsible for hyper-proliferative epidermis was further explored by immunofluorescent staining. Ki67 is a representative marker of cell proliferation, and cytokeratin 14 (K14) is the intermediate filament protein of basal keratinocytes. From the microphotographs, the expression level of ki67 showed remarkable upregulation in the DT and DTP group. After merging both ki67 and K14 staining with DAPI, the hyperplasia of the epidermis arising from basal keratinocytes was seen which was alleviated by KWM-EO topical treatment (Figure 4B). In addition, the paradoxical MAPK activation that could lead to cell proliferation in *RAS* mutant cells treated with BRAF inhibitors was also investigated. The IHC staining result revealed considerable p-ERK protein between the dermis and papilloma, especially in the group with PLX4032 stimulation; and this activation was significantly diminished by KWM-EO treatment (Figure 4C).

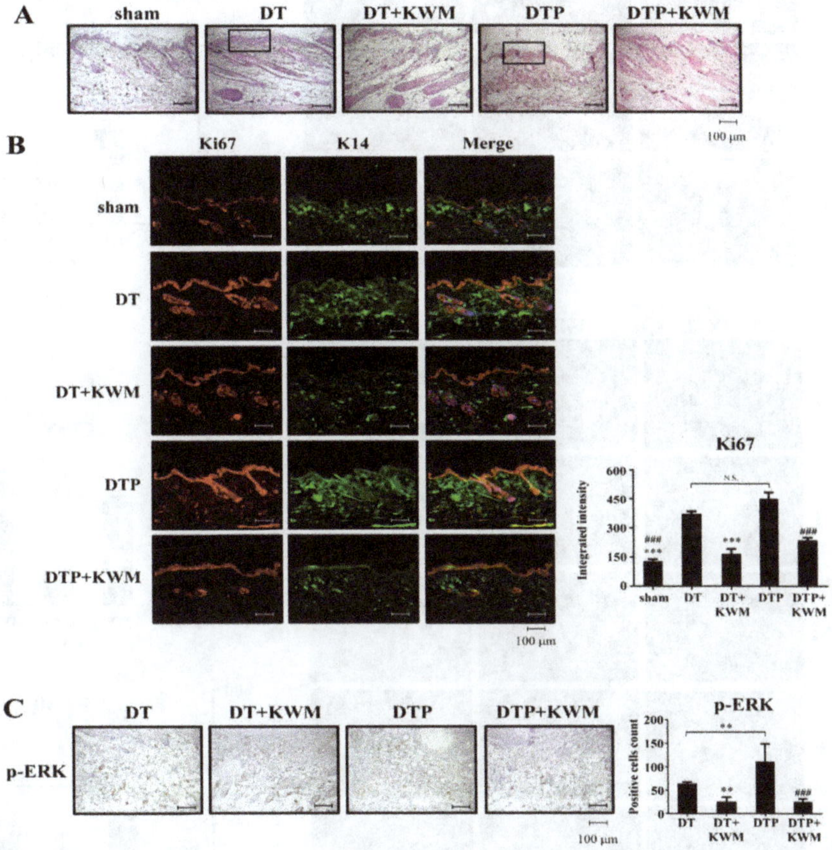

Figure 4. Effect of KWM-EO on skin and papilloma tissue from mice. (**A**) Skin morphology was examined by H&E staining. (**B**) Abnormal epidermal proliferation was detected by immunofluorescent staining of ki67 (red). Basal keratinocytes were stained with K14 (green), and nuclei were stained with DAPI (blue). (**C**) Histological images of papilloma indicated the paradoxical activation of p-ERK. Representative images are shown. The data are representative of three independent experiments and are expressed as mean ± SD. N.S. means non significance; $P^{**} < 0.01$, $P^{***} < 0.001$ compared to DT group; $P^{\#\#\#} < 0.001$ compared to DTP group (ANOVA). Scale bar: 100 μm.

2.6. *Anti-Inflammatory Effect of KWM-EO*

Inflammation is a vital element in the progression of two-stage skin carcinogenesis. COX-2, a pro-inflammatory enzyme commonly observed in inflamed cells or tissues was counter-stained with pro-inflammatory immune cells, neutrophils (neutrophil elastase+) and macrophages (F4/80+). The overexpression of COX-2 was increased in both DT and DTP mouse dorsal skin. Interestingly, most of the COX-2 proteins were observed colocalized with infiltrated neutrophils, but not macrophages (Figure 5A,B). Upon treatment with KWM-EO, the neutrophil and macrophage infiltration and upregulation of COX-2 were alleviated (Figure 5A,B).

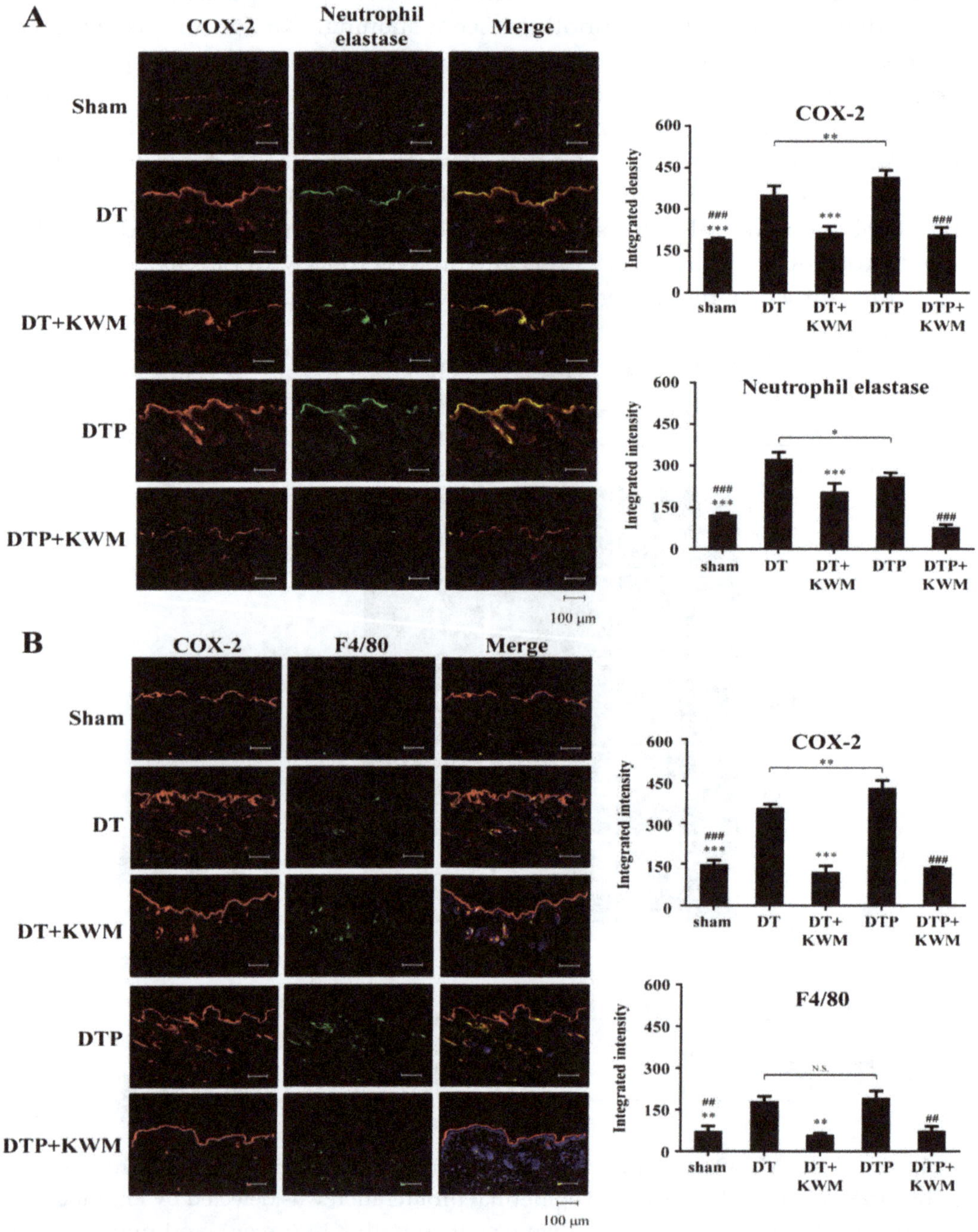

Figure 5. Effect of KWM-EO on the inflammatory immune system in skin tissue from the mice two-stage skin carcinogenesis. Immunofluorescent staining of inflammatory mediator COX-2 (red) with neutrophil elastase (green) (**A**) and macrophage marker, F4/80 (green) (**B**). Nuclei were counterstained with DAPI (blue). Representative images are shown. The data are representative of three independent experiments and are expressed as mean ± SD. N.S. means non significance; $P^{*} < 0.05$, $P^{**} < 0.01$, $P^{***} < 0.001$ compared to DT group; $P^{\#\#} < 0.01$, $P^{\#\#\#} < 0.001$ compared to DTP group (ANOVA). Scale bar: 100 μm.

3. Discussion

EOs have been utilized as fragrances, food flavorings, and folk medicines, among other applications throughout human history. In recent decades, a large number of studies have reported chemical constituent analysis of EOs and investigated their bio-efficacy and the responsible bioactive compounds. EOs from *Mentha* species have been reported to have anti-inflammatory, anti-oxidant, anti-fungal, and anti-bacterial activities [14–18]. The ethanolic extract of *Mentha×piperita* L., a cross-species of watermint and spearmint, at 50 and 100 μg/mL, suppressed LPS-induced nitric oxide production in macrophages by 18.85% and 41.88% inhibition, respectively [22]. Anti-cancer cell activity has also been reported for mint EOs. For example, *Mentha×piperita* L. extract showed more potent activity against proliferative activity of human MDA-MB-231 breast cancer cells (cell inhibition ratio = 46.53% at 150 μg/mL) than human A375 melanoma cells (cell inhibition ratio = 25.08% at 150 μg/mL) [14]. This study is the first to investigate and observe that KWM-EO can prevent two-stage skin carcinogenesis chemically induced by DMBA/TPA and its acceleration by BRAF inhibitor drug PLX4032. The two-stage skin carcinogenesis mouse model established by DMBA and TPA irritation is considered to be a representative study system through which to explore the pathology and underlying mechanisms of human squamous cell carcinomas [23]. It has also been used to evaluate the $BRAF^{V600E}$ inhibitor drugs, such as vemurafenib-induced cutaneous side-effects, including SCC and KA in patients [3]. We, thus, established this two-stage skin carcinogenesis mouse model, and the bioactivities of KWM-EO were examined. Our results indicated that KWM-EO treatment significantly inhibited papilloma incidence and number in DT and DTP mice. According to the histopathological analysis of skin tissue sections, KWM-EO not only attenuated the abnormal proliferation and hyperplasia of the epidermis but also decreased the inflammatory neutrophil and macrophage infiltration and COX-2 overexpression in neutrophils. Moreover, this study is the first to observe that abnormal epidermis proliferation in DT and DTP mice was mainly contributed by keratinocytes as a co-positively stained marker protein K14 and proliferation marker ki67. Topical administration of KWM-EO can reverse the over proliferation of K14 keratinocytes in DT- or DTP-irritated mouse skins.

A previous review article published by Pandey et al. [24] summarized that EOs of some *Ocimum* species exhibited anti-inflammatory and anti-cancerous properties which contain pinene, β-ocimene, and linalool, the chemical constituents present in KWM-EO. α-Pinene present in KWM-EO by 10.49% was reported to induce cell apoptosis and disrupt mitochondrial potential in B16F10 cells, and it also effectively reduced melanoma lung metastasis [25]. β-Caryophyllene accounted for 2.8% in KWM-EO was a major compound in the EO of *P. missionis*. Pavithra et al. demonstrated that EO from *P. missionis* induced cell death through intrinsic mitochondrial and extrinsic apoptotic pathways in A431 and HaCaT cells [26]. The results from these studies might potentially support part of our observations for the anti-inflammatory and chemopreventive activities of KWM-EO against two-stage skin carcinogenesis.

PDV keratinocytes harboring *HRAS* mutation are commonly found in DT-induced mouse SCC [27]. We adapted this cell model to investigate the in vitro effect and modes of action of KWM-EO. Our data revealed that KWM-EO treatment significantly diminished PDV cell colony formation ability and suppressed reactivation of MEK-ERK signaling stimulated by PLX4032. The PDV cell invasive and migratory abilities were promoted by PLX4032, which were suppressed by KWM-EO treatment. KWM-EO also induced G_2/M arrest in PDV cells through deregulating p-cdc2, p-cdc25C, and cyclin B1 proteins. The cell apoptosis induced by KWM-EO was through activation of caspase 3 and PARP-1 after cells were treated for 6 h. These in vitro data support in part the inhibitory activity of KWM-EO in the DT and DTP mouse skin on keratinocyte proliferation and papilloma formation.

In an open-label phase 2 study using a combination of BRAF inhibitor dabrafenib and MEK inhibitor trametinib in patients, the rate of skin lesions was not significantly reduced although a slight decrease in proliferative skin lesions was observed [28]. A previous study revealed that tumor multiplicity and incidence of skin tumors in DT-induced two-stage skin carcinogenesis accelerated by BRAF inhibitor was decreased when a COX-2 inhibitor celecoxib was orally administrated [29]. Our current data show that topical application of KWM-EO attenuated the formation of cutaneous papilloma in mice induced by DMBA/TPA or by DMBA/TPA/PLX4032. The paradoxical MAPK activation induced by PLX4032 in vitro in PDV keratinocytes and in skin of DT and DTP mice was suppressed by KWM-EO. Taken together, the results of this study demonstrate the novel chemopreventive activity of the essential oil of *Mentha aquatica var. citrata Kenting Water Mint* which can be potentially used in preventing BRAF inhibitor drug-induced cutaneous side-effects in cancer patients.

4. Materials and Methods

4.1. Mint Cultivation and Distillation of Essential Oils

A variety of *Mentha aquatica* (Lamiaceae), named *M. aquatica var. Kenting Water Mint* was cultivated in an experimental field at the Taichung District Agricultural Research and Extension Station, Taichung, Taiwan for 2 years. Mature shoots were harvested and subjected to water vapor distillation to collect essential oils. Two kilograms of fresh shoots were distilled with 4 L of water. Mint essential oil was evaporated, passed through a condenser then the oil and hydrosol were collected with a separating funnel. After 1 L of the hydrosol/essential oils were collected, the distillation ended. The hydrosol and essential oil were then separately collected for use in the following experiments. The mint essential oils were stored at −20 °C in sealed vials. Essential oils used in in vitro cell-based assays were diluted into different concentrations with DMSO and those used in in vivo animal studies were diluted in acetone.

4.2. Chemical Profiling of KWM-EO Composition by GC×GC−TOF MS

The samples were analyzed using LECO Pegasus 4D GC×GC−TOF MS (St Joseph, MI, USA). The first dimension capillary column was Restek Rtx-5MS (30 m × 0.25 mm × 0.25 μm) and the second capillary column was Restek Rtx-200 (2 m × 0.25 mm × 0.25 μm). The GC temperature program was set as follows: injection temperature: 280 °C; oven temperature: 40 °C maintained for 1 min, and increased at a rate of 10 °C/min to 310 °C and held constant for 8 min. The helium flow rate was set at 1 mL/min. The mass spectrometry temperature was set at 320 °C. The ion source temperature was 200 °C, and the analysis mass range was 50-800 m/z. KWM-EO was ran in hexane with a dilution of 1 mg/mL. Hexadecane solution, 64.25 μg/mL, was used as an internal standard to monitor the shift of retention time. Compounds were identified by matching the mass spectra fragmentation patterns, and the results were compared with LECO/Fiehn and Wiley Registry 9th Edition mass spectral library and NIST. Linear Kovats index of n-alkanes (C_7-C_{40}, C_7-C_{30}) were calculated for each compound and compared with the literature to identify the compound ID [30].

4.3. Cell Lines and Cell Culture

PDV cells, which harbor the $HRAS^{Q61L}$ mutation were obtained from CLS Cell Lines Service (Eppelheim, Germany). Cells were cultured at 37 °C in DMEM supplemented with 10% FBS, containing 100 units/mL penicillin and 100 μg/mL streptomycin in a humidified 5% CO_2 incubator. Cells were used within 10 passages for this study.

4.4. Measurement of Cell Viability

Cells (5 × 10^3 cells/well in 96-well plates) were treated with vehicle (0.5% DMSO) or 20, 40, 60, 80, and 100 μg/mL KWM-EO for 24 h. Cell viability was determined by 3-(4,5-Dimethylthiazol-2-yl)-2,5-diphenyl tetrazolium bromide (MTT)-based colorimetric assays according to Scudiero et al. [31]. The viability of the cells treated with vehicle-only was defined as 100% viable. The viability of the cells after treatment with KWM-EO was calculated using the following formula: $cell\ viability\ (\%) = \left[OD_{570\ (treated\ cells)} \div OD_{570\ [vehicle\ control]}\right] \times 100$ empty. The data are presented by three independent experiments with six replicates per experiment.

4.5. Colony Formation Assay

Colony formation was obtained by growing PDV cells (250 cells/well in 24-well plates) treated with 10 and 40 μg/mL KWM-EO in the presence or absence of 0.5 μM PLX4032 for 6 days. The culture medium was refreshed once on day 3. Cells were fixed with chilled methanol and stained with 0.1% crystal violet. Cells retaining crystal violet were dissolved with 20% acetic acid and quantified by measuring absorbance at 595 nm [32]. The data are presented by three independent experiments with three replicates per experiment.

4.6. Cell Invasion Assay

The cell invasion assay was performed by Millicell Cell Culture Inserts (Merck Millipore, United States). For invasion assay, 100 μL Matrigel (300 μg/mL) was applied to an 8-mm polycarbonate membrane filter and incubated in 37 °C for 2 h. PDV cells (5×10^4) were seeded to Matrigel-coated filters in 200 μL of serum-free medium in triplicate for 16 h. The bottom chamber of the apparatus contained 1 mL medium with 10% FBS as a chemoattractant and 50 and 75 μg/mL KWM-EO, in the presence or absence of 2 μM PLX4032. Cells were allowed to migrate for 24 h at 37 °C. After incubation for 24 h, the non-migrated cells on the apical side of the membrane were removed with cotton swabs. The migrated cells on the basal side of the membrane were fixed with cold 100% methanol for 20 min and washed 3 times with PBS. The cells were stained with 0.1% crystal violet and then washed with PBS to remove extra dye solution. Images were captured using a reverse-phase microscope (Zeiss Axiovert 200M). Cells retaining crystal violet were dissolved with 20% acetic acid and quantified by measuring absorbance at 595 nm. The data are presented by three independent experiments with three replicates per experiment.

4.7. Wound Healing Assay

The wound healing assay was performed by using Culture-Insert (ibidi GmbH, Germany). Culture-Inserts were inserted in 24-well plates before cells were seeded. PDV cells were seeded in Culture-Inserts at a density of 5×10^5 cells/mL in 70 μL medium. After 16 h, Culture-Inserts were removed which created two cell-free gaps of 500 ± 50 μm. Undetached cells were washed away by PBS, then the remaining attached cells were immersed in 1 mL medium with 50 μg/mL KWM-EO, in the presence or absence of 2 μM PLX4032. Cell migration was observed using a reverse-phase microscope (Zeiss Observer D1) every 6 h. The data are presented by three independent experiments with three replicates per experiment.

4.8. Cell-Cycle Analysis

PDV cells were seeded in 6-well plates at a density of 1×10^5 cells/well with respective medium containing 10% FBS for 16 h. To synchronize the cell-cycle, cells were washed with PBS and incubated with fresh medium containing 5% FBS for 8 h, followed by washing with PBS and incubation with fresh medium containing 0.5% FBS for 24 h. The synchronized PDV cells were then treated with 75 μg/mL KWM-EO, 0.5 μM PLX4032, and 0.5 μM PLX4032+75 μg/mL KWM-EO in the medium containing 10% FBS for 12 and 24 h. Both adherent and floating cells were collected, washed with PBS, and fixed with 500 μL ice-cold 70% ethanol overnight at 4 °C. Cells were stained with 500 μL propidium iodide (PI) solution, which contained 20 μg/mL PI, 20 μg/mL RNase A, 0.1% Triton X-100 for 30 min at room temperature in the dark and then analyzed by flow cytometry (Flow cytometry BD Accuri C6, United States).

4.9. Apoptosis Assay

Cells were seeded in 6-well plates at a density of 1.5×10^5 cells/well for 16 h and then treated with 75 μg/mL KWM-EO, 0.5 μM PLX4032, and 0.5 μM PLX4032+75 μg/mL KWM-EO. After 24 h, both adherent and floating cells were collected and washed with PBS. Apoptotic cells were analyzed by using FITC Annexin V Apoptosis Detection Kit (BD Bioscience, United States) according to the manufacturer's instructions.

4.10. Western Blot Analysis

Cells were treated with KWM-EO at the indicated concentrations in the presence or absence of PLX4032 and lysed in RIPA lysis buffer. Protein concentrations were measured by *DC* protein assay (Bio-Rad, United States). Western blotting was performed as described by Shyur et al. [33]. Primary antibodies ERK 1, cyclin B1, p-cdc2 p34, p-cdc25C, and PARP-1 were purchased from Santa Cruz (Texas, United States). Antibodies phospho-p44/42 MAPK (Erk1/2), MEK1/2, and phospho-MEK1/2 were purchased from Cell Signaling Technology (Massachusetts, United States). Caspase 3 antibody was purchased from GeneTex (Texas, United States).

4.11. Two-Stage Skin Carcinogenesis Study

Female FVB/NJNarl mice (5–6 weeks old) were purchased from the National Laboratory Animal Center (Taipei, Taiwan) and bred in the Laboratory Animal Core Facility (Agricultural Biotechnology Research Center, Academia Sinica, Taiwan). Animals were given a standard laboratory diet and distilled H_2O *ad libitum* and kept on a 12-h light/dark cycle at 22 ± 2 °C with humidity 55 ± 5%. All experimental protocols were approved by the Institutional Animal Care and Utilization Committee (IACUC: Protocol #18-08-1221), Academia Sinica, Taiwan. Mice were randomized and had their back hair shaved three days before topical application of 25 μg DMBA in 200 μL acetone. The first week after tumor initiation, 4 μg of TPA in 200 μL acetone was topically applied twice a week to the shaved dorsal skin for 12 weeks [5]. Mice were treated with the indicated concentration of KWM-EO (in 200 μL acetone) twice a week by topical application the day after TPA treatment for 12 weeks (Supplementary Figure 1). Tumor size of more than 1 mm diameter was counted every week.

4.12. Histopathological and Immunohistochemical Analysis

Tissues were fixed with 10% formalin, hydrated, and embedded in paraffin. Tissue sections were cut at 4 μm thickness, then deparaffinized following rehydration in a descendant ethanol bath. H&E staining, immunohistochemistry, and immunofluorescent staining followed the previously published protocols [30]. An upright microscope (Carl Zeiss Axio Imager, Z1) was used to observe the expression of targeted proteins. Primary antibodies cytokeratin 14 and CD163 were purchased from Proteintech (Illinois, United States). Ki67 and neutrophil elastase were purchased from Abcam (Cambridge, United Kingdom). Antibody against COX-2 was purchased from Cayman (Michigan, United States). Antibody against F4/80 was purchased from Biolegend (California, United States). Antibody against iNOS was purchased from BD transduction Laboratories (California, United States).

4.13. Statistical Analysis

All the data are expressed as mean ± standard deviation (SD). Statistical analyses were conducted by the Predictive Analysis Suite Workstation (PASW Statistics, United States), and the significant difference between different treatment groups was determined by analysis of variance (ANOVA). *P* values of less than 0.05 were considered statistically significant.

5. Conclusions

This study is the first to prove that KWM-EO has potential for prevention of chemically induced two-stage skin carcinogenesis. Topical application of KWM-EO significantly attenuated the number of papillomas in DMBA-initiated and TPA-promoted mouse skin, with or without co-stimulation with PLX4032. KWM-EO suppressed epidermal hyperplasia and over proliferation of keratinocytes in DMBA/TPA and DMBA/TPA/PLX4032 mice. Notably, KWM-EO treatment diminished MAPK pathway reactivation, pro-inflammatory immune cell infiltration, and COX-2 expression in both DMBA/TPA and DMBA/TPA/PLX4032 mouse skin tissues. Overall, the results in this study provide strong support for the development of KWM-EO into chemopreventive agents for squamous cell carcinoma patients or cancer patients taking BRAF inhibitor therapy.

Author Contributions: Conceptualization, L.-F.S.; methodology, L.-F.S., C.-T.C., Y.-H.C. and W.-N.S.; validation, C.-T.C. and L.-F.S.; formal analysis, C.-T.C., W.-N.S. and L.-F.S.; investigation, C.-T.C., W.-N.S., Y.-H.C. and L.-F.S.; resources, L.-F.S.; data curation, C.-T.C. and L.-F.S.; writing—original draft preparation, C.-T.C. and L.-F.S.; writing—review and editing, C.-T.C. and L.-F.S.; visualization, C.-T.C. and L.-F.S.; supervision, L.-F.S.; project administration, L.-F.S.; funding acquisition, L.-F.S.

Acknowledgments: The authors thank the Metabolomics Core Facility and the Laboratory Animal Facility of Agricultural Biotechnology Research Center, Academia Sinica, Taiwan for their services, and Ms. Miranda Loney, Agricultural Biotechnology Research Center English Editor's Office, Academia Sinica, Taiwan, for English editorial assistance.

References

1. Sosman, J.A.; Kim, K.B.; Schuchter, L.; Gonzalez, R.; Pavlick, A.C.; Weber, J.S.; McArthur, G.A.; Hutson, T.E.; Moschos, S.J.; Flaherty, K.T.; et al. Survial in BRAF V600-mutant advanced melanoma treated vemurafenib. *N. Engl. J. Med.* **2012**, *366*, 707–714. [CrossRef] [PubMed]
2. Gibney, G.T.; Messina, J.L.; Fedorenko, I.V.; Sondak, V.K.; Smalley, K.S.M. Paradoxical oncogenesis-the long-term effects of BRAF inhibition in melanoma. *Nat. Rev. Clin. Oncol.* **2013**, *10*, 390–399. [CrossRef] [PubMed]
3. Zhang, C.; Spevak, W.; Zhang, Y.; Burton, E.A.; Ma, Y.; Habets, G.; Zhang, J.; Lin, J.; Ewing, T.; Matusow, B.; et al. RAF inhibitors that evade paradoxical MAPK pathway activation. *Nature* **2015**, *526*, 583–586. [CrossRef] [PubMed]
4. Doma, E.; Rupp, C.; Varga, A.; Kern, F.; Riegler, B.; Baccarini, M. Skin tumorigenesis stimulated by Raf inhibitors relies upon Raf functions that are dependent and independent of ERK. *Cancer Res.* **2013**, *73*, 6926–6937. [CrossRef] [PubMed]
5. Su, F.; Viros, A.; Milagre, C.; Trunzer, K.; Bollag, G.; Splesis, O.; Reis-Filho, J.S.; Kong, X.; Koya, R.C.; Flasherty, K.T.; et al. RAS mutations in cutaneous squamous-cell carcinomas in patients treated with BRAF inhibitors. *N. Engl. J. Med.* **2012**, *366*, 207–215. [CrossRef] [PubMed]
6. Caulín, C.; Bauluz, C.; Gandarillas, A.; Cano, A.; Quintanilla, M. Changes in keratin expression during malignant progression of transformed mouse epidermal keratinocytes. *Exp. Cell Res.* **1993**, *204*, 11–21. [CrossRef]
7. Abel, E.L.; Angel, J.M; Kiguchi, K.; DiGiovanni, J. Multi-stage chemical carcinogenesis in mouse skin: Fundamentals and applications. *Nat. Protoc.* **2009**, *4*, 1350–1362. [CrossRef]
8. Thomas, G.; Tuk, B.; Song, J.Y.; Truong, H.; Gerritsen, H.C.; Gruijl, F.R.D.; Sterenborg, H.J. Studying skin tumourigenesis and progression in immunocompetent hairless SKH1-h mice using chronic 7,12-dimethylbenz(a)anthracene topical applications to develop a useful experimental skin cancer model. *Lab. Anim.* **2017**, *51*, 24–35. [CrossRef]
9. Gonda, T.A.; Tu, S.; Wang, T.C. Chronic inflammation, the tumor microenvironment and carcinogenesis. *Cell Cycle* **2014**, *8*, 2005–2013. [CrossRef]
10. Korniluk, A.; Koper, O.; Kemona, H.; Dymicka-Piekarska, D. From inflammation to cancer. *Ir. J. Med. Sci.* **2017**, *186*, 57–62. [CrossRef]
11. Mantovani, A.; Allavena, P.; Sica, A.; Balkwill, F. Cancer-related inflammation. *Nature* **2008**, *454*, 436–444. [CrossRef] [PubMed]
12. Pollard, J.W. Trophic macrophages in development and disease. *Nat. Rev. Immunol.* **2009**, *9*, 259–270. [CrossRef] [PubMed]
13. Weber, C.; Telerman, S.B.; Reimer, A.S.; Sequeira, I.; Liakath-Ali, K.; Arwert, E.N.; Watt, F.M. Macrophage infiltration and alternative activation during wound healing promote MEK1-induced skin carcinogenesis. *Cancer Res.* **2016**, *76*, 805–817. [CrossRef] [PubMed]
14. Alexa, E.; Dauciu, C.; Radulov, I.; Obistioiu, D.; Sumalan, R.M.; Morar, A.; Dehelean, C.A. Phytochemical screening and biological activity of *Mentha x piperita* L. and Lavandula angustifolia Mill. Extracts. *Anal. Cell Pathol.* **2018**. [CrossRef] [PubMed]
15. Ogaly, H.A.; Eltablawy, N.A.; Abd-Elsalam, R.M. Antifibrogenic influence of *Mentha piperita* L. essential oil against CCl4-induced liver fibrosis in rats. *Oxid. Med. Cell Longev.* **2018**. [CrossRef]
16. Tsai, M.L.; Wu, C.T.; Lin, T.F.; Lin, W.C.; Huang, Y.C.; Yang, C.H. Chemical composition and biological properties of essential oils of two mint species. *Trop. J. Pharm. Res.* **2013**, *12*, 577–582. [CrossRef]

17. Bouyahya, A.; Et-Touys, A.; Bakri, Y.; Talbaui, A.; Fellah, H.; Abrini, J.; Dakka, N. Chemical composition of Mentha pulegium and Rosmarinus officinalis essential oils and their antileishmanial, antibacterial and antioxidant activities. *Microb. Pathog.* **2017**, *111*, 41–49. [CrossRef]
18. Zu, Y.; Yu, H.; Liang, L.; Fu, Y.; Efferth, T.; Liu, X.; Wu, N. Activities of ten essential oils towards *Propionibacterium acnes* and PC-3, A-549 and MCF-7 cancer cells. *Molecules* **2010**, *15*, 3200–3210. [CrossRef]
19. Hara, M.; Abe, Y.; Tanaka, T.; Yamamto, T.; Okumura, E.; Kishimoto, T. Greatwall kinase and cyclin B-Cdk1 are both critical constituents of M-phase-promoting factor. *Nat. Commun.* **2012**, *3*, 1059–1067. [CrossRef]
20. Gray, D.C.; Mahrus, S.; Wells, J.A. Activation of specific apoptotic caspases with an engineered small-molecule-activated protease. *Cell* **2010**, *142*, 637–646. [CrossRef]
21. Hall-Jackson, C.A; Eyers, P.A; Cohen, P.; Goedert, M.; Boyle, F.T.; Hewitt, N.; Plant, H.; Hedge, P. Paradoxical activation of Raf by a novel Raf inhibitor. *Chem. Biol.* **1999**, *6*, 559–568. [CrossRef]
22. Li, Y.X.; Liu, Y.B.; Ma, A.Q.; Bao, Y.; Wang, M.; Sun, Z.L. In vitro antiviral, anti-inflammatory, and antioxidant activities of the ethanol extract of *Mentha piperita* L. *Food Sci. Biotechnol.* **2017**, *26*, 1675–1683. [CrossRef] [PubMed]
23. Neagu, M.; Caruntu, C.; Constantin, C.; Boda, D.; Zurac, S.; Spandidos, D.A.; Tsatsakis, A.M. Chemically induced skin carcinogenesis: Updates in experimental models (Review). *Oncol. Rep.* **2016**, *35*, 2516–2528. [CrossRef] [PubMed]
24. Pandey, A.K.; Singh, P.; Tripathi, N.N. Chemistry and bioactivities of essential oils of some *Ocimum* species: An overview. *Asian Pac. J. Trop. Biomed.* **2014**, *4*, 682–694. [CrossRef]
25. Matsuo, A.L.; Figueiredo, C.R.; Arruda, D.C.; Pereira, F.V.; Scutti, J.A.B.; Massaoka, M.H.; Travassos, L.R.; Sartorelli, P.; Lago, J.H.G. α-Pinene isolated from Schinus terebinthifolius Raddi (Anacardiaceae) induces apoptosis and confers antimetastatic protection in a melanoma model. *Biochem. Biophys. Res. Commun.* **2011**, *411*, 449–454. [CrossRef] [PubMed]
26. Pavithra, P.S.; Mehta, A.; Verma, R.S. Induction of apoptosis by essential oil from *P. missionis* in skin epidermoid cancer cells. *Phytomedicine* **2018**, *50*, 184–195. [PubMed]
27. Katsanakis, K.D.; Gorgoulis, V.; Papavassiliou, A.G.; Zoumpourlis, V.K. The progression in the mouse skin carcinogenesis model correlates. *Mol. Med.* **2002**, *8*, 624–637. [CrossRef] [PubMed]
28. Flaherty, K.T.; Infante, J.R.; Daud, A.; Gonzalez, R.; Kefford, R.F.; Sosman, J.; Hamid, O.; Schuchter, L.; Cebon, J.; Ibrahim, N. Combined BRAF and MEK inhibition in melanoma with BRAF V600 mutations. *N. Engl. J. Med.* **2012**, *367*, 1694–1703. [CrossRef]
29. Escuin-Ordinas, H.; Atefi, M.; Fu, Y.; Cass, A.; Ng, C.; Huang, R.R.; Yashar, S.; Comin-Anduix, B.; Avramis, E.; Cochran, A.J.; et al. COX-2 inhibition prevents the appearance of cutaneous squamous cell carcinomas accelerated by BRAF inhibitors. *Mol. Oncol.* **2014**, *8*, 250–260. [CrossRef]
30. Schomburg, G.; Dielmann, G. Identification by means of retention parameters. *J. Chromatogr. Sci.* **1973**, *11*, 151–159. [CrossRef]
31. Scudiero, D.A.; Shoemaker, R.H.; Paull, K.D.; Monks, A.; Tierney, S.; Nofziger, T.H.; Currens, M.J.; Seniff, D.; Boyd, M.R. Evaluation of soluble tetrazolium/formazon assay for cell growth sensitivity in culture using human and other tumor cell lines. *Cancer Res.* **1988**, *48*, 4827–4833. [PubMed]
32. Franken, N.A.P.; Rodermond, H.M.; Stap, J.; Haveman, J.; Bree, C.V. Clonogenic assay of cells in vitro. *Nat. Protoc.* **2006**, *1*, 2315–2319. [CrossRef] [PubMed]
33. Apaya, M.K.; Lin, C.Y.; Chiou, C.Y.; Yang, C.C.; Ting, C.Y.; Shyur, L.F. Simvastatin and a plant galactolipid protect animals from septic shock by regulating oxylipin mediator dynamics through the MAPK-$cPLA_2$ signaling pathway. *Mol. Med.* **2016**, *21*, 988–1001. [CrossRef] [PubMed]

Permissions

All chapters in this book were first published by MDPI; hereby published with permission under the Creative Commons Attribution License or equivalent. Every chapter published in this book has been scrutinized by our experts. Their significance has been extensively debated. The topics covered herein carry significant findings which will fuel the growth of the discipline. They may even be implemented as practical applications or may be referred to as a beginning point for another development.

The contributors of this book come from diverse backgrounds, making this book a truly international effort. This book will bring forth new frontiers with its revolutionizing research information and detailed analysis of the nascent developments around the world.

We would like to thank all the contributing authors for lending their expertise to make the book truly unique. They have played a crucial role in the development of this book. Without their invaluable contributions this book wouldn't have been possible. They have made vital efforts to compile up to date information on the varied aspects of this subject to make this book a valuable addition to the collection of many professionals and students.

This book was conceptualized with the vision of imparting up-to-date information and advanced data in this field. To ensure the same, a matchless editorial board was set up. Every individual on the board went through rigorous rounds of assessment to prove their worth. After which they invested a large part of their time researching and compiling the most relevant data for our readers.

The editorial board has been involved in producing this book since its inception. They have spent rigorous hours researching and exploring the diverse topics which have resulted in the successful publishing of this book. They have passed on their knowledge of decades through this book. To expedite this challenging task, the publisher supported the team at every step. A small team of assistant editors was also appointed to further simplify the editing procedure and attain best results for the readers.

Apart from the editorial board, the designing team has also invested a significant amount of their time in understanding the subject and creating the most relevant covers. They scrutinized every image to scout for the most suitable representation of the subject and create an appropriate cover for the book.

The publishing team has been an ardent support to the editorial, designing and production team. Their endless efforts to recruit the best for this project, has resulted in the accomplishment of this book. They are a veteran in the field of academics and their pool of knowledge is as vast as their experience in printing. Their expertise and guidance has proved useful at every step. Their uncompromising quality standards have made this book an exceptional effort. Their encouragement from time to time has been an inspiration for everyone.

The publisher and the editorial board hope that this book will prove to be a valuable piece of knowledge for researchers, students, practitioners and scholars across the globe.

List of Contributors

Chao-Yu Loung and Wasundara Fernando
Department of Pathology, Faculty of Medicine, Dalhousie University, Halifax, NS B3H 4R2, Canada

H.P. Vasantha Rupasinghe
Department of Pathology, Faculty of Medicine, Dalhousie University, Halifax, NS B3H 4R2, Canada
Department of Plant, Food, and Environmental Sciences, Faculty of Agriculture, Dalhousie University, Truro, NS B2N 5E3, Canada

David W. Hoskin
Department of Pathology, Department of Microbiology and Immunology, Department of Surgery, Faculty of Medicine, Dalhousie University, Halifax, NS B3H 4R2, Canada

Danielly C. Ferraz da Costa
Departamento de Nutrição Básica e Experimental, Instituto de Nutrição, Universidade do Estado do Rio de Janeiro, Rio de Janeiro 20550-013, Brazil

Luciana Pereira Rangel
Faculdade de Farmácia, Universidade Federal do Rio de Janeiro, Rio de Janeiro 21941-902, Brazil

Mafalda Maria Duarte da Cunha Martins-Dinis, Giulia Diniz da Silva Ferretti and Jerson L. Silva
Programa de Biologia Estrutural, Instituto de Bioquímica Médica Leopoldo de Meis, Instituto Nacional de Ciência e Tecnologia de Biologia Estrutural e Bioimagem, Universidade Federal do Rio de Janeiro, Rio de Janeiro 21941-902, Brazil

Vitor F. Ferreira
Departamento de Tecnologia Farmacêutica, Faculdade de Farmácia, Universidade Federal Fluminense, Rio de Janeiro 24241-000, Brazil

Nejat Düzgüneş and Krystyna Konopka
Department of Biomedical Sciences, Arthur A. Dugoni School of Dentistry, University of the Pacific, 155 Fifth Street, Room 412, San Francisco, CA 94103, USA

Yu Zhang
Key Laboratory of Phytochemistry and Plant Resources in West China, Kunming Institute of Botany, Chinese Academy of Sciences, Kunming 650201, China
Natural Product Research Laboratories, UNC Eshelman School of Pharmacy, University of North Carolina, Chapel Hill, NC 27599, USA

Masuo Goto, Pei-Ling Hsu and Susan L. Morris-Natschke
Natural Product Research Laboratories, UNC Eshelman School of Pharmacy, University of North Carolina, Chapel Hill, NC 27599, USA

Akifumi Oda
Graduate School of Pharmacy, Meijo University, 150 Yagotoyama, Tempaku-ku, Nagoya, Aichi 468-8503, Japan

Ling-Li Guo, Yan-Hui Fu and Xiao-Jiang Hao
Key Laboratory of Phytochemistry and Plant Resources in West China, Kunming Institute of Botany, Chinese Academy of Sciences, Kunming 650201, China

Ernest Hamel
Screening Technologies Branch, Developmental Therapeutics Program, Division of Cancer Treatment and Diagnosis, Frederick National Laboratory for Cancer Research, National Cancer Institute, Frederick, MD 21702, USA

Kuo-Hsiung Lee
Natural Product Research Laboratories, UNC Eshelman School of Pharmacy, University of North Carolina, Chapel Hill, NC 27599, USA
Chinese Medicine Research and Development Center, China Medical University and Hospital, 2 Yuh-Der Road, Taichung 40447, Taiwan

Yu-Ning Teng
Department of Medicine, College of Medicine, I-Shou University, 8 Yida Road, Kaohsiung 82445, Taiwan

Charles C. N. Wang
Department of Bioinformatics and Medical Engineering, Asia University, 500 Lioufeng Rd., Wufeng, Taichung 41354, Taiwan

Wei-Chieh Liao and Yu-Hsuan Lan
Department of Pharmacy, College of Pharmacy, China Medical University, 91 Hsueh-Shih Road, Taichung 40402, Taiwan

Chin-Chuan Hung
Department of Pharmacy, College of Pharmacy, China Medical University, 91 Hsueh-Shih Road, Taichung 40402, Taiwan
Department of Pharmacy, China Medical University Hospital, 2 Yude Road, Taichung 40447, Taiwan

Ashana Puri, Sonalika A. Bhattaccharjee and Ajay K. Banga
Center for Drug Delivery Research, Department of Pharmaceutical Sciences, College of Pharmacy, Mercer University, Atlanta, GA 30341, USA

Wei Zhang, Meredith Clark, Onkar N. Singh and Gustavo F. Doncel
CONRAD, Department of Obstetrics and Gynecology, Eastern Virginia Medical School, Arlington, VA 22209, USA

Haitao Yang, Jing Li and Sravan Kumar Patel
Department of Pharmaceutical Sciences, School of Pharmacy, University of Pittsburgh, Pittsburgh, PA 15261, USA
Magee-Womens Research Institute, Pittsburgh, PA 15213, USA

Kenneth E. Palmer
Center for Predictive Medicine and Department of Pharmacology and Toxicology, University of Louisville School of Medicine, Louisville, KY 40202, USA

Brid Devlin
International Partnership for Microbicides, Silver Spring, MD 20910, USA

Lisa C. Rohan
Department of Pharmaceutical Sciences, School of Pharmacy, University of Pittsburgh, Pittsburgh, PA 15261, USA
Magee-Womens Research Institute, Pittsburgh, PA 15213, USA
Department of Obstetrics, Gynecology and Reproductive Sciences, University of Pittsburgh, Pittsburgh, PA 15261, USA

Simayijiang Aimaiti, Yohei Saito and Shuichi Fukuyoshi
School of Pharmaceutical Sciences, College of Medical, Pharmaceutical and Health Sciences, Kanazawa University, Kanazawa 920-1192, Japan

Katsunori Miyake
Tokyo University of Pharmacy and Life Sciences, Hachioji, Tokyo 192-0392, Japan

David J. Newman
NIH Special Volunteer, Wayne, PA 19087, USA

Barry R. O'Keefe
Natural Products Branch, Developmental Therapeutics Program, Division of Cancer Treatment and Diagnosis, National Cancer Institute, NCI at Frederick, Frederick, MD 21702-1201, USA
Molecular Targets Program, Center for Cancer Research, National Cancer Institute, NCI at Frederick, Frederick, MD 21702-1201, USA
Chinese Medicine Research and Development Center, China Medical University and Hospital, Taichung 40447, Taiwan

Kyoko Nakagawa-Goto
School of Pharmaceutical Sciences, College of Medical, Pharmaceutical and Health Sciences, Kanazawa University, Kanazawa 920-1192, Japan
Natural Products Research Laboratories, UNC Eshelman School of Pharmacy, University of North Carolina at Chapel Hill, Chapel Hill, NC 27599-7568, USA

Mohammad Bagher Majnooni
Student Research Committee, Kermanshah University of Medical Sciences, Kermanshah 6714415153, Iran

Sajad Fakhri and Mohammad Hosein Farzaei
Pharmaceutical Sciences Research Center, Health Institute, Kermanshah University of Medical Sciences, Kermanshah 6734667149, Iran

Antonella Smeriglio and Domenico Trombetta
Department of Chemical, Biological, Pharmaceutical and Environmental Sciences, University of Messina, Viale Palatucci, 98168 Messina, Italy

Courtney R. Croley and Anupam Bishayee
Lake Erie College of Osteopathic Medicine, Bradenton, FL 34211, USA

Piyali Bhattacharyya
Escuela de Ciencias de la Salud, Universidad Ana G. Méndez, Recinto de Gurabo, Gurabo, PR 00778, USA

Eduardo Sobarzo-Sánchez
Laboratory of Pharmaceutical Chemistry, Department of Organic Chemistry, Faculty of Pharmacy, University of Santiago de Compostela, 15782 Santiago de Compostela, Spain
Instituto de Investigación e Innovación en Salud, Facultad de Ciencias de la Salud, Universidad Central de Chile, Santiago 8330507, Chile

Koji Wada and Hiroshi Yamashita
Department of Medicinal Chemistry, Faculty of Pharmaceutical Sciences, Hokkaido University of Science, 4-1, Maeda 7-jo 15-choume, Teine-ku, Sapporo 006-8590, Japan

Michael Kahnt, Sophie Hoenke, Lucie Fischer and René Csuk
Organic Chemistry, Martin-Luther-University Halle-Wittenberg, Kurt-Mothes-Str. 2, D-06120 Halle (Saale), Germany

Ahmed Al-Harrasi
Natural and Medical Sciences Research Center, University of Nizwa, Birkat Al-Mauz, Nizwa 616, Oman

Elena-Alina Moacă and Cristina-Adriana Dehelean
Department of Toxicology and Drug Industry, Faculty of Pharmacy, "Victor Babes" University of Medicine and Pharmacy, 2 Eftimie Murgu Square, 300041 Timisoara, Romania

Ioana Zinuca Pavel, Corina Danciu and Daliana Minda
Department of Pharmacognosy, Faculty of Pharmacy, "Victor Babes" University of Medicine and Pharmacy, 2 Eftimie Murgu Square, 300041 Timisoara, Romania

Zorin Crăiniceanu
Department of Plastic and Reconstructive Surgery, Faculty of Medicine, "Victor Babes" University of Medicine and Pharmacy, 2 Eftimie Murgu Square, 300041 Timisoara, Romania

Florina Ardelean and Diana Simona Antal
Department of Botany, Faculty of Pharmacy, "Victor Babes" University of Medicine and Pharmacy, 2 Eftimie Murgu Square, 300041 Timisoara, Romania

Roxana Ghiulai
Department of Pharmaceutical Chemistry, Faculty of Pharmacy, "Victor Babes" University of Medicine and Pharmacy, 2 Eftimie Murgu Square, 300041 Timisoara, Romania

Andreea Cioca and Mihnea Derban
Department of Pathology, CFR Clinical Hospital, 13-15, Tudor Vladimirescu, 300173 Timisoara, Romania

Sebastian Simu
Department of Physical Chemistry, Faculty of Pharmacy, "Victor Babes" University of Medicine and Pharmacy, 2 Eftimie Murgu Square, 300041 Timisoara, Romania

Raul Chioibaş
CBS Medcom Hospital, 12 Popa Sapca Street, 300047 Timisoara, Romania

Camelia Szuhanek
Department of Orthodontrics, Faculty of Dentistry, "Victor Babes" University of Medicine and Pharmacy, 2 Eftimie Murgu Square, 300041, Timisoara, Romania

Chih-Ting Chang
Agricultural Biotechnology Research Center, Academia Sinica, Taipei 115, Taiwan
Department of Biological Science and Technology, National Taiwan University, Taipei 106, Taiwan

Wen-Ni Soo
Agricultural Biotechnology Research Center, Academia Sinica, Taipei 115, Taiwan

Yu-Hsin Chen
Taichung District Agricultural Research and Extension Station, Council of Agriculture, Executive Yuan, Taichung 515, Taiwan

Lie-Fen Shyur
Agricultural Biotechnology Research Center, Academia Sinica, Taipei 115, Taiwan
Department of Biological Science and Technology, National Taiwan University, Taipei 106, Taiwan
Graduate Institute of Pharmacognosy, Taipei Medical University, Taipei 110, Taiwan

Index

www.ingramcontent.com/pod-product-compliance
Lightning Source LLC
LaVergne TN
LVHW082132200926
848484LV00008B/2041